W0106637

WERNER'S SYNDROME
AND HUMAN AGING

ADVANCES IN EXPERIMENTAL MEDICINE AND BIOLOGY

Editorial Board:

NATHAN BACK, *State University of New York at Buffalo*

NICHOLAS R. DI LUZIO, *Tulane University School of Medicine*

EPHRAIM KATCHALSKI-KATZIR, *The Weizmann Institute of Science*

DAVID KRITCHEVSKY, *Wistar Institute*

ABEL LAJTHA, *Rockland Research Institute*

RODOLFO PAOLETTI, *University of Milan*

A Continuation Order Plan is available for this series. A continuation order will bring delivery of each new volume immediately upon publication. Volumes are billed only upon actual shipment. For further information please contact the publisher.

WERNER'S SYNDROME AND HUMAN AGING

Edited by

Darrell Salk

School of Medicine
University of Washington
Seattle, Washington

Yoshisada Fujiwara

Kobe University School of Medicine
Kobe, Japan

and

George M. Martin

School of Medicine
University of Washington
Seattle, Washington

SPRINGER SCIENCE+BUSINESS MEDIA, LLC

Library of Congress Cataloging-in-Publication Data

United States-Japan Cooperative Seminar on Werner's Syndrome and Human Aging
  (1982: Kobe-shi, Japan)
  Werner's Syndrome and Human Aging.

  (Advances in experimental medicine and biology; v. 190)
  "Proceedings of a United States–Japan Cooperative Seminar on Werner's Syndrome
and Human Aging, held December 10–12, 1982, in Kobe, Japan"—T.p. verso.
  Includes bibliographies and index.
  1. Werner's syndrome—Congresses.   2. Cells—Aging—Congresses.
3. Aging—Congresses.   I. Salk, Darrell.   II. Fujiwara, Yoshisada.   III. Martin,
George, 1927–   IV. Title.   V. Series.   [DNLM: 1. Aging—congresses.
2. Werner's Syndrome—pathology—congresses. W1 AD559 / QZ 45 U58w 1982]
  RC580.W47U55 1982   618.97   85-19426

  ISBN 978-1-4684-7855-6   ISBN 978-1-4684-7853-2 (eBook)
  DOI 10.107/978-1-4684-7853-2

Proceedings of a United States–Japan Cooperative Seminar on
Werner's Syndrome and Human Aging, held December 10–12, 1982,
in Kobe, Japan

© Springer Science+Business Media New York 1985
Originally published by Plenum Press, New York in 1985
Softcover reprint of the hardcover 1st edition 1985

All rights reserved

No part of this book may be reproduced, stored in a retrieval system, or transmitted
in any form or by any means, electronic, mechanical, photocopying, microfilming,
recording, or otherwise, without written permission from the Publisher

PREFACE

In keeping with the traditions of developmental biology and gerontology, there was a long incubation period before full expression of the plans for an International Conference on the Werner Syndrome and the publication of the present monograph based upon the proceedings of that conference. The initial concept emerged at the XIth International Congress of Gerontology, which took place in Tokyo in 1978. Drs. G.M. Martin, Y. Fujiwara and Y. Mitsui met on that occasion to discuss ways of accelerating the pace of research on this important disorder, including banking and sharing of cell cultures, establishment of patient registries, and planning of joint conferences and publications.

In November 1979, under the auspices of the Gerontological Society of America and a conference grant from the National Institute on Aging of the U.S. National Institutes of Health, a group of Japanese investigators (Drs. Fujiwara, Mitsui, M. Goto, T. Ishii, K. Oota and T. Matsumura) met with Drs. Martin, D. Salk and W. Ted Brown to develop plans to implement the goals discussed at the initial Tokyo meeting. A workshop focused on the needs of cell banking and led to an accumulation of research materials both in Japan (mainly under the leadership of T. Matsumura) and in the U.S.A. (with the cooperation of Dr. Arthur Greene of the Institute of Medical Research).

In 1981, Drs. Martin, Salk and Fujiwara developed joint proposals to the U.S. National Science Foundation and the Japan Society for the Promotion of Sciences for a U.S.-Japan Cooperative Seminar on the Werner Syndrome. The conference took place in Kobe, Japan in December, 1982. This was the first major conference exclusively devoted to a comprehensive examination of the natural history and experimental studies of the Werner syndrome. In the subsequent two years, the conference members participated in the preparation of this volume which brings together most of of what is known about the Werner syndrome, including pervious major reviews and the first English translation of Otto Werner's original description. Unfortunately we seem to be a long way from elucidating the primary biochemical genetic defect, presumably an enzyme deficiency. There is, therefore, tne promise

of future joint efforts to understand this experiment of nature.
All of the conference participants were enthusiastic in agreeing
to a second International Conference on the Werner Syndrome some
years hence, perhaps in Germany, where Otto Werner first
recognized and described the syndrome that bears his name.

We are grateful to the N.S.F. and the J.S.P.S. for having
generously funded the conference. Additional support was provided
by the Poncin Foundation, the Sanyo Electric Company Fund, the
Naito Grant (1982), and several Japanese pharmaceutical companies.
Colleagues and students in the Department of Radiation Biophysics,
Kobe University School of Medicine provided invaluable assistance
in organizational matters during the conference. Special thanks are
due Kathy Hall for editorial and organizational assistance with the
preparation of this book, and to Marie Walters for coordinating so
much. Several other persons contributed to editing and manuscript
preparation, and we express our appreciation: Allison Ross, Ginny
Walters, Christy Cota, Suzanne Simmons, Linda Lawson and Ginny
Wejak.

CONTENTS

CONTENTS

GENE ACTION, DEVELOPMENT AND AGING:
NEW DIRECTIONS FOR RESEARCH IN THE WERNER SYNDROME

OPENING REMARKS

Kunio Oota

Director Emeritus, Tokyo Metropolitan Institute of
Gerontology, Shiroyama 2-31-2, Bunkyo-ku, Tokyo 112,
Japan

This morning, I have the honor to say a few words on behalf of
the Committee on Aging Research, the parent committee of the
Japanese organizer of this seminar, as a part of the government-
supported national project of life-science studies in Japan,
welcoming to Japan and to the City of Kobe all of you participating
in the U.S.-Japan Seminar on Pathogenetic Mechanisms of Werner's
syndrome.

As you are well aware, not a great number of the world's
scientists are deeply committed to aging research. It is not
because gerontology is being regarded as unimportant, but because
of difficulties in finding effective approaches to this most
interesting problem. Mechanisms involved in the senescence of
living bodies seem to be in a great big black box, the guarded wall
of which has been penetrated only by so many theories and
hypotheses. One expects, however, that if only a tiny hole could
be dug deep enough, we might possibly insert glass-fiber optics and
inspect the inside.

One of the most hopeful candidates of such pioneering attempts
may be the elucidation of the mechanisms involved in the
pathogenesis of human progeroids. As it happens, our colleagues
here have been successful in collecting data from a number of cases
with the Werner syndrome, now called segmental progeroid, and in
analyzing them from various aspects. I congratulate the U.S.
National Science Foundation and the Japan Society for Promotion of
Sciences for selecting this subject as a topic of the U.S.-Japan
Cooperative Research Project.

To be very frank, we did not expect too much when the group was first formed in Japan a few years ago to study progeroid. We had the very good luck to find enthusiastic scientists among the members and an extremely able leader in Professor Fujiwara, and now we are grateful to the members and proud of their accomplishments.

I am convinced that the fruits to be reaped from the preeminent gerontologists of the world during the three-day seminar will make a distinguished and valuable contribution, not only to the study of the Werner syndrome per se, but also to the basic knowledge of gerontology in general. I personally expect, especially, that the discussions will point out the future direction of the aging study. Some of us even expect to hear choice discussions on whether we could regard senescence as a biological expression of extended differentiation or as a sequence of stochastically occurring errors among the biological molecules.

I was born in Kobe some 70 years ago, and I may be allowed to add a few words concerning the history of the land on which we are now standing. The city was almost completely destroyed by bombing during World War II. A very imaginative mayor with his background in technology proposed that the city be rebuilt with a new idea. His plan, as now realized, presents to you spacious lots of new land reclaimed from the sea. The work took over 30 years to complete. In completing it, the citizens of Kobe City moved earth from the mountains in the background into the sea, expanding the living and working spaces in both the background and the foreground of the city.

I hope you enjoy your seminar and also your stay in the City of Kobe, which is very beautiful.

Thank you.

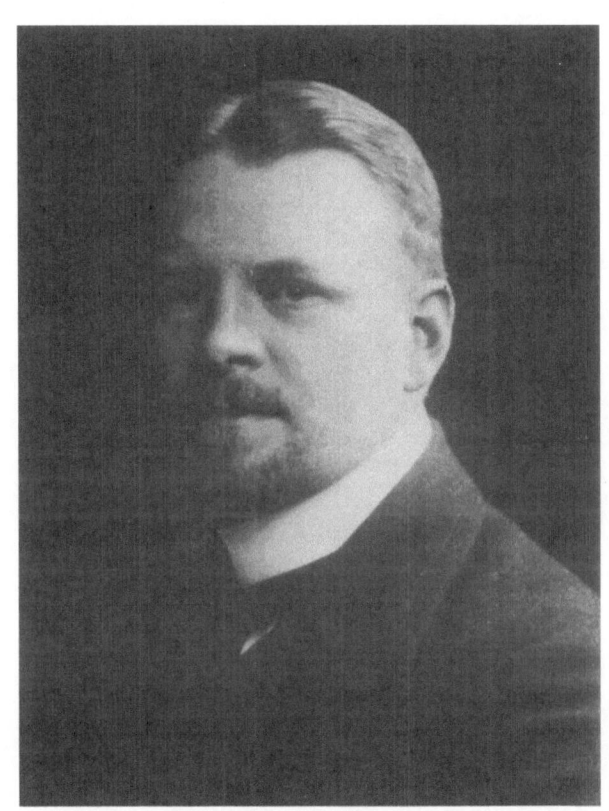

Carl Wilhelm Otto Werner
1879 - 1936
(Kiel, 1904)

ON CATARACT IN CONJUNCTION WITH SCLERODERMA

Otto Werner
Doctoral Dissertation, 1904, Royal Ophthalmology Clinic
Royal Christian Albrecht University of Kiel

Translated by Holger Hoehn

Professor and Chairman, Department of Human Genetics
University of Wuerzburg, Federal Republic of Germany

TRANSLATOR'S NOTE:

While a medical student at the ophthalmology clinic at the University of Kiel, Otto Werner had occasion to examine four siblings in a family who all had cataracts, premature greying and loss of hair, and skin changes that he referred to as scleroderma. He assumed that there must be an inherited disposition for the condition, although he found no evidence of the condition in earlier generations and no evidence for consanguinity that might have resulted in "a degenerative process." With the support of his teacher, Professor Voelkers, he presented the cases in his "Inaugural-Dissertation" for his medical degree, which he received when he was twenty-five years old. The twenty-six-page dissertation was published in 1904 (Schmidt and Klaunig, Kiel) and came to the attention of Oppenheimer and Kugel in the United States when they presented a similar case in 1934 (Trans. Am. Assn. Phys., 49:358-370). The latter authors gave the condition the eponym "Werner's syndrome."

With the assistance of Dr. Gundolf Keil in the Department of the History of Medicine, University of Wuerzburg, I obtained a copy of Werner's dissertation from the library at the University of Cologne and was able to correspond with his daughter, a physician in Hamburg. Dr. Werner's daughter, Dr. Gertrude Pehmoeller-Werner, kindly provided one of the few remaining photographs of her father, this one taken in 1904; most other family documents were burned in Hamburg in 1944.

Little is known of the life of Otto Werner beyond the brief curriculum vitae he wrote to precede his dissertation:

> "I, Carl Wilhelm Otto Werner, of Protestant confession, was born in Flensburg on February 1, 1879. My father is the University Provost Kanzleirat Gotthold Werner. I received my undergraduate education at the Royal Gymnasium in Kiel from which I graduated in 1899. From Easter of 1899 until Easter of 1904 I attended medical school, passing the first exam on Easter of 1901, and taking the state boards during the winter of 1903/4. From April 1 until September 31, 1901 I served in the infantry, regiment Herzog von Hostein (Holsteinisches) no. 85 in Kiel. On March 14, 1904 I received my medical license. On April 1 I was commissioned for a one year voluntary term as medical officer with the 1st naval division."

According to his daughter, Werner served as a naval medical officer in Kiel from April 1 to September 30, 1904. On October 27, 1906 he married the daughter of a physician in Kiel and subsequently set up a general medical practice in the village of Eddelak, Sueder-Dithmarshen/Holstein, a rural area northwest of Kiel, close to the Danish border. During the First World War, Werner once again served in the Navy. From August 1, 1914 to February 23, 1915 he was an officer in a medical evacuation unit and aboard the S.M.S. Thetis. Until 1919 he served in the naval defense unit and the 13th naval artillery command in Kiel. From 1919 until his death from liver cancer on June 5, 1936, Otto Werner took care of his extensive rural medical practice in Eddelak. His daughter writes: "He worked as a physician in the best and most comprehensive sense of the word. To me and to my brother he serves as an ever present example for the performance of our medical profession."

The style of Werner's original German is rather dry, although there is an antique charm to it that I fear has been lost in translation. I have tried to make the translation as literal as possible, which accounts for some of the odd-sounding English. A portion of the odd-sounding English may be due to my years of language training in an environment of fast foods, television, academic politics and Jello.

Owing to many investigations and experiments our knowledge of cataract formation has greatly progressed during the past decades. Indeed, the etiology of this disease has received plenty of attention, and the prevailing opinion to date is that every cataract arises in principle as a consequence of a nutritional impairment of whatever kind.

In order to briefly characterize the nutrition of the lens it should be noted that it occurs via osmosis from the anterior and posterior chamber fluids, from the vitreous body, and, most probably, also by way of the canalis petiti. The intracapsular epithelial layer thereby has the physiologic function of modifying the chamber fluid substances such that they become suitable for the nutrition of the lens.

A nutritional derangement may arise if these conditions are perturbed, either via purely traumatic, via inflammatory or via otherwise pathologic events such as iridocyclitis and chorioiditis. These events interfere with the functional capacities of said cell layer. The portions of the lens adjacent to afflicted epithelial cells hence suffer from malnutrition and thus develop partial cataracts. A different category from such cataracts caused solely by local events are those which arise as a consequence of constitutional changes involving, for example, the composition of the blood as is the case in diabetes. To the latter category also belong cataracts which arise during general albuminuria, or during the course of generalized senile degeneration. Yet another category would be cases which develop as a result of epileptic or hysterical convulsions, or as a sequelae of muscular contractions after ergot-poisoning.

In very rare instances, however, cataracts were also observed in conjunction with acute or chronic skin afflictions. In such cases one must assume that one is dealing with a disease entity which involves a common cell type, since both the epidermis and the lens are derivatives of the ectoderm. As in the case described by Rothmund in 1868, the cause for the disease would then have to be sought in a defective anlage with variable temporal manifestation.

To the latter category I should like to add an interesting observation from the Royal Eye Clinic whose publication has become possible through the kindness of Herrn Geheimrat Volckers. The observation concerns four of five siblings who developed, during their third decades of life, scleroderma of the extremities and cataracts. In addition, these patients manifest other signs of senile degeneration such as greying of hair, etc. To the best of my knowledge the literature to date contains only a single similar, albeit not exactly comparable case, namely the one mentioned above which was published by by Rothmund in 1868. I will first recall the important features of that case before reporting my own observations.

*TRANSLATOR'S NOTE: The next five pages of the dissertation
deal with the families described by Rothmund ("Uber
Kataract in Verbindung mit einer eigentumlichen
Hautdegeneration"). With this rather extensive
introduction Dr. Werner probably intended to emphasize the
differences in clinical manifestation, clinical course, and
pattern of inheritance (as conceived by him) between the
families described by Rothmund and his own observations.
The last paragraph on page 11 of the original thesis serves
as a rejoinder by which the author introduces his personal
observations. Dr. Werner writes:*

Whereas Rothmund, at least in one of his families, regards
consanguinity as an acceptable explanation for the etiology of the
disease, and thereby implies the notion of its degenerative nature,
and whereas such a concept is quite plausible for the other
families in his study in view of the geographic isolation of the
alpine valley ("Walsertal") where they live, the family history of
the following cases from the Royal Department of Ophthalmology in
Kiel, in spite of detailed field research, do not only fail to
yield clues for a similar explanation, but on the contrary
emphasize that we are dealing with an otherwise extremely vigorous
family. I will now proceed with the presentation of the personal
histories and physical examinations of said family members:

CASE I

Carl K., 40 years of age, had diphtheria as a child, otherwise
was reportedly healthy. As early as age 20 he suffered from
"corns" forming at his heels and his big and small toes, which
rendered walking difficult for him. When they were removed, they
reappeared within rather short intervals, and in spite of all
efforts on the part of the patient could not be eradicated. The
existence of other skin abnormalities was reportedly not noted by
the patient at that time. At approximately 28 years of age the
patient noted a beginning deterioration of his visual capacity
which worsened rapidly at age 33 and led to his presentation in
Kiel during the spring of 1900. His pre-operative status is as
follows:

Bilateral visus = quantitative light sensitivity only. Both
eyes affected by moderate chronic conjunctivitis. Lacrimal duct
patent. Bulbi not irritated. Cornea normal. Pupillar reflexes
within normal limits. Anterior chamber of normal size. Iris
normal. Completely turbid lenses on both sides except a few clear
spots on the anterior corticalis. Retina not visible. Projection
within normal limits. Surgery consisted of modified linear

extraction. Right eye (5-21-1900): formation of a mid-size
coloboma leaving only minor remnants of the corticalis. A shallow
anterior chamber is formed by May 25, and primary healing occurs
three days later with the anterior chamber assuming normal depth.
A corresponding procedure is performed on the left eye on May 31
which is likewise successful. Testing of visual capacity on
6-16-1900 yields the following results:

R with +10.0 S = 4/15
L with +10.0 S = 4/50

After discission of emerging bilateral thin secondary
cataracts on 6-20:

R with +9.0 stenop.S = 8/15
L with +10.0 stenop.S = 8/20

bilateral with +13.0 Nieden 7. The patient is released on 6-21
with glasses +10 (distance) and +13 (proximity).

As early as during 1896 the patient had noticed greying of his
hair. One and a half years after discharge the epidermis began to
thicken at several circumscript sites of his lower shanks and feet.
This took place mostly but not always at exposed areas. When those
thickenings lacerated, or opened spontaneously (which happened
frequently), an open lesion remained which sometimes extended down
to the bone. The lesions healed only with greatest difficulty.
First, these events involved chiefly the terminal phalanx of the
third toe; the resulting defect took 1 and 1/2 years to heal. It
was succeeded by two similar defects, approximately penny-size, at
the dorsum pedis which however healed within a relatively short
period of time. A ten penny-piece sized lesion at the malleolus
externus healed after 1 and 1/2 years; a somewhat larger lesion
formed where the Achilles tendon ends; two smaller ones appeared
over the terminal phalanges of the 2nd and 4th toes, respectively;
finally, during last winter a large defect appeared inside and up
from the malleolus internus.

The involvement of the patient's right leg was somewhat less
extensive. 1 1/2 years ago a 10 penny-piece sized lesion appeared
at the lateral right ankle which healed during the winter. While
this defect was healing, smaller defects appeared at the 2nd and
5th toes with involvement of the terminal phalanges of the 2nd and
3rd, and the middle phalanges of the 4th and 5th toes,
respectively. In all these instances the appearance of open
lesions was preceded by a marked cornification of the epidermis
without prior exposure to unusual amounts of localized pressure,
since the patient had stayed in bed without wearing shoes when
these lesions appeared.

Within certain intervals the feet showed signs of an inflammatory process accompanied by such intolerable itching, piercing, burning and paresthesias that the patient at times cried like a child. Such episodes of inflammation were regularly followed by intense de-cornification.

Presently, the patient by and large evokes the impression of senility. His hair is snow-white, scarce and thin; his nutritional status is quite good even though the lower limb musculature is poorly developed and atrophic which may be the result of prolonged immobilization. Both feet are swollen and feel hot. The pedal vaults are well formed; the big toe is bent backwards and rather immobile, as are the remainder of the toes due to tight skin. There is only minor pain upon pressure. Up to the middle third of the lower leg the skin appears smooth, somewhat glossy and atrophic. The remainder of skin displays a close to normal color. The lower leg and the areas behind and below the malleoli are covered with epidermal scales. There are venectasias around the medial malleoli, while their outside is covered by a prominent layer of cornified epidermis. Likewise, major cornifications are found to the left of each heel, the big and small toes (which are extremely pressure sensitive), and over the entire 2nd toe. The terminal phalanx of the 3rd toe appears "capped" by such cornifications. The right foot displays similar changes on the dorsal aspect of the 4th and 5th toes, respectively, over parts of the planta, the plantar portion of the big toe, and involving the tip of the little toe.

On the left foot there are scars at the sites of healed ulcers; the toes are extremely atrophic, in particular the terminal phalanges, whose nails have completely vanished from the 3rd and 4th, while rudiments thereof are left on the 2nd toe. There is also a scar of a healed lesion to the right of the middle phalanx of the 3rd toe. The middle phalanx of the 2nd and the terminal phalanges of the 4th and 5th toes show granulating, darkly covered defects. The toes are generally atrophic with the big toe being least affected; the toe nails lack on the 4th and 5th toes, and only rudiments are left on the 2nd and 3rd toes, respectively. The mobility of all toes is severely limited. The affected areas lack any growth of hair. Following surgery the patient's eyes are stable and he sees well.

CASE II

Marie K., age 38, was not particularly ailing as a child and is said to have grown nicely. She started menstruating at age 13, and her periods were regular up to age 20 when they became sporadic (1-2 times a year) and finally ceased without having returned to this date. At age 23 the patient noted that her eyesight

deteriorated, first on the right and within a year's time also in
the left eye. A cataract was diagnosed, but it took six years to
mature. The patient underwent successful cataract surgery in 1896.
The eye exam at that time was as follows:

> Right: quantitative light sensitivity
> Left: finger-counting at a distance of 0.5 m

Projection well perserved in both eyes. Conjunctivae and lacrimal
apparatus without complications. Following modified linear
extraction and subsequent discission the status is as follows:

> Right: 4/36 with +10.0
> Left: 8/36 with +10.0

Nieden with +15.0 o.k. on both sides; the ophthalmologic
examination revealed slightly atrophic papillae and chorioditis
aequatorialis manifesting as small pigmented spots. The patient
was discharged with glasses +10.0 (distance) and +15.0 (proximity).

Already a year prior to her noticing the worsening of her
eyesight the patient had become aware of "hardening" of her left
foot and of the distal portion of her left lower leg. Soon
thereafter this hardening was also noted on the right side. As
time passed these changes progressed, although without bothering
her too much. Approximately 10 years later, in 1898, an ulcer
appeared over the lateral aspect of her left ankle which took 2
years to heal. In 1902 the patient noted a defect on her left
lower leg which reached the size of a walnut, and which presently
is in the process of healing. The patient denies any itching or
pain in the affected areas. A number of years ago she developed a
struma; she denies having any disturbances of the nervous system,
nor having ever experienced palpitations.

Physical examination: The patient is a small, delicate person
with a fine bone structure, weak musculature and only moderate
amounts of adipose tissue. The general impression is that of a
fairly degenerate body. The skin appears overall normal, but there
are numerous venous ectasias throughout the face which render it
rather red. Her hair is largely grey, sparse, and individually
thin. Psyche and intelligence are completely normal. Her frontal
neck area is covered by a fist-sized tumor that proved to be a well
developed struma. Pulse rate 104, reasonably strong and regular.
Palpitations were never noted by the patient; there is no hand
tremor, no exophthalmus or any other signs which could speak for a
"morbus Basedowii." The skin of the right foot and of the distal
lower leg is shiny, smooth and atrophic, spotted with small grey
and brownish discolorations even though the overall color does not
deviate substantially from that of normal skin. Low-grade shedding
of cornified materials is limited to the border between healthy and

affected skin, the latter being completely void of hair as noted previously.

A walnut-sized lesion extends above the plantar insertion of the Achilles tendon with re-epithelialization noticeable at the peripheral margins. There is a slight protrusion from the medial pedal margin, discharging small amounts of putrid-serous liquid. Additional ulcers exist in the vicinity of the lateral malleolar region, and at the border between the lower and the middle third of the tibial aspect of the lower leg. These are in the process of healing. At the lateral foot margin and near the phalangeal joints "epidermoidal" thickenings exist that are not pressure sensitive. These skin alterations are most prominent in the toe areas, with all toes being cramped tightly together. As a consequence of the epidermoidal skin thickenings and the resulting tension of the skin the mobility of the toes is reduced to zero.

On the left side up to the border between middle and upper third of the lower leg the skin is completely atrophic, smooth and shiny. There is no sharp demarcation between diseased and healthy areas, and the skin cannot be lifted from its supporting structures. It appears rather transparent, allowing for easy visualization of underlying vessels and their smaller ramifications. Sensation is not impaired. Somewhat below the middle portion of the lower leg and lateral to the frontal tibial margin one finds a clean, healing ulcer which is of 10 penny-piece size and surrounded by strongly reddish and shiny skin; there are more or less extensive but circumscript epidermal thickenings throughout the foot at sites which correspond to points of support. Moreover, such changes can be seen also in the middle portion of the plantar vault in an area lateral to and below of the insertion of the Achilles tendon. Three further thickenings follow the lateral foot margin, one near the middle of the medial margin, and, finally, there are rather numerous changes spread over the dorsal aspects of all toes whose tips appear "capped" by translucent (one can see vessels underneath) epidermoidal hyperplasias. Desquamation is limited to a few isolated sites. As before, the worst changes involve the toes which are extremely atrophic, covered by reddish, tightly stretched, and smooth-shiny skin, and which appear crowded together. Toes number 2 to 5 lack nails altogether, while that of the first toe is in a rudimentary state. The movement of all toes is severely impeded, and almost exclusively limited to the tarsometatarsal joints. Movement of the talocrural joint is similarly restricted.

In this case the situation of the upper extremities closely corresponds to what was found at the lower extremities.

The skin of the left hand is of normal color with the exception of the exposed areas (as the wrist) where it is reddish-

blue. It can be lifted only with difficulty from the back of the
hand in small, meagre folds. The skin feels hardened and tight,
especially around the fingers. The fingers themselves have a
similar appearance as the toes: their skin is reddish, shiny,
smooth, atrophic. A particularly severe involvement is found of
the little finger whose terminal phalanx is hardly recognizable and
fixed in flexed position. Its nail or remnants thereof can hardly
be distinguished. All other finger joints between the end and
middle phalanx are "ankylotic," and the fingers are fixed in a
medium-flexed position since neither complete flexion nor extension
are possible anymore.

The right hand shows essentially the same picture with the
exception of even more pronounced epidermoid thickenings. Such
thickenings are found over the metacarpophalangeal joints of the
2nd and 5th fingers, and extending to the interphalangeal joints of
the 2nd finger. Vestiges of healed rhagades can clearly be
recognized at these sites. The fifth finger is likewise most
severely affected, and the entire hand is held in a medium-flexed
position whereas the mobility appears to the somewhat better than
on the left.

CASE III

Heinrich K., age 36, was affected by diphtheria at age 8 which
required tracheotomy. Ever since he suffers from bronchitis which
however does not bother him too much. Otherwise, he has been
always healthy and vigorous, supporting himself as a farmer and
being well capable of ploughing. However, soon after leaving
school he noticed interspersion of his capital hair with greyish
strands, a very prominent such strand extending to the middle of
the os frontale. Approximately 12 years prior to this admission,
i.e. since age 24, the entire capital hair began to turn grey. At
age 29 the patient became convinced that he could not see well
anymore, which had been his impression all along for several years.
Four years later, at age 33, his eyesight had deteriorated so badly
that he presented himself for surgery. The eye-exam at that time
revealed the following:

Bilateral quantitative light sensitivity only;
Bilateral chronic conjunctivitis.
Bulbus w/o inflammation, corneae clear, moderately sized
anterior chamber; iris normal; prompt and symmetrical
pupillar reflexes; lens almost completely cloudy; minor iris
shadow; pressure normal, projection o.k., lacrimal duct
patent.

Successful surgery was via the modified linear extraction procedure
yielding a fairly large, shrunken and flat lens nucleus. The

resulting bilateral secondary cataracts were eliminated via
discission on May 3 and May 8, respectively. After that, the
patient's eye status was as follows:

    Right with +11.0 = 8/20
    Left with +10.0 = 8/25.

He is able to read with +16.0 Nieden 1 in 20 cm. He was discharged
with glasses +10 (distance) and +16 (proximity).

    At the same time when the loss of his eyesight had reached its
peak, i.e. around the year 1900, the patient noted changes at his
feet which began with swellings accompanied by burning and itching.
First the medial aspect of the right ankle presented with
epidermoidal thickening leading to ulceration which took 1 1/2
years to heal. Next the medial aspect of the big toe became
involved with thickening and subsequent ulceration which has not
resolved to this date. The tip of the small toe has been affected
for the last two years with intermittent healing and relapse after
renewed thickening of the affected skin areas.

    On physical examination the patient gives the impression of
extreme senility. His build is delicate, his musculature only
moderate, and there is almost no panniculus adiposus. With the
exception of the affected foot, the withered skin is plied into
senile folds. There is obvious arteriosclerosis with prominent
winding of the arteries.

    On the right side, the disease process involves primarily the
proximal part of the entire foot and the lower third of the shank.
Throughout the affected areas the skin is reddish, smooth and shiny
while being thin and atrophic. Sensation is not impaired. There
is increased desquamation from underneath a bandage. A nicely
granulating lesion is present at a finger-width below the malleolus
medialis which is of walnut size and secretes a purulent liquid.
Otherwise, the skin around the toes is fairly normal, and there is
little atrophy.

    However, atrophy is more distinct at the left foot where the
toes are red and their skin appears shiny, smooth and tight.
Similar changes, albeit less noticeable, occur throughout other
parts of the foot and extending up to the lower half of the shank
where the skin appears blueish and feels cold (this is also what
the patient says). There is also minor desquamation in this area.
The medial aspect of the big toe displays a 5 penny-piece sized
smeary defect whose center secretes a small amount of purulent-
serous liquid.

    On both feet and lower legs the disease is accompanied by
intermittent swellings as well as itching, the latter leaving

distinct scratch marks. The right elbow displays thickenings of
cornified epidermis around the olecranon area which looks like a
small tent. Within a palm-sized area this site is surrounded by
reddish skin which is smooth, shiny, thin and atrophic.

The patient's eye status has not changed since his dismissal
from our hospital.

CASE IV

Minna K., age 31, had measles, scarlet fever, diphtheria and
german measles; otherwise, her childhood development is said to
have been normal. During puberty she experienced brief and
irregular menstruations which ceased at age 19. During the winter
of 1895 when the patient was 22 years of age, the epidermal layer
of the 2nd and 3rd toes on her left foot began to thicken. This
ultimately resulted in a capsule-like structure that was extremely
painful upon pressure. Removal of these capsules left a skin
defect through which the bone could be reached with a probe. Both
toes had to be removed. 1 1/2 years later the same process started
at the 4th toe of the left foot, and 3 years ago the 2nd toe of the
right foot became likewise affected. Both had to be removed.
Three years ago the patient also noted bad vision beginning in the
right eye where all she has left now is quantitative light
sensitivity. The other eye became involved during last fall and
has meanwhile progressed to a stage where the patient can only
perform rough-machine work. She cannot read the newspaper anymore.
She will undergo surgery in the near future. Her status praesens
is as follows:

The patient gives the impression of being degenerate by all
measures. She is very small, of extremely delicate build, with
small bones, meagre musculature, and very moderate amounts of body
fat. Her hair is very grey. Skin and mucous membranes appear
normal, as do her hands. Her feet, however, are severely
disfigured. The bony vault of the left foot is exaggerated. The
middle portion of the lateral foot margin shows prominent bony
bossing extending downward and outward. While being of near normal
color, the pedal skin appears shiny, smooth and atrophic with
spotty desquamations. The exposed areas of the dorsal foot and
around the malleoli display numerous venectasias. The mobility is
restricted due to tight skin. The thenar area of the planta shows
unusual amounts of cornified epidermis whose middle portions
display brownish-red invaginations. The 2nd to 4th toes are
absent; the remainder are grossly atrophic, particularly their
terminal phalanges, where the nails have completely vanished. At
all affected areas the skin spans the bone tightly, shows a red
color, and is very shiny and smooth.

On the right side, the patient has a typical flat-foot. The middle portion of the lateral foot margin displays bony bossing which is covered by thickened skin. The dorsal aspect of the right foot shows likewise bony bossing and, in addition, venectasias and epidermoidal cornifications. The behaviour of the skin in these areas is quite analogous to what has been described for the other side, including the toe areas, but with the exception of partially preserved nails. The entire process does not seem to have progressed as far as on the left. The second toe is missing. The mobility of the foot is likewise restricted but not quite as severely as on the other side. There is also less desquamation.

Otherwise, the patient displays a fist-sized neck tumor which turns out to be a struma. There are no discernible palpitations or tremor. However, the patient is quite irritable; she frequently bursts out in sudden tears being closely followed by bursts of laughing. She is distrustful, and an extremely nervous person who is reluctant towards any examination.

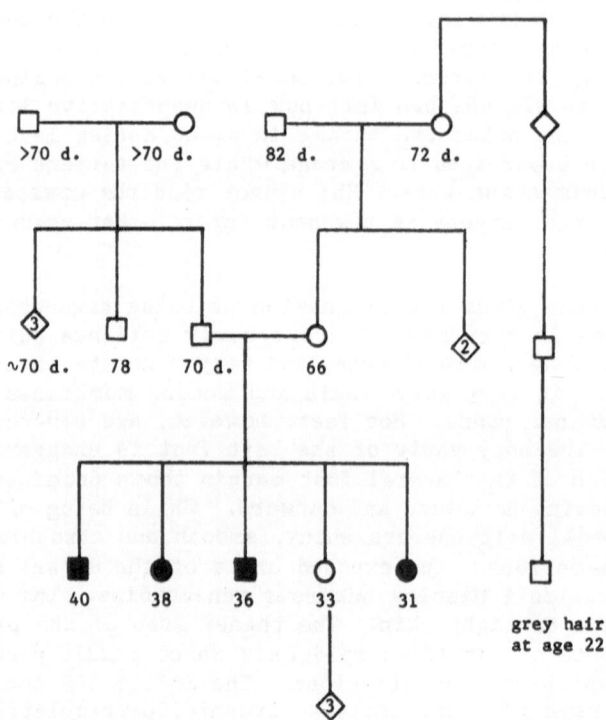

Pedigree constructed from Dr. Werner's thesis.
(d = died at age indicated)

Her eye-exam yields the following:

Right eye with nearly complete cataract; iris shadow greatly reduced. Only quantitative light sensitivity; normal pupillar reflexes, normal projection; left eye with strongly reduced visual acuity; bare inspection, however, does not reveal signs of lens changes. In contrast, the ophthalmoscopic examination shows irregular opacities scattered throughout the entire lens with special prominence in the upper medial quadrant area.

FAMILY HISTORY

The family history does not yield any substantial clues which might explain the disease in this family. The patients' father died at age 70 from cancer of the stomach while having been healthy and vigorous before. Three paternal siblings died in their seventies, and one brother is alive and well at age 78. The paternal grandparents likewise reached old age. The patients' mother is still alive and 66 years old. With the exception of scoliotic deformation of the spine the mother is healthy. In spite of her age she is extremely active and mobile. The maternal grandparents died at ages 82 and 72, respectively; the maternal grandmother suffered from varices and ulcera cruris. Otherwise, the family history provides no indication for skin afflictions or cataracts, in particular not for those with early onset. The only positive finding was greying of the hair, in his twenties, of a maternal cousin twice removed. The patients deny knowledge of any marriage among relatives during the last generations.

A sister of the four patients, born as the 4th of five siblings, is presently 33 years old and completely healthy: she is married and has three vigorous, exceptionally well developed children who bear not the least sign of abnormality.

In spite of all this, and even though the family history does not yield any clues for the possibility of inheritance nor, more specifically, for a degenerative process resulting from consanguinity, we nevertheless must assume that we are dealing with an inherited disposition for the disease at hand. It is conceivable that the acquisition of this disposition, and the occurrence of other potentially affected family members took place so long ago that these events are no longer remembered by the family. The cause of the disease would thus have to be found in a faulty embryonic anlage of the ectoderm created by said disposition. As a consequence, the vigor of the ectodermal cells is reduced. This reduction involves the epidermis including glands, hair, etc., as well as the lens which is derived from an invagination of the ectoderm. In any case, we cannot postulate that we are dealing with a condition that has just been acquired by

the patients themselves, since it would be highly unlikely that
such a disease should have been picked up independently by each of
the four affected sibs, and then taken such an identical course.

ACKNOWLEDGEMENT

In winding up this report it is a pleasant duty to gratefully
acknowledge my highly esteemed teacher, Herrn Geheimrat Prof. Dr.
Voelckers, who entrusted me with these cases and who lent his kind
support to this writing.

REFERENCES

Rothmund, Uber Katarakte in Verbindung mit einer eigentumlichen
     Hautdegeneration.
Becker, Pathologie und Therapie des Linsensystems.

WERNER'S SYNDROME (PROGERIA OF THE ADULT) AND ROTHMUND'S SYNDROME:

TWO TYPES OF CLOSELY RELATED HEREDOFAMILIAL ATROPHIC DERMATOSES
WITH JUVENILE CATARACTS AND ENDOCRINE FEATURES; A CRITICAL STUDY
WITH FIVE NEW CASES

S.J. Thannhauser
Boston, MA, 1944

*(Editor's note: The original version of Thannhauser's article
was divided into three sections; only Section I is reproduced
here. We have not reproduced Thannhauser's original
photographs, but the figure legends are given in an appendix.)*

INTRODUCTION

Observations on these rare and apparently heredofamilial
disorders are scattered throughout the different branches of
medical literature according to the particular interest of the
individual author specializing in involvement of the eye or the
skin or the nervous system.

B.S. Oppenheimer and V.S. Kugel (1934) have the distinction of
first reporting this condition in American medical literature,
renaming it "Werner's syndrome." The characteristics of this
syndrome are:

> Shortness of stature, characteristic habitus
> Canities (i.e., premature graying of the hair)
> Premature baldness
> Scleropoikiloderma
> Trophic ulcers of the legs
> Juvenile cataracts

*Reprinted from Annals of Internal Medicine, 23:559 (1945)
with permission of the American College of Physicians.*

Hypogonadism
Tendency to diabetes
Calcification of the blood vessels
Osteoporosis
Metastatic calcifications
Tendency to occur in brothers and sisters

The cases published in the literature under different titles
have been purposely selected and grouped. It seems necessary to
quote and discuss in detail the pertinent literature in order to
prove the actual existence of Werner's as well as Rothmund's
syndrome and to justify their separation. Observations of our own
cases should show that the classification of the skin changes as
"scleroderma" or "scleropoikiloderma" is not appropriate, since we
are dealing with heredofamilial dermatoses of a special nature.
The pathogenesis of the ulcers occurring in Werner's syndrome,
either "trophic" or due to "pressure," will be discussed.   In
addition, the relationship of the syndrome under discussion to other
clinical syndromes will be demonstrated.

I.   Werner's syndrome (progeria of the adult)
II.   Rothmund's syndrome
III. Cases related to Werner's syndrome (progeria of the
      adult) and Rothmund's syndrome
      A.   Cataracta dermatogenes (neurodermitis) Type Andogsky
      B.   Progeria of children (Hutchinson-Gilford's syndrome)
      C.   Myotonic Dystrophy
      D.   Hereditary ectodermal dysplasia of the hydrotic
           type. Dystrophy of the hair and nails (Type McKay-
           Davidson)

I.   WERNER'S SYNDROME (PROGERIA OF THE ADULT)

In 1904 Otto Werner (1) described in his Doctor's thesis from
Ophthalmological Clinic in Kiel, a peculiar disorder, under the
title "Cataract in Connection with Scleroderma," occurring in four
brothers and sisters, two males 40 years and 36 years old, and two
females, 38 years and 36 years old (a fifth sister, 33 years old,
was healthy). The grandfather and grandmother and parents of the
patients lived to an old age. There were no interfamilial
marriages and no blood relationship. It was only reported that a
cousin of the patients, on the mother's side, already showed
graying of the hair at the age of 20.

Case reports

Case 1. Carl K., 40 years old. Normal birth. Normal development in childhood. Short in stature. No measures of height were reported. The appearance was atrophic and senile. Hairs started to turn gray at 20. At 40 they were snow white and very scarce. Nothing is reported concerning eyebrows, eyelashes or pubic hair at the age of 20. Areas of hyperkeratosis were first noted under the large toe, under the fifth toe and on the heels. After removal they recurred in a short time. At the age of 40 hyperkeratotic areas were noted over the malleoli, heels, and on almost all toes, especially the end phalanx of the left second toe, which was covered with a cap of horny tissue. The skin over the lower extremities and on both feet became thickened at 30. Ulcers appeared at this time, first on the left third toe and on the skin of the dorsal surface of both feet. The ulcers were as large as a dime. Later ulcers developed on the external malleoli and on the skin over both Achilles tendons. In almost all instances areas of inflammation were observed, especially on the dorsum of the feet. These places were so painful that the patient cried like a child. The taut skin was stretched over the underlying structures which were lacking in subcutaneous fat. In some places fine scales covered the shiny, thin skin. The skin changes were only noted on the lower legs and feet. Because of the tightness of the skin, motion in the ankle and phalangeal joints of the feet was considerably restricted. There were no hairs in the afflicted skin areas. Unlike his brother, this patient did not complain of pain in his legs. The muscles and subcutaneous fat tissue on both lower legs were underdeveloped. On the forearms and hands, also, muscles as well as subcutaneous fat tissue were atrophic, but to a lesser degree than on the lower legs and feet. The toenails were lacking on the left third and fourth toes and on the other toes the nails were atrophic. A similar condition of the nails was noted on the right foot. There is no report on the character of the voice. Cataracts developed at the age of 28 and were operated upon at the age of 36. Endocrine features: Other than the senile atrophic appearance, there was no report on the sex organs or his sexual life. The fact that he was not married hints at a sexual deficiency.

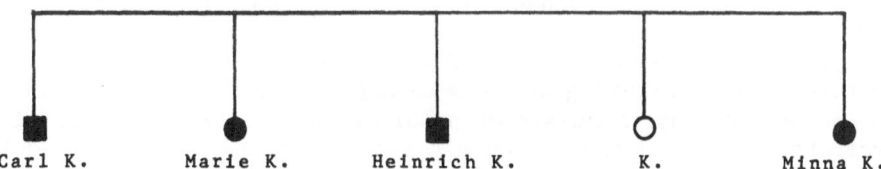

Pedigree of Family K

    Case 2. Marie K., 38 years old. Normal development as a
child. She was very short in stature and gave the general
impression of being an underdeveloped, degenerated person, with
thin muscles and very little subcutaneous fat tissue. Hairs were
fine, gray and scarce. Psyche and intelligence were normal. Skin:
At the age of 22, the patient noted that the skin of both lower
legs and feet had already become taut and fixed on the underlying
structures. The veins under the thin atrophic skin became visible
in their smallest ramifications. There were no hairs on the
affected parts of the skin. Because of the tightness of the
stretched skin, motion of the ankle joints and phalangeal joints
was almost impossible. The color of the skin was normal, except
that the face had a reddish hue due to severe acne. When she was
32, an ulcer developed on the skin covering the left outer
malleolus, which did not close for two years. When she was 34, an
ulcerative skin defect, the size of a walnut, developed on the left
lower edge of the shin bone, which, after several years, had not
yet healed. At the time this 38-year-old patient was first seen,
the skin of both lower legs was taut, glossy and atrophic. The
skin on the affected parts showed patches of grayish brown
discoloration beside normal skin of normal color. Slight scaling
was noted on sharply defined places where the normal skin bordered
the affected parts. Areas of thick hyperkeratosis were present
over both heels, under the large toes, on the lateral sides of the
feet and on the dorsum pedis on several toes. Ulcers and scars of
ulcers were seen on all parts exposed to pressure on both lower
legs. Especially large ones were located over both Achilles
tendons, on both shins, on the malleoli and on the lateral sides of
the feet and on the back of some toes. On the large toe of the
left foot only a rudimentary nail had developed. On all other toes
of the left foot nails were lacking. Of special interest was the
severe involvement of the skin of both lower arms and hands. The
thin, reddish, atrophic skin over both hands was so tightly
stretched over the bony structures that the first and second
phalangeal joints on all fingers were ankylosed. The patient could
not move her fingers. The fifth finger of the left hand was
contracted in a flexed position. Defined areas of hyperkeratosis
similar to the condition on the feet were noted over the
metacarpophalangeal and over some interphalangeal joints. The
fingernails were normal except that of the left fifth finger, which
was atrophic. The muscles of both lower arms were atrophic and
meager. The subcutaneous fat tissue was almost lacking on both
lower arms and hands. Tendon reflexes were normal. Cataracts
developed on both lenses at the age of 23. The cataracts matured
six years later and were successfully operated upon. Endocrine
features: The thyroid gland was enlarged to the size of a fist.
The patient did not complain of palpitation or other symptoms of
hyperthyroidism. Menstruation had started at the age of 13 and had
been regular until the age of 20. Thereafter, the patient
menstruated only twice a year for a few years, then menstruation
ceased altogether.

Case 3. Heinrich K., 36 years old. He was a farmer and was able to work until his eyesight deteriorated at the age of 33. As a child, his development was normal. No record of his height was reported. At the time of his first examination, his appearance was senile. After he graduated from high school, his hair began to turn gray. At the age of 24, all the scalp hair was grayish. There was no report of the presence or absence of pubic hairs. His bony structure was very thin. The skin was of senile texture and shrivelled. A withered condition was especially noted on the skin of the face. Tightness of the skin in Heinrich K. was observed only on both feet and the lower third of the lower legs. The skin in these areas was taut and atrophic and of a reddish hue. Some areas of the feet were puffy and itching. Slight scaling on some areas was noted. The mobility of ankle and phalangeal joints was not restricted. Only over the olecranon of the right elbow circumscribed areas of hyperkeratosis were seen. Ulcers were present only on two areas, namely, on the skin over the right malleolus and over the medial side of the large toe. Cataracts developed at the age of 29. The patient was operated upon at the age of 33. The arterial blood vessels exhibited definite signs of arteriosclerosis. Endocrine features: Other than his senile, atrophic appearance, no remarks concerning endocrine symptoms were made.

Case 4. Minna K., 31 years old. Her development in childhood was normal. At the time of her examination, she gave the impression of a degenerated and infantile person. She was of very short stature. Her psyche was abnormal. She cried and laughed without reason. She was suspicious and refused at first to be examined. Her scalp hairs were entirely gray. The first skin changes were observed at the age of 22. The skin over the second and third left toes became thickened and covered these toes like a horny "capsule," After the horny layer was removed, an ulcer remained. Both toes had to be amputated. Two years later the same condition resulted in the amputation of the fourth left and second right toes. At the time of her examination, at the age of 31, both feet were deformed because of the previous operations. The arches were abnormally high. Exostoses were present on lateral parts as well as on the dorsal parts of the feet. There was slight scaling of the skin over the lower legs and feet and it was taut and atrophic, but of normal color. The skin was so tightly stretched over the bony structures of the feet that the mobility in both ankle joints was almost completely restricted. Numerous telangiectases of the skin covering the malleoli and the exotoses were noted. Areas of circumscribed hyperkeratosis were outstanding on both heels and over the exostoses. The nails of the two remaining toes of the left foot had completely disappeared; the end phalanges of these toes were atrophic. The nails of the four

remaining toes of the right foot were present only in rudimentary
form. The muscles of both lower legs were extremely thin and
underdeveloped. The panniculus adiposus in this part of the legs
was almost completely absent. Although the bony structures of the
whole body were extremely thin and fragile, spontaneous fractures
had never occurred. Cataracts developed at the age of 27, first on
the right eye and, two years later, on the left eye. Endocrine
features: The thyroid was enlarged forming a goiter the size of an
apple. No signs of hyperthyroidism were noted. During her
adolescent years the menstruation was rare and scanty. At the age
of 19 the menses stopped completely. Her presenile appearance was
outstanding.

Comment

There is no question that Werner's observations on four
brothers and sisters represent the first description of a unique
clinical entity. Werner, a medical student in the ophthalmological
ward, was concerned chiefly with the juvenile cataracts, but the
description of the appearance of these patients, especially the
detailed appearance of the skin changes, at once gives the
impression that the described disease is of general medical
interest and significance since it involves not only the eyes but
the whole body. All the symptoms of these brothers and sisters
developed during the second and third decades of life. Birth was
normal, development in childhood was normal, but in the adolescent
age they remained short in stature. It is remarkable how similar,
almost to the last detail, the other features likewise appeared in
these patients. They became gray around the age of 20, later the
skin on the lower legs became taut, atrophic and stretched over the
underlying tissues, which consisted of a very meager subcutaneous
fat tissue and thin atrophic muscles. Areas of circumscribed
hyperkeratosis were painful and after the horny layer was torn off
or removed by the pressure of shoes or clothes, ulcers resulted. At
the same time, in the second decade of life, cataracts developed in
both eyes. The whole appearance became more and more senile. The
patient became incapacitated for heavy work, partly owing to the
immobilization of the ankle joints and feet as a result of the
tightness of the skin and the ulcers, and partly owing to general
weakness and to the reduced nutritional status of the whole body.
Signs of arteriosclerosis became evident and completed the picture
of presenility.

Werner has classified the skin changes as scleroderma because
the skin of these patients in the affected areas was taut and
tightly stretched over the underlying tissues, as in true
scleroderma. He did not consider that the circumscribed
hyperkeratosis and ulcer formation are not observed as features of
true scleroderma nor did he make biopsies to prove his
classification histologically. Unfortunately this designation, as

will be noted, was used in similar familial cases later published.
On the basis of our own observations, an effort will be made to
classify the nature of the skin changes simulating scleroderma in
Werner's syndrome. Werner, himself, relates the observations made
on the four adult members of the family K. to observations
published by Rothmund 61 years ago, describing young people of
three different families in whom peculiar skin changes, together
with cataracts, occurred. The difference, and the relationship of
the syndromes described by Rothmund on the one side and by O.
Werner on the other will be pointed out in the second part of this
paper.

Other Case Reports

    A. Vossius, (2) in 1920, reported two cases with scleroderma and
cataract.

    Case 1 was a 57-year-old, intelligent woman, with a small
skull. The scalp hair was snow white and scarce. Proptosis of the
eyes was noted. The voice was high pitched and hoarse.
Scleroderma developed at the age of 20 and bilateral cataracts at
the age of 31. No similar disorder in the family was reported.

    Case 2 was a 35-year-old male who was short in stature. The
muscles and adipose tissue were underdeveloped. The voice was high
pitched and hoarse. Scleroderma started at 20 and cataract at 30.
One sister was reported to be of the same small stature as the
patient.

    G. Guillain, J.T. Alajouanine and R. Marquezy (3) (1923)
reported a male patient, 28 years old, under the title
"Sclerodermie progressive avec cataracte double precoce chez un
infantile."

    No other members of the family were afflicted. He was short
in stature (148 cm) and his growth stopped at the age of 10. The
extremities were short and thin in contrast to the chest and
abdomen. Hands and feet were small. The fingers showed nodular
deformities as in arthritis. Hair: Face and chin were hairless
with the exception of a few fine mustache hairs. Pubic hairs were
scarce and of a female distribution. The skin was tight and
not pliable on the lower part of the legs, especially on the toes.
The skin was fine in texture on the dorsum of the feet. Under the
great toes, areas of hyperkeratosis were found. Ulcers were also
present under the great toes as well as on points of pressure. The
muscles on the lower part of the legs were atrophic. Above the
knee the muscles were normal. On the face, chin and arms, the skin
was also tight but less so than on the feet. There was some
difficulty in opening the mouth wide. No telangiectases were
noted. Cataracts developed in both eyes when he was 25. The voice

was harsh and high pitched. The heart was normal. Blood pressure
was 140 mm Hg systolic and 90 mm diastolic. Endocrine features:
Gynecomastia of both breasts. Although the genital organs were
very small and the testes were only the size of those of a 10-year-
old boy, the patient claimed to have had intercourse three to four
times in a single night. He had married at the age of 24 but had
no children. Sella turcica was normal. Roentgenograms of the
bones showed the epiphyseal fuges closed.

     N. Manjukowa, (4) in 1923, in a paper concerning the relation of
cataract to endocrine disturbances, described a 36-year-old man
whose features apparently belong to the syndrome under discussion,
whereas a patient, reported in 1922 by C. Papastratiyakis, (5) with
complete alopecia, atrophy of the nails and cataracts, should not
be registered as Werner's syndrome, but rather as "hereditary
ectodermal dysplasia."
     E.M. Barbot, (6) in a These of Paris in 1925 (the same cases
were later republished by Monier-Vinard and Barbot (7)) discussed in
a paper entitled "La sclerodermie associe a la cataract (affection
familial)" a family in which the grandfather had early canities,
and cataracts at the age of 40. The mother observed graying of the
hair at the age of 20 and cataracts between the ages of 20 and 30.
She did not have any skin changes. This woman had five children.
One child died of intestinal troubles. Two sons were healthy. Two
daughters showed skin changes, canities and cataracts.

     Case 1. Miss Marie C., age 46, height 160 cm. Shell-like
plaques of hyperkeratosis on both soles beneath the great toe were
noticed at the age of 20. The skin over the lower legs and ankles
was tightly stretched. At the age of 22 the voice became hoarse.
She was a singer and had to give this up. At the same time the

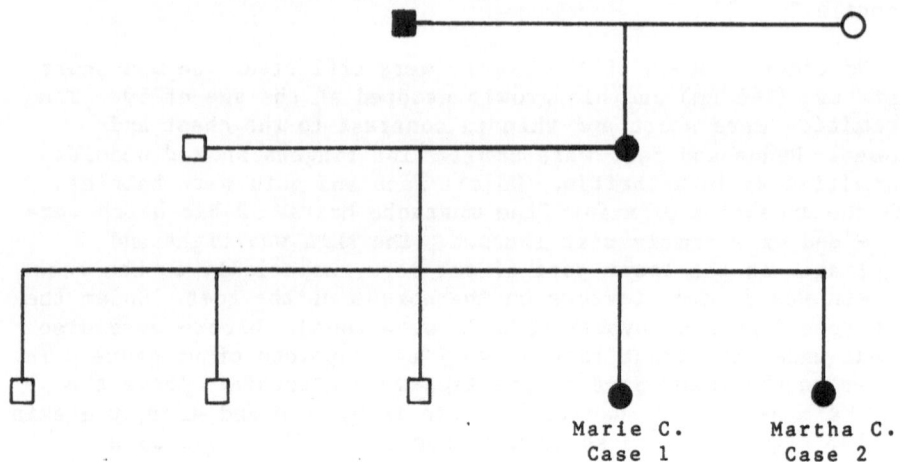

Pedigree of Family C

scalp hair began to turn gray and become sparse. The pubic hairs
almost disappeared. When she was 25, cataracts developed. At the
time of the last examination, 1931, the skin over the ankles and
feet was taut and tight. She had difficulty in moving. On the
points of pressure on both lower legs ulcers and scars of ulcers
were present. Both lower legs were very thin, almost like a
skeleton (Cadavre congele). Above the knees skin was normal and
the muscles better developed. Toenails were atrophic.
Menstruation started at 12 and stopped at 44. Tendon reflexes of
the lower extremeties could not be elicited. Triceps were normal.

Case 2. Miss Martha C., 42 years old. Short in stature. The
skin changes developed at the age of 25. The ulcers are the same
even in small details, as seen in her sister. When she was 30,
bilateral cataracts were evident. Menstruation began at the age of
13 and was still regular at 42. Her voice was clear.

S. Bau-Prussak (8) reported in 1926, in his paper entitled "La
degenerescence genito-sclerodermique," the case of a 36-year-old
woman. At the age of three the patient's vision was defective.
Menstruation started at 18 and stopped at 20. The general habitus
of the patient was underdeveloped.

M. Sainton and Mamou (9) described, in 1927, under the title
"Syndrome pluriglandulaire avec sclerodermie et cataracte" a 25-
year-old male metal worker. He had only one brother, who was
normal. He was short in stature, 149 cm. He looked much younger
than his age. Hairs were rare and gray; there was no mustache.
Eyebrows and eyelashes were sparse as were, also, the pubic hairs.
The ears stood out from the head and were flat. The skin was of
waxy color, thin and adherent to the underlying tissue. The motion
of both feet was inhibited by the taut, sclerodermatous skin. On
the feet were several ulcer scars. On the right great toe an
active ulcer was present. In contrast to the globulous abdomen the
extremities were slender and thin. The toenails were atrophic and
deformed. Bilateral cataracts developed at the age of 22. The
voice was hoarse. Endocrine features: The penis was small. The
testes descended at the age of 13 and were small in size. Sella
turcica was normal in size. The thyroid was difficult to palpate.
There was gynecomastia of the right breast.

T. Hashimoto (10) reported, in 1930, the case of a 44-year-old
man who developed cataracts and scleroderma. Penis, testes and
epididymis were very small.

H. Eguchi (11) published, in 1930, two isolated cases, without
history of familial incidence, which belong to this group. A 32-
year-old man and a 30-year-old woman had identical symptoms: 1.
Disturbance of growth; height 148 cm. 2. Scleroderma-like skin
changes on hands and feet. 3. Canities (grayness of the scalp

hair). 4. Cataracts showed at the age of 28 in the man and at the age of 26 in the woman, star-like densities on the posterior cortex of the lens. 5. Hoarse voice. 6. Retarded development of the sex organs in both cases. 7. Both patients had high blood sugar values. In addition, a goiter was present in the female.

The cases reported by A. Sezarry, Favory and H. Mamou, (12) published also in his These de Paris, 1931, by H. Mamou (13) alone, under the title "Some rare symptoms of scleroderma", do not belong to the group of Werner's syndrome. They do not show shortness in stature, canities, ulcers or presenility, but true scleroderma with melanosis of the skin and cataracts.

The most impressive evidence of the heredofamilial occurrence of the syndrome under discussion is found in the description of E. Krebs, E. Hartmann and F. Thiebaut (14) of "un cas familial de syndrome de sclerodermie avec cataracte, troubles endocriniens et neurvovegetatifs associes."

Case 1. Mrs. Germaine G., nee P.; 35 years old; married; no children. Short stature, very slender; scanty gray hair in contrast to her young appearance. Scalp hairs started to turn gray when she was 18. There were almost no eyebrows and only a few eyelashes. Secondary pubic hairs were short and straight. Skin: Scleroderma developed slowly without premonitory edema on the lower legs and feet. The hue of the skin was waxy. For a long time the patient had been able to walk only with difficulty because the skin was very tightly stretched over the ankles and the dorsum of the feet. The feet gave the impression of solid blocks. The skin over both Achilles tendons, over both heels and on the soles under the large toes showed circumscribed areas of extreme hyperkeratosis of a corn-like nature. After the hyperkeratotic areas peeled off, deep, non-healing ulcers developed. Both large toes were in hallux valgus position. The insteps were very high and the toes were fixed in extensor position. The reflexes were normal. Cataract on both eyes. Operation performed on cataract of the right eye. There was slight exophthalmos; slight tremor of the hands. The thyroid was not enlarged. Endocrine features: Menstruation was always irregular. It started at 12. There were complaints of hot flashes. Basal metabolic rate +11. No disease of internal organs found. Fasting blood sugar, 88 mg. per cent. Sugar tolerance curve was normal. Cholesterol 170 mg. per cent; calcium 11 mg. per cent. There was no report of roentgenograms of the blood vessels or bones.

Case 2. Miss Fernande P.; 38 years old; aunt of case 1. Short in stature. Presenile appearance. Hair was already gray at 18. There were almost no eyebrows or eyelashes. Pubic hairs were very scarce and straight. Skin: The same changes with circumscribed hyperkeratosis and ulcers as described in case 1 were

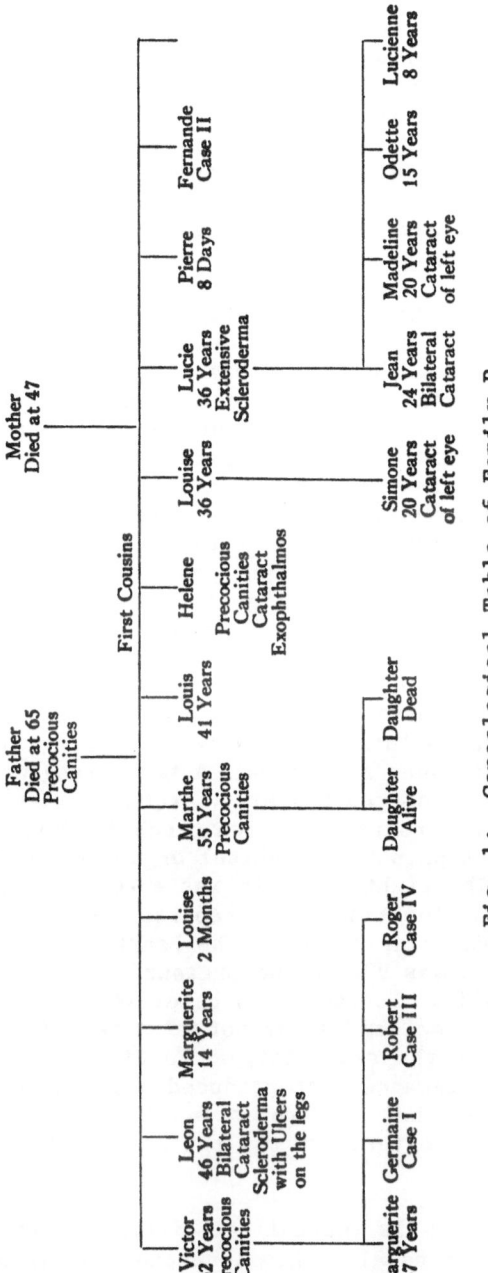

Fig. 1: Genealogical Table of Family P

found. The phalanges of the toes were fixed in a flexed position
in contrast to the extensor position of case 1. Both large toes
were in hallux valgus position. The skin was more scaly and
itching. Bilateral cataracts were operated upon at the age of 30.
Endocrine features: Slight exophthalmos. Palpitation at a rate of
100 was noted. Thyroid was not enlarged. Basal metabolic rate
+16. Menstruation was regular. Mammae very small. Hot flashes.
Sella turcica normal in size. Vascular system: Heart -- no
disease was noted. Roentgenogram showed the aorta distended and
slightly sclerotic. Wassermann reaction was negative. Fasting
blood sugar, 88 mg. per cent. Sugar tolerance normal. Total
cholesterol 260 mg. per cent.

Case 3. Robert P.; 29 years old; brother of Germaine, case 1.
Short in stature, 151 cm. Weight 45 kg. Gray, scarce scalp hairs.
Pubic hairs very rare. Body hairless. The nose was beaked. The
chin was small and retracted. The ears were very small; the
auricles were flat but projected from the head. The skin over the
forehead was taut, without folds. The skin on the forearm and
hands was tightly stretched. The hands were small and the fingers
were short and crooked and of nodular appearance. A similar shape
of the fingers was also observed in cases 1 and 2. The skin over
the lower legs and feet was atrophic and of a wax-like appearance.
The skin on these parts was so tightly stretched that any motion in
the ankle joints was difficult. The underlying muscles were so
thin they gave the lower legs and feet a skeleton-like appearance.
Both large toes were in hallux valgus position. The toes were
fixed in extension position. Numerous ulcers, old and new ones,
were present on the points of pressure. An especially large ulcer
was located on the inner malleolus. A few telangiectases were
observed on the base of the thorax. Cataracts were present in both
eyes. The voice was hoarse and high pitched. Endocrine features:
The thyroid was not palpable. Genital organs were small and
underdeveloped. The right testicle was ectopic; the left testicle
was small. Genital functions were reported as normal, but probably
developed late. Vascular system: The heart was reported as
normal. Pulse rate was 90. Blood pressure was 130 mm. Hg systolic
and 80 mm. diastolic. No report on calcification in the arterial
wall was made. The spleen was of normal size. Tendon reflexes
were normal, as was the sensibility. Fasting blood sugar 116 mg.
per cent. Sugar tolerance test produced glycosuria. Sugar
tolerance curve was that of a potential diabetic. Calcium 9.9 mg.
per cent. Total cholesterol 90 mg. per cent. Basal metabolic rate
+13.

Case 4. Roger P. is the tallest of his family -- 167 cm. He
presented the same general presenile aspect as his brother. The
forehead was smooth, without wrinkles, the nose was thin, the chin
was small and retracted, the ears were flat and projecting. The
face resembled that of a mummy. The skin had features similar to

those of his brother Robert, but to a lesser degree. Scars of ulcers were visible on the points of pressure (over elbows, heels and ankles). On the lower part of the thorax the skin showed the same telangiectases as did that of his brother. Scalp hairs were of an indefinite grayish color and scarce. Eyebrows were present. Pubic hairs were almost absent. Cataracts were developing in both eyes. Teeth showed malformation, especially on the superior incisors. Endocrine features: The penis and the testicles were very small. Puberty was late. Intercourse was sometimes carried out. Slight exophthalmos. Vascular system: The heart was normal. Blood pressure was 130 mm. Hg systolic and 80 mm. diastolic. Pulse rate was 102. The skin changes were the same as in all the cases reviewed above and characteristic for the heredofamilial dermatosis in Werner's syndrome, but not of true scleroderma. All cases of family P. were short in stature and abnormally lean. Especially the lack of subcutaneous tissue in the distal parts of the extremities gave the lower legs a skeleton-like appearance. Hallux valgus formation was noted in all members of this family. Hands and feet were abnormally small and short. The chin was small and retracted. The small size of the hands and feet and the small retracted chin, in contrast to their large size in acromegaly, is justifiably called acromicria. Slight exophthalmos with and without goiter formation, but without definite signs of hyperthyroidism, is reported in some members of family P. Hypogonadism, however, is observed in all four cases exhibiting the complete syndrome under discussion.

Comment

In addition to these four cases of the family P., examined by the authors personally, the history of the whole family is revealed in the family tree.

The syndrome under discussion was present in all its features in three members of the second generation (Leon, Louis, Fernande) and in three members of the third generation, but some features of the syndrome (canities, scleroderma-like skin changes and cataracts) occurred interchangeably as abortive features (forme fruste) also in other members of the family in three generations. These observations are of great importance since they prove: first, a recessive inheritance of the syndrome; second, that abortive features of the syndrome may occasionally occur as "forme fruste" easily overlooked by physicians not familiar with this peculiar heredofamilial disorder.

B.S. Oppenheimer and V.H. Kugel (15) reported, under the title "Werner's syndrome," three cases with photographs and autopsy findings. Two of these were brothers.

Case 1. D.G., male, 48 years old. Grandparents and parents were first cousins. Stature was short; height 149 cm. Weight was 118 pounds. At the age of 12 premature graying of the scalp hairs and a loss of scalp hair were noticed. At 48 he was bald, only sparse hairs being present on the scalp. Pubic hairs were sparse. Chest hairs were abundant, but gray. On the extremities hairs were absent and sweating was diminished. The skin of the entire face, part of the scalp and back of the ears was distinctly abnormal but not so markedly altered as in the extremities. The normal luster, smoothness and pliability were replaced by a thickening, roughness and loss of normal elasticity. The mouth was abnormal, small, surrounded by fine rhagades, and could not be opened easily. In the extremities the changes were most marked distally and gradually regressed to merge imperceptibly into apparently normal skin, at the upper third of the legs and forearms. There were circumscribed areas of hyperkeratosis on the plantar surfaces of both feet and over the very taut scar at the site of the amputation of the left foot. The skin of the feet was atrophic, smooth, glistening and taut and impeded the motion of the joints of the toes. There was an edematous appearance of the feet, but no pitting on pressure.

There were numerous scars of old ulcerations, some surrounded by areas of pigmentation, over both malleoli and plantar surfaces of the toes. There was an indolent, non-erythematous ulceration, the size of a quarter, over the right external malleolus, and there were several other ulcerations around the right ankle and over the dorsal surface of the toes of the right foot. There were also a few fine telangiectases. The skin of the hands and fingers was more typically "sclerodermatous." It was thickened, wrinkled, in places adherent with marked loss of elasticity. Over the olecranon were patches of hyperkeratinization. On the forearm the skin was atrophic and taut. The nails of the toes showed advanced atrophic changes, i.e., hyperkeratinization, deformation and discoloration. The nails of the fingers were brittle and revealed numerous longitudinal striations. Biopsy of the skin "shows marked atrophy of the epidermis. Papillae are flattened. Underlying tissue is hyalinized. Calcium stain is negative. Histological picture is consistent with the diagnosis of scleroderma" (Dr. Perla).

Joints: The small joints of both feet were immobile owing to the taut skin stretched over them. There was limited motion of the ankle joints. There was normal mobility of the larger joints of the body. Left foot showed productive arthritis. Small exostoses were present. Both feet were flat and everted with hallux valgus formation. The contrast between the well developed chest and trunk and the thin slender "juvenile" extremities was striking. The bones of the arms and legs were thin. The subcutaneous fat and the muscles were underdeveloped (especially on both lower limbs and forearms, according to the photograph). Osteoporosis of the osseous system was seen by roentgenogram.

Blood vessels: Calcification of the medium-sized arteries was visible in different parts of the extremities in roentgenograms. Eyes: Cataracts in both eyes had been operated upon. The cataracts developed at the age of 36. Teeth were normal and not decalcified. Voice was high pitched and husky.

Larynx: (S.R. Kramer) "Overhanging epiglottis. On the upper surface of the vocal cords there are white areas, irregular in size and shape, separated from one another by bands of varying width of pinkish red mucosa. These reddish strands are made up of dilated vessels in the midst of congested mucosa and extend into the ventricles and on the free edges of the vocal cords. The whole picture is a bizarre one of variegated shape and color. There is slight thickening of the edge of the right cord in its midportion, due to an area of injection."

Vascular system: The patient complained of precordial pain relieved by nitroglycerin. A blowing systolic murmur was heard over the cardiac area. Blood pressure was 168 mm. Hg systolic and 90 mm. diastolic. Roentgenogram showed cardiac enlargement and calcified deposits in the arch of the aorta.

Endocrine glands: The thyroid was not enlarged. Basal metabolic rate was -12, -19, -5. Fasting blood sugar was 85 mg. per cent. Sugar tolerance test showed a flat curve. No glycosuria. Blood calcium was 9.9 - 10.0 mg. per cent, phosphorus 2.5 - 4.2 mg. per cent, phosphatase 7 Bodansky units. Calcium balance was normal. Testes were normal in contour and consistency, but reduced in size. The penis was underdeveloped. Libido and potency were claimed to be normal. Neurologic status showed no abnormality.

Case 2: A.G., a 30-year-old man, brother of D.G., was short in stature. Height was 147 cm., weight 131 pounds. In general appearance he resembled his brother so closely that they were often taken for twins. Although six years younger than his brother, on the whole he looked older. The general habitus, premature senility, thin, slender extremities, flat and everted feet, hallux valgus formation, were the same in both patients. Scalp hairs started to turn gray at the age of eight. At the age of 20 he began to lose his scalp hair and at 22 he was noticeably bald. Hair over the chest and abdomen was sparse. The distribution of the pubic hair was feminine in type.

Skin: Although the distribution of the changes of his skin was identical with that of his brother, the predominating features were atrophy and telangiectases, so that dermatologists, from inspection of his skin alone, would emphasize the poikilodermatous rather than sclerodermatous character of the change, whereas in his brother the scleroderma predominated. In his lower extremities he

also presented cutis marmorata. The ulcerations were more
numerous, more extensive and more persistent than those of his
brother. There was a shallow ulcer, due to pressure, over his left
elbow, about 3 cm. by 1.5 cm., exposing the periosteum.
Telangiectases on knees and scrotum were prominent. He was
admitted to the hospital several times because of his ulcers.
Secondary infection and cellulitis made an amputation of the right
big toe and metatarsal bone necessary.

Skin biopsy: (S.M. Peck) "The epidermis is thin throughout
most of the section. The normal rete pegs have disappeared. There
is a moderate hyperkeratosis with no parakeratosis. The epidermis
has for the most part been reduced to six layers. The stratum
granulosum is only one layer thick. The basal cell layer shows
scattered areas of edema; many of the cells are reduced in size,
seem shrunken, whereas others show intracellular edema and even
formation of vacuoles in the cytoplasm. Many of the basal cells
contain a fairly good amount of melanine arranged in 'cap'
formation over the nuclei. No dendritic cells are seen. The
papillary bodies are flat. Scattered through the upper layers of
the cutis are a few dilated capillaries with very little, if any,
perivascular infiltration consisting mostly of lymphocytes. The
sebaceous and sweat glands are reduced in number but appear
unchanged. The cutis is very poor in cellular elements. the
elastic tissue has mostly disappeared and where it is present it is
fragmented and torn. In places the collagen fibers themselves take
a basophilic stain and seem to have undergone degenerative changes.
The sections certainly seem to fit in with the picture of
poikilodermia atrophicans. But there are also some elements which
fit in with the picture of scleroderma, especially the atrophic
stage of that disease. The histologic picture which I have
described seems to parallel that of Bloch in his cases."

Joints: Lower and upper extremities, especially on the
phalanges of the small hands and feet, ankles and wrists, showed
productive arthritic changes similar to those of his brother.
Slight arthritic changes were also seen on the roentgenograms of
pelvis and spine. Osseous system: Diffuse osteoporosis like that
of his brother. Blood vessels: Calcification of the medium sized
arteries, in different parts of his extremities, was even more
marked than in the roentgenograms of his brother. Cataracts had
developed in both eyes. The left eye had already been operated
upon. Marked proptosis of both eyes was noted, without signs of
hyperthyroidism. He lost 20 teeth in the last year; the remaining
teeth were loose owing to absorption of the alveolar bone rather
than to caries. The voice was high pitched and husky like that of
his brother. Also the bizarre and characteristic laryngoscopic
picture was the same as in his brother. Vascular system: Blood
pressure was 140 mm. Hg systolic and 90 mm. diastolic to 170 mm.
systolic and 100 mm. diastolic. Electrocardiogram showed left axis

deviation but no other changes. On his first admission no
enlargement of liver and spleen was found. On his third admission
liver and spleen were found to be greatly enlarged. Ascites was
present. The diagnosis of a hepatic neoplasm was made and verified
at necropsy. Endocrine features: The thyroid was not enlarged.
Metabolic rate was between −24 and −6. Fasting blood sugar was
153 mg. per cent. Sugar tolerance curve was characteristic of
potential diabetes. There was no glycosuria. Blood calcium was
10.6 − 13.1 mg. per cent. Hamilton test was positive. Blood
phosphatase showed 4 − 8 Bodansky units. Calcium balance was
within the range of normal. Both testes were small. Hypogonadism
was evident. In contrast to his brother, he was of normal
intelligence. The patient died of terminal pneumonia. The autopsy
confirmed the diagnosis of a primary liver carcinoma and is
reported in detail in B.S. Oppenheimer and V.H. Kugel's paper (16).
The chief abnormal findings were calcification of the mitral and
aortic valves, diffuse arteriosclerosis of Monckeberg's type,
status after bilateral cataract extraction, diffuse osteoporosis,
moderate metastatic calcification in skin, kidneys and vessels.

Endocrine glands: (examined by D. Marine) "The testes,
seminal vesicles and prostate gland were very small. The
aspermatogenesis and atrophy of the testes were premature. The
adrenals are large with multiple cortical adenomata, the glomerular
zone is active (whereas the glomerular zone in older people is
usually ill-defined). The thyroid must have passed through cycles
of increased and decreased activity to account for the multiple
adenomata. The pituitary showed no abnormality. Parathyroids
showed increased activity." Skin showed the same findings as
reported in the previous biopsy.

Case 3. H.T., male, 38 years old. Parents were first
cousins. The father's sister had a daughter with short
extremities. The patient was born in Hungary in a district not far
removed from the place where the ancestors of both brothers (case 1
and case 2) lived, but the families were not related as far as
could be ascertained. He was well until 1926. Injury to his left
heel caused a foot drop. At this time he developed various cracks
in the skin of the foot which took a long time to heal. By 1937
ulcers of the left foot appeared with shortening of the Achilles
tendon. In 1937 he had an ulcer on the right heel. The toes of
his feet gradually became immovable and the skin became hard, dry
and shiny. In 1937 a new growth on the radius of the left forearm
was detected. The mass was removed in 1938 and histologically
diagnosed as fibrosarcoma.

Appearance: Although actually 38 years old, he was generally
taken for 45. He was short in stature. His height was 157 cm.;
his weight 52 kg. The same bizarre discrepancy in the size of the
large and even fat torso and the thin and gracile extremities could

be seen in the published photograph. The hands were very small.
The graying of the hair began at 18. At 38 he was partly bald and
gray. The hair over the chest and abdomen was sparse. The
distribution of pubic hair was feminine in type. The skin was
drawn tightly over the shins and wrists and presented many areas of
pigmentation, discoloration and dry scales. There were a few
telangiectases of the skin over the knees and feet. A foul-
smelling necrotic mass overlaid the left radius. A pressure ulcer
was found over the right elbow and a crusted ulcer was seen over
the right malleolus. Severe ulcerations and pigmentations were
present on both feet. The skin of the toes was dry, hard and so
taut that the toes could not be moved. The left ankle was fixed in
extension, the knee could not be fully extended and the right ankle
had slight power and movement. There were prominent veins over the
thorax and extremities.

The vascular system showed advanced sclerosis of the blood
vessels of the upper and lower extremities. No pulsation of the
dorsalis pedis or posterior tibial arteries could be felt. The
heart was not enlarged. There was a systolic murmur over the
aortic area. Blood pressure was 180 mm. Hg. systolic and 108 mm.
diastolic. Electrocardiogram showed a left axis deviation. The
eyes were prominent and staring. The sclarae were blue. There was
bilateral postoperative coloboma of the iris. Cataracts in both
eyes were present. They appeared at the age of 31. The cataract
of the right eye was operated upon at the age of 38; the cataract
of the left eye was operated upon earlier. The teeth began to
loosen at the age of 33. The remaining teeth were carious. The
voice was high pitched. Liver and spleen were not enlarged.
Osseous system: Generalized osteoporosis was found by
roentgenogram.

Endocrine features: The thyroid was not enlarged. Basal
metabolic rate was −5 and −8. Total cholesterol 167 mg. per cent,
cholesterol esters 111. Fasting blood sugar 87 mg. per cent.
Glucose tolerance curve was rather flat but within normal limits.
Serum calcium was 10.3 mg. per cent, serum phosphorus 3.9 mg. per
cent and phosphatase 6 Bodansky units. Hamilton test was positive.
The genitalia were small. The prostate was very small and smooth
and felt about one-third normal size. A mild degree of
gynecomastia was present.

Comment

Oppenheimer and Kugel published a family tree of both brothers
D.G. and A.G. Like the genealogic table of the family P. reported
by E. Krebs, E. Hartmann and F. Thiebaut, the occurrence of the
syndrome in some members with incomplete features (forme fruste) is
evident. In the family G. usually canities appeared in members of
different generations as the outstanding feature, whereas in the

family P. reported by the French authors, the juvenile cataracts
occurred in members of different generations as the outstanding
symptom. The skin changes of the three cases of Oppenheimer and
Kugel are designated as "sclerodermatous" as the earlier authors
did in their cases, or as "poikilodermatous," especially in the
case of the younger brother, A.G.

The question of the presence of true scleroderma is of great
importance, since this type of skin disease was ascribed to a
primary hyperfunction of the parathyroids. The present conception
of the etiology of true scleroderma is based on the histological
picture of skin biopsies which exhibit as characteristic features:
1. Homogenization and sclerosis of the subcutaneous tissue, and 2.
Inflammatory changes of the arteries of the subcutaneous tissue
revealing perivascular infiltration and obliterative vascular
changes. Neither of these charactersistics was prominent.
Vascular infiltration and obliterative changes were absent. The
pathogenetic connection of diffuse scleroderma with hyperfunction
or hypertrophy of the parathyroids is abandoned in the newer
literature in favor of a pathogenesis due to inflammatory
involvement of the blood vessels of the subcutaneous tissue. Even
if the tight and taut appearance of the skin simulates scleroderma
in the cases under discussion the histologic features do not bear
out the presence of true scleroderma. In case 2, A.G., the
histological diagnosis pointed to poikiloderma vasculare. Indeed
the lesions with telangiectases are very suggestive of this type of
skin disorder first described by Jacobi. B. Bloch, however (see
page 605. *Editor's note: The original page 605 is in Section II
and is not reprinted here.*) hesitated to designate this skin lesion
as identical with real poikiloderma or poikiloscleroderma. It is
possible, therefore, only to designate these peculiar atrophic skin
lesions by a simple descriptive name such as "atrophic
heredofamilial dermatosis with skin ulcers." It does not seem
appropriate to attach a dermatological classification already in
use for the designation of well defined inflammatory skin diseases
to a heredofamilial disorder.

Oppenheimer and Kugel (16) express the opinion that the
syndrome described by Rothmund in 1868 is essentially different
from the cases of Werner and their own cases. We agree with the
authors that there are definite differences between the adult cases
of Werner and the children described by Rothmund, but one is bound
to admit that the follow-up study by R. Seefelder of Rothmund's
cases during their adult life, as well as the later description of
other adult cases of Rothmund's syndrome, bears out the close
relationship of Werner's and Rothmund's syndrome. Further
classification of the differences and similarities in Werner's and
Rothmund's syndromes will be offered in the second part of this
paper.

Own observations

The brothers, Sidney O., 38 years old, and Nathan O., 34 years old, were born in the United States of Russian Jewish parents. Both parents were healthy. They came from different towns in southern Russia and were not related. Both paternal and maternal grandparents were healthy and lived to an old age. No interrelationship of any ancestors or any occurrence of a similar disorder in this family is known.

Case 1. Sidney O. was born a normal child. He went to high school and later to a pharmaceutical school. After graduation he practiced pharmacy. He was very intelligent, well read, and wrote poetry. Appearance: He was short in stature -- five feet three inches (168 cm.); weight 120 pounds. There had been no recent weight loss. He looked like an old man, about 20 years older than his actual age. The scalp hairs began to turn gray at the age of 15. They became sparse at the age of 20. They now looked like the hairs of a mouse suffering from food deficiency, being fine, sparse and of an indefinite grayish color. He had fine, scarce hairs on the upper lip and on his face. He shaved twice a week. The hairs on his body were scanty and gray. On the lower arms and legs, where the skin changes were most outstanding, there were no hairs at all. On these hairless areas of the extremities perspiration did not occur. The sex hairs were scarce and rudimentary, most of them being straight like bristles. At the age of 21 he noticed circumscribed areas of hyperkeratosis under his big toes, under his heels, on both lateral parts of his feet, as well as on his insteps. At the time of his admission to the hospital these areas of hyperkeratosis were slightly elevated above the surface of the skin and consisted of cornified, horny layers, which gave these areas a shell-like appearance. The patient reported that the removal of these "corns" resulted always in an ulcer which did not heal for a long time. The skin of the face was taut but not tightly fixed on the underlying structures. Beneath the eyes, especially on the nose and nostrils, the skin was not tightly stretched, as was seen in true scleroderma. The opening of his mouth was not hampered although the aperture was small. On both sides of the face there were two distinct, symmetrical areas of fat accumulation. A similar fat deposit was found in the region of the parotid gland and over the horizontal part of the mandible. The subcutaneous fat in other parts of the face was rather poorly developed.

The skin over his lower legs and feet showed the most characteristic changes. Starting downward from the knees the skin appeared taut and tightly stretched over the underlying structures and over the ankles and insteps became so tightly adherent to the underlying tissue that the motion in the ankle joints and phalangeal joints was grossly impaired. Large ulcers, the size of

a silver dollar, were present over both Achilles tendons. Several
smaller ulcers were found over the malleoli, the lateral surfaces
of the feet and between the large and second toes. The ulcers
seemed to be located on parts exposed to pressure. The patient
himself reported that the ulcers appeared first at the age of 24
and healed very slowly or not at all, draining a thick fluid. Most
of the ulcers were covered with a thick, greenish, fibrinous
membrane. The ulcers had been painful, especially at night, to
such a degree that morphine had to be given. Besides the active
ulcers there were many scars from healed ulcerations. Both large
ulcers over the Achilles tendon were grafted by Dr. E. Cooney; the
grafts healed. (After six months a new ulcer started on the edge
of the graft). Slight linear pigmentation of a light brownish
color together with some scaling along the pigmented lines was
noted. There were no telangiectases. The skin over the phalanges
had a reddish hue, whereas the color on all other areas involved
was whitish and waxy. There was no pitting on pressure. The skin
on the lower parts of the arms and hands was also taut, but not so
tightly stretched over the underlying tissue as on the lower legs
and feet. On the dorsal surface of the hands the thin, atrophic
skin was even pliable, like tissue paper, whereas over both wrists
the skin was tightly drawn. The circumference of the wrist was 14
cm.; of the upper arms 20 cm.; of the calf 24 cm.; and of the
ankles 16 cm. In these parts of the body the subcutaneous fat
tissue was extremely scanty. One got the impression that this lack
of subcutaneous fat paralleled the atrophy and tightness of the
skin. The muscles of the distal parts of the extremities were thin
and poorly developed, but there was no restriction of motion due to
paresis or paralysis of the muscles. Where there was restriction
of motion it was the result of the tightly stretched skin. Both
feet were extremely flat and everted with hallux valgus formation.
The phalangeal joints of the hands and feet showed thickening of
the periarticular tissue as seen in arthritis. All the toes were
small and immobile. The toenails were present but atrophic. The
fingernails were short. The patient reported that they grew very
slowly. The arms and legs, as a whole, appeared extremely thin and
gracile. The small hands and feet, lacking any fat tissue, in
contrast to a rather round abdomen, gave the extremeties a
grotesque appearance. Roentgenograms of the bones, especially of
the arms where the dermatosis is evident, showed severe
osteoporosis. In the same roentgenograms the arteries of the lower
legs and feet showed calcification due to arteriosclerosis. The
arterial pulse could not be felt in either dorsalis pedis artery.
Arteriosclerosis, but to a lesser degree, also involved the
arteries of the upper arm.

   Eyes: (Note of Dr. J.J. Skirball) "Cataract extraction, left
eye, 1936, eight years ago. Right eye, 1939, five years ago. Some
capsular remnants. Patient has had a secondary iridotomy. Fundus:
Disk is of good color, the margin is clear, no elevation of the

disk is seen. The arteries are moderately narrowed and slightly
angulated, also veins are slightly narrowed. The changes on the
arteries indicate early arteriosclerosis. There is definite
proptosis of both eyes; no lid lag."

The nose was small and beak-shaped; the nostrils were freely
movable. The chin was small but not retracted. The ears were
small, but flat and protruding laterally from the head. The drums
were very thin and almost atrophic. Hearing was good in both ears.
Voice was high pitched. Laryngoscopic findings did not show any
abnormal change. Teeth had all developed and were in fairly good
condition. The chest was of normal diameter. The lungs were
normal. The heart was normal in size; no murmurs were heard.
Blood pressure was 125 mm. Hg systolic and 85 mm. diastolic.

Endocrine features: The short stature, the general senile
appearance and canities have already been mentioned. The thyroid
was not enlarged. The proptosis of the eyes was not a true
exophthalmos. There was no lid lag. There were no features of
hyperthyroidism. Basal metabolic rate was -15. Total cholesterol
was 172 mg. per cent; free cholesterol 39.5 mg. per cent; ester
cholesterol 132.5 mg. per cent. The penis was very small in size.
The two testes were descended but were of small size. The prostate
was small. His sexual desire was not very strong. He sometimes
had ejaculations. He was not married. Follicular stimulating
hormone in blood was reported negative; 3.24 mg. of 17 ketosteriods
per 24 hours were excreted. Creatine was 0.8 - 0.61 mg. per cent
in 24 hour urine. Sugar was present in traces. Sugar tolerance
curve: fasting 150 mg. per cent; one-half hour 274 mg. per cent;
one hour 286 mg. per cent; two hour 278 mg. per cent; three hour
272 mg. per cent. Calcium was 11.8 mg. per cent; phosphorus, 3.6
mg. per cent; alkaline phosphatase, 2.2 Bodansky units. Other
laboratory findings: Total serum protein was 8 gm. per 100 c.c.;
albumin, 5.5 gm.; globulin 3.2 gm. Blood sedimentation rate was 28
mm. in 20 minutes, 74 mm. in one hour. (Blood sedimentation rate
was increased, probably owing to ulcers of the leg.) Wassermann
and Hinton reactions were negative. Hemoglobin was 75 per cent,
red blood cell count 2.24 million per c.c.; color index 0.9.
Leukocytes were 10,000 per mm. Differential count: Band forms 5
percent, adult neutrophiles 63 per cent, eosinophiles 3 per cent,
basophiles 1 per cent, lymphocytes 16 per cent, monocytes 12 per
cent. Platelets were normal. The appetite of the patient was
excellent. In the hospital he consumed a diet of 2500 to 3000
calories without gaining weight.

Case 2. Nathan O., 34 years old, had the same schooling as his
brother Sidney. He also graduated from a pharmaceutical school in
Providence and practiced thereafter with his brother, as a
pharmacist in his own drug store. He was intelligent, also, but
had less literary ambition than his brother. As a boy, until he

was 16, his maximum weight was 140 pounds. At the age of 20 he
lost considerable weight. This weight loss was believed to be due
to hyperthyroidism. The patient was told that he had an internal
goiter, but only a slight external one. A subtotal thyroidectomy
was done when he was 21. After the operation he lost further
weight. It was then discovered he had diabetes. He was put on
insulin and his diet was regulated. He controlled his treatment
himself and the urine was sugar free for years.

In July 1943 his left foot became infected and gangrene of the
second and third digits developed. It was thought that this
infection was due to a diabetic gangrene, but apparently the
infection and gangrene developed from an infected ulcer. An
amputation below the left knee was performed by Dr. L.S.
McKittrick. The pathological report (Dr. B. Castleman) was:
"Advanced arteriosclerosis, thrombosis and recanalization.
Gangrene with fistula formation." After the patient came under our
observation Dr. McKittrick sent us the following note: "His whole
appearance is unusual. His skin is inelastic . . . almost that of
a patient with scleroderma. He did not do as well after his
amputation as most patients do in that there was a small area that
necrosed." He was put on an 1800 caloried diet with 25 units
protamine zinc and 10 units regular insulin. Six months later the
patient was admitted to our hospital. At this time the 24 hour
urine contained 8 - 10 gm. sugar.

Appearance: He was short in stature, five feet and three-
quarters inches (144 cm.); weight: 93.5 pounds. His likeness to
his brother was surprising. Many people considered the brothers
twins. His face, however, was not as full as his brother's. The
fat pads over the parotid and on the lower mandibular region, as
seen on Sidney, were not present on Nathan's face. He looked much
older than his actual age. The general impression was that he
appeared even more senile than his brother. The scalp hairs began
to turn gray at the age of 16. They were now the same indefinite
grayish color as seen on his brother. They were also fine in
texture but very scarce. The hair of his face was more abundant
than that on his brother's face. He had to shave almost every
other day. Also, the hair on chest and abdomen was better
developed. The distal parts of both extremities were hairless.
The pubic hairs were poorly developed, not curled, but straight and
short.

The patient noticed the first changes in his skin at the
age of 20. "Corns," i.e., circumscribed areas of hyperkeratosis,
developed on both heels, on the lateral parts of his feet and under
the large toes. The hyperkeratotic areas were prominent over the
skin and had a shell-like configuration consisting of horny layers.
Skin ulcers appeared on the points of pressure on the malleoli, on
the lateral parts of his feet and on the left instep and over the

left second and third toes. Apparently a secondary infection
developed in 1943 from the ulcers of the toes which resulted in a
amputation below the knee of the left leg. At present a large
ulcer, the size of a quarter, was present on the inner side of his
right foot, causing excruciating pain, usually during the night.
Opiates were necessary every night to relieve this pain. The skin
over the Achilles tendon, unlike that of his brother, was not
ulcerated. A smaller ulcer developed on the skin of the right
second digit where it pressed against the skin of the large toe.

The skin of his face was taut but wrinkled. Long, stiff,
nasolabial folds gave his face an old appearance. The aperature of
his mouth was small. The skin over the stump of his left leg was
normal on the thigh but around the knee, just over the amputation,
the skin was atrophic. The pressure of the prosthesis had caused
reddening of the skin. (Ulcer formation on the lower end of the
stump was feared.) The skin over the right lower leg showed the
same characteristics as his brother's. The skin from the knee down
was taut, atrophic, and stretched over the ankle and metatarsal
joints. Scaling and slight linear pigmentation were visible.
Motion of the right foot was limited because of the tightness of
the skin. He was able to walk with the help of two sticks, when
the prothesis was in place. The subcutaneous fat tissue and the
muscles of the right leg from the knee down were extremely poor.
Circumference of the right ankle was 18 cm. Circumference of the
left calf was 23 cm. The skin on both upper arms and hands was
taut, but not so tightly pulled over the wrist that it could not be
wrinkled. The texture of the skin was thin and atrophic. The
subcutaneous fat was almost lacking on both upper arms and the
muscles were very thin. Circumference of the wrists was 12.5 cm.
Circumference of the upper arms was 20 cm. The joints had the same
appearance as presented by his brother Sidney. Roentgenograms of
the osseous system, especially of the extremities, showed
osteoporosis. The arteries of the right leg were extremely
calcified. That those of the left leg were in a similar state was
confirmed by the pathological examination after amputation.
Arteriosclerosis was more advanced than in the case of his brother
Sidney.

Both cataracts had been extracted. The patient had had a
secondary iridotomy. The fundi showed changes characteristic of
arteriosclerosis. The ears were small and flat, protruding
laterally from the head. The inner ears were normal. His nose was
somewhat longer than his brother's. The nostrils were freely
movable. The chin was small and slightly retracted. The voice was
high pitched and husky.

Laryngoscopic findings: (Dr. Kelemann) "Even after
anesthesia only two-thirds of the larynx is seen because the large,
flat epiglottis covers the other third. The right side of the

larynx is normal. At the left side the vocal cord is covered in
its central part by a diffuse red structure moving with the vocal
cord. This structure may consist of distended veins or may consist
of a hemangiomatous structure. The mucosa of the left ventricle is
prolapsed. The arytenoid movements are free as are the other
movements of the larynx."

Vascular system and heart: As has already been stated, the
roentgenograms showed sclerosis of the arteries of the right leg.
The examination of the amputated left leg showed, as above stated,
severe arteriosclerosis. The heart was of normal size. There were
no murmurs. Action was regular. Blood pressure was 160 mm. Hg
systolic and 90 mm. diastolic. Liver and spleen were not enlarged.

Endocrine features: His short stature and presenile
appearance have already been described. His thyroid was not
palpable; the scar of a partial thyroidectomy was visible. His
eyes were protruding but there was no lid lag or other symptoms
which would indicte hyperthyroidism. Basal metabolic rate was +0.
The testicles were descended but small. The scrotum was very
small, the size of that of a 10-year-old boy. The penis was short.
(Sexual desire was minimal but ejaculations did occur. He had
never had intercourse.) The excretion of total 17 ketosteroids was
5.8 mg. per 24 hours. Sella turcica was within normal limits. His
fasting blood sugar ranged between 205-251 mg. per cent. The
patient excreted 8 - 10 gm. of sugar, in spite of receiving 25
units of protamine zinc and 10 units of regular insulin, and a diet
of 1800 calories (170 gm. carbohydrates; 85 gm. protein; 87 gm.
fat). Other laboratory findings were: 75 per cent hemoglobin;
4.44 million red blood corpuscles per cu. mm.; color index 0.87;
leukocytes 9,800 per cu. mm. The differential count was normal.
Total serum protein, 8.08 gm. per 100 c.c., albumin, 5.26 gm.,
globulin, 2.82 gm. Blood sedimentation rate was 75 mm. in one
hour. Blood Hinton reaction was negative. Creatine excretion was
1 gm. in 24 hours. Blood calcium was 11.8 mg. per cent, phosphorus
3.6 mg. per cent, alkaline phosphatase 2 Bodansky units.

Comment

The two brothers not only looked alike but had the following
characteristics in common: (1) Shortness of stature; (2) atrophy
of the subcutaneous fat tissue and the muscles of the lower arms
and lower legs, hands and feet; (3) small hands and feet; (4)
canities (premature graying of scalp hair); (5) scarce scalp hairs;
(6) atrophic dermatosis of lower legs, feet, upper arms and hands,
partially on face; (7) pressure ulcers on exposed parts of the
feet; (8) circumscribed areas of hyperkeratosis on feet and
insteps; (9) arteriosclerosis of the arteries in the extremities;
(10) osteoporosis; (11) diabetes or potential diabetes; (12)
hypogonadism and reduced sexual desire. The description of other

cases in the literature is so similar in most of the detailed
features that there is no doubt that this syndrome first described
by O. Werner is a clinical entity. It is evident from the family
trees, especially from that published by E. Krebs, E. Hartmann and
F. Thiebaut (14) that this syndrome may, also, occur as an
incomplete form, so-called "forme fruste."

    The study of the cases of brothers S.O. and N.O., however,
leads us to doubt whether or not one of the outstanding symptoms of
Werner's syndrome is correctly described by the term "scleroderma"
or "poikiloscleroderma." To the best of our knowledge there is no
case of true scleroderma described in the literature in which this
disease occurs in families as a recessive familial disorder.
Diffuse scleroderma usually involves the skin and tissue beneath
the lower eyelid, the skin covering the nose and nostrils and the
skin around the mouth and chin. In most of these cases the skin of
the neck, of the thorax and of the abdomen as well as the skin of
the extremities is involved. In many cases of true scleroderma an
intensive melanotic pigmentation is seen in some areas of the body,
especially on the neck, in the axilla, on the trunk and buttocks.
Areas of circumscribed hyperkeratosis, however, occurring on feet,
insteps and elbows are not a feature of true scleroderma. In
Werner's syndrome, in contrast to scleroderma, the skin changes
begin with circumscribed areas of hyperkeratosis beneath the heels,
beneath the large toes, on the lateral parts of the feet as well as
on the instep and over the Achilles tendon. In Werner's syndrome
areas of melanotic pigmentation are never observed. Scaling,
however, along very fine, faintly yellowing brown stripes may be
found in some cases. As a whole the skin in Werner's syndrome is
white and waxy in color and has a reddish hue only on the parts of
the extremities where it is exposed to pressure from clothes and
shoes. These distinct differences in clinical features of true
scleroderma and the "pseudo" scleroderma in Werner's syndrome are
strikingly supported by the histological examination of the skin
biopsies obtained from both brothers O. The histology of true
scleroderma is characterized by edema, homogenization, fibrosis and
sclerosis of the collagen fibers and obliterative changes in the
vessels of the cutis. Lymphocytic infiltration of the subcutaneous
tissue especially about the blood vessels is a characteristic
histologic feature. These characteristics of true scleroderma are
not found in the biopsies of our cases. In the histological
examination of the skin biopsy of Sidney O. the horny layer seemed
to be of normal thickness and structure. The pars papillaris was
either somewhat flattened or definitely flattened. There was no
homogenization or sclerosis of the connective tissue underlying the
papillae nor homogenization of connective tissue of the pars
reticularis. The hair follices and the sweat glands were not
numerous and, if present, were not well developed. No
proliferative nor necrotizing arteritis was visible in the arteries
of the subcutaneous tissue. The subcutaneous veins were more

distended than usual. The elastic fibers of the corium were loose and appeared essentially unaltered. Fat cells were almost absent in the subcutaneous tissue.

We are indebted to Dr. H. Montgomery, of the Mayo Clinic, Section on Dermatology, for examination of our slides of S.O. He was kind enough to give the following opinion: "I would guess that the biopsy and slides of Sidney O. (N. 6018) were taken from the leg, probably the lower part of the leg, because of the large varicose veins present in the subcutaneous tissue. Some atrophy of the hair follicles is present, but this often occurs in skin taken from the legs and areas where the skin has been subject to friction, as from socks and garters. There is no evidence of so-called senile skin, such as tinctorial changes in the staining of the collagen or basophilic staining of the elastic tissue, which can be seen in polychrome methylene-blue and hematoxylin-eosin stained sections. The slides of the skin show practically no inflammatory reaction, no appreciable obliterative changes in any of the vessels. The connective tissue fibers appear essentially normal and there is no decrease in thickness of the cutis. All this speaks against scleroderma.

"Pseudosclerodermatous infiltrations with ulceration, especially in the vicinity of the ankles, and poikiloderma-like changes are often seen in the relatively rare skin condition known as 'acrodermatitis chronica atrophicans.' Clinically, however, there usually is no systemic disturbance or evidence of systemic disease, and, histopathologically there is a rather specific picture with marked atrophy of the epidermis and flattening of the rete ridges with partial to almost complete loss of the cutis, the cutis being replaced by a dense infiltrate that is separated from the epidermis by a normal 'grenz' or border zone. Unless the sections were taken from a pseudosclerodermatous area, one can rule out acrodermatitis chronica atrophicans on the basis of these sections."

The skin biopsy taken from Nathan O. showed more flattening of the pars papillaris than that of his brother Sidney. The histological pattern, however, was the same as described in the slides of Sidney O. Here, also, the connective tissue of the pars reticularis was not homogenized or sclerosed. There was no inflammatory reaction in the rete. A few lymphocytes were occasionally found around some blood vessels. In sections stained for elastic tissue no abnormal conditions were found either in the case of Sidney or Nathan O. The muscle biopsies taken from Sidney O. and Nathan O. showed no cellular infiltration or specific changes.

It is evident from these histological findings that the skin changes in Werner's syndrome are not identical with the skin

changes found in diffuse or localized scleroderma. Such a
classification of the skin disorder in Werner's syndrome is not
justified since neither the clinical picture nor histological
examination coincides with scleroderma or poikiloscleroderma. It
seems more appropriate to designate the skin lesions in Werner's
syndrome by a simple descriptive name such as "heredofamilial
atrophic dermatosis with skin ulcers."

Case 3. George W. St., 39 years old, was studied on the
Medical Service of the Massachusetts General Hospital. (I am
indebted to Dr. Fuller Albright for letting me examine this
patient). Mother and father were direct cousins. Both were
normal. He had two married sisters, 46 years old and 40 years old.
The older sister had two healthy boys in the Navy. The younger
sister had a healthy girl, 17 years of age. The patient was born a
normal child but was delicate. He graduated from high school and
from a school of architectural drafting. Appearance: He was short
in stature -- five feet. He had grown very little since the age of
nine. Weight was 75 pounds. His maximum weight was 100 pounds, at
the age of 22, when he entered the Navy, but at the time of his
discharge he weighed 85 pounds. He looked older than his actual
age. He did not know when his hair started to turn gray. At the
age of 33 he was completely gray. The scalp hairs were now scarce,
fine, and of an indefinite grayish color. His eyebrows were
normal. He had only a few eyelashes. He shaved about twice a
week. His beard was gray. His body hairs were almost absent. His
pubic hairs were scarce and straight, not curled. The skin of his
face was taut, but movable over the underlying structures. The
nasolabial folds were distinct and formed taut, longitudinal lines.
The aperture of his mouth was small but the opening of the mouth
was not hampered. The skin of his neck and thorax was thin,
transparent and movable. The skin of his upper arms and lower legs
was taut and tightly stretched over the underlying tissue. The
skin above the knees and elbows was normal. Although the skin on
the dorsal parts of his hands was pliable, the skin over both
ankles and both feet was so tightly pulled over the bones that the
motion of both ankle, metatarsophalangeal, and phalangeal joints
was limited. He walked with stiff ankle joints and everted feet.

Skin biopsy: "There is slight superficial keratosis. The
rete pegs have disappeared. The pars papillaris is flat. The zone
of prickle cells is reduced. No inflammatory changes of the
subcutaneous tissue are seen. There is no cellular infiltration
around or within the arteries. The walls of the arterioles are
somewhat thickened. The subcutaneous tissue is loose. Neither
homogenization nor sclerosis of the subcutaneous tissue is seen.
The subcutaneous fat is very scarce. Some veins of the
subcutaneous tissue are distended. The elastic fibers are
essentially unaltered. Hairs and sebaceous glands are almost
absent in this section. Areas of hyperkeratosis on his feet were

the first signs of skin changes the patient had noticed. He
reported that at the age of 17 he became aware of calluses on both
soles under the large toes and both heels. No ulcers were present
at this time. The first ulcers developed at the age of 37 on the
lateral parts of both feet. He now had circumscribed areas of
hyperkeratosis under both large toes, under both heels, and on the
lateral margins of his feet. The ulcers were almost healed but the
scars of former ulcers were visible on both feet. The subcutaneous
fat tissue, as well as the muscles of upper arms, hands, lower
legs and feet, were underdeveloped. The lower parts of arms and
legs were so thin that they had a skeleton-like appearance.
Circumference above the wrists was 13 cm.; above the ankle joints
it was 15 cm. Hands and feet were very small in size. The fingers
seemed somewhat deformed because the interphalangeal joints were
prominent, as in an arthritic person. The roentgenograms of the
bones in the parts where the dermatosis of the skin was evident
showed osteoporosis due to decalcification. In the roentgenograms
made at the Massachusetts General Hospital, November 30, 1941,
small areas of calcium deposits were seen in the soft tissue close
to the right fifth metacarpal phalangeal joint and of the proximal
phalanx of the fourth right finger. Similar areas of calcium
deposits were also seen around both ankles. At present
calcification was noted only in the Achilles tendon. Calcification
of the arteries was not visible in the roentgenograms of both lower
legs.

Eyes: At the age of 30 cataracts developed in both lenses.
The cataracts were successfully extracted at the age of 34 by Dr.
Chandler of the Massachusetts General Hospital. Both eyes were now
aphacic and showed scars of a healed iridocyclitis. There was no
proptosis of the eyes. The nose was fine in contour and somewhat
elongated. The chin was small but not retracted. The ears were
small and flat but did not protrude laterally from the head. The
voice was high pitched and hoarse. The teeth were all developed
but carious. The roentgenogram of the lungs showed thickening of
the apical pleura on the right side. Vascular system: The heart
was normal. Blood pressure was 130 mm. Hg systolic and 80 mm.
diastolic. There was no visible arteriosclerosis. Electrocardiogram was normal. The reflexes were normal. A myotonic
reaction could not be elicited. Endocrine features: The shortness
of stature and the senile appearance with graying of the scalp
hairs has already been discussed. The thyroid was not palpated.
Basal metabolic rate in 1941 was -14; in 1943, -32. The sexual
organs were very small. The penis was short. The scrotum was
small in size. The testes, although descended, were of the size of
those of a 12-year-old boy. In 1941 the 17-ketosteroids in the 24
hour urine were 13.3 mg.; in 1943, 5.7 mg. The sella turcica, on
roentgen-ray examination, was normal. Laboratory findings: Total
serum protein, sodium and potassium and calcium determination in
the serum were normal.

Comment

This patient was the child of first cousins, but as far as could be ascertained there was no similar case in his ancestry. The features of Werner's syndrome present in George St. were: Presenile appearance, shortness of stature, canities, skin changes consisting of stretching of the taut skin over the underlying structures on the lower legs and feet, skin ulcers, areas of hyperkeratosis, atrophy of subcutaneous tissue as well as muscles of the upper arms and lower legs, hands and feet; small chin, hands and feet; osteoporosis; sexual underdevelopment. Although potential diabetes and arteriosclerosis were not evident in this case the other features are convincing that this case belongs to the group of Werner's syndrome. In 1941 our patient underwent a lumbar sympathectomy because it was thought that the skin changes were due to scleroderma and the ulcers were due to trophic disturbances of the skin. A follow-up note of the Massachusetts General Hospital, in the case history, reads as follows: "I cannot see that any benefit was obtained from this operation. Since that time his condition has remained essentially unchanged." It seems, therefore, that the ulcers are not the result of a trophic disorder. The good healing of the ulcers after grafting, in the case of Sidney O., supports the opinion that the ulcers are due to the vulnerability of the atrophic and stretched skin to outside pressure from shoes and clothes. The gross skin changes are the same as in all cases reported. The histological examination of the skin biopsy concurred with the biopsies of the brothers Sidney and Nathan O. in that the characteristics of true scleroderma were not found. Homogenization and sclerosis of the subcutaneous tissue as well as inflammatory reactions consisting of lymphocytic infiltration in the subcutaneous tissue and proliferative arteritis were absent. These negative findings on three patients with Werner's syndrome demonstrate that the taut and stretched skin is not the result of true scleroderma but rather a part of the general abiotrophic process which involved the endocrine glands as well as the whole body. It is highly suggestive that such an abiotrophic degenerative process which manifests itself in the second and third decades of life may originate in a recessively transmitted hereditary defect of the germ plasm.

Case 4. Miss M.F., 29 years old. There was no history of intermarriage in her ancestry. No similar cases were known in the family. The family was highly intellectual. Father and brother were outstanding professors in medical schools in Germany. A maternal uncle was one of the great physiologists of the past century. The girl was mentally retarded, having the mentality of a 12-year-old child. She graduated, however, from a private school. Her appetite became very poor at age 17. Instead of eating her meals she hid her food and threw it away when she was unobserved.

Appearance: She was very short in stature and considerably
underweight. She looked like an old woman, about 20 years older
than her actual age. The scalp hairs began to turn gray around the
age of 20. They were sparse, fine and of an indefinite grayish
color. The eyebrows as well as the eyelashes were scarce. The
axillary hairs were completely absent. Only a few short pubic
hairs were found. The skin of the face was wrinkled, but taut.
Longitudinal firm nasolabial fat gave the face an old appearance.
The skin on the chest and abdomen was thin and atrophic. No
pigmentation or telangiectases were present. The skin of the upper
arms and hands was atrophic and thin. Over both hands the skin was
pliable like tissue paper. In contrast to the skin on the forearms
and hands the skin over both lower legs was taut and adherent to
the underlying structures, the latter especially noticeable over
the ankles and insteps. The motion in the ankle joints was
moderately impaired by the stretched skin, and she walked with
everted feet.

She complained of pain in circumscribed areas of
hyperkeratosis under both large toes, both heels and on the
external sides of the feet. She reported that she had ulcers on
the lateral malleolus and on the instep from pressure of her shoes.
The ulcers healed only after a long time. Ulcer scars, but not
active skin ulcers, were visible. Nails on hands and feet were
poorly developed, but all were present. The subcutaneous fat
tissue and the muscles on both lower legs and upper arms were thin
and poorly developed. The lower legs had a skeleton-like
appearance. Roentgenograms of the bones were not made. The
phalangeal joints on both hands had the appearance of arthritic
joints with thickened periarticular tissue. The patient did not
complain of pain in her joints. At the age of 24 she noticed
difficulty in reading. Beginning cataracts were found. At the
time she was observed, at 29, the cataracts had almost matured.
Her nose and chin were small. The ears were small and flat, but
did not protrude laterally from the head. The voice was high
pitched and slightly hoarse. The lungs were normal. The heart was
normal in size. Blood pressure was 130 mm. Hg systolic and 90 mm.
diastolic. There was no note in regard to the arteries.

Endocrine features: Senile appearance, canities and the very
short stature have already been described. The thyroid was not
enlarged. No proptosis of the eyes was noticed. Basal metabolic
rate was not recorded. The patient first menstruated at the age of
16. After that menstruation was sparse, occurring only a few times
during the year, and ceased at the age of 25. Gynecological
examination reported by a gynecologist (Dr. Weber): "External
genitalia normal; hymen intact. By rectal examination neither
uterus nor ovaries could be felt distinctly; probably
underdeveloped." No records of laboratory examinations were
available.

Comment

        The patient was seen almost every year, from the age of 29 to
37. The cataracts were operated upon at the age of 31. At the
time she was under observation I did not make the diagnosis of
Werner's syndrome because I was then not aware that such as
syndrome had been described. Since in later years I have become
familiar with the literature there is no doubt that the features of
this patient, i.e., short stature, canities, cataracts, atrophic
dermatosis with taut and stretched skin, sexual underdevelopment,
justify in retrospect the diagnosis of Werner's syndrome. Stunted
growth resulting in short stature and sexual underdevelopment was
reported by R.F. Varney, A.T. Kenyon and F.S. Koch (17) and by F.
Albright, P.H. Smith and R. Fraser (18). L. Wilkins and W.
Fleischmann (19) designated this syndrome as "ovarian agenesis"
because they demonstrated in their cases, by their histological
studies, that the ovaries did not develop. Wilkins and Fleischmann
suggest that ovarian agenesis as well as stunted growth is due to
defects of the germ plasm and not to endocrine deficiencies of
normally developed organs. "It is well recognized that multiple
germinal defects frequently occur in the same individual."

        We are inclined to explain Werner's syndrome as the result of
multiple germinal defects because it presents recessive
characteristics and is of heredofamilial occurrence and because its
endocrine manifestations, namely stunted growth and sexual
underdevelopment, are only a part of its multiple features.
Wilkins and Fleischmann tabulate 32 cases published by different
authors in which they suggest the presence of ovarian agenesis.
Only one of these cases (case 10 by F. Albright, P.H. Smith and R.
Fraser (18)) exhibited progeria and cataracts in addition to
ovarian agenesis. Although skin changes and heredity are not
reported, it seems possible that this case is related to the group
of Werner's syndrome. When in the future we have better learned
how to differentiate the features of functional endocrine
deficiencies from the endocrine features resulting from germinal
defects, reports of Werner's syndrome and related syndromes will
become more numerous.

II. *ROTHMUND'S SYNDROME*

        *Editor's note: This 21-page section has not been reprinted
        because of space considerations.*

III. *Diseases Related to Werner's Syndrome (Progeria of the Adult),
        and Rothmund's Syndrome*

        *Editor's note: This 8-page section has not been reprinted
        because of space considerations.*

GENERAL COMMENT

As seen from various publications quoted from the world's literature, there is considerable confusion in recognizing Werner's and Rothmund's syndromes as different, although related, clinical entities. This is the more astonishing for the striking resemblance of cases of one family affected with one of the syndromes to cases of another family. The striking differences of Werner's syndrome and Rothmund's syndrome are as follows:

1. Werner's syndrome starts at the age of 20 to 30, beginning with graying of the hair. Later, skin changes and cataracts develop. Rothmund's syndrome begins in early childhood. The skin changes are already visible three to six months after birth. Cataracts develop also in childhood, namely, from three to five years of age.

TABLE I

Symptoms	Werner's Syndrome	Rothmund's Syndrome	Cataracta Dermatogenes with Neurodermitis	Progeria of Children with Nanism	Myotonic Dystrophy	Ectodermal Dysplasia with Dystrophy of Hair and Nails
Heredofamilial occurrence	+++	+++	±	0 ·	++	+++
Age at the beginning of disorder	20–30 y	3 mo.–3 y	3–20 y	2–5 mo.	20–30 y	shortly after birth
Shortness of stature	+++	+	0	++++	+	0
Skin changes	++++	++++	++++	+	+	++
a) Tightly drawn over underlying tissue	++++ 20–30 y	0	0 3–20 y	+ 2–5 mo.	+ 20–30 y	0 shortly after birth
b) Atrophic and thin skin	++++	++	++	++	++	+
c) Telangiectases	+	++++ 3 mo.	0	0	0	0
d) Scaling	++	++++	++++	+	0	0
e) Pigmentation and depigmentation	+	+++	++	+	+	0
f) Ulcers	++++	0	0	0	+	0
Canities of scalp hairs Age	++++ 20–30 y	± 40 y	0	++++ 2–5 mo.	+++ 20–30 y	Bald
Sparse sex hairs	+++	++	0	+++	+++	0
Muscular atrophy on distal parts of extremities	+++	±	0	+++	+++	0
Atrophy of the subcutaneous fat tissue	+++	±	0	+++	+++	0
Bilateral cataracts	++++ 20–30 y	++++ 3–4 y	±	0	+++ 20–30 y	0
Diffuse arteriosclerosis	+++	±	0	++++	++	0
Osteoporosis	+++	0	0	++	+	0
Joint deformities	+++	+	0	+++	+	0
Thyroid	+	0	0	0	+ ，	0
Proptosis	+++	0	0	++++	0	0
Sexual underdevelopment	++++	++	0	+++	+++	0
Myotonic reaction	0	0	0	0	++	， 0

2.   The shortness of stature is more outstanding in Werner's
syndrome than it is in Rothmund's syndrome.

3.   The skin changes are different in their features in both
syndromes. In Werner's syndrome the most striking feature is
tightening of the skin over the underlying structures which are
very poor in subcutaneous fat tissue. The skin changes are
localized on the lower legs and feet and, to a lesser degree, on
the forearms, hands and face. The ears are only slightly deformed
and there is little involvement of the skin over the ears.
Circumscribed hyperkeratotic areas of shell-like appearance are
present on the soles beneath the great toes and heels. Ulcers
develop mainly on the points of pressure on heels and toes, over
the ankles and, especially, over the Achilles tendon. The fact
that skin can be successfully grafted on the ulcerated areas
demonstrates that the ulcers are not entirely trophic in origin,
but due to pressure on areas where the skin is tightly drawn over
the bone without any padding of subcutaneous fat tissue. The
classification of these skin disorders in the literature as
"scleroderma" or "scleropoikiloderma" does not correspond to the
clinical or histological findings. The characteristics of true
scleroderma, namely, sclerosis of the skin and homogenization of
the subcutaneous tissue, are not present, but there is atrophy of
the skin, flattening of the rete and of the papillae. The most
impressive feature, however, is the poorly developed panniculus
adiposus beneath the involved areas in the distal parts of the arms
and legs. It seems that the disappearance of the subcutaneous fat
tissue which apparently occurs simultaneously with the atrophy of
the superficial layers of the skin results in tightening of the
skin over the underlying structure and simulates scleroderma.
Inflammatory changes of the blood vessels (arteries) which are
found in true scleroderma are not present. Calcium deposits in the
walls of the subcutaneous blood vessels, however, are seen in the
most progressed cases. Since the skin changes in Werner's syndrome
only simulate true scleroderma but are in no way identical with
this disease, the classification as scleroderma should be rejected.
A descriptive name as "heredofamilial atrophic dermatosis with skin
ulcers" seems to be more approporiate.

In Rothmund's syndrome the skin lesions are in evidence five
months after birth. In contrast to Werner's syndrome there is
neither stretching of the skin nor the presence of ulcers. The
first changes occur on the skin of the face, ears, on the cheeks,
on the buttocks, and later the skin over the knees and extensor
surfaces of the extremities is involved. The flexor surfaces show
lesions late, or not at all. The vola manus and the bend of elbows
and knees remain free. In the first stages the skin changes
correspond to the livedo reticularis and exhibit, therefore, a
reddish hue. Reddish striae, round reddish spots with
telangiectases, appear later on. The color of the lesion changes

to a yellowish scar tissue which scales slightly. Normal skin encircled by such yellowish scar tissue acquires a characteristic areolated appearance. The areas of the skin not involved are extremely fine, soft, and translucent, causing the smallest ramifications of the skin veins to become visible. The skin on the hands and feet is pliable and thin as tissue paper. Some scattered telangiectases are also seen in these areas. Pigmented and depigmented areas are more pronounced than in Werner's syndrome. The classification of these skin changes as scleropoikiloderma does not coincide with the features as described. A descriptive designation of the skin lesions in Rothmund's syndrome as "heredofamilial atrophic dermatosis with telangiectasis" seems more appropriate.

4. Histological examination of the skin shows, in both cases, atrophy of the mucous layer, flattening of the papillae, even complete disappearance of the rete pegs. The changes typical of scleroderma and scleropoikiloderma were absent; there were neither inflammatory changes of the subcutaneous tissue and of the blood vessels nor sclerosis or homogenization of the collagenous tissue. The difference between the histological changes in Werner's and Rothmund's syndromes is the distention of the veins. In Werner's syndrome only occasional distention of the veins is found in the subcutaneous tissue whereas in the affected parts of the skin in Rothmund's syndrome the veins are generally distended and may even form small pools.

5. The muscles and the subcutaneous fat tissue of the distal parts of the extremities in Rothmund's syndrome are less atrophic than in Werner's syndrome. In childhood the muscles of Rothmund's syndrome are, in this respect, normally developed. In the few cases of Rothmund's syndrome observed at a later age muscular atrophy occurs on forearms and lower legs. Fingers and hands remain small and short in both syndromes.

6. Cataracts are of the same kind in both syndromes. They develop as star-like opacities in the periphery of the lens, mostly on the posterior pole. However, the age at which the cataracts begin to develop is significant. In Rothmund's syndrome they are already formed in early childhood, that is, at the age of three to five; in Werner's syndrome they develop in adult life, between the ages of 20 and 30.

7. Canities is the earliest feature of Werner's syndrome. It appears in the early twenties. The children exhibiting Rothmund's syndrome have abundant scalp hairs of normal color; even in the cases observed at a later age canities is not an outstanding feature.

8. Diffuse arteriosclerosis is evident in Werner's syndrome in
all cases and results in early complications involving the
circulatory system, such as gangrene or heart failure. In
Rothmund's syndrome diffuse arteriosclerosis is not observed in
young patients. Patients exhibiting Rothmund's syndrome in
childhood may reach an old age, as Seefelder's follow-up study of
Rothmund's cases shows. In some cases, however, as in Bloch and
Stauffer's case, arteriosclerosis developed in the fourth decade of
life.

9. Osteoporosis occurred in all cases of Werner's syndrome in
which roentgen-ray studies of the bones were made. In Rothmund's
syndrome osteoporosis was not observed.

10. Dysfunction of the thyroid was noticed in some patients
exhibiting Werner's syndrome. In some patients a goiter was found;
in some patients the thyroid could not be palpated at all.
Symptoms of hyperthyroidism were not present in any of these
patients. Proptosis of the eyes found in most of these patients is
not due to hyperthyroidism. In Rothmund's syndrome dysfunction of
the thyroid was not observed. These patients do not show
proptosis.

11. Underdevelopment of the sex organs and of the pubic hair is
found in all cases of Werner's syndrome. In males, however,
erections and the ability to have intercourse seem to have been
preserved for some time. Most of the females described did not
marry but had menstruated at least for some time. The patients
exhibiting Rothmund's syndrome showed, in most cases, normal sexual
development during puberty. In some male cases, however,
retardation of sexual development and, later, atrophy of the
testes, was noted. Those females of the families described by
Rothmund who exhibited both skin changes and cataracts were
childless, whereas those females who had only skin changes produced
children.

12. The bizarre changes of the epithelium of the vocal cords
causing a hoarse, high pitched voice, were found only in patients
exhibiting Werner's syndrome. High pitched voices may occur in
Rothmund's syndrome due to sexual retardment, but the
characteristic changes of the surface of the vocal cords were never
observed in cases with Rothmund's syndrome.

13. Tendency to diabetes or diabetic glycosuria is observed in
cases of Werner's syndrome but not in Rothmund's syndrome. The
tendency to diabetes seems to parallel the progress of arteriosclerosis. The occasional observation of gangrene of the lower
legs is the result of a secondary infection of the ulcers but
aggravated by the presence of arteriosclerosis.

The comparison of features of both syndromes under discussion shows that Werner's, and Rothmund's, syndromes are heredofamilial disorders with atrophic dermatosis, bilateral cateracts and endocrine features. Striking differences, however, are evident in the skin changes, as well as in the time and in the site of their occurrence. The difference in the appearance of the patient, especially in respect to the symptoms of presenility (progeria) justify separating Werner's and Rothmund's syndromes into two different but related clinical entities.

14. Both syndromes may not develop in all their features and may occur as "forme fruste." Intimate acquaintance with the syndromes under discussion may facilitate their recognition even as forme fruste. Thus, more families stricken with these heredofamilial disorders will be discovered, bearing out my contention that the disorders are not so rare as now believed.

ETIOLOGY

The survey of all cases demonstrates clearly that Werner's, as well as Rothmund's syndrome, is a recessive hereditary disorder. This conception cannot be altered by the occasional occurrence of cases with a normal family history. It is a special feature of these particular heredofamilial disorders that they occur collaterally in one generation. Werner, as well as Rothmund, suggested that we are dealing with a disorder of the ectodermal layer, since both skin and lens are derived from the ectoderm. Such a theory is not substantiated by the multiplicity of symptoms, involving blood vessels, subcutaneous fat tissue, muscles and endocrine glands; especially not since we know the symptom complex of a heredofamilial disorder involving only the ectodermal layer -- "ectodermal dysplasia of the anhydrotic and hydrotic type," which is entirely different from the syndromes under discussion.

Such authors as Bloch and Stauffer favor a primary endocrine disorder which is reflected in the skin as an explanation of the pathogenesis of the syndromes. Oppenheimer and Kugel, who reported an autopsy of a case of Werner's syndrome, found the parathyroid hyperactive. The Hamilton-Schwartz test was positive during life. These authors were inclined to attribute an etiological significance to the hyperactivity of the parathyroids. Oppenheimer, however, in a personal communications, states that he no longer adheres to the opinion that the parathyroid gland is predominately involved.

It is not unusual that in chronic diseases of young individuals the functions of the endocrine glands are impaired. The physical development of the body, growth as well as sexual

maturity, suffers if other organs, like heart, lungs or kidneys,
are congenitally underdeveloped. This may be so in our syndromes.
The endocrine dysfunction may then be secondary to the
heredofamilial constitutional skin disorder.

The heredofamilial character of the syndromes under
discussion, however, is indicative of a more basic nature of its
pathogenesis. This points to a defective germ plasm which
manifests its multiple defects at different periods of life. The
multiple defects result in abiotrophic processes not only of organs
which originate from the ectodermal layer, but also of organs which
originate from the other germinal layers. The only certain fact
bearing on the etiology of these syndromes is its heredofamilial
nature. For this reason the occurrence of defects of the entire
germinal plasm, recessive in heredity, seems the most plausible
explanation of the pathogenesis of Werner's as well as Rothmund's
syndrome.

SUMMARY

1.   The symptomatology of Werner's syndrome is established and
demonstrated in cases from the literature and in four of our own.
With the exception of Oppenheimer and Kugel's cases, the cases of
Werner's syndrome in the literature are published under the
misleading designation "Scleroderma and Cataracts."

2.   The skin changes in Werner's syndrome are not those of true
scleroderma. Because of its recessive heredofamilial occurrence it
is suggested that the skin changes, as the other symptoms of
Werner's syndrome, are the result of a defective germ plasm not
manifesting itself until the second and third decades of life. A
general term for the designation of the disorder as "progeria of
the adult" is suggested since all symptoms of Werner's syndrome
result in presenility of the patient.

3.   The designation of the skin changes with a purely descriptive
name, as "heredofamilial atrophic dermatosis with skin ulcers"
seems more appropriate.

4.   The skin ulcers in Werner's syndrome are not entirely trophic
in origin since they appear only on exposed parts and are probably
the result of pressure upon the thin, atrophic and stretched skin.
The healing of the ulcers by grafting skin upon the skin defects
supports such an opinion.

5.   The symptomatology of Rothmund's syndrome is illustrated by
cases selected from the literature and by a case of our own.

6. The skin changes of Rothmund's syndrome are classified in the literature as "poikiloderma" or "scleropoikiloderma." Such a classification does not accord with the heredofamilial occurrence of the skin disorder nor with the histological findings. In conformity with the designation of the skin disorder in Werner's syndrome it seems appropriate to use for the skin changes in Rothmund's syndrome a simple descriptive name such as "heredo-familial atrophic dermatosis with telangiectases."

7. Both syndromes may occur as incomplete forms, so called "forme fruste."

8. The heredity in both forms is recessive. The collateral occurrence in brothers and sisters of one generation is often observed. Rothmund's syndrome starts usually in childhood; Werner's syndrome in the second and third decades.

9. Clinical syndromes related to Werner's and Rothmund's syndromes are discussed. A chart tabulating the features of Werner's and Rothmund's syndromes in comparison with related clinical entities is presented to aid in the differential diagnosis of these syndromes.

10. For the pathogenesis of Werner's syndrome and Rothmund's syndrome a purely ectodermal dysplasia as well as primary endocrine functional disturbance is rejected. The recessive heredity of both syndromes suggests as an explanation for its etiology the existence of multiple germ plasm defects manifesting themselves in abiotrophic features of various organs at different periods of life.

APPENDIX

Editor's note: The legends for the photographs contained in the original Thannhauser article are reproduced here.

Fig. 2: Case 1. Germaine: Gray scarce scalp hairs; scanty eyebrows; no eyelashes. Presenile appearance.

Fig. 3: Shell-like hyperkeratosis on both heels, under the large toe. Ulcers under the fifth toe; hallux valgus.

Fig. 4: Case 2. Fernande: Note same areas of hyperkeratosis only this time small ulcer under left toe.

Fig. 5: Skin tightly stretched over ankles and toes. Note healed ulcer under the left malleolus.

Fig. 6: Case 3. Robert. Large ulcer on left inner malleolus.

Fig. 7:   Case 4. Roger. Small hands; deformed phalangeal joints.
            Presenile appearance.

Fig. 8:   Picture of vocal cords. (Reproduced from B.S. Oppenheimer
            and V.R. Kugel.)

Fig. 9:   Nathan O. and Sidney O. Short stature; presenile
            appearance.

Fig. 10:   Fine, scarce, gray scalp hairs, beaked noses; small
            mouths.

Fig. 11:   Sidney O. The small, thin upper arms and lower legs in
            direct contrast to globulous abdomen.

Fig. 12:   Sidney O. Taut skin tightly stretched over underlying
            tissue; motion impaired in both ankle joints; hallux
            valgus. Ulcers on left inner malleolus, on lateral sides
            of feet.

Fig. 13:   Large ulcers on Achilles tendons.

Fig. 14:   Healed ulcers of Achilles tendons after grafting.

Fig. 15:   Nathan O. Amputated left leg. Taut skin tightly
            stretched over the right lower leg. Ulcer on the inner
            side of the foot.

Fig. 16:   Skin biopsy of Sidney O. Papillae fairly well preserved;
            subcutaneous tissue normal; no proliferative necrotizing
            arteritis visible.

Fig. 17:   Skin biopsy of Nathan O. Papillae are definitely
            flattened; subcutaneous tissue not homogenized; some
            veins distended. No inflammatory infiltration of
            arteries or tissues.

Fig. 18:   Higher magnification of figure 17.

Fig. 19:   George St. General leanness, extremely thin legs and
            arms.

Fig. 20:   Skin under lower eyelids wrinkled (in contrast to
            scleroderma). Aperture of mouth small. Hairs are fine
            and gray. Presenile appearance.

Fig. 21:   Skin over both ankles tightly pulled; motion in ankle-
            joints impaired. Ulcers on left malleolus and sides of
            feet. Areas of hyperkeratosis.

Fig. 22:   Skin biopsy of George St.   Papillae are entirely
           flattened.   Small mucous layer.   Prickle-cells reduced in
           number.   Subcutaneous tissue normal; not homogenized.   No
           inflammatory infiltration around arteries or in
           subcutaneous tissues.   Some distended veins.

Fig. 23:   Higher magnification of Figure 22.

REFERENCES

1.   Werner, C.W.O., Uber Katarakt in Verbindung mit Sclerodermie,
     Inaug. Disseft., Kiel, 1904.
2.   Vossius, A., Zwei Falle von Katarakt in Verbindung mit
     Sclerodermie, Ztschr. f. Augenh., 1920, xliii, 640.
3.   Guillain, G., Alajouanine, T. and Marquezy, R., Sclerodermie
     progressive avec cataracte double precoce chez un infantile,
     Bull. et mem. Soc. med. d. hop. de Paris, 1923, xxxix, 1489.
4.   Manjukowa, N., Zur Frage uber den Zusammenhang der
     Linsentrubungen mit Storungen der inneren Sekertion, Ruski
     Ophth. Jour. 2, Klin. Monatbl. f. Augenh, 1923, lxx, 785.
5.   Papastratiyakis, C., Un nouveau syndrome dystrophique
     juvenile, Paris med. 1922, xlv, 475.
6.   Barbot, E.M., La sclerodermie associe a la cataracte, These de
     Paris, 1925.
7.   Monier-Vinard, and Barbot, E.M., Sclerodermie et cataracte,
     syndrome familial, Bull. et mem. Soc. med. d. hop. de Paris,
     1928, lii, 708.
8.   Bau-Prussak, S., La degenerescence genito-sclerodermique, Rev.
     Neurol., 1926, Tome I, 316.
9.   Sainton, M. and Mamou, H., Syndrome pluriglandulaire avec
     sclerodermie et cataracte, Bull. et mem. Soc. med. d. hop. de
     Paris, 1927, li, 1685.
10. Hashimoto, T., Ein Fall von Sklerodermie kombiniert mit
     Katarakt, Zentralbl. f. Hautkrankh, 1930, xxxvii, 205.
11. Eguchi, H., Uber Cataracte bei pluriglandularem Infantiilismus
     mit Sklerodermie, Art. Soc. Ophth. Jap. 35, Ref. Zentralbl.
     f. d. ges. Opth., 1931, xxv, 507.
12. Sezarry, A., Favory, A., and Mamou, H., Syndrome tardif de
     sclerodermie avec cataracte, associe a des troubles
     endocriniens, Bull. et mem. Soc. med. hop. de Paris, 1930,
     xlvi, 358.
13. Mamou, H., Sclerodermie et cataracte, maladie de Rothmund,
     These de Paris, 1931.
14. Krebs, E., Hartmann, E. and Thiebaut, F., Un cas familial de
     syndrome de sclerodermie avec cataracte, troubles endocriniens
     et neurovegatatifs associes, Rev. Neurol., 1930, i, 606, 775,
     Rev. Neurol., 1930, ii, 121.
15. Oppenheimer, B.S. and Kugel, V.H., Werner's syndrome, a

heredofamilial disorder with scleroderma, bilateral juvenile
cataract, precocious graying of the hair and endocrine
stigmatization, Trans. Assoc. Am. Phys., 1934, xlix, 358.

16. Oppenheimer, B.S. and Kugel, V.H., Werner's syndrome, report
of the first necropsy and of findings in a new case, Am. Jr.
Med. Sci., 1941, ccii, 629.

17. Varney, R.F., Kenyon, A.T. and Koch, F.S., Association of
short stature, retarded sexual development and high urinary
gonadotropin titers in women, Jr. Clin. Endocrinol., 1942, ii,
137.

18. Albright, F., Smith, P.H., and Fraser, R., A syndrome
characterized by primary ovarian insufficiency and decreased
stature, Am. J. Med. Sci., 1942, cciv, 625.

19. Wilkins, L. and Fleischmann, W., Ovarian agenesis, Jr. Clin.
Endocrinol., 1944, iv, 357.

WERNER'S SYNDROME: A REVIEW OF ITS SYMPTOMATOLOGY, NATURAL
HISTORY, PATHOLOGIC FEATURES, GENETICS AND RELATIONSHIP TO THE
NATURAL AGING PROCESS

Charles J. Epstein,[1] George M. Martin,[2]
Amelia L. Schultz,[3] and Arno G. Motulsky [3]

1.   Laboratory of Chemical Biology, National Institute of
      Arthritis and Metabolic Disease, Bethesda, MD

2.   Department of Pathology, University of Washington
      Seattle, WA

3.   Division of Medical Genetics, Department of Medicine
      University of Washington, Seattle, WA

INTRODUCTION

    Werner's syndrome was first described in 1904 by Otto Werner
in his doctoral thesis, "Uber Katarakt in Verbindung mit
Sklerodermie" ("Cataract in combination with scleroderma") (137).
He reported four sibs with similar clinical findings: shortness of
stature; senile appearance; graying of the hair beginning at about
age 20; cataracts appearing during the third decade; skin changes
(tautness, atrophy, hyperkeratoses and ulceration) designated as
scleroderma and primarily involving the feet and, to a lesser
degree, the hands; joint deformities associated with the skin
abnormalities; atrophy of the muscles and connective tissues of the
extremities; and early cessation of menstruation. Werner was
impressed principally by the cataracts, skin changes, senile
appearance, and graying of the hair and attributed the condition to
a "failure" of the cells derived from the ectoderma. Although he knew
that the features displayed by the affected members of the family

---

*Reprinted from Medicine 45:177-221, 1966, with permission
of the Williams & Wilkins Co., Baltimore.*

represented a new and distinct entity, he related this condition to
one described by Rothmund (106) in which juvenile cataracts were
found together with skin changes. The implied association of these
two syndromes and the identification of the skin alterations in
Werner's cases as scleroderma were sources of confusion for many
years, and it was not until the appearance of the paper by
Oppenheimer and Kugel in 1934 (94) and of the comprehensive study
by Thannhauser in 1945 (131) that the two syndromes were clearly
delineated and the character of the skin changes defined.

In his paper, Thannhauser listed twelve principal characteristics of Werner's syndrome: 1) shortness of stature with a
characteristic habitus; 2) canities (premature graying of the
hair); 3) premature baldness; 4) scleropoikiloderma; 5) trophic
ulcers of the legs; 6) juvenile cataracts; 7) hypogonadism; 8)
tendency to diabetes; 9) calcification of the blood vessels; 10)
osteoporosis; 11) metastatic calcifications; and 12) tendency to
occur in brothers and sisters. Since the time of Werner's original
report, over a hundred cases which fulfill these criteria have been
described. In many, the descriptions and investigations are
fragmentary, and only by considering the information available in
all of the reports is it possible to gain a reasonably clear
picture of the nature of the syndrome.

In this study, we shall describe a new sibship containing
three individuals affected with Werner's syndrome. The various
features of the disease as derived from analysis of these and 122
other definite cases will be discussed and the formal genetics of
the syndrome will be analyzed. The possible relationship of
Werner's syndrome to the processes of natural aging and to various
disease states will be discussed.

CASE REPORTS

The sibship designated M8 has already been referred to in a
preliminary communication by Motulsky et al. (90). It consists of
nine American-born individuals of Japanese parentage, three of whom
present the classic features of Werner's syndrome. The three
affected sisters are the first, second and seventh children in a
family that is otherwise healthy (see Fig. 13). The parents and
the non-affected sibs are all short in stature (ranging from 147 to
166 cm), but, except for early graying of the hair of one brother,
have none of the stigmata of the syndrome. The parents are not
known to be consanguineous, but did come from the same town in
Japan, Okayama, not far from Hiroshima. The eldest affected
sister, H. McG (M8a), cooperated in several extensive studies, and
will be described in detail. The second affected sister, C.I.
(M8b), died before the inception of these studies, but we were able
to obtain the record of a previous hospitalization at the Deaconess

Hospital, Spokane, Washington. The youngest patient, M.I. (M8c), was only seen once.

Case 1 - (M8a)

History

H. McG. (UWH #077-54), a 48 year old Japanese-American housewife, was first seen at the University of Washington Hospital in 1960 (at age 44) for treatment of foot ulcers. She was in good health as a child, but noted that her growth ceased at about age 13. At an age between 20 and 25 her weight reached 38.6 kg, but it then decreased to 30 kg without loss in height. Cataracts were diagnosed at the age of 22 and were removed 5 years later. The right eye was subsequently enucleated after an attack of acute glaucoma.

In the early part of the third decade, the patient noted graying and loss of hair, and a generalized increase in skin pigmentation. Glycosuria was first detected at age 31, but the patient never received insulin or oral anti-diabetic agents. Ulcerations of the skin of the feet and ankles occurred at age 36, and since then there have been recurrent, poorly healing ulcers of the malleoli and Achilles tendons bilaterally. Ulcers also appeared on the elbows.

The menstrual periods began in her early "teens" and were regular until age 44, at which time they ceased abruptly. However, hot flashes had begun 13 years earlier, and libido was always poor. The patient married late and had no pregnancies. At age 46, her voice, which had been hoarse and high pitched for many years, became completely inaudible, but returned to its previous quality of squeaky hoarseness six months later.

Physical examination

The patient was a diminutive but alert and intelligent Japanese woman who appeared to be about 70 years old (Fig. 1). Her height was 142 cm, weight 30.2 kg, and blood pressure 170/80 mm Hg. The head was grossly normal. The external ears were quite stiff, with a hyperkeratosis on the left ear and patchy white areas, possibly containing calcium, on the right. There was ptosis of the right eyelid and a prosthesis for the right eye; the left eye was aphakic and there was some increase in pigmentation of the fundus. The teeth, pharynx, neck, thyroid, and chest were normal, but the breast tissue was underdeveloped. The heart was not enlarged; there was a grade 2/6 blowing, early systolic murmur at the base. There was no enlargement of abdominal organs, and the panniculus adiposus was of good thickness. The extremities were extremely thin, but strength was good despite marked muscle atrophy. Movement at the ankle joints was severely restricted.

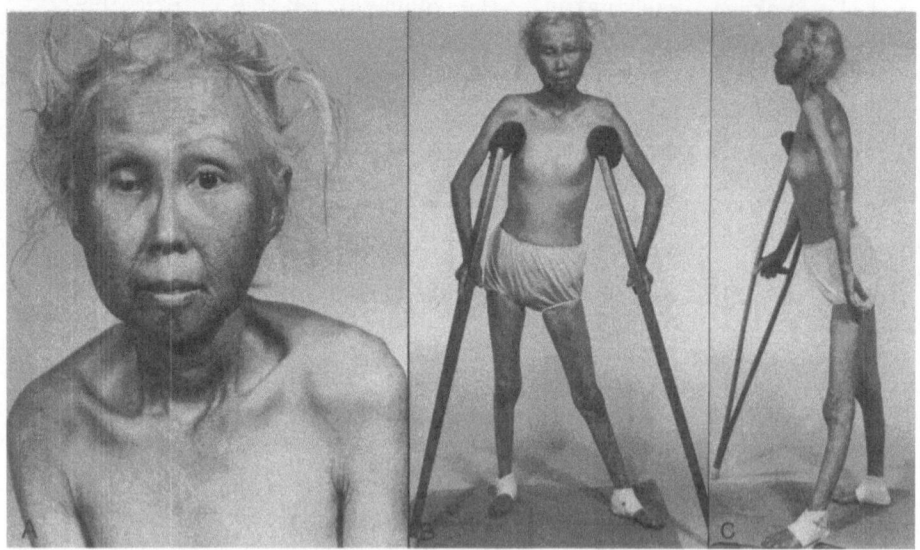

Fig. 1 :   Case 1 at the age of 48 years. The general
           appearance of senility is well illustrated, as are the
           loss and graying of hair, the thinness of the extremities
           with a relatively normal trunk, the poor breast
           development, and the healed ulcer on the left elbow.

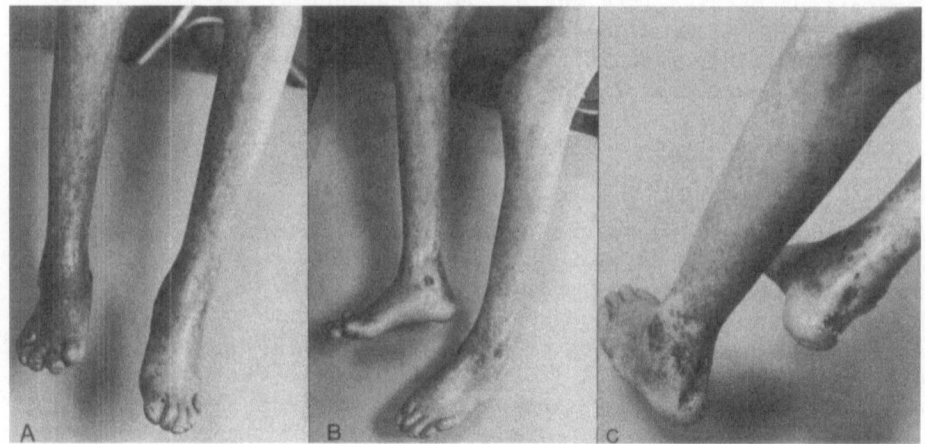

Fig. 2 :   The feet and legs of case 1, illustrating the chronic
           ulcerations over the ankle and heels, the contractions of
           the toes, the areas of hyperpigmentation and
           depigmentation on the legs, and the abnormal toenails.

The skin of the body was thin and hyperpigmented, and there were numerous freckled areas. The skin over the lower legs and feet, in particular over the toes, was smooth, shiny, and tight (Fig. 2); the fifth toes of both feet were pulled superiorly and medially. There was blotchy, brown pigmentation with intermingled areas of depigmentation over the feet and lower legs, and ulcers were present over the Achilles tendons and the malleoli bilaterally (Fig. 2). The skin was also tightly adherent to the elbows, and scars of healed ulcers were present. The hair on the scalp was very sparse and steel gray in color; there was no axillary or pubic hair. The clitoris was normal, but the labia and vaginal mucosa were atrophic. The uterus and ovaries could not be palpated. On neurologic examination, the deep tendon reflexes were brisk. Sensation was intact except for a slight diminution of vibration sense and two-point discrimination in the toes and feet; in these areas, there was also hyperesthesia to pinprick.

Laboratory Data

a) Hematologic: Hematocrit 38%, hemoglobin 11.7 g/100 ml, red blood cell count 4.41 million/mm^3, mean corpuscular volume 86 μ^3, mean corpuscular hemoglobin 87 $\mu\mu$g , mean corpuscular hemoglobin concentration 31%. Peripheral blood smear: slight aniocytosis and microscytosis; adequate number of platelets. White blood cell count and differential: normal. Serum iron 34 μg/100 ml, iron binding capacity 307 μg/100 ml; serum haptoglobin 1350 mg of bound hemoglobin. Plasma iron turnover 0.51 mg/100 ml/day (normal); red cell iron utilization: day 3-67%, day 6-100% (normal). Bone marrow smears; slight erythroid hyperplasia, adequate iron stores, moderate increase in eosinophils.

Red cell carbohydrate and glutathione metabolism: (studied by Dr. E. R. Simon): Abnormalities in glutathione (GSH) metabolism in red cells have been associated with shortening of red cell life and with cataract formation (76). Since both red cells and the lens fibers are anucleate cells which share some features of carbohydrate and glutathione metabolism, certain aspects of these metabolic pathways were studied in the red cells of this patient in the hope of finding a metabolic lesion. The "pentose shunt" pathway of carbohydrate metabolism was investigated. This pathway generates TPNH, a substance required for the production of reduced glutathione (GSH) by GSH reductase, i.e. GSSG + TPNH $\xrightarrow{\text{GSH reductase}}$ GSH + TPN (119). The findings are summarized in Table 1. GSH and GSH stability were normal. There was evidence of increased glycolytic activity affecting both the Embden-Meyerhof cycle (i.e. increased $C^{14}O_2$ production from glucose-1-C^{14}, increased enzyme levels for glucose-6-phosphate dehydrogenase [G-6-Pd] and 6-phosphogluconate dehydrogenase [6-P-Gd] and increased $C^{14}O_2$ from glucose-2-C^{14}. Stimulation of the shunt pathway with methylene blue showed no blocks in this metabolic route. As with control red cells, no

significant amount of $C^{14}O_2$ was evolved from glucose-6-C^{14}.
Methemoglobin reduction with glucose or inosine as substrates was
normal. In the presence of methylene blue and glucose,
methemoglobin reduction was definitely elevated while a normal rate
of methemoglobin reduction was found with methylene blue and
inosine.

These data show no deficiency or block in red cell carbohydrate
metabolism and also document normal values for GSH and GSH
stability. The finding of increased methemoglobin reduction with
glucose and methylene blue is compatible with similar data on iron
deficiency. At the time of testing, the patient had a saturation of
transferrin of 10% - a finding indicative of iron deficiency. It is
possible that the elevated values of some other parameters of red
cell carbohydrate metabolism can also be explained by the mild iron
deficiency, but detailed studies with these methods have not yet

Table 1:   Studies on red cell metabolism of case 1[a]

	Normal	±2 SD	Patient
	(μmoles/g hemoglobin/hour)		
Glucose catabolism			
Glucose disappearance	7.0	0.8	8.7, 9.6, 9.5
Lactate formation	11.6	0.9	15.8, 18.1, 18.7 (high)
C^1O_2 formation	0.21	0.05	0.80, 0.55, 0.66
C^2O_2 formation	0.023, 0.015, 0.13		0.13
C^6O_2 formation	0.015	0.009	0.029, 0.025
With methylene blue			
Glucose disappearance	8.6	1.0	10.6, 10.3
Lactate formation	12.7	1.5	17.3, 19.2 (high)
C^1O_2 formation	4.7	1.0	5.1, 4.5
C^2O_2 formation	1.4	0.5	1.1
Methemoglobin reduction			
With glucose	1.1	0.46	1.4
With inosine	1.3	0.46	1.8
Glucose with MB	13.2	2.2	21.6 (high)
Inosine with MB	15.3	3.7	14.4
	(μmoles/g hemoglobin)		
Glutathione	7.5	2.6	8.4
GSH stability	91%	12.8%	99%
	(units/g hemoglobin)		
Enzymes			
G-6-PD	4.87	0.24	6.4 (high)
6-PGD	2.97	0.22	4.0 (high)

• Performed by Dr. E. R. Simon; methods as described in Simon and Ways (119).

been performed in iron deficiency. A red cell population enriched
with young cells would give similar metabolic findings, but no
direct measurements of red cell lifespan were performed.

b. Endocrine: Serum butanol extractable iodide 5.2 μg/100 ml
(normal, 3.2-6.4); 24 hour radioactive iodine uptake 8%; 24 hour
urinary excretion of gonadotropins, >100 (8/5/60) and 50-100 mouse
units (8/11/60) (normal, to 50).

   Glucose metabolism: The results of glucose and tolbutamide
tolerance tests (performed by Drs. M. Nydick, E. Samols, and T.
Kazuya), in which levels of serum insulin were assayed
immunochemically (110), are shown in Fig. 3. Glucose (25 g) was
rapidly given intraveneously and produced a typically diabetic
response in the blood sugar level; the final serum insulin level
attained was greater than has been seen in normal subjects. When
tolbutamide (1 g) was administered intravenously, the serum insulin
level tripled within the first ten minutes and then declined;
however, the maximal fall in blood sugar did not occur for 60

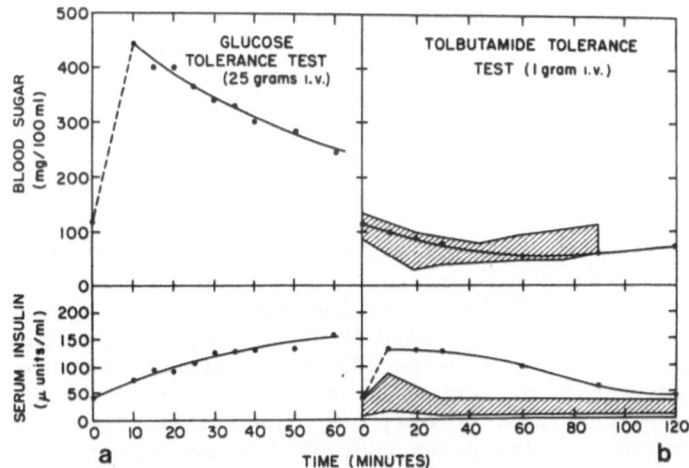

Fig. 3a. (Left). Response of blood glucose and serum insulin levels
         to the intravenous infusion of glucose. The serum
         insulin level, which is higher than normal even in the
         fasting state, rises very slowly and the elevation is
         very prolonged. 3b (Right). Response of blood glucose
         and serum insulin levels to the intravenous infusion of
         tolbutamide. The normal responses are indicated by the
         hatched areas. Although the blood sugar response fall
         within the normal area, the shape of the curve is
         abnormal, with the maximum response being delayed and
         prolonged. The insulin response is excessive and very
         prolonged.

minutes (normal: 20-30 minutes). The response in insulin levels
to tolbutamide was again far in excess of that seen in normal
individuals, and resembled that of typical "late onset" diabetics.
Therefore, both studies were interpreted as being compatible with a
diagnosis of the adult type of diabetes (see below). On dietary
control alone, the patient's urine was free of glucose except in
the late evening samples when it averaged + to ++ (Testape, glucose
oxidase).

Adrenal function: (evaluated by Drs. S.H. Waxman and V.C.
Kelley) (136). The patient was given 25 units of ACTH
intraveneously over a four hour period, and the plasma cortisol and
11-desoxyeortisol levels determined. The former rose from 10
mg/100 ml to 57 mg/100 ml; the latter, which was very low, did not
increase. These responses were considered to be normal.
Metapyron (SU-4885) (30 mg/kg), an inhibitor of 11-beta-
hydroxylation of adrenal steroids, (i.e. of the conversion of 11-
desoxycortisol to hydrocortisone) was given intravenously. Plasma
cortisol rapidly decreased and desoxycortisol greatly increased
during the period of drug administration, the latter indicating
that the pituitary was able to respond to the decrease in cortisol
precursors. When the SU-4885 was discontinued, the levels of both
steroids returned to normal values. Half-lives of cortisol and 11-
desoxycortisol were 102 minutes (normal 95-130) (101) and 16
minutes (normal 18-40 minutes), respectively. Despite the slightly
short half-life of desoxycortisol, it was concluded that none of
the studies indicated any basic dysfunction in the production or
metabolism of the adrenal hydroxycorticoids.

c) Genito-urinary and electrolytes: Urinalysis: normal except
for trace of protein and 2-3 white cells per high powered field.
Blood urea nitrogen 20 mg/100 ml (normal 8-18); serum creatinine
0.6 mg/100 ml (normal 0.6-1.3); 24 hour urinary excretion of
creatinine 484 mg, of creatine 352 mg; creatine clearance 54.9
ml/min. (corrected for surface area of 1.73 m2). Urinary excretion
of mucopolysaccharides, normal; one-dimensional paper chromatography of urinary amino acids, normal. Serum sodium 145 mEq/1;
potassium 4.8 mEq/1; bicarbonate 33 mEg/1; chloride 103 mEq/1;
calcium 11.0 mg/100 ml, phosphorus 4.8 mg/100 ml.

d) Gastro-intestinal: Serum amylase 79 Somogyi units (normal 40-
160); alkaline phosphatase 4.95 SJR units (normal 2.8-8.6);
glutamicpyruvic transaminase 26 Frankel units (normal 5-35);
glutamic-oxalacetic transaminase 25 Frankel units (normal 10-40);
lactic dehydrogenase 285 Wroblewski units (normal 100-350);
aldolase 10 SL units (normal 10-12). Serum cholesterol 202 mg/100
ml (normal 120-260); bilirubin 0.2 mg/100 ml (normal 0.1-1.0);
thymol turbidity 1.0 (normal 0.12-1.3); serum mucoprotein (as
tyrosine) 2.7 mg/100 ml (normal 1-5); serm triglycerides 246 mg/100
ml (normal 50-200); esterfied fatty acids 450 mg/100 ml (normal

250-500); phospholipids 248 mg/100 ml (normal 50-350).
Prothrombin, 100%. Serum protein paper electrophoresis (g/100 ml):
total 9.1, albumin 4.3, globulins: alpha1 0.4, alpha2 1.0, beta
1.1, gamma 2.3.

e) X-rays: Feet (Figure 4, see appendix II) -- small, deformed
and osteoporotic throughout, with multiple areas of soft tissue
calcification; fusion of metatarsal-phalangeal joints and atrophy of
distal halves of 5th metatarsals; destruction of left talo-navicular
joint with resorption of articulating surfaces. Wrists and hands --
sclerotic shafts of digits; tiny areas of calcification in region of
capsular attachments in interphalangeal joints. Knees -- extensive
calcification of quadriceps tendon. Elbows -- calcification in
tendinous attachments to olecranon and capsule of joint. Skull,
pelvis, lumbar and thoracic spine -- normal. Chest -- marked
calcification of costal cartilages.

f) Electrocardiography and electromyography: An electrocardiogram
was normal. Electromyographic fibrillation potentials suggesting
denervation were observed in the extensor digitorum brevis and
tibialis anterior muscles of the leg; normal patterns were found in
the gastrocnemius, quadriceps and opponens muscles. Nerve
conduction times: left median nerve 64 meters/sec and left
peroneal nerve 60 meters/sec (both normal).

Case 2 (M8b)

     C.I., who was said to have been healthy as a child, ceased
growing in her early teens. Axillary and pubic hair never
developed, and there were no menses. Bilateral cataract
extractions were performed at age 9 years. At age 28 she developed
infected areas which failed to heal properly on both feet.

     On physical examination (at age 29 years) the patient was a
very small, "infantile" appearing woman who weighed 22.7 kg. Her
blood pressure was 180/118 mm Hg. She had very little scalp hair
and no pubic or axillary hair. The pupils were irregular and the
lenses were absent. The genitalia were infantile and secondary sex
characteristics were absent. Numerous small furuncles were present
over both feet.

     Hemoglobin 12.3 g/100 ml white blood cell count and
differential normal. Urinalysis: reducing sugar (3+), but no
acetone or protein. The blood sugar on admission was 370 mg/100 ml
and, with therapy, ranged from 53 to 114 mg/100 ml.

     The final impression was of diabetes mellitus with endocrine
imbalance suggestive of hypophyseal dwarfism. The patient died
unmarried at the age of 31 of unknown causes, and no autopsy was
performed. Her death was attributed by the family to "diabetes."

Case <u>3</u> - <u>(M8c)</u> (evaluated with the assistance of Dr. Merton Proctor)

M.I., (UWH #054-75) allegedly had a normal childhood but was always quite small. Her maximum weight was 36.5 kg, and declined to about 28 kg at the age of 20. Her menses, which began at age 10, were painful and very irregular and ceased at age 32. The onset of graying of the hair was noted at age 14-18, and the hair gradually became completely white. The voice became high pitched and rasping in her early 20's, and bilateral cataract extractions were performed at age 25.

Hyperpigmentation and dryness of the skin were thought to have been always present. The skin of the distal extremities, particularly the feet, was quite taut and large calluses on the feet developed at age 20-23. At age 32, ulcers appeared on the ankles and the bony prominences of the feet. The ankle joints became immobile and a flexion contracture of the right knee developed.

On physical examination at age 34 the patient had a blood pressure of 80/40 mm Hg and weighed 26.9 kg. She was a short, white-haired woman who appeared to be in her 60's. The skin was hyperpigmented throughout, and there was perioral tightening and cheilosis; facial movements were not restricted. Except for palmar thickening, the skin on the hands was thin and taut. The skin of her feet and legs below the knees was taut, shiny, thin and smooth. There were 0.5 to 1.0 cm diameter open ulcerations on the mallioli bilaterally, and an ulcerated callus on the medial aspect of the right foot. Several other calluses were present on the soles. The nails were brittle and there were longitudinal ridges. The hair of the scalp was pure white and decreased in amount. Axillary and pubic hair were sparse, as were eyebrows and eyelashes.

The eyes were aphakic, and the fundi showed an increase in pigmentation and mild arteriosclerotic changes. The teeth were in poor condition, and there was redness and denudation of the mucosa of the tip and lateral margins of the tongue. The ears, nose, and pharynx were normal, but several firm nodules were palpated in the thyroid. The breasts were very small and no glandular tissue was palpable. Examination of the chest, heart, and abdomen was negative.

All extremities showed marked muscle atrophy and there was a flexion contracture of the right knee. Marked scoliosis of the spine was noted. Examinations of the cranial nerves and sensory modalities were normal, but deep tendon reflexes could not be elicited.

Rectal and vaginal examinations were not performed.

Laboratory Data

Hematocrit: 38.5%; peripheral blood smear: slight
microcytosis. White bood cell count and differential were normal.
Urinalysis: normal. Serum electrolytes, calcium, phosphorus,
prothrombin, alkaline phosphatase, and thymol turbidity were
normal. Serum cholesterol, 268 mg/100 ml. Serum protein paper
electrophoresis (g/100 ml): total protein 8.6, albumin 4.8,
globulins: $alpha_1$ 0.3, $alpha_2$ 0.7, beta 0.9, gamma 1.9.
Electrocardiogram: normal.

X-rays: Skull (including sella turcica) and lumbar spine,
normal; abdominal aorta not visible. Ankles: focal soft tissue
calcifications. Knee (right): calcification of the quadriceps
tendon, but normal joint. Hands: resorption of the phalangeal
tufts with sclerosis of the shafts of the distal phalanges and
generalized osteoporosis; no joint abnormalities. Chest:
scoliosis of the spine and calcification of the costal cartilages;
no vascular calcifications noted.

III. CHRONOLOGY AND SYMPTOMATOLOGY

Including the three cases reported above, we have been able to
examine the original reports of 125 definite cases of Werner's
syndrome. Each of these patients had cataracts and skin changes,
and in addition, all or most of the other signs and symptoms listed
in the introduction and described in greater detail below. Several
other cases, totaling eleven in number, have been considered as
probable since they lacked one of the two cardinal signs but
appeared otherwise to satisfy the criteria of the syndrome.

The pertinent information relating to the identification of
the patients and sibships is listed in Table 2.

The mean age at which patients were first recognized as having
Werner's syndrome was 38.7 years, with a range of 21 to 58 years
(Fig. 5). All signs and symptoms generally appeared several years
earlier, indicating that there was a significant delay in the
establishment of the correct diagnosis. This is not surprising
since Werner's syndrome is not well known and is often confused
with other disease entities and with premature but "normal" aging.

A. Chronology

On the basis of the data presented above the time of appearance of the various signs and symptoms are as shown in Fig. 6.

Table 2:   Summary of sibships with Werner's syndrome

Sibship[a]	Authors	Total Sibs[b]	Nationality	Parental Consanguinity	Case	Initials[d]	Sex	Age[e]
A1	1, 56, 95, 142, 145	3 (1)	Hung. (Jew)[f]	1	A1a	HT	M	38
B1	3, 4	—	Dutch	—	B1a (B1b)[g, h]		M M	41 37
B2	6	8	U. S.	—	B2a B2b	EC	F F	44
B3	8	—	Ital.	—	B3a	GA	M	29
B4	9, 138	—	Ital.	2 (prob)	B4a		M	21
B5	11	4	Eng.	0	B5a	SG	F	29
B6	14, 82, 100	7 (5)	U. S.	2	B6a B6b B6c	ER OA KE	M F F	45 49 42
B6′	82	11 (10)	U. S.	2	B6′a B6′b	MK LS	F M	>52 37
B7	15, 49	4	Irish	—	B7a		M	55
B8	16	12 (4)	Afrikaans	1	B8a	SF	F	58
(B9)[g]	17, 66	7 (-)	Puerto Rico	(0)	(B9a)[i]	SS	F	28
B10	18	4	Dutch	0	B10a B10b[h]		M M	38 41
C1	20	4	Negro	—	C1a C1b		M F	43 45
C2	23	1	Polish	—	C2a	PH	F	33
C3	24	—	U. S.	0	C3a C3b	P	M M	30 27
D1	29	—	German	0	D1a	RH	F	32
D2	30	2	Ital.	+	D2a	A	F	35
D3	31	5	Eng.	—	D3a D3b	AR	F F	56 41
D4	32	—	N. Zeal.[j]	—	D4a		M	49
E1	35	5	Jap.	0	E1a E1b		M F	32 30
E2	36	10 (8)	Eng.	—	E2a E2b (E2c)[h]	IV-7 IV-10 IV-2	F F M	51 42
F1	37	11 (6)	Ital.	—	F1a	EC	F	44
F2	38	5	U. S. (Jew)	0	F2a	JB	F	42

Table 2 -- continued

Sibship[a]	Authors	Total Sibs[b]	Nationality	Parental Consanguinity	Case	Initials[d]	Sex	Age[e]
M8	90[f]	9	Jap.	(0)	M8a	HMcG	F	47
					M8b	CI	F	29
					M8c	MI	F	34
M9	92	4	Swed.	0	M9a	AR	M	36
					M9b	AL	F	36
O1	56, 94, 95, 126, 145	11 (3)	Hung.	1	O1a	DGr	M	42
					O1b	AGr	M	36
O2	96	8	Norw.	0	O2a	OO	M	33
P1	102	14 (11)	U. S.	0	P1a	ER	F	30
					P1b	RS	F	30
					P1c	Vu	F	
					P1d	By	M	
P1'	102	8 (–)	U. S.	0	P1'a	JM	M	
P2	103	3	U. S.	—	P2a	LK	F	35
R1	104	—	Eng.	0	R1a	TR	M	46
R2	105	5	U. S.	1	R2a	RG	F	42
R3	=	3 (–)	U. S.	—	R3a	CW	M	42
R4	106	4 (3)	Ital.	—	R4a	SD	M	36
S1	111	4	Ital.	—	S1a		M	36
S2	112	2	Argen.	—	S2a	NP	F	29
S3	113	7 (3)	U. S.	1	S3a	MB	F	45
					S3b	RW	F	41
S4	114	5	Hung.	—	S4a	BL	M	35
					S4b	BJ	M	30
S5	115	3	Czech.	—	S5a		M	42
S6	118	7	U. S.	—	S6a	CS	M	42
					S6b	LS	M	50
(S7)	122	2	U. S.	—	(S7a)[f]		M	27
(S8)	122	7 (–)	Negro	—	(S8a)[f]		F	27
S9	123	—	French	1	S9a		F	34
S10	125	1 (–)	Bulg.	—	S10a		F	42
S11	127	3	Pol.	0	S11a		M	36
S12	128	—	Hung.	—	S12a		M	27
T1	130	2	French	0	T1a	ML	M	46
T2	131	—	Russ. (Jew)	0	T2a	NO	M	34
					T2b	SO	M	38
T3	131	—	Germ.	0	T3a	MF	F	29
T4	131	3	U. S.	1	T4a	GSt	M	39
V1	133	7	Persian (Jew)	1	V1a		M	39
V2	134	—	Hung.	2	V2a	ER	M	41

(continued)

Table 2 -- continued

Sibship[a]	Authors	Total Sibs[b]	Nationality	Parental Consanguinity	Case	Initials[d]	Sex	Age[e]
F3	38, 141	5	Russ.	1	F3a	BL	M	37
F4	41, 109	—	French	—	F4a		M	25
(F5)	42	5 (−)	U. S.	—	(F5a)[i]	FB	M	45
F6	45, 80	7 (5)	Swiss	1	F6a	LS	F	49
					F6b	GS	M	31
G1	50	—	Germ.	—	G1a	WH	M	28
G2	51	±	French	—	G2a	Le	M	28
H1	54	—	Jap.	—	H1a		M	44
I1	58	2	Eng.	0	I1a	MA	F	42
I2	59	—	Turk.	0	I2a		M	38
I3	60	8	U. S.	—	I3a	AM	M	47
I4	60	3	U. S.	—	I4a	EH	F	39
J1	61, 62	. —	Pol.	—	J1a	AZ	F	55
J2	61, 62	5	Pol.	—	J2a	MS	F	45
J3	65	—	Czeck.	0	J3a	VK	M	44
K1	67	10 (7)	Yugo.	0	K1a		M	50
					K1b		F	52
					K1c		M	47
K2	69	—	Iraq (Jew)	—	K2a		M	38
K3	70, 96	—	Norw.	—	K3a	EH	M	37
K4	71	—	Germ.	0	K4a	L.Sch.	F	28
K5	73	4	French	—	K5a	GG	F	35
					K5b	Rob.P.	M	29
					K5c	Rog.P.	M	23
K5′	40, 73	11 (8)	French	1	K5′a	FR	F	38
					K5′b	Leon	M	
					K5′c	Lucie	F	
L1	74	5	Belg.	—	L1a	A	M	45
L2	78, 79	7	Danish	—	L2a		F	43
L2′	107	10	Danish	0	L2′a	AF	F	47
					L2′b	AaP	M	42
					L2′c	ARP	M	56
M1	81	5	Austral.	0	M1a	RS	M	38
					M1b	ES	F	39
M2	82	5	U. S.	0	M2a	WG	M	52
M3	84	—	Jap.	—	M3a		F	35
(M4)	84	—	Jap.	—	(M4a)[k]		F	23
M5	86	6	Danish	1.5	M5a		F	34
M6	87	—	French	—	M6a	Marie	F	46
					M6b	Martha	F	42
M7	88	—	Russ.	—	M7a		M	36

Table 2 -- continued

Sibship[a]	Authors	Total Sibs[b]	Nationality	Parental Consanguinity	Case	Initials[d]	Sex	Age[e]
V3	135	—	Germ.	—	V3a	RH	F	37
V4	135	6 (3)	Germ.	—	V4a	LF	M	35
W1	137	5	Germ.	—	W1a	MiK	F	31
					W1b	HK	M	36
					W1c	MK	F	38
					W1d	CK	M	40
W2	139	5	U. S.	0	W2a		M	42
					W2b		F	
					W2c		F	
W3	143	—	Germ.	—	W3a	BS	F	34
W4	144	2 (-)	U. S.	—	W4a		M	44
Z1	145	10 (8)	U. S.	0	Z1a	AGa	M	57
					(Z1b)[i, k]		M	47
					(Z1c)[i, k]			
Z2	145	11 (9)	Ital.	0	Z2a	CC	F	34
					Z2b		F	54
Z3	145	2	U. S.	0	Z3a	EW	F	40
Z4	145	—	U. S.	0	Z4a	RG	F	38
Z5	145	—	U. S. (Jew)	0	Z5a	JB	M	51
(Z6)	145	2 (-)	U. S. (Jew)	(0)	(Z6a)[i, k]		F	50

[a] The symbol *prime* (') indicates a separate but related sibship.

[b] The numbers in parentheses refer to the numbers of sibs used in segregation analyses; these numbers represent the total sibs less those who died young. A dash in the parenthesis indicates that the sibship was not used for analysis because of insufficient data or inclusion after completion of calculations.

[c] Degree of consanguinity: 0, none; +, present, degree unknown; —, no information; ( ), uncertain; 1, first cousins; 1.5 first cousins, once removed; 2, second cousins.

[d] Initials or other identification of cases.

[e] Age at ascertainment.

[f] Jewish.

[g] Parentheses indicate probable cases or sibships.

[h] Incomplete information on signs of Werner's syndrome.

[i] No cataracts.

[j] Caucasian.

[k] No ulcerations.

[l] This report.

[m] Rosen, S., Personal communication.

Graying of the hair, at a mean age of 20 years, is the earliest sign, followed in order by skin changes (25.3 years), loss of hair (25.8 years), alterations of the voice (26.6 years), visual symptoms or detection of cataracts (30.0 years), skin ulcers (33.0 years), and lastly diabetes at a mean age of 34.2 years. It is apparent that the range of the age of appearance of these features is wide, and that this specific order is not necessarily obeyed.

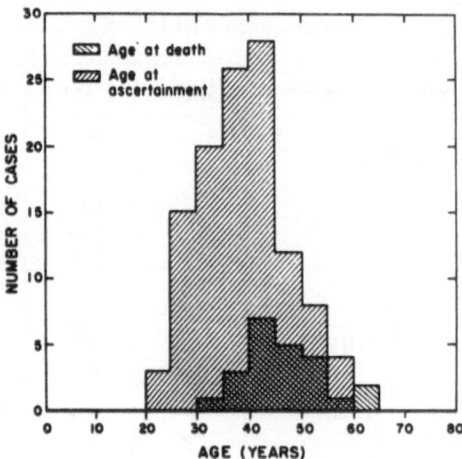

Fig. 5.   Distributions of the ages of ascertainment (diagnosis)
           and death of patients with Werner's syndrome.

This may be due, in part, to the fact that information of this type
is often subjective and retrospective and is subject to error.
However, it probably also indicates that many factors, environmental
or hereditary, in addition to the underlying genetic defect
influence the appearance and progression of the various features of
the syndrome.

B. Symptomatology

1. Growth and Stature

     Shortness of stature, which results from a failure of growth,
is a constant feature in Werner's syndrome. The mean height for
males is 157 cm (5'1") and for females 146 cm (4'9 1/2"), with a
range of 129 to 173 for both sexes. The weights are likewise
decreased, males averaging about 45 kg (99 lb) and females about 40
kg (88 lb); no patient weighed more than 75 kg (165 lb). Many
patients were described as being small as children, and cessation of
growth was noted to occur at ages ranging from 10 to 18 (average 13-
14 years). The extremities of several of these individuals were
noted to be thin even in childhood, but atrophy was not noted in
others until ages as high as 46. A few patients recalled a loss of
weight amounting to as much as 10-15 kg which occurred in the third
and fourth decade. This was sometimes, but not always, related to
the onset of diabetes.

     The general habitus of the patients is characteristic (Fig. 1).
Although the parts of the body are roughly proportional in size, the

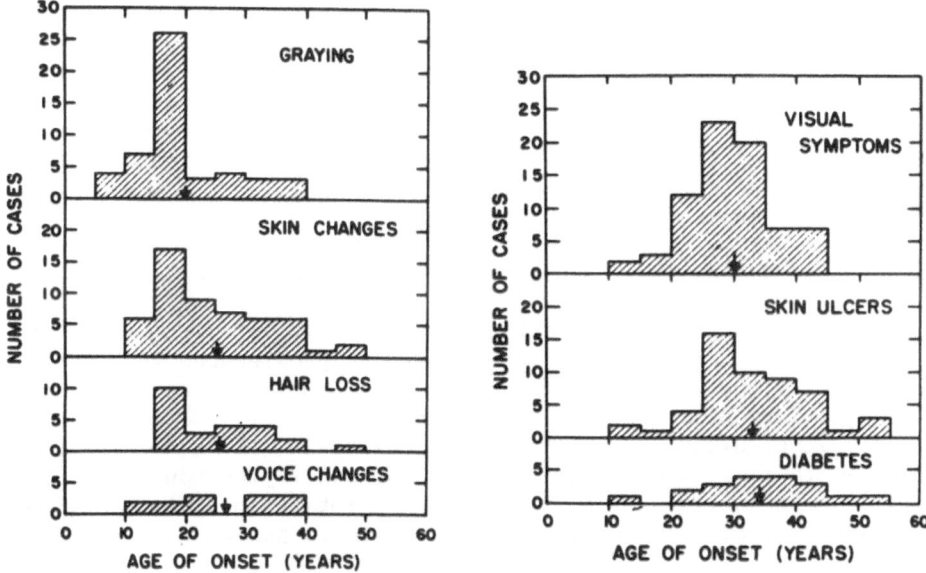

Fig. 6.   Distributions of the ages of onset of the various major
signs and symptoms of Werner's syndrome. The means for
each feature are indicated by arrows.

thinness of the extremities is out of proportion to the moderately
well-developed, sometimes stocky trunk, and the patients are often
underweight relative to their height. The hands and feet are
diminutive, and their smallness, as well as the generally spindly
appearance of the extremities, is accentuated by soft tissue
atrophy. The combination of the habitus with the facies, skin
atrophy, and graying and loss of hair produces an impression of
senility or premature aging, and these individuals are often
described as looking 20-30 years older than their age.

2.   Skin

Thannhauser (131) was the first clearly to differentiate the
skin changes in Werner's syndrome from those of Rothmund's
syndrome and of scleroderma. He pointed out that atrophy of the
skin over areas in which the subcutaneous adipose tissue is
depleted results in a shiny, smooth skin which cannot be lifted up
from or is actually adherent to the underlying tissue. The
principal areas of skin involvement are the face and distal
extremities, especially the feet. In addition, there is atrophy of
the underlying connective tissue, musculature, and fat.

The involvement of the face usually produces a thinning and sharpening of the nose, giving it a "pinched" or "beaked" appearance. Sometimes, the skin around the mouth is radially ridged but fixation of the mouth as seen in scleroderma does not occur. There may be loss of circumorbital tissue, making the eyes appear protuberant and staring (a pseudo-exophthalmos). Not infrequently, the skin of the ears is also atrophic and tight. The sum of the facial features produces the effect of a "bird-like" visage, although other terms, such as "moon-like" (referring to relative fullness of the cheeks) and "mask-like," have also been applied.

An early but prominent feature of the skin involvement is the development of hyperkeratoses over the bony prominences and on the soles of the feet. The hyperkeratoses frequently become ulcerated, producing large indolent lesions which heal poorly and tend to recur. These ulcers commonly overlie the heels, toes, malleoli, and Achilles tendons, and often extend to the underlying bones and joints. The combination of skin atrophy, ankylosis or bone destruction, and ulceration may produce severe pain and difficulty in walking.

While the skin changes discussed above are restricted to specific parts of the body, more widespread alterations are also present. In addition to areas of localized hyper- or depigmentation in the extremities, a generalized hyperpigmenta-tion, both of a diffuse nature and in the form of freckles or lentigenes, has often been noted. Moreover, the body skin is frequently described as thin and dry, and telangiectases are sometimes recorded.

3. Eyes

The cataracts that are a cardinal feature of Werner's syndrome have been variously described as juvenile, diabetic, endocrine, tetanic, complicated, and rarely, embryonal. The pathologic process is usually one of posterior cortical and subcapsular opacities, generally striate or homogeneous in nature. The presence of vacuoles and punctate opacities and involvement of other parts of the lens, including, but only occasionally, the nucleus, have also been described.

Of the lens changes found in aged individuals, only nuclear sclerosis is considered to be the result of the "normal" processes of aging (47, 76). Other changes, referred to as "senile" cataracts, are of unknown etiology but are considered to be pathologic (33). In many instances the cataracts described in patients with Werner's syndrome are indistinguishable from the "pathologic" cataracts of aging. However, in other cases the descriptions do not fit into this category, and it would appear that, as a group, the cataracts of Werner's syndrome are different from those associated with "normal" aging.

The eye disease in Werner's syndrome is nearly always bilateral, although the process may be at different stages in the two eyes. Once opacities do appear, maturation of the catarcts seems to be rapid. The response to surgery is usually good, but keratopathy, other corneal changes, and glaucoma occur not infrequently and may cause persistent difficulty with vision or even lead to loss of an eye.

Several ocular abnormalities, other than cataracts, have also been found. Retinis pigmentosa has been described in two unrelated oriental Jews (K2a, V1a). Blue sclerae (A1a, O1b), telangiectasia of the iris (T1a), and vitreous opacities have also been noted. Two sibs (B6'a, B6'b) were found to have retinal diseases (a healed chorioretinitis and a macular degeneration) which were probably unrelated to Werner's syndrome.

4. Hair

Among the earliest of the characteristic signs in Werner's syndrome are the loss and graying of the hair. The graying process, which generally begins with the hair of the scalp and the eyebrows, often extends to the point of complete whiteness and may require from 5 to 20 years for maximal loss of color.

The loss of hair is generalized. It is most commonly described as occurring in the scalp, eyebrows, and eyelashes, but body hair is also decreased. Loss of axillary and pubic hair is common as is a decrease in facial hair in males. It is not clear, however, whether these changes are part of the overall alopecia or whether they are, in many cases, more directly related to hypogonadism.

5. Voice and Vocal Cords

Almost half of the patients had an abnormally thin, high-pitched, or hoarse voice and only five patients were specifically said to have normal voices. The onset of the changes in speech ranged from early childhood (i.e. "always" abnormal) to the middle of the fourth decade.

Examinations of the larynx and vocal cords by direct or indirect laryngoscopy was performed in about one-quarter of the cases. The findings were normal in half of these (6 of whom had abnormalities of phonation). In the others, there were atrophy, dilated or prominent superficial vessels on or adjacent to the cords, and/or poor movement or faulty approximation of the cords.

6. Muscle

    Although profound wasting of the musculature of the legs,
feet, and hands has long been recognized as part of Werner's
syndrome, little investigation of this tissue has taken place.
Electromyography has been carried out in only three patients: one
(F3a) had greatly reduced action potentials in the legs, while two
others (M8a, S2a) were essentially normal. Of various chemical
tests related to muscle function and disease, measurements of serum
enzymes (LDH, SGOT, aldolase) did not suggest any acute dystrophic
process, although the loss of muscle mass was reflected in a high
urinary creatine/creatinine ratio.

7. Osteoporosis, Calcium Metabolism, and Soft Tissue
Calcification

    Osteoporosis of either a generalized or patchy nature was
observed radiologically in at least half of the cases. It was found
most frequently to affect the feet, ankles, and lower legs, less
often the hands, forearms, and the spine, and almost never the
skull. Deformities of the feet, often with joint destruction, were
frequently seen. Osteoarthritis of the peripheral joints
(Heberden's nodes) and spondylitis deformans were also observed (64)
but frank vertebral collapse was noted only once (M2a).

    Jacobson et al. (64), in a discussion of the radiological
features of Werner's syndrome, commented on neurotrophic bone
changes in the feet, the feet, with "spindling," thinning, and
narrowing of the terminal tufts of the phalanges. They also noted
lesions with destructuve changes of the bones that were or closely
resembled those of osteomyelitis, and felt that these lesions were
related anatomically and perhaps causally to metastatic
calcifications and ulcerations.

    Because of the frequency of osteoporosis and of soft tissue and
vascular calcification, a disturbance in calcium metabolism was, for
a while, felt to be a significant factor in the pathogenesis of
Werner's syndrome. However, the levels of serum calcium,
phosphorus, and alkaline and acid phosphatases were rarely abnormal.
Calcium balance studies showed a negative balance in two patients
(B10a, O1b) and negative but probably normal or positive balance in
four others (I3a,I4a,O1a,Z5a). One other case (L1a) was described
as having transient hypocalcemia with tetany that responded to
parathormone and remitted spontaneously. The blood parathormone
level, as assayed by the unreliable Hamilton-Schwartz assay, was
normal in O1a and elevated in A1a and O1b (142).

    Soft tissue calcification was observed in about one-third of
the patients. The major areas of involvement were the tendons and
ligaments of the knee, elbow, and ankle joints, and the tissues

immediately adjacent to these areas. The soft tissues of the feet
and sometimes of the hands were also frequently involved.
Occasionally the skin (R3a), the conjunctivae (B10a), the
diaphragmatic pleura (D4a) or the falx cerebri (B4a) contained areas
of calcification.

8.   Cardiovascular System: A prominent feature of Werner's
syndrome is the severe, often generalized, vascular disease found in
many of the patients. Vascular calcification of the Moenckeberg
type was noted radiologically in at least 31 patients, with the
vessels of the legs most frequently involved. However,
calcification of most of the other major vessels has also been
noted. Aortic calcification was observed radiologically in 14
patients, but in only 4 was the root or ascending aorta specifically
mentioned as being involved.

The clinical manifestations of the peripheral vascular disease
range from diminished or absent pulses (by palpation or
oscillometry) to severe vascular insufficiency resulting in
gangrene. The latter, although not common, has frequently
necessitated amputation. It is not possible from the clinical
reports to distinguish between necrosis resulting from vascular
disease and that due solely to the atrophy of the skin and the
attendant ulcerations (if, indeed, the two processes are
distinguishable). Sympathectomy has occasionaly been employed, but
without demonstrable benefit.

Clinical evidence of coronary artery disease is common and is
of several types: abnormal electrocardiograms, congestive heart
failure, coronary artery calcifications by x-ray, and frank coronary
pain and infarction. Calcifications of the rings or cusps of the
mitral and/or aortic valves were frequently detectable
radiographically (64).

Reproductive organs - Male

The size of the external genitalia is described for 54 of the
65 males with Werner's syndrome, and of these, only two (M7a, Z5a)
were reported as having normal genitalia. Most of the men had small
testes and a small penis, with the testes often likened in size to
those of 10-13 year-old boys. In several instances the prostate was
small, but in one case (B10a) large seminal vesicles, claimed to
have been detected by rectal palpation, were described. Many of the
patients had diminution in the amount of pubic hair and at least 11
had the female type of pubic hair distribution. Gynecomastia was
noted in eight cases, most of whom also had small genitalia. The
status of patients' libido and potency was described in only a few
instances: four of nine had diminished potency and eight of ten had
a diminution in libido starting at an age between 27 and 38 years.

In some patients libido and potency were never great. The time of puberty was only stated a few times, and was given as 15-16 years.

Eleven men fathered a total of 19 children, and at least seven of these men had small genitalia at the time of examination. The ability to have children did not appear to be related to the time of onset of the general symptoms of the disease.

Measurements of the urinary excretion of pituitary gonadotropins or of FSH were made in ten individuals, all with small genitalia: in two (B10a, C3a) the values were high, in five (I3a, O2a, R3a, S6a, V1a) normal, and in two (B7a, T2b) low. One patient (D4a) had high levels which later declined to normal. Estrogen levels in the urine were measured in three patients and were found to be normal in two (I3a, O2a) and possible slightly elevated in a third (R3a). "Androgenic" activity in the urine of one of the patients (O2a) was low. The semen of one patient (K1a) was low in volume and in sperm count and mobility. That of another (R3a), whose testicular biopsy showed early tubular hyalinization, had a reduced sperm count -- 13 x 10^6/ml (57).

The levels for 24 hour excretion of urinary 17-ketosteroids were determined in many instances and when plotted as a function of age are generally in the low to low normal range. In two instances the 17-ketosteroid were fractionated. In one (F3a), the 17-ketosteroid value was normal, but the dehydroisoandrosterone level was suggestive of gonadal failure. In the other case (K1a), the total 17-ketosteroid excretion was low, and fractions attributed to both adrenal and sex hormones were diminished. The authors concluded that the results were compatible with adrenal hypofunction.

One patient (C3a) was treated with "hormones" for six months after a diagnosis of hypopituitarism was made. This regimen did not produce any alteration in the size of the small genitalia. Except for increased libido in one (D4a), two other patients (D4a, S10a) have also been reported as not responding to therapy with testosterone.

Hypogonadism may be divided into two categories: hypergonadotropic and hypogonadotropic (72, 97). In the former category are included those conditions in which there is presumed to be a primary defect in testicular function (e.g. Klinefelter's syndrome, castration or testicular injury, Leydig cell "failure," seminiferous tubule "failure," and myotonic dystrophy). Hypogonadotrophic hypogonadism on the other hand, is generally related to pituitary failure. Although the resemblance to hypergonadotrophic hypogonadism is perhaps greater, it is impossible to definitely assign the "hypogonadism" in males with Werner's syndrome to either category. However, the fact that many affected

men probably do not ever develop normal secondary sexual
characteristics indicates that the "hypogonadism" may begin as early
as the first decade, although many patients do have children and do
not experience loss of libido or potency until later in life.

10. Reproductive Organs – Females

Many of the 60 women with Werner's syndrome were desribed as
having poorly developed genitalia. Specific information was given
on 21 women, and of them only 2 (S3b, Z3a) were desribed as having
normal genitalia. The remainder had infantile or atrophic external
genitalia and in a few instances, the uterus was found to be small.
Breast development was commented on in 25 cases; over half had
small, atrophic, or underdeveloped breasts while the breasts of
others were described as "well-developed" (although varying in size
from small to large). Although it is rarely explicitly stated in
the case reports, it would appear that many of the women failed to
develop normal secondary sex characteristics.

In 35 instances the age of onset of the menses was recorded
and ranged between 9 and 20 years, the average being 13.9 years.
At least one patient (M8b) never menstruated. The menstrual
periods were frequently sparse and irregular, and 26 women ceased
menstruating at ages ranging from 18 to 45 years (mean 33 years).
However, menopausal symptoms were mentioned only twice (K5a, M8a).
In a few cases the patient's libido was either normal or
diminished.

At least 16 of the women never married, and the number is
probably considerably greater. Nevertheless, 19 women did have a
total of at least 53 recorded pregnancies, and 10 gave birth to 30
children who survived the perinatal period. The other 23 known
pregnancies ended either in abortions, stillbirths, premature
deliveries, or deaths at delivery. Two cases, B6a and I4a, are of
unusual interest since they had a total of six and nine children
respectively. Except for absence of ulcerations, they had all of
the stigmata of Werner's syndrome, and there is no reason to
question the diagnosis. The earliest symptoms of one were observed
at the age of 34, although growth had ceased at age 13; the other's
symptoms had begun at age 11.

The urinary excretion of gonadotropins of FSH was normal in
seven women, three of whom were no longer having menstrual periods
and might therefore have been expected to have elevated levels. An
elevated level was found in an amenorrheic woman (I1a) and a low
level of FSH was found in another (D1a) who was still menstruating.
Estrogen assays were performed in seven women and two of them, one
the woman with six children (I4a), had definitely low levels.

As in the case of male hypogonadism, it is not possible to
assign the hypogonadism in affected females to a definite category
(77). Moreover, the facts that patients usually menstruate
regularly for a period of at least a few years and that some do
have children indicates that hypogonadism is not always present.
Thus, whatever degree of hypogonadism does exist probably develops
during the course of the disease and not to the same degree or at
the same rate in all patients.

11. Diabetes Mellitus

Diabetes has been recognized in 55 of the 125 definite cases
(44.4%) under discussion. Of these, 28 were males and 27 females.
Diabetes was tested for but not found in 21 patients ranging in age
from 28-56 years. In only five cases (E2b, F2a, M1b, O1b, R2a)
were significant symptoms of polyuria, polydipsia, pruitus, and
weight loss present, and in only two was "diabetic coma" (M8b, O1b)
recorded; the former allegedly died in a coma, but this finding
could not be confirmed.

Many patients had normal blood sugar levels, but diabetic
glucose tolerance tests were observed following oral or intravenous
administration of glucose. On several occasions, the fall in blood
sugar was very slow and plateaued at levels as high as 300-400
mg/100 ml, sometimes lasting for several hours. In general the
patients were managed by dietary restriction of calories. Insulin,
given in amounts ranging from 15 to 100 units daily, was often
ineffective in controlling the hyperglycemia or even in producing a
significant fall in blood sugar. Despite this general
unresponsiveness to insulin, the diabetes was usually mild, and
ketonuria was not observed even with massive glycosuria. Except
for one report of diabetic retinopathy (M1b) and one of
Kimmelstiel-Wilson lesions in the kidney (R2a), the usual
complications of diabetes (nephropathy, retinopathy, and
neuropathy) have not been demonstrated. Furthermore, the vascular
disease and the diabetes are not well correlated with one another.

In two cases reported by Field and Loube (F2a, F3a) (38)
significant decreases in blood sugar occurred after the ingestion
of 1 to 4 grams of tolbutamide. Both patients responded to
intravenous insulin, 0.1 u/kg with slow falls to about 50% of the
fasting blood sugar level.

In only one case prior to the present report were serum
insulin levels determined. Daweke et al (29) measured serum
insulin-like activity (ILA) using the epididymal fat pad method and
found that the fasting ILA level was "358% of normal" and that the
"insulinogenic reserve," during a glucose tolerance test, was only
17.2% of normal. In two separate oral glucose tolerance tests, the

ILA either peaked at 30 minutes and then remained elevated for the next 2 1/2 hours, or it rose slowly throughout the entire duration of the test (3 hours).

Both Field and Loube (38), and Daweke et al (29) interpreted their results as indicating a defect in the utilization of carbohydrate, probably related to deficiencey of muscular and adipose tissue. They likened the diabetes of Werner's syndrome to lipoatrophic diabetes. However, as Field and Loube mentioned, and has already been discussed above in relation to the investigation of carbohydrate metabolism in case M8a (case 1 of the present report), all findings are compatible with the "late-onset" type of diabetes such as is commonly seen in post-menopausal females, and do not suggest that the diabetes of the Werner syndrome is, in any way, special. Karem et al (68) have recently suggested that the prolonged insulin response to glucose could be the result of a peripheral antagonism to insulin activity, but no studies have, as yet, been made in Werner's syndrome of serum insulin antagonists or of bound and free forms of insulin.

In view of the controversy about the etiology and mode of inheritance of diabetes mellitus (120), the occurrence of diabetes in a genetically well-defined disease such as Werner's syndrome is especially interesting. Its frequent occurrence indicates that it must be considered an intrinsic part of the syndrome and that a predisposition to develop "late onset" diabetes may be inherited in an autosomal recessive manner in this syndrome. Its failure to appear in all of the cases suggests (as was mentioned above with reference to the chronology of Werner's syndrome) that other factors, both external and internal, are probably also involved in its pathogenesis.

12. Fat Metabolism

Serum cholesterol levels generally ranged between 150 and 300 mg/100 ml. Measurements of various other serum lipid components were carried out in a few patients, usually with normal results in one (I3a), a reduced level of high density lipoproteins in one (R3a) and elevated mal results in one (I3a), a reduced level of high-density lipoproteins in three others (Dla, F2a, I4a). One of the latter patients (F2a) was diabetic and had elevated levels of total and free cholesterol, phospholipids, and triglycerides. Another (Dla), who was also diabetic, had elevated levels of total and polyunsaturated fatty acids, cholesterol, and phosphatides, even after restriction of fat intake, and an oral fat tolerance and heparin clearance test was interpreted as showing delayed absorption from the gut and a poor response to heparin. The authors (29) suggested that there is a defect in endogenous fat utilization specifically related to the lack of adipose tissue in Werner's syndrome, but similar aberrations in lipid levels were not found in

all cases investigated. Furthermore, the marked diminution in
total fat stores sometimes observed is by no means a universal
finding.

13. Adrenal Cotrex

Because several features of Werner's syndrome are similar to
manifestations of adrenal hyperactivity (wasting of extremities
with loss of fat and muscle; relatively mild, insulin insensitive
diabetes; osteoporosis; alopecia; atherosclerosis and hypertension;
and, in children, retardation of growth) (12, 43, 83), Bauer and
Conn (6) suggested that a defect in the inactivation of
glucocorticoids might be present. On the basis of their
investigations, they postulated an impairment in the metabolism of
11-desoxycortisol and, by inference, of other glucocorticoids,
producing a state of chronic, though mild, hyperadrenalism.

The conclusions were later disputed by Boyd and Grant (15)
whose findings, however, were similar. They felt that the data
were more compatible with hypopituitarism and secondary
hypoadrenalism than with hyperadrenalism. The detailed
investigation of the adrenal-pituitary axis undertaken in the study
of case M8a has already been discussed and did not show evidence of
a disturbance of adrenal function or of the pituitary production of
ACTH. Furthermore, in opposition to the results of Bauer and Conn,
the disappearance of 11-desoxycortisol was, if anything, more rapid
than normal. ACTH tests alone were carried out in three other
cases (D1a, D4a, I1a) and again the responses did not indicate
adrenal aberrations.

The low to low normal excretion of 17-ketosteroids by males
has already been mentioned. The values of excretion by females
were generally in the normal range, although occasional low values
were observed. Measurements of 17-hydroxysteroid excretions were
performed in but a few instances and were normal, in both sexes, in
all but one individual (in whom the levels were low).

14. Thyroid

Investigation of thyroid activity had been carried out in many
patients, and the results were generally within the normal range.
In most cases, the basal metabolic rate ranged from -20 to +20%,
with the average in the range of 0 to +5%. The average value of
the serum protein-bound iodine was 5.6 with only two patients (K4a,
V1a) having subnormal levels. Likewise, measurements of the uptake
of radioactive iodine by the thyroid were usually found to be
normal.

One patient (J2a) had "exophthalmos", a basal metabolic rate
of +67% and was thought to be hyperthryoid.

15. Pituitary

Investigations of specific aspects of pituitary function have been discussed under the headings of the various end organs. To summarize briefly, there is as yet no evidence of either generalized hypopituitarism or of over- or under-activity of any specific component system. Nevertheless, Werner's syndrome does, to some extent, approximate acquired hypopituitarism as exemplified by the Sheehan's and posthypophysectomy syndromes (28). In these syndromes, atrophy of the genitalia and diminution of libido and potency occur without (in females) menopausal symptoms. There is also a generalized loss of body, axillary, and pubic hair. However, in panhypopituitarism there is the gradual development of hypothyroidism, adrenal insufficiency, a decrease in melanin pigmentation, low blood glucose levels, and a difficulty in excreting water (post-hypophysectomy). None of these are features of Werner's syndrome. In Sheehan's syndrome, the skin may appear waxy and the patient may appear prematurely aged.

So far, nothing is known about the secretion, metabolism, or action of growth hormone in patients with Werner's syndrome. This would be of considerable interest since the growth spurt, which is usually attributed to the activity of growth hormone and/or adrenal androgens (129, 140), usually fails to occur.

Examinations of the sella turcica by X-ray have not revealed any consistent changes, although small ones were occasionally seen. Hyperostosis frontalis interna was noted in 6 cases.

16. Kidney Function and Blood Pressure

In general, no evidence of gross impairment of renal function was found by measurements of phenolsulfonthalein (PSP) excretion, blood urea nitrogen, or creatinine clearance. However, occasional patients did have poor function, and one with widespread vascular disease (Vla) died in uremia.

Blood pressure measurements are difficult to interpret because of the severe muscular wasting exhibited by many of the patients. However, values are given for about half of the patients listed, and of these, approximately 45% had systolic pressures of 150 mm Hg or greater. At least nine patients had significant elevations of both systolic (>150 mm Hg) and diastolic (>100 mm Hg) pressures, and all but one was 41 years of age or younger. It would appear, therefore, that systolic hypertension, possibly the result of the "stiff" sclerotic vessels, is common and that "true" hypertension is also significantly increased. The basis of the latter has not been clearly delineated.

17. Gastrointestinal Tract

   Liver function tests performed in several patients did not
suggest hepatic dysfunction. Likewise, investigations of the
esophagus, stomach and small intestine by x-ray were usually normal,
though "scleroderma-like" changes of the esophagus of one patient
(B6b) were described.

18. Neurologic and Psychiatric Status

   Reports of neurologic examinations are available on about 25%
of the patients with Werner's syndrome. Approximately 1/3 of these
had mild defects, predominantly involving loss of distal deep tendon
reflexes; paresthesias were reported in one patient (L2a). As will
be discussed below, meningiomas were found in three others.

   Intelligence is commented on 19 cases, and 9 of these were
regarded as retarded. Moreover, several other patients were felt to
be normal in intelligence, but to be "infantile" emotionally. The
meaning of a diagnosis of infantilism is difficult to interpret. It
may be related to the fact that because of the small stature the
overall physical impression is often one of infantilism (as well as
a premature senility). Two patients (F6a, Plc) were psychotic.

19. Hematopoietic and Lymphoid Systems

   Measurements of red cell volume and hemoglobin, of white cell
numbers and differential counts, and bone marrow examinations did
not, in general, indicate any difficulty with hemato- or
leucopoiesis. Ferrokinetic measurements in our patient, M8a, were
normal. Likewise, serum electrophoretic patterns were unremarkable
except for an increase, probably attributable to chronically
infected ulcers, in the gamma-globulin fraction.

20. Serum and Urine Constituents

   Serum electrolytes and uric acid levels were usually normal,
although occasionally elevated uric acids were noted.
Determinations of such serum components as magnesium, various
enzymes (including glutamic-oxalacetic and pyruvic transaminases,
lactate dehydrogenase, aldolase, amylase), mucoproteins, and
clotting factors did not reveal significant abnormalities.

   Analysis of the excretions of urinary amino acids have been
performed on eight patients: of these, six were normal (B5a, D4a,
M8a, Pla, Pl'a), one showed aspartic aciduria (E2a) and one had an
elevated excretion of taurine (B7a). The most probably explanation
of the latter finding is the fact that the patient was receiving
ACTH, a substance known to increase taurine excretion (99), at the
time of the urine collection.

21. Neoplasia

It has long been felt that the occurence of tumors is increased in Werner's syndrome, but the striking preponderance of non-carcinomatous neoplasms has not been fully emphasized. Seven patients, with ages ranging from 35-47 had malignant tumors which were sarcomatous in nature: fibroliposarcoma (Ala), osteogenic sarcoma (B6b), sarcoma of nerve sheath origin (B6'b); melanotic sarcoma (E2b), hemanogiolipoma with occasional mitosis (Ila), spindle cell sarcoma (Mlb), and uterine myosarcoma (M9b). Meningiomas were found in three patients (M5a, R2a, Z5a), and carcinomas in four: adenocarcinoma of hepatic duct origin (Olb), carcinoma of the liver (R2a), carcinoma of the breast (S3b), and papillary adenocarcinoma of the thyroid (V1a). In six of these cases, death was directly attributable to the tumors (Ala, B6b, B6'b, E2b, Olb, R2a). "Adenomas" of the thyroid or adrenals were also noted in several patients, and a large uterine myoma in one (F2a). Including these, significant tumors, predominantly of connective tissue or mesenchymal derivation were found in 13 of the 125 patients (10%), and one of the patients (R2a) had two.

Despite the chronic ulcerations and atrophic changes of the skin, skin cancer, a neoplasm common in aged skin, has never been reported in a patient with Werner's syndrome.

22. Attempts at Therapy

Most therapy in this disease has been directed toward specific management of the cataracts, the skin lesions, and the diabetes. More general treatment has usually not be employed, although various preparations were tried. A few patients were reported as showing subjective improvement or softening of the skin (W3a). Other remedies said to lead to improvement were intravenous Koch's salts, intramuscular novocaine (C2a), subcutaneous oxygen (J3a), and a combination of isonicotinic acid hydrazide, testosterone proprionate, calciferol, and cortisone (B3a).

23. Death

Data relating to the age and cause of death was available on only 23 of the cases. The ages of death varied from 31 to 63, the average being 47 years (Fig. 5). The two principal causes of death were malignancies and vascular accidents (myocardial and cerebrovascular), claiming six and three individuals respectively. Other causes were "diabetes," "liver trouble," anemia, and "cachexia, edema, and anemia."

IV. PATHOLOGIC ANATOMY

In addition to the biopsy material from our own case, M8a, we were able, through the cooperation of several physicians, to obtain the original microscopic slides or tissue blocks (from which new slides were prepared) of eight definite and one probable case (Table 3). All sections were stained with hematoxylin and eosin. Autopsy protocols, either complete or in abstract form, were available for an additional four patients, and histological descriptions of specific tissue biopsies were available for several more.

A summary of the pathologic findings in several cases which were studied at the Montefiore Hospital in New York has already appeared in the paper by Jacobson et al (64) and further studies (including pathologic observations) by the same group are soon to be reported (145). These authors pointed out the high incidence of generalized vascular disease and valvular calcification, of neoplastic disease and of testicular atrophy in the patients with Werner's syndrome.

1. Skin and Subcutaneous Tissue

Review of sections of the skin and subcutaneous tissue from various sites revealed the following salient features.

Table 3: Sources of material for review of the pathology of Werner's syndrome [a]

Case	Sex	Age	Hospital	Hospital Number	Autopsy Number	Biopsy Number	Type of Material[b]	References
A1a	M	43	Montefiore, N. Y.	30303	9004		S, R	95, 145
B6a	M	49	Georgetown Univ., Wash. D. C.		55A309		S, R	100
B6b	F	49	" "				R	82
B7a	M	62	Belfast City		57-4429		P, S, R	15
F2a	F	26	Sibley, Wash. D. C.			28972	P	
M8a	F	47	Univ. Washington	077-54		S-640174	P, S, R	
O1a	M	50	Montefiore, N. Y.	22676	9041		S, R	95, 145
O1b	M	42	" "	2080212	8213		P, S, R	145
R2a	F	42	Memorial, Hollywood, Florida		A-57-94		P	105
R3a	M	42	National Institutes of Health	04-31-78		S63-402 S63-418	S	
V1a	M	39	Rambam, Haifa		G-85-58		R	133
Z1a	M	59	Montefiore, N. Y.	90039	15376	553851	P, S, R	145
Z5a	M	54	" "	67706			R	145
[Z6a]	F	53	" "	50241	13329	545033	P, S, R	145

[a] Does not include descriptions of biopsies contained within case reports.
[b] P = autopsy or surgical protocol, S = slides (microscopic), R = references.

There was atrophy of subcutaneous fat (Fig. 7, see appendix II), the earliest indication being the disappearance of the normal finger-like "extensions" of areolar connective tissue into the dermis where they characteristically encircle skin appendages.

The skin appendages and epidermis were atrophic, and although loss of appendages was never complete, hair follicles and sebaceous glands were probably less in evidence than sweat or apocrine glands (Fig. 7). The epidermis was reduced to a thickness of two or three cell layers in some areas (Fig. 8), and the rete pegs were rarely conspicuous. However, there was frequently mild or diffuse hyperkeratosis, although on occasion this was found to be sharply focal (Fig. 8). The basal layer of the epidermis was generally focally hypermelanotic (Fig. 8) and, in one case ([Z6a]) melanin pigment was present within the more superficial layers of the epidermis. Focal lymphocytic infiltrates were occasionally observed in the dermis and subcutaneous tissues, often in relation to small blood vessels or skin appendages.

Dermal fibrosis (Fig. 7) tended to be variable and ranged from mild sub-epidermal hyalinization to a striking scleroderma-like picture ([Z6a]). Fibrosis or sclerosis of small blood vessels in the skin and subcutaneous tissues, even in severely affected areas, was not impressive. Wound repair following the biopsy of skin and muscle of our patient (M8a) was excellent, with the formation of a fine scar.

In general, these findings are consistent with the histological descriptions given in the literature, with the following additions or exceptions: the dermal collagen has been variously described as hyalinized, thickened, frayed, or disorganized, and the elastic tissue as either normal or decreased in amount. Descriptions of the dermal blood vessels have also been contradictory. In several instances they were normal, but abnormalities such as obliterative endarteritis (F3a) and thickened walls (R1a, S2a, T4a) have been observed.

One electron microscopic investigation has been carried out (R1a), and the collagen fibrils were found to be coated with amorphous debris which could be removed by treatment with trypsin; the underlying fibrils appeared to be normal. It has been suggested that the debris represents deposits of calcium (122), probably in a protein matrix, and interstitial calcification has also been observed by light microscopy (B3a).

2. Muscle

The most consistent histological finding in the sections reviewed was the relative scarcity of associated areolar connective tissue. One specimen (M8a) showed evidence of arteriosclerosis.

Of the cases reported in the literature, the muscle from four (S2a, S5a, T2a, T2b) were reported as normal, while two others (B6a, F3a) showed an increase in connective tissue with abnormalities in the muscle fibers (swelling, loss of striations, irregularity in size and shape).

3. Respiratory

Three patients had evidence of pulmonary emphysema at autopsy. In several patients there was a terminal pneumonitis and/or chronic passive congestion of the lungs, and squamous metaplasia was occasionally noted in the bronchial mucosa. Sections from the larynx in three cases (Fig. 9, see appendix II) showed evidence of focal squamous metaplasia (O1a, [Z6a]), marked hyperplasia of seromucous glands, submucosal fibrosis and chronic inflammation (O1a, Z1a, [Z6a]), atrophy of skeletal muscle (all three), bony metaplasia of cartilage with extramedullary hematopoiesis (Z1a), and sub- and intramucosal telangiectasia.

4. Cardiovascular

All of the autopsy material that we examined revealed arteriosclerosis of a severity not regularly encountered in this age group. There were no morphologically unique aspects of any of these lesions. Atherosclerosis was the principal variety and had the typical distribution including involvement of coronary arteries with myocardial infarction (4 patients) and/or interstitial fibrosis (3 patients). Monckeberg's sclerosis (medial calcinosis) was also observed (O1b, Z1a, [Z6a]), and hyaline arteriosclerosis was found frequently, but not regularly. Perhaps the most striking of the cardiovascular lesions was the severe calcification of the aortic and/or mitral valve leaflets and rings (Fig. 10, see appendix II). Sections from the valve rings (O1b, Z1a, [Z6a]) showed a remarkably similar picture of extensive replacement of the tissues with masses of calcium. In one case (Z1a) there was bony metaplasia of the mitral valve ring, with focal extra-medullary hematopoiesis. All patients had some type of valvular pathology, and three patients had extensive involvement of both aortic and mitral valves. The myocardium showed varying degrees of hypertrophy, atrophy, and fibrosis, but lipofuscin pigment was not unusually abundant.

5. Genito-Urinary

Male reproductive organs: Perhaps the most striking pathologic feature of Werner's syndrome involved the testes (Fig. 11, see appendix II).

All of the male patients for whom histologic sections or descriptions were available had evidence of moderate to severe testicular atrophy. Many (B6a, V1a) to virtually all (B7a) seminiferous tubules were completely hyalinized and devoid of spermatogenic activity. Only in case (B6a) could moderate numbers of mature spermatozoa be found.

The slides from these patients with Werner's syndrome were compared with a group of 13 control autopsy sections from the atrophic testes of aged men in their 7th, 8th and 9th decades, and except for the fact that the lesions in the senile group were generally less severe, they could not be differentiated from each other. The type of tubular hyalinization was identical: the distorted, variably shrunken tubules had walls which were greatly thickened by pale eosinophilic homogeneous material. Furthermore, the general frequency of Leydig cells was the same for the two groups, although in view of the variation of the quality of fixation and staining, it was difficult to perform accurate counts of these cells. Lipochrome pigment was not conspicuous in these cells.

There was evidence of some degree of prostatic epithelial atrophy in at least five patients (Ala, B6a, B7a, Ola, Olb), and none of the patients had benign prostatic hypertrophy. The epithelium of the epididymis was well preserved in one case (Olb) but moderately atrophic in another (Ola).

Female reproductive organs: Pathological examination of the ovary was performed in one autopsy ([Z6a]), and it was described as atrophic. An ovarian cyst was surgically removed from another patient (K4a), following which a cyst developed in the other ovary. At the time of resection of the first cyst, the remaining ovarian tissue was described as showing macroscopic cystic degeneration, and the uterus was said to be the size of a "pigeon's egg." Two years of cyclic hormone therapy did not restore normal menstruation. A third patient (F2a) had a supracervical hysterectomy and a right salpingo-oophorectomy performed at age 26, one year after a miscarriage at 6 1/2 months gestation. The histologic sections were not available for review, but the surgical pathology protocol described a normal sized uterus with an atrophic endometrium, fibrosis of the myometrium, and large fundal fibroids with interstitial hemorrhage. The ovary was normal in size with a narrow tunica albuginea, loose fibrotic cortex, and a large corpus luteum cyst.

Renal: A review of the available histologic material revealed varying degrees of hyaline arteriolosclerosis and arteriosclerosis. There were also interstitial fibrosis, patchy hyalinization of glomeruli, occasional calcified tubules, and mild chronic pyelonephritis. Kimmelstiel-Wilson glomerular lesions were described in R2a, but "wire loop" lesions were never seen in any case.

6. Endocrine Glands

Adrenals: There was a variability in size, from atrophy to adenomatous hyperplasia. The glomerulosa zone was more or less conspicuous (sometimes focally) in at least five cases (Ala, B6a, B7a, Ola, Olb), being most conspicuous in Olb (Fig. 12, see appendix II). Small clusters of plasma cells and/or lymphocytes were noted within the cortices of three cases (Ala, Ola, [Z6a]), and in two the glands were involved by malignant tumors originating in other sites.

No abnormalities of the adrenal medulla were noted.

Thyroid: At autopsy there was evidence of some degree of atrophy in the three cases (Olb, Zla, [Z6a]) in which gross weights were available. The histology usually showed interstitial fibrosis and an epithelium which was flat to cuboidal.

Parathyroid: Our review of the parathyroid histology in four cases (Ala, B6a, B7a, Ola) showed a predominance of chief cells in all; aggregates of water clear cells were present in one (Ola). Oxyphil cells were not abundant.

Pituitary: With the exception of case B6a, there has been no careful histologic study of the pituitary. In this case, normal differential counts were reported for the anterior lobe. However, since the extent of sampling was not stated, it is difficult to evaluate the results. A pinhead chromophobe adenoma was found in an apparently normal-sized pituitary in Vla, and small cysts of the anterior lobe were noted in two cases. Of possible interest was an "invasion" of the posterior lobe by acidophiles and chromophobes in two cases (Ala, B7a); more commonly, basophiles are found to infiltrate into the contiguous posterior lobe.

7. Gastrointestinal

Various changes in the liver were noted, but none appeared characteristic of Werner's syndrome. The amount of lipochrome pigment was variable, but never unusually abundant. An unidentified, slightly refractile, non-birefringent pale grey-brown pigment was noted in the Kupfer cells in Olb.

In case M8a, biopsies of the small bowel and stomach (Dr. C.E. Rubin) were normal. The histologic sampling of esophagus, stomach, and intestine of available necropsy material was not adequate for a coherent evaluation. However, further evidence against the interpretation of the skin pathology as manifestations of scleroderma is the fact that involvement of the esophagus, so characteristic of scleroderma, has never been observed.

Sections of pancreas from several patients showed relatively good preservation of lobular architecture, with essentially normal appearing acini and islets. Not a single focus of islet hyalinization could be found in nine generous sections of pancreas from five cases (Ala, B6a, B7a, Ola, Olb) and none have been reported in the literature.

8. Lymphatic

There was evidence of lymphoid depletion in all available autopsy material. Atrophic spleens were recorded in two cases (B7a, Vla), but there was gross splenomegaly in three others (Olb, B6a, R2a). Varying degrees of interstitial fibrosis were seen in all spleens, with a diagnosis of Banti's splenomagaly having been made in case Olb.

Three generous sections were taken from the thymic bed in Ola, but there was not a trace of thymic tissue. Only minute remnants of thymus were noted in a section from the thymic area in Ala.

9. Neurologic

There was evidence of some degree of cerebral cortical atrophy in at least five cases (B6a, B7a, R2a, Zla [Z6a]). This atrophy may have been related to various forms of cerebral arteriosclerosis. There did not appear to be a remarkable amount of lipofuscin pigment or of corpora amylacea. No lesions of the peripheral nerves were noted.

V. TISSUE CULTURE AND CHROMOSOME STUDIES

On two separate occasions, unsuccessful attempts were made to establish fibroblast cultures from 1.0 mm pinch biopsies of forearm skin of case 1 (M8a). To determine whether this inability to establish cultures was significant, a surgical biopsy of skin and subcutaneous tissue from the proximal anterior thigh was obtained. Cell cultures were established with portions of this tissue in two different laboratories (Drs. S.M. Gartler and G.M. Martin), and the following results were obtained.

In one laboratory, in which Waymouth's medium with 15% newborn calf serum was used, one of two cultures was established after an unusually long latent period of a few weeks. This culture did not continue to proliferate after the first two to three passages.

In the other laboratory, nine cultures, each consisting of about a dozen fragments 1-3 mm in diameter, were successfully established in Waymouth's medium containing 10% heat treated (56°C for 30 minutes) newborn calf serum. Cultures of subcutaneous tissue grew out more rapidly than those from the epidermis and

dermis. After the rapid initial period of growth, mitotic activity
ceased rather abruptly in the former and mitotic figures could
rarely be found after six weeks. Although the cultures were split
only into halves or thirds, most could be passaged no more than two
or three times, at most five times, before entering the
"degenerative" phase. The phase of diminished growth was also
associated with alterations in cellular morphology, and large PAS
positive perinuclear inclusions, similar to those found in other
human skin fibroblast cultures entering the "degenerative" phase,
were observed.

Electron micrographs (by Dr. M.A. Lutzner, University of
Washington) of trypsinized fibroblasts from Werner's syndrome
cultures showed groups of perinuclear cytoplasmic granules,
probably lysosomes, but there was no evidence of virus infection.

These results must be contrasted with those obtained with
other cultures established in the same laboratories at the same
time. Several were from middle aged women and proliferated
actively for more than 20-36 weeks (9-14 transfers, cultures split
in fifths) before being terminated. Other cell cultures from
foreskins of newborns and skin biopsies of infants have been
passaged 17-24 times (split in fifths) for periods of 40-52 weeks.
Thus it appears that the cells of this patient with the Werner
syndrome have a sharply restricted life-span in vitro.

Unsuccessful attempts were made to stimulate the growth of
these cells with media supplemented with either 30% heated calf
serum, non-essential amino acids, sodium pyruvate, or with
refiltered, pooled "conditioned" media (i.e. media in which
actively proliferating fibroblasts had grown for three to four days
from an initial inoculum of 50,000 cells/ml). Conversely, the
medium from the patient's cultures did not influence the growth or
morphology of normal fibroblast cultures for periods of up to seven
days.

Attempts to obtain karotypes of the cultured skin fibroblasts
(during the degenerative phase) were not successful. However,
adequate metaphase plates were obtained from phytohemagglutinin
treated cultures of peripheral blood leukocytes. Eleven cells with
46 chromosomes were karyotyped (by Dr. J. Priest) and exhibited
normal morphology.

Jacobs et al. (63) have recently demonstrated a tendency to
increased aneuploidy, primarily hypodiploidy ($\leq$45 chromosomes),
occurring in both sexes with increasing age. In females 65 years
and older, the average proportion of hypodiploid cells is 13%, with
the missing chromosome(s) generally being from the 6-12, X group.
In males, the proportion of hypodiploidy is not as great, and the
missing chromosome is usually from the 21-22, Y group. The

Table 4:   Chromosome counts of cells from patients with Werner's syndrome

Case	Age	Sex	44	Number of Cells		47 Chromosomes
				45	46	
C3a..............	30	M		"normal"		
I1a..............	42	F	5	5	21	1
M8a.............	48	F		2[a]	196[b]	2[c]
P1b.............	30	F			8	
Patient of Frac-caro et al (44)..	46	F	1	4	26	
Patient of Lear-ner et al (75)..	36	F			19	1

[a] C-group chromosome missing from one cell; G-group chromosome from another.

[b] Includes 2 cells with a Philadelphia chromosome.

[c] One cell contained 46 chromosomes plus a fragment; the other, an additional chromosome 2 and 3 extra C-group chromosomes.

suggestion has been made that in both sexes, the missing chromosome is most likely to be one of the sex chromosomes. In a second study (by Mrs. J. Bryant), 200 cells of M8a were counted to allow for the detection of aneuploid cells, and the results shown in Table 4 were obtained. No consistent abnormality was noted in the aneuploid cells. However, among the 196 cells with the modal number of 46 chromosomes, at least 2 were found to demonstrate a typical Philadelphia chromosome with 1/2 to 2/3 of the long arm of a G-group chromosome deleted.

A summary of the results of all of the chromosome studies known to have been performed on leukocyte cultures from various patients with Werner's syndrome are given in Table 4 (two patients included in this table have not been fully reported in the literature and are not listed in Table 2). In all, the modal number was 46, and the sex chromosome distribution was as expected. In two cases in which several cells were counted, there were a significant number of aneuploid cells, but karyotypes done on the cells with 45 chromosomes from one of these patients did not demonstrate any chromosome to be consistently absent.

VI.   GENETICS

All of the patients listed in Table 2 belong to 94 sibships, 6 of which contain only probable patients. The pertinent family data have been subjected to several types of analysis. All of the results are compatible with an autosomal recessive mode of inheritance.

A. Proportion of Sibs Affected

(See Appendix I for pertinent equations.)

If a disease is inherited in a recessive manner, one would expect that, on the average, 25% of the children from marriage of two heterozygotes would be affected. Unfortunately, this theoretical ratio is rarely attainable in practice, and the observed values are related to the method by which the cases are ascertained. If this is known, it is possible to employ rather precise corrections to derive the proportion of affected offspring expected according to the recessive hypothesis. However, in the absence of such information (as is the case in the present heterogenous group of cases culled from the literature) two different types of correction methods are commonly employed and it is expected that the correct value should lie betwen the two estimates obtained.

For such calculations, it is necessary to know both the size of the sibship and the number of affected sibs. In the present series, sufficient information was available in 53 sibships and is shown in Table 5. For purposes of analysis, the probable cases [B1b], [B10b], [E2c], [Z1b], and [Z1c] in families with at least one other patient were counted as affected and sibs who died young (< 25 years) or who were less than 25 years of age were eliminated.

Table 5: Summary of genetic data

Size of Sibship	Number of Sibships (N_s)	Total Sibs (N_t)	Total Affected (N_a)	Bias (B)	$N_s \cdot B$	From Finney's Tables	
						Weight (W)	$N_s \cdot W$
2	5	10	6	5.224	26.120	3.483	17.415
3	9	27	11	5.049	45.441	7.480	67.320
4	8	32	14	4.815	38.520	11.948	95.584
5	14	70	26	4.533	63.462	16.833	235.662
6	2	12	2	4.214	8.428	22.071	44.142
7	4	28	7	3.872	15.488	27.598	110.392
8	6	48	13	3.517	21.102	33.347	200.082
9	2	18	5	3.160	6.320	39.258	78.516
10	2	20	5	2.810	5.620	45.274	90.548
11	1	11	4	2.476	2.476	51.530	51.530
Totals:	$\Sigma N_s = 53$	$\Sigma N_t = 276$	$\Sigma N_a = 93$	$\Sigma N_s \cdot B = 232.977$		$\Sigma N_s \cdot W = 991.227$	

The simple sib method of correction (124) for ascertainment bias is based on the assumption that the chance of finding a sibship is proportional to the number of affected individuals in the sibship. If this is not entirely the case, the simple-sib method will produce an underestimate of the proportion of sibs affected. When this method is used for the present series of cases, a value of $17.9 \pm 2.5\%$ is obtained--somewhat less than expected on the autosomal recessive hypothesis.

The second method of correction (truncate ascertainment method) makes the assumption that ascertainment of a sibship is independent of the number of affected sibs and, in most series tends to result in an overestimate. In this technique it is necessary to correct for those children (of two heterozygotes) who are not detected because their sibship does not happen to have any affected members. Several ways of performing such calculations are available, and for this paper, the maximum-likelihood method with Finney's tables has been used (39). The value arrived at is $26.5 \pm 3.2\%$ affected. Thus, by the two methods employed, the proportion of affected sibs ranges from $17.9 \pm 2.5\%$ to $26.5 \pm 3.2\%$, and the correct estimate probably lies between these values. It must be pointed out, however, that both estimates are probably somewhat low since it is likely that at least a few of the so-called "normal" sibs were or would become affected. Nevertheless, it is unlikely that the estimates, both reasonably close to 25%, would be greatly altered.

B. Consanguinity and Gene Frequency

In recessively inherited diseases, the frequency of consanguineous marriages among the parents is expected to be increased, with the fraction of such marriages being inversely related to the frequency of the recessive genes in the population (89). Of 87 sibships (N_s) in the present series of cases, there was consanguinity in 17 (N_c), no consanguinity in 30 (N_o), and no information in 40. Of the consanguineous marriages, 11 were of first cousins, 5 were of first cousins once removed or of second cousins, one was not stated.

Minimal and maximal estimates of the frequency of consanguineous marriages can be made as follows:

$$\text{Minimal} = N_c/N_s = 17/87 = 19.3\%;$$

for 1st cousin marriages, 12.6%.
$$\text{Maximal} = N_c/(N_o+N_c) = 17/(30+17) = 17/47 = 36.2\%;$$

for 1st cousin marriages, 23.4%. Although the rate of consanguinity for the general population cannot be accurately determined, the present series being derived from many countries and over period of 60 years, there is little question that the proportion of consanguineous marriages is far in excess of consanguinity rates observed in the relevant populations.

From the frequencies (k) of 1st cousin marriages among the parents of patients with recessive genes and in the general population (c) it is possible to estimate the frequency (q) of rare recessive genes by Dahlberg's formula (24),

$$q = \frac{c(1-k)}{16K-15C-ck}.$$

The difficulties of this method are discussed by Neel et al. (93) and Hamilton et al (53). Although the value of c is not known, it may be assumed to be in the range of 0.05 to 0.1 (from the data of Bell on England and Wales (7), and Nell et al. on Japan (93)). With these data, crude minimal estimates of q may be calculated and are, respectively, 0.0010 and 0.0047. The corresponding homozygote frequencies, q^2, are 1.0×10^{-6} and 22.1×10^{-6} (i.e. 1-22 cases per million people). For a country the size of the United States, with approximately 100 million people over 30, there should be between 100 and 2200 recognizable patients with Werner's syndrome.

C. Sex Ratio, Birth Order, and Fertility

Of the total of 125 definite cases, 64 were males and 61 females, giving a sex ratio very nearly 1:1. X-linkage and sex limitation are therefore ruled out.

In autosomal recessive diseases, the chance of an individual being affected is independent of his position within the birth order. To test this, the method of Haldane and Smith (52) has been used to calculate the expected mean birth order (See Appendix I). The difference between the expected and observed means was not statistically significant, and it is inferred that no birth order effect is present.

Of the 125 patients with Werner's syndrome, 45 are known to have been married and 30 single. The total number of children known to have survived the perinatal period is 51 and the net fertility for the whole group is 0.4 children per patient (or 1.1 children per known married patient). Although no precise control figures are available, this appears to represent a reduction in fertility. Several factors probably enter into this decrease: lower occurrences of marriage, descrease in libido and potency (especially male), decrease in count and viablity of sperm, inablity to conceive and to carry pregnancies to successful completion.

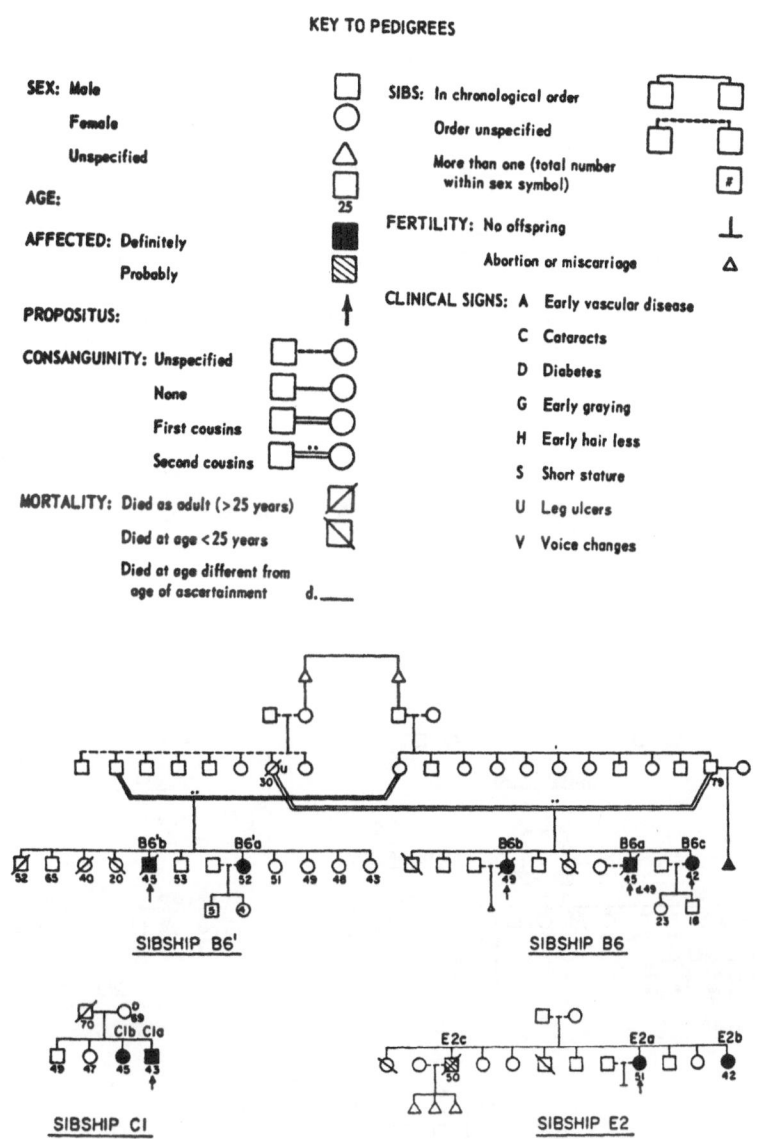

Figure 13: Pedigrees of patients with Werner's syndrome. The meanings of the various symbols are shown in the key.

D. Analysis of Pedigrees: Possible Heterozygote Manifestations

Seventeen representative pedigrees encompassing 21 sibships,
are shown in Figure 13. All of these, with one possible exception
to be discussed, are compatible with the recessive mode of
inheritance. The frequent occurrence of consanguinity is well
illustrated, and the tendency for the disease to appear in more
than one branch of a family may be caused by in-breeding.

Direct vertical transmission of the disease has been suggested
only once (pedigree Z1) (145). The patient's mother, who did not
have cataracts, was described as "having been very short with tiny
hands and feet...gray (hair) and as long as the patient could
remember...(with) painful ulcerated feet." There are three
possible explanations for this apparent dominant transmission: (1)
The mother did not have Werner's syndrome. (2) The mother was a

WERNER'S SYNDROME

Fig. 13--continued

heterozygote with strong manifestations (unlikely, see below). (3)
The mother was homozygous, i.e. had the Werner, syndrome and the
father was a heterozygote. At the present, it is impossible to
distinguish among these alteratives, although the latter may be the
most likely.

The existence of "formes frustes," "abortive forms," and
heterozygote manifestations has frequently been claimed (61, 92,
100, 102). The use of the first two terms has been somewhat
confused, since it has been applied both to presumed homozygotes

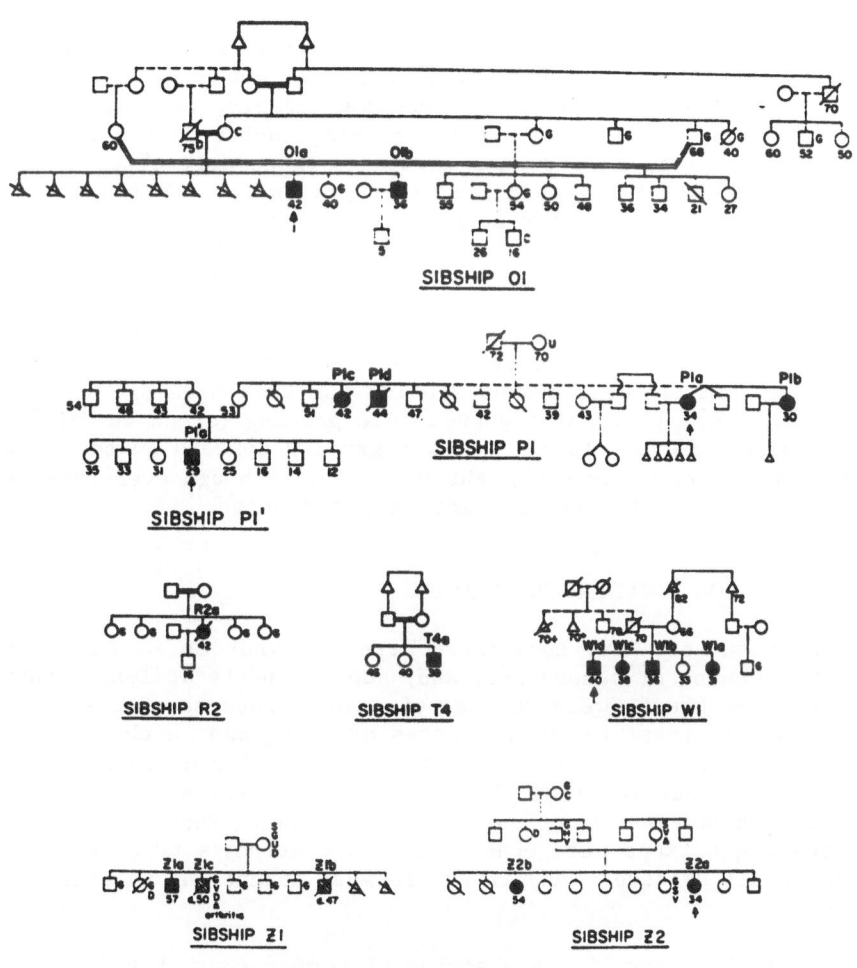

Fig. 13--continued

who lack one or more of the major features of the syndrome, and to
heterozygotes with a few stigmata such as cataracts, premature
graying, or diabetes. The question of whether homozygous
individuals may incompletely express the syndrome is difficult to
decide, but the "probable" causes such as those in sibship Z1,
suggest that this may, in fact, occur. For this reason, isolated
cases [B9a], [F5a], [S7a], and [Z6a], have been designated as
probable, even though they lacked cataracts, and it likely that
many more such cases exist. The apparent incompleteness of
expression may be related, in large measure, to the great
variability in the ages of onset of the various symptoms.

The existence of heterozygote manifestations is even more
difficult to decide upon, since nearly all of the manifestations of
Werner's syndrome may occur in normal individuals in an isolated
fashion. The best individuals in which to detect such
manifestations are the parents of the patients, sicne they are
obligate heterozygotes (children of patients would be also, but
would be too young for study). Data were scanty, but vascular
disease, diabetes, and "premature" graying each occurred in about
ten parents, short stature and cataracts (generally of the "senile"
type) each in about five and leg ulcers or early hair loss in
fewer. Since those figures do not significantly depart from what
would be expected in normal population, they do not support the
notion of heterozygote manifestations.

The other group who should display such manifestations, if
they do occur, is composed of the patients' sibs, 2/3 of whom would
be heterozygotes. Here again, mention has been made of various
manifestations, particularly premature graying (often in "all"
sibs) and cataracts. Of these, only graying appears to be somewhat
excessive in frequency and might possibly, although even this is
unlikely, represent a heterozygote manifestation.

VII. COMPARISON WITH NATURAL AGING

Many authors have considered Werner's syndrome as a form of
premature aging or senescence, and, superficially at least, there
is a resemblance between the two entities. Because of the
widespread interest in the processes of aging and in the
pathological events associated with it, any relevant information
that could be derived from the study of a condition such as the
Werner syndrome would, of course, be valuable. Therefore, the
following questions were considered. Are Werner's syndrome and
aging at all related? And if so, to what extent and in what
manner?

In Table 6 are listed a series of comparisons, based mainly on
athological observations, between Werner's syndrome and aging.

Table 6:   Comparison of features of Werner's syndrome with those of aging.

	Werner's syndrome	Aging
A. Similar findings		
1. Atherosclerosis, arterio-sclerosis and medical calcinosis		
2. Graying of the hair		
3. Hypermelanosis		
4. Cerebral cortical atrophy		
5. Lymphoid depletion and thymic atrophy		
B. Similar findings, but differences in degree		
*1. Calcification of valve rings and leaflets	Very severe	Moderate
*2. Hyalinisation of semi-niferous tubules	Very severe	Severe only in very aged
*3. Atrophy of skin appendages	Severe	Moderate
*4. Osteoporosis	Generalised, but found particularly in distal extremities	Generalised, spine particularly vulnerable
*5. Loss of hair	Generalised	Principally scalp
C. Features characteristic of Werner's syndrome		
*1. Cataracts	"Dystrophic" type: subcapsular and cortical	"Senile" type: cortical or nuclear (probably different from those of Werner's syndrome)
*2. Ulcerations and atrophy of extremities	Non-trophic, very frequent	Trophic, infrequent
*3. Short stature	Primary	Acquired
*4. Laryngeal atrophy	Common	Unusual
*5. Proportion of sarcomas and connective tissue tumors among neoplasms	High	Low
*6. Soft tissue calcification	Common	Unusual
7. Prostate	Atrophic epithelium	Benign prostatic hypertrophy
8. Adrenal glomerulosa	Conspicuous	Poorly demarcated
9. Parathyroid	Chief cell predominant	Oxyphils predominant

* Differences considered to be of principal significance.

There is little question that some features are common to both. In particular, the involvement of the blood vessels, although occurring earlier and sometimes with greater severity in Werner's syndrome, is qualitatively similar in character and distribution in the two conditions. In this comparison, no distinction has been made between the "normal" and "pathological" aspects of aging (72). If such a distinction were made atherosclerosis would then represent a further point of difference between Werner's syndrome and "normal aging."

However, if features such as valvular calcification,
testicular atrophy and atrophy of the skin appendages are
considered, a somewhat different pattern of relationships emerges.
The pathological processes are, as has already been discussed, very
similar in Werner's syndrome and aging, but the extent of
involvement in the former is, in all cases, much more severe.
Thus, in the case of hyalinization of seminiferous tubules, such
severe involvement is seen only in very aged individuals, and even
then it is not a constant finding. Likewise, the calcification of
the cardiac valve rings in Werner's syndrome is a very striking
and, in the autopsy material reviewed, constant finding, again
occurring to a degree far greater than that associated with the
"normal" aging processes.

The major contrast between aging and Werner's syndrome occurs
in relation to certain of the signs which are considered
pathognomonic of Werner's syndrome: cataracts, ulcerations,
laryngeal pathology, atrophy of the distal extremities, and the
high incidence of non-carcinomatous neoplasms. The pathologic
processes and/or the frequencies of these lesions are not at all
comparable in the two situations, and, as is shown in Table 6,
alterations in several other organs are also different. On the
other hand, certain features commonly associated with aging occur
to a much lesser degree or not at all. These include senile
keratoses and other malignant lesions of the skin (basal and
squamous cell carcinoma), senile elastosis (basophilic degeneration
of dermal collagen), hyalinization of pancreatic islets, deposition
of lipofuscin pigment (in hepatic cells, myocardial fibers and
neurones), and the presence of corpora amylacea in the brain and
spinal cord.

In a recent review on aging, Casarett (21) cited three
idealized critera for premature aging: 1) An earlier increase in
mortality, without alteration of the shape of the mortality curve.
2) Proportional advancement in time of all diseases or causes of
death, without alterations of degree, sequence, or absolute
incidence, and without induction of disease. 3) Proportional
advancement in time of all morphological and physiological
manifestations of the aging process. Casarett's criteria, while
possibly too rigid in detail, serve as a basis for evaluating the
relationship between Werner's syndrome and aging. Taken in the
aggregate, these and the foregoing considerations indicate that
Werner's syndrome is certainly not merely a process of precocious
(earlier onset) or accelerated (more rapid progression) aging.
There are too many differences in the degree and nature of the
various features of the two entities to allow them to be closely
identified with each other. Werner's syndrome may be better
considered a "caricature" of aging, exaggerating, although not
necessarily by the same mechanisms, some of the clinical and
pathologic features which connote aging. If one takes the view

that both Werner's syndrome and aging represent the results of
generalized metabolic processes, or aberrations thereof, and that
the various tissues of the human organism have only a limited
number of reactions to such processes, then the overlap between the
two entities is not surprising. Their relationship may be similar
to the relationships among Werner's syndrome and the various
models (to be discussed below) which mimic it to a greater or
lesser extent. Many of the similarities may be fortuitous, with
the convergence of the various pathological processes occurring
only at the level of the various affected end organs. However,
other similarities may denote a more fundamental identity, with
common biochemical and physiological mechanisms actually being
involved. Therefore, even if Werner's syndrome and aging are
considered to be distinct entitites, an analysis of those features
that they have in common could conceivably be useful in achieving
and understanding of both.

VII. COMPARISON WITH RELATED HEREDITARY AND NON-HEREDITARY
      DISEASES OF MAN

     There are many other diseases which have, in the past, been
considered as related to Werner's syndrome. These include
cataracta dermatogenes, anhidrotic ectodermal dysplasia,
poikiloderma atrophicans congenita (Thompson's syndrome),
acrogeria, scleroderma, and the Hallerman-Streiff and Cockayne
syndromes. Their relationship to Werner's syndrome is tenuous
and they will not be discussed here. However, several other
entities do deserve comment.

A. Progeria (Hutchinson-Gilford's Syndrome (27)

     This condition, which might be recessively inherited (46),
begins early in life. Although the head is near normal in size
(but abnormal in shape), there is severe dwarfing and the limbs
are thin, the mandible receding, the eyes prominent, and the nose
beaked. The joints are large, and periarticular changes may lead
to contractures. Subcutaneous fat is almost absent, and the skin
is thin and often sclerotic (especially over the abdomen and
extremities), pigmented, and deficient in hair follicles and
sebaceous glands. Moderate generalized osteoporosis has been
observed, as have atrophic changes in the distal extremities.
Perhaps the most stiking feature is the severe generalized
atherosclerosis which is found to involve all of the major
vessels, including the aorta and coronary arteries, even in
patients autopsied as young as nine years of age. This vascular
disease is the principal cause of death. Hypercholesterolemia
has been frequently observed and is thought to be somehow
involved in the pathogenesis of the atherosclerosis.

While many of these features of progeria are similar to
features of Werner's syndrome, cataracts, hyperkeratoses, skin
ulcers, and diabetes are not characteristically found in
progeria. Therefore, while progeria, of all the conditions to be
discussed, bears the closest resemblance to Werner's syndrome,
the metabolic defect in the two diseases must be considered to be
distinct.

B. Rothmund's Syndrome

Thannhauser (131), in his review of Werner's and Rothmunds'
syndromes, clearly indicated the differences between these two
diseases. The onset of the skin and eye (cataract)
manifestations of Rothmund's syndrome occurs during the first
four years of life. Telangiectasia, scaling, and disorders of
pigmentation are more characteristic of the skin changes than are
the atrophy, tightening and ulceration found in the Werner
syndrome. Premature graying, shortness of stature, atrophy of
the extremities, osteoporosis, diabetes, and arteriosclerosis are
not present. However, some degree of hypogonadism in males, with
testicular atrophy, has been described, and cases thought to be
Rothmund's syndrome have been seen in which ulceration of the
skin, short stature, and abnormal glucose tolerance tests exist
(Dr. J. Bass, personal communication). With these possible
exceptions, and except for the fact that both syndromes represent
recessively inherited conditions in which the skin and lens of
the eye are affected, there is little reason to consider the two
as related.

C. Myotonic Dystrophy (22)

Although this condition with its myotonia and dominant mode
of inheritance is obviously different from Werner's syndrome,
there are several significant features in which they overlap.
The disease usually begins in the second or third decade, and
cataracts are a frequent manifestation.

In males, testicular atrophy with degeneration and
hyalinization of the seminiferous tubules may occur, although the
external genitalia are normal in size. Gonadal disturbance in
females has been less well documented, and it is not clear whether
female hypogonadism occurs at all. Abnormal ("diabetic") glucose
tolerance tests are found in 20-30% of the patients, but few cases
of frank diabetes have been reported. Premature frontal baldness is
common in males and sometimes occurs in females, and atrophy of skin
(with thinning, roughness, and dryness) on the eyelids and backs of
the hands has been noted (34).

The muscle atrophy in myotonic dystrophy involves principally
the muscles of the face, jaw, neck, and some groups in the

extremities; generalized atrophy of the distal musculature does not occur.

D. Triparanol Intoxication

For a short while, Triparanol (MER-29), a drug which principally blocks the conversion of desmosterol to cholesterol (48), was employed therapeutically to reduce cholesterol levels. Among the complications resulting from its use were cataracts (especially posterior subcapsular), loss of hair, change in hair color, impotence, and drying and rashes of skin (85). The resemblance of many of these still unexplained side effects to features of Werner's syndrome is intersting and raises the possibility, when considered in light of the analogies to hypogonadism and hyperadrenalism, that some aberration in steroid hormone metabolism or action may indeed be present in Werner's syndrome.

IX. ANIMAL MODELS

A. Hereditary Premature Senescence of the Rabbit (98)

A hereditary disease that seems to bear a more than superficial resemblance to Werner's syndrome is a condition of Belgian hares that has been termed hereditary premature senescence of the rabbit. Because of the deaths of the investigators who were studying the disease, only a clinical description is available; the exact mode of inheritance (which may be recessive by the descriptions available) is unknown.

The rabbits were dwarfed and had a generally senile appearance resulting from coat, skin, and eye lesions. The coat was dry, thin, lax, and inelastic, and there were calluses or ulcerations of the feet. Conjunctivitis and a granulomatous keratitis were common. Both sexes tended to be infertile and the females had difficulties with pregnancy, parturition, and lactation. Toward the end of life, there was generalized degeneration with muscle wasting and loss of body fat. No mention has been made of cataracts, vascular lesions, or bone disease, and there are no pathological descriptions.

Many of the features of the rabbit disease are directly analogous to Werner's syndrome, and some of the differences could be due, in part, to a species variation. It is not inconceivable that the two conditions represent the same, or closely related, genetic defects. As in the case of Werner's syndrome itself, the manifestations of hereditary premature senescence appear to mimic, rather than to represent, true prematurity of the aging process.

B. The Progeria-like Syndrome of the Rat

Selye and his collaborators (116), by the chronic administration of low doses of dihydrotachysterol (DHT) to young adult rats, have produced a syndrome that closely resembles Werner's syndrome. The life-span is shortened, and there is a generalized tissue wasting with atrophy of the sex organs and viscera. The skin becomes thin and pigmented, and there is loss of hair, fragmentation of elastic fibers, and trophy of the dermal collagen and hair follicles. Severe calcification of the intervertebral discs and of the costal, laryngeal, and tracheal cartilages develops. In addition, there is generalized calcification (of the Moenckeberg type) of the blood vessels, both large and small. Unlike Werner's syndrome, osteosclerosis, rather than osteoporosis, develops, and soft tissue calcification appears only in the stomach. Cataracts occur only rarely, but the administration of DHT sensitizes the lens to the production of cataracts by agents such as 5-hydroxytryptamine. All of the effects of DHT are prevented by the administration of methyltestosterone or ferric dextran.

Although many attempts to implicate abnormalities in calcium metabolism to the pathogenesis of Werner's syndrome have been unsuccessful, the combination of pathologic features in "experimental progeria" still makes it an interesting animal model for the disease.

C. Radiation-induced "Aging"

Another animal model which mimics several of the features of Werner's syndrome is the "aging" produced by the irradition of experimental animals, particularly mice. As in the case of Werner's syndrome, it is thought that the late effects of irradiation do not represent a true acceleration of the aging process, although this point is still being debated (2, 21). Nevertheless, the life-span of the animals is shortened, cataracts appear early and with a high frequency, and graying and loss of hair may ensue. Certain tumors (such as of the lung) appear earlier than usual, but their incidence is not increased. (In man exposed to moderate amounts of radiation, the frequency of leukemia rather than of mesenchymal tumors, except when there has been prolonged localized radiation, is increased (55, 132).)

The chief difficulty in equating the effects of radiation with Werner's syndrome is that the cells that appear most vulnerable to radiation, namely those that are rapidly dividing (such as in the gastrointestinal mucosa, the blood forming cells, and the lymphoid system), do not appear to be seriously affected in Werner's syndrome.

D. Vitamin Deficiences

In a remarkable paper published over 20 years ago, the similarity of Werner's syndrome to certain experimentally produced conditions in rats was pointed out by Buschke (19). He and others were able to produce "dystrophic" cataracts (anterior and posterior subcapsular and cortical) similar to those of Werner's syndrome by the administration of diets deficient in "riboflavin" or "tryptophan" and by chronic thallium poisoning. In addition to the cataracts, which could be induced only in young animals, these treatments resulted in arrest of body growth, testicular atrophy, alopecia and other cutaneous lesions, and corneal vascularization with keratitis and iritis. Thallium poisoning also affected several of the endocrine glnds, the mucosa of the gastrointestinal tracts, and, on occasion, caused rickets.

In referring to the significance of these experimentally produced cataracts, Bushke expressed the hope that they would "serve, at least partially, to delimit the field in which (the) metabolic links ...between the endogenous (i.e. hereditary) and the exogenous (i.e. induced) forms of dystrophic cataracts...would be sought." This hope was based on the assumption, "that the same group of tissues may be affected either by the absence in food of an exogenous (extrinsic) factor or by a genotypical defect of the endogenous (intrinsic) part of the same metabolic system."

It is for this reason that we have devoted attention to those conditions of man and animals which appear relevant to Werner's syndrome. It is possible, as Buschke implies, that one or more of these conditions may, at some level, be truly related to Werner's syndrome and will provide a clue to the ultimate elucidation of the primary defect.

X. POSSIBLE PATHOGENETIC MECHANISMS

The fact that Werner's syndrome is characteristically expressed only in the homozygous state might suggest, in analogy with many other recessively inherited condtiions, that it results from a deficient or defective enzyme (15, 89, 102, 133). However, considerations introduced by a study of control mechanisms in lower organisms suggest that this need not be the case, and that derangements of more complex genetic regulatory mechanisms may be involved. Nevertheless, whatever mechanism is ultimately postulated must be compatible with the recessive mode of inheritance. For the present, it seems reasonable to assume as a working hypothesis that an enzyme defect is responsible for the syndrome. But, whatever the nature of the gene lesion, neither the genetic analysis nor the examination of the presently available clinical or pathological data specifies its location. In particular, it is not known whether the defect is present in all (or many) of the tissues that are affected, or whether it occurs at some site distant from all of these. Possibly there is a failure in the production of some material important for function of the affected tissues. Or, as occurs in phenylketonuria (10), there may be an accumulation of substances toxic to these tissues.

Some of the diseases and animal models already discussed in sections VIII and IX indicate that a single defect could easily produce the wide variety of manifestations found in Werner's syndrome, but models of this type may not necessarily be relevant in pointing to a specific site for the lesion.

As discussed above, Werner's syndrome is not primarily an acceleration of the normal aging process. Even though the grosser manifestations of the syndrome do not appear until the second and third decades, the retardation of growth and the early onset of the skin manifestations suggest that the disease starts much earlier. Growth, in particular, is a sensitive indicator of the overall status of the body's metabolic pathways, and a wide variety of disorders will interfere with it. Nonetheless, unlike most other recessive conditions, Werner's syndrome can be considered as a disease which causes or permits the degeneration of tissues that had apparently been functioning adequately for many years.

Virtually nothing is known about the mechanisms of abiotrophies, or of aging in general, although many possible mechanisms, again including the accumulation of toxic materials, have been suggested (13, 24, 26, 121). Recent studies on Pompe's disease (type II glycogenosis) (5) indicate that these absence of a specific enzyme may result in the gradual accumulation of glycogen within lysosomes and provide a good example of how such a mechanism could operate. Perhaps a more cogent analogy is provided by ochronotic arthropathy, a late complication of alkaptonuria--one of Garrod's original "inborn errors of metabolism." This condition apparently results from the deposition in cartilage of metabolites of homogentesic acid, substances which are thought to eventually affect the integrity of the tissue (91).

Alternative mechanisms for abiotrophies are also possible. Enzymes involved in a biochemical reaction not operative until puberty might be defective, so that the appearance of the enzyme deficit is delayed. Normal reparative mechanisms concerned with the preservation or the integrity of intracellular and extracellular constituents, such as the chromosomes,

mitochondria, or even structural proteins, may be impaired.
Enzymes capable of repairing induced lesions in bacterial
deoxyribonucleic acid (DNA) have been described (117) and could
conceivably exist in man. Lesions in such repair systems might
be of particular importance in tissues in which cell replacement
does not occur (as, for example, in certain parts of the nervous
system) and in tissues subject to severe stress. And, in fact,
many of the areas of major involvement in Werner's syndrome--the
heart, blood vessels, tissues of the feet, tendons and ligaments,
and larynx--are exposed to significant stresses. Therefore,
while certain relatively protected tissues (notably the lens and
testes) are also affected, it is conceivable that a defect in the
repair of certain tissues or in the synthesis or repair of
particular connective tissue elements could be a factor in the
pathogenesis of Werner's syndrome. Of interest in this regard is
the relatively high incidence of mesenchymal tumors, again
suggesting the possibility of an aberration in the control and
function of connective tissue. The tissue culture studies
reported in this paper, indicating a sharply restricted in vitro
lifespan of fibroblasts, may also point in this direction.

XI. SUMMARY AND CONCLUSIONS

In this report we have presented the results of a series of
investigations carried out on a patient with Werner's syndrome
and of a review of the present state of knowledge concerning this
hereditary disease. On analysis of 125 definite cases with
Werner's syndrome (including three reported in detail here) the
clinical picture had the following pattern. In usual order of
the appearance, the principal manifestations of the syndrome were
a symmetrical retardation of growth with absence of the
adolescent growth spurt, graying of the hair, atrophy and
hyperkeratosis of the skin, generalized loss of hair, alterations
of the voice, cataracts (subcapsular and cortical, usually
posterior), ulcerations of the skin of the feet, and, in about
half of the cases, mild diabetes. Other features which were
usually present were atrophy of the muscle, fat and bone of the
extremities, vascular calcification, soft-tissue (usually
periarticular) calcification, and generalized osteoporosis.
"Hypogonadism," manifested by small genitalia, female hair
distribution, and decreased libido and potency in males and by
oligomenorrhea or early menopause, small genitalia and breasts,
and decreased libido in females, was frequently present. The
fertility of both sexes was reduced. Ten per cent of the cases
had serious neoplasms. Of these, the majority were not
carcinomas, but sarcomas and meningiomas.

Several special studies were undertaken on a patient with
typical Werner's syndrome to elucidate specific aspects of the

disease. In contrast to the results obtained by earlier workers, no evidence for abnormalities of adrenal cortical steroid production or metabolism were obtained. The results of studies of the effects of glucose and tolbutamide on circulating insulin levels were similar to those obtained in patients with the mild "adult" form of diabetes mellitus (delayed and prolonged response with elevated fasting levels of serum insulin). Glucose and glutathione metabolism in erythrocytes was not impaired, and levels of numerous serum and urinary constituents were normal.

In vitro cell cultures were prepared from a surgically obtained piece of skin and subcutaneous tissue. Unlike control cultures, which proliferated rapidly and survived numerous passages and changes of medium, the skin fibroblasts from this patient divided slowly and were viable for only a few passages. These results raise the possibility that an in vitro cell culture approach may be useful in studying the disease.

On review of histologic sections and pathology protocols from autopsies or biopsies performed on several patients, several salient features were noted: severe calcification of the cardiac valve rings and to a lesser extent, valve leaflets; severe hyalinization of the seminiferous tubules; severe atrophy of skin appendages and subcutaneous fat; atrophic prostatic epithelium; and conspicuous adrenal glomerulosa. Arteriosclerosis, including atherosclerosis, was severe. While some of these lesions, such as the arteriosclerosis and testicular atrophy, are only quantiatively, rather than qualitatively different from those seen in the very aged, the features of Werner's syndrome, taken in the aggregate, are different from those of aging.

A genetic analysis of the family data on Werner's syndrome gives results that are wholly compatible with an autosomal recessive mode of inheritance. A crude gene frequency calculated from the consanguinity data is of the order of 1-5 per thousand and 2-10 persons in a thousand are presumably carriers. With the possible exception of early graying of the hair, there is no evidence for heterozygote manifestations.

Even though Werner's syndrome differs from many other recessive diseases in being slow and somewhat variable in its progresssion, this type of inheritance immediately suggests the possibility that a single protein or enzyme defect is responsible for all of its manifestations. There are several clinical and experimental conditions which resemble Werner's syndrome in various respects and may be considered as models for it. Although the models indicate the wide variety of metabolic sites in which the lesion of Werner's syndrome could reside, none has yet provided any real clue into the nature of the disease. There is evidence to suggest an impairment in the development and metabolism of connective tissue, but it is unlikely that the metabolic defect is restricted to this tissue.

The elucidation of the primary defect of Werner's syndrome and tracing of its diverse ramifications thus remains a tantalizing challenge. In one hereditary disorder are combined two major diseases of modern man--vascular disease and neoplasia, as well as others of widespread importance--diabetes, cataracts, and osteoporosis. The solution of the puzzle of the Werner syndrome may, therefore, provide us with clues to the pathogenesis of many diverse problems.

Addendum

Since the preparation of this paper, several additional case reports have appeared: Jilek, M. and Kuta, A., Werneruv Syndrom. Sbornik Lekarsky, 66:55, 1964; Tanenbaum, M.H., Werner's syndrome. Progeria of the adult.   Arch. Intern. Med. 116:499, 1965 (two unrelated patients, one of whom had an affected sister who had had a total hysterectomy at age 22 for "uterine tumors"); and Riley, T.R., Weiland, R.G., Markle, J., and Hamwi, G.J., Werner's syndrome. Ann. Intern. Med. 63:285, 1965 (this patient, a 34 year old male, was found to have normal amounts of circulating growth hormone).

We have had the opportunity to evaluate another case (P.N., NIH #06-16-12) at the National Institutes of Health. He was a 47 year old father of two who presented with partial bladder and ureteral obstruction and was found to have an undifferentiated carcinoma, presumably prostatic in origin, and moderate testicular atrophy. Pathological material on a previously undescribed case has also been examined. The patient, GMB (Armed Forces Institute of Pathology #1081995), died at age 37 years and was found at autopsy to have: severe generalized atherosclerosis; partial calcification of the aortic valve ring; pancreatic islet cell hyperplasia (diabetes); small ovaries with numerous dilated and atretic follicles, luteinized stromal and thecal cells, but only one promordial follicle in two microscopic sections; and two paragangliomas (one submucosal in the bladder, one adjacent to the left adrenal). Again, the appearance of uncommon tumors in patients with Werner's syndrome is striking.

Finally, the patient listed in Table 2 as case F2a died at age 47 of an acute myocardial infarction.

ACKNOWLEDGMENTS

We are particularly indebted to Dr. Lorenz Marquis of Marysville, Washington, who originally referred case 1 to us and whose generous coopertion and close medical supervision has made her investigation possible.

We wish to thank the many individuals who assisted in the evaluation of cases 1, 2, and 3 or who made available to us clinical information, pathologic materials, or their helpful comments. These include: Drs. W. Bateille, M.W. Boyd, S.M. Gartler, T. Kazuya, V.C. Kelley, M.A. Lutzner, J. Mickley, J. Morison, M. Nydick, J. Priest, M. Proctor, A.S. Rogers, S.W. Rosen, C.E. Rubin, E. Samols, E.R. Simon, G.L. Spaeth, S.H. Waxman, and Mrs. J. Bryant.

We are also grateful to Drs. D. Zucker-Franklin and H. Rifkin who made available to us, prior to publication, the detailed case histories of several patients from Montefiore Hospital, New York. Pathologic material on several of these patients was kindly made available by Dr. H.M. Zimmerman.

APPENDIX I: STATISTICAL METHODS

Editor's note: Appendix I, which is not reproduced here, explains the methods for segregation analyses and birth order calculations.

APPENDIX II: PHOTOGRAPHS

Editor's note: The Epstein review contained several photographs that were not available for reproduction here. The legends below provide a guide for the photographs contained in the original review.

Fig. 4:   X-ray view of the feet of case 1, showing diffuse osteoporosis, soft tissue calcification, bony atrophy, and joint destruction and fusion.

Fig. 7:   Pubic skin. a. Case B7a: Atrophy of subcutaneous tissue and skin appendages; fibrosis (x 19.6). b. Control autopsy section from 48-year-old white male who died of malignant hypertension and uremia (x 19.6).

Fig. 8:   Skin. a. Case (Z6a): Sharply focal hyperkeratosis; site unknown (x 125). b. Case M8a: Focal hyperkeratosis; epidermal atrophy. From anterior of thigh (x 528). c. Case M8a: Hypermelanosis with prominence of "clear cells" (x 528).

Fig. 9:   Larynx. a. Case (1a: Telangiectasia; thickened squamous epithelium (x 110). b. Case 0la: Peri- glandular lymphocytic infiltrates (x 33). c. Case B7a: Lymphoid nodule (x 63).

Fig. 10: Heart. Case Z1a: Calcification and bony metaplasia of mitral valve ring; the metaplastic bone (lower left) includes hematopoietic tissue (x 44).

Fig. 11: Testis. a. Case B6a: Representative of best preserved areas from this case, which showed the least severe testicular pathology; there is diminished spermatogenic activity and slight thickening of the tubular wall (x 301). b. Case A1a: Complete hyalinization of seminiferous tubules; prominent clusters of interstitial cells (x 301).

Fig. 12: Adrenal cortex. Case B6a: Hyperplasia of zona glomerulosa with giant cell (arrow)(x 110).

REFERENCES

1. Agatston, S.A. and Gartner, S.: Precocious cataracts and scleroderma (Rothmund's syndrome; Werner's syndrome). Arch. Ophthal. 21:492, 1939.
2. Alexander, P. and Connell, D.I.: Differences between radiation-induced life span shortening in mice and normal aging as revealed by serial killing, in Cellular Bases and Etiology of Late Somatic Effects of Ionizing Radiation, ed. by Harris, R.J.C., Academic Press, New York, 1963, p. 277.
3. Bakker, B.J.: Syndrome von Werner. Dermatologica (Basel), 109:230, 1954.
4. Bakker, B.J.: Syndroom van Werner. Ned. Tschr. Geneesk. 98:1662, 1954.
5. Baudhuin, P., Hers, H.G. and Loeb, H.: An electron microscopic and biochemical study of type II glycogenosis. Lab. Invest. 13:1140, 1964.
6. Bauer, J.M. and Conn, J.W.: Werner's syndrome. A study of adrenocortical and hepatic steroidal metabolism. Texas J. Med. 44:882, 1953.
7. Bell, J.: Determination of the consanguinity rate in the general hospital population of England and Wales. Ann. Eugen. 10:370, 1940.
8. Bellafiore, V.: Su un caso di sindrome di Werner. Ann. Ital. Derm. Sif. 14:53, 1959.
9. Bennedeti, G.: Zur Psychopathologie des Wernerschen Syndrome. Confina Neur. (Basel) 13:27, 1953.
10. Bessman, S.P.: Some biochemical lessons to be learned from phenylketonuria. J. Pediat. 64:828, 1964.
11. Blau, J.N. (for Earl, C.J.): Werner's syndrome. Proc. Roy. Soc. Med. 55:328, 1962.
12. Blodgett, F.M., Burgin, L., Iezzoni, D., Gribetz, D. and Talbot, N.B.: Effects of prolonged cortisone therapy on the

statural growth, skeletal maturation and metabolic status of children. New Engl. J. Med. 254:636, 1956.

13. Blumenthal, H.F. and Berns, A.W.: Autoimmunity and aging. Adv. Gerontological Res. 1:289, 1964.

14. Boatwright, H., Wheeler, C.E. and Cawley, E.P.: Werner's syndrome. A.M.A. Arch Intern. Med. 90:243, 1952.

15. Boyd, M.W. and Grant, A.P.: Werner's syndrome (progeria of the adult). Further pathological and biochemical observations. Brit. Med. J. 2:920, 1959.

16. Brink, A.J. and Findlay, G.H.: Werner's syndrome. Ulcerating atrophodermia, cataracts and premature senility. Report of a case. South Afr. Med. J. 24:318, 1950.

17. Brodey, A. and Ruppe, J., Jr.: Werner's syndrome. Arch. Dermat. Syph. 69:243, 1954.

18. Brouwer, K.: Het syndroom van Werner. Ned. Tschr. Geneesk. 99:2056, 1955.

19. Buschke, W.: Dystrophic cataracts and their relation to other "metabolic" cataracts. Arch. Ophthal. 30:751, 1943.

20. Carney, J.W.: Werner's syndrome. Arch. Derm. 87:756, 1963.

21. Casarett, G.W.: Similarities and contrasts between radiation and time pathology. Adv. Gerontological Res. 1:109, 1964.

22. Caughey, E. and Myrianthopoulos, N.C.: Dystrophia Myotonia and Related Disorders. Thomas, Springfield, Ill., 1963.

23. Chorazak, T., Kochanowicz, T. and Pietrzykowska, A.: Das Werner-Syndrom in der Gruppe der Kongenitalen Hautatrophien mit einem Bericht uber einen eigenen Fall. Hautarzt 12:116, 1961.

24. Cohen, M. and Shelley, W.B.: Ankle ulcer sign of Werner's syndrome. Arch. Derm. 87:86, 1963.

25. Comfort, A.: Ageing, the biology of senescence. Routledge and Kegan Paul Ltd., London, 1964, p. 216.

26. Curtis, H.J.: Biological mechanisms underlaying the aging process. Science, 141:686, 1963.

27. Danowski, T.S.: Progeria in chidren and adults, in Clinical Endocrinology, Vol. 1, Williams and Wilkins, Baltimore, 1962, p. 244.

28. Daughaday, W.H.: The adenohypophysis, in Textbook of Endocrinology, 3rd Ed., ed. by Williams, R.H., W. B. Saunders Company, Philadelphia & London, 1962, p. 11.

29. Daweke, H., Jahnke, K. and Zimmerman, H.: Untersuchungen des Kohlenhydrat-und Fettstoff-wechsels beim Werner-Syndrom. Deut. Arch. Klin. Med. 208:553, 1963,

30. De Berardinis, E: Contributo allo studio delle cataratte sindermatotiche. Un case tipico di sindrone di Werner. Giorn. Ital. Oftalmol. 7:3, 1954.

31. Deuchar, D.C.: Werner's syndrome. Proc. Roy. Soc. Med. 49:316, 1956.

32. Doak, P.B. and Eyre, K.E.D.: Werner's syndrome. New Zeal. Med. J. 59:574, 1960.

33. Dobree, J.H.: Cataract, in Modern Opththalmology, ed. by

Sorsby, A., Butterworth and Co., Washington, 1964, p. 598.

34. Dumaine, L. and Lozeron, P.: Contribtion a l'etude clinique et genetique de la dystrophie myotonique (Steinert) et de la myotonie congenitale (Thomsen). J. Genet. Hum. 10:221, 1961.

35. Eguchi, H.: Uber Katarakte bei pluriglandularen Infantilismus mit Sklerodermie. Acta Soc. Opththal. Jap. 34:167 (in Japanese), 185 (in German), 1930.

36. Ellison, D.J. and Pugh, D.W.: Werner's syndrome. Brit. Med. J. 2:237, 1955.

37. Fedrizzi, G.: Sumorbo di Werner--studio clinico. Soc. Ophthal. Lombarda. Atti. (Milano).11:276, 1956.

38. Field, J.B. and Loube, S.D.: Observations concerning the diabetes mellitus associated with Werner's syndrome. Metabolism, 9:118, 1960.

39. Finney, D.J.: The truncated binomial distribution. Ann. Eugen. 14:319, 1949.

40. Flandin, C., Poumeau-Delille, G. and Olivier, J.: Un noveau cas familial de maladie de Rothmund. Bull. Soc. Med. Hop. Paris, 24:1181, 1936.

41. Flandin, C., Poumeau-Delille, G. and Perreau, R.: Syndrome pluriglandulaire, maladie de Rothmund. Bull. Soc. Med. Hop. Paris, 24:1184, 1936.

42. Force, B.P. and Powell, C.F.: Progeria in the adult (Werner's syndrome). U.S. Armed Forces Med. J. 1:578, 1950.

43. Forsham, P.H.: The adrenals, in Textbook of Endocrinology, 3rd Ed., ed. by Williams, R.H., W. B. Saunders Company, Philadelphia, & London, 1962, p. 282.

44. Fraccaro, M., Bott, M.G. and Calvert, H.T.: Chromosomes in Werner's syndrome. Lancet, 1:536, 1962.

45. Franceschetti, A. and Maeder, G.: Cataracte et affections cutanees du type poikilodermie (syndrome de Rothmund) et du type sclerodermie (syndrome de Werner). Schweiz. Med. Wschr. 79:657, 1949.

46. Gabr, M.: Progeria, a pathologic study. J. Pediat. 57:780, 1960.

47. Goldman, H.: Senile changes of the lens and the vitreous. Amer. J. Ophthal. 57: 1, 1964.

48. Goodman, D.S., Avigan, J. and Wilson, H.: The metabolism of desmosterol in human subjects during triparanol administration. J. Clin. Invest. 41:962, 1962.

49. Grant, A.P.: Werner syndrome (progeria in the adult). Ulster Med. J. 26: 65, 1957.

50. Greither, A.: Uber das Rothmund- und das Werner-syndrom. II. Die Symptomatologie des Werner-syndroms. III. Die Abgrenzung beider Zustande gegeneinander. Arch. Klin. Exp. Derm. 201:423; 431 , 1955.

51. Guillaine, G., Alajouanine, F. and Marquezy, R.: Sclerodermie progressive avec cataracte double precoce chez un infantile. Bull. Soc. med. Hop. Paris, 47:1489, 1923.

52. Haldane, J.B.S. and Smith, C.A.B.: A simple exact test for

birth order. Ann. Eugen. 14:117, 1948.

53.   Hamilton, H.B., Neel, J.V., Kobara, T.Y., and Ozaki, K.:
      Frequency in Japan of carriers of the rare "recessive" gene
      causing acatalasemia, J. Clin. Invest. 40: 2199, 1961.

54.   Hasimoto, T.P.: Ein Fall von Sklerodermie Kombiniert mit
      Katarakt. Jap. J. Derm. 30:90 (in Japanese), 130 (in German),
      1930.

55.   Hempelmann, L.H. and Hoffman, J.G.: Practical aspects of
      radiation injury. Ann. Rev. Nucl. Sci. 3:369, 1953.

56.   Herstone, S.K. and Bower, J.: Werner's syndrome. Amer. J.
      Roentgenol. 51:639, 1944.

57.   Hotchkiss, R.S.: Infertility in the male, in Urology, Vol. I,
      ed. by Campbell, M.F., Saunders, Philadelphia, 1963, p. 643.

58.   Illis, L.: A case of Werner's syndrome. Post-grad. Med. J.
      38:286, 1962.

59.   Incedayi, C.K.: Bir "Werner syndrome" u vak'asi. Instanbul.
      Univ. Tip fakultesi. Mecmua (Bull. Fac. Med. Istanbul),
      16:503, 1953.

60.   Irwin, G.W. and Ward, P.B.: Werner's syndrome, with report of
      two cases. Amer. J. Med. 15:266, 1953.

61.   Jablonska, S. and Segal, P.: Das Wernersche Syndrom und
      dessen atypische Formen, beziehungsweisse Verwandte Syndrome.
      Minerva Derm. 34:259, 1959.

62.   Jablonska, S., Segal, P. and Kukasiak, B.: Zespol Wernera
      (Werner's syndrome). Przegl. Derm. 8:277, 1958.

63.   Jacobs, P.A., Brunton, M., Court-Brown, of human chromosome
      count distributions with age: evidence for a sex difference.
      Nature, 197:1080, 1963.

64.   Jacobson, H.G., Rifkin, H. and Zucker-Franklin, D.: Werner's
      syndrome: a clinical roetgenological entity. Radiology,
      74:373, 1960.

65.   Jelek, M.: Pripad Wernerova syndromu leceny oxygenotherapii
      (A case of Werner's syndrome treated by oxygen). Cseck. Derm.
      (Praha), 32:263, 1957.

66.   Kallos, A. and Ruppe, J.P., Jr.: Werner's syndrome. New York
      J. Med. 54:2180, 1954.

67.   Kansky, A. and Franzot, J.: Werner's syndrome. Acta
      Dermatovener. 43:44, 1963.

68.   Karam, J.H., Grodsky, G.M., Pavlatos, F.C. and Forsham, P.H.:
      Critical factors in excessive serum-insulin response to
      glucose. Obesity in maturity onset diabetes and growth
      hormone in acromegaly. Lancet, 1:286, 1965.

69.   Kleeberg, J.: A case of Werner's syndrome. Acta Med. Orient
      (Tel Aviv) 8-9:145, 1949.

70.   Knap, J.: A case of Rothmund's disease. Acta Dermatovener.
      25:302, 1945.

71.   Knowth, W., Baethke, R., and Hoffman, L.: Uber das Werner-
      Syndrom. Ein Beitrag zur Kenntniss der Schilddruesenfunktion
      nach Radiojodstudium, der symptomatologie der
      Schrifttumsfaelle and der histologischen Differentialdiagnose

zum Rothmund-syndrom. Hautarzt 14:145; 193, 1963.

72. Korenchevsky, V.: Physiological and Pathological Aging.
Hafner, New York, 1961.

73. Krebs, E., Hartman, E. and Thiebaut, F.: Un cas familial de
syndrome de sclerodermie avec cataracte, troubles endocriniens
et neurovegetatifs associes. Rev. Neurol. 53:606, 1930.
Addendum in Rev. Neurol. 54:121, 1930.

74. Lapiere, S. Syndrome de Werner. Arch. Belges Derm. Syph.
9:315, 1953.

75. Learner, N., Day, H.J., Weiss, L. and Di-George, A.:
Chromosomes in Werner's syndrome. Lancet, 1:536, 1962.

76. Lerman, S.: Cataracts. Thomas, Springfield, Ill., 1963.

77. Lloyd, C.W.: The ovaries, in Textbook of Endocrinology, 3rd
Ed., ed. by Williams, R.H., W.B. Saunders Company,
Philadelphia & London, 1962, p. 446.

78. Louw, A.: Rothmund-Werner's disease. A case with internal
frontal hyperostosis. Acta Med. Scand. 121:333, 1945.

79. Louw, A.: To tlfaelde af Rothmund-Werner's sygdom (Two cases
of Werner's syndrome). Nord. Med. 37:2067, 1946.

80. Maeder, G.: Le syndrome de Rothmund et le syndrome de
Werner. (Etude clinique et diagnostique). Ann. Ocul.
182:809, 1949.

81. Matras, A. and Kohler, J.: Ein Beitrag zum Werner-
Syndrome. Wien. Med. Wschr. 106:437, 1956.

82. McKusick, V.: Medial Genetics 1962. J. Chron. Dis. 16:600,
1963.

83. Miller, M.: Diabetes associated with acromegaly,
hyperadrenocortecism, hemochromatosis, pancreatitis,
pancreatectomy, and cancer, in Diabetes, ed. by Williams,
R.H., Hoeber, New York, 1960, p. 710.

84. Minami, M., Kimura, S. and Matsumoto, K.: Two cases of
cataract by endocrine disturbance. J. Clin. Ophthal.
(Tokyo) (Ganka Rinsho Iho) 11:758, 1957.

85. Minton, L.R. and Bounds, G.W., Jr.: Ectodermal side effects
of MER-29. Ophthalmologic findings in patients with
ectodermal side effects while on MER-29. Amer. J. Ophthal.
55:787, 1963.

86. Mogensen, E.F.: Konveksitetsmeningeon hos en patient med
Werner's syndrome. Ugesk. Laeger. 155:18, 1953.

87. Monier-Vinard and Barbot, E.M.: Sclerodermie et cataracte.
Syndrome familial. Bull. Soc. Med. Hop. Paris, 52:708,
1928.

88. Monjukowa, N.: Zur Frage uber den Zusammenhang der
Linsentrubungen mit Storrungen de inneren sekretion. Russki
Opth. Zh. 2:174, 1923, and Klin, Mbl. Augache. 70:785,
1923.

89. Motulsky, A.G. and Gartler, S.M.: Consanguinity and
marriage. The Practitioner, 183:170, 1959.

90. Motulsky, A.G., Schultz, A. and Priest, J.: Werner's
syndrome: chromsomes, genes, and the ageing process.

Lancet 1:160, 1962.

91. Mueller, M.N., Sorenson, L.B., Stranjord, N. and Kappas, A.:
    Alkaptonuria and ochronotic arthopathy. Med. Clin. N. Amer.
    49:101, 1965.

92. Mueller, L. and Anderson, B.: Werner's syndrome: a survey
    based on two cases. Acta. med. Scand. Suppl 283:3, 1953.

93. Neel, J.V., Kodani, M., Bruer, R. and Anderson, R.C.: The
    incidence of consanguineous matings in Japan. Amer. J. Hum.
    Genet. 1:156, 1949.

94. Oppenheimer, B.S. and Kugel, V.H.: Werner's syndrome – a
    heredo-familial disorder with scleroderma, bilateral
    juvenile cataract, precocious graying of hair and endocrine
    stigmatization. Trans. Ass. Amer. Physicians, 49:358, 1934.

95. Oppenheimer, G.S. and Kugel, V.H.: Werner's syndrome:
    report of the first necropsy and of findings in a new case.
    Amer. J. Med. Sci. 202:629, 1941.

96. Ostensjo, B.: Werner's syndrome. Progeria genito-
    dystrophicum. Acta dermatovener. 33:497, 1953.

97. Paulsen, C.A.: The testes, in Textbook of Endocrinology.
    3rd Ed. ed. by Williams, R.H., W.B. Saunders Company,
    Philadelphia & London, 1962, p. 395.

98. Pearch, L. and Brown, W.H.: Hereditary premature senescence
    of the rabbit. I. Chronic form: general features. II.
    Acute form: general features. J. Exp. Med. 111:485; 505,
    1960.

99. Pentz, E.I., Moss, W.T. and Denko, C.W.: Factors
    influencing taurine excretion in human subjects. J. Clin.
    Endocr. 19:1126, 1959.

100. Perloff, J.K. and Phelps, E.T.: A review of Werner's
     syndrome, with a report of the second autopsied case. Ann.
     Intern. Med. 48:1205, 1958.

101. Peterson, R.E. and Wyngaarden, J.B.: The miscible pool and
     turnover rate of hydrocortisone in man. J. Clin. Invest.
     35:552, 1951.

102. Petrohelos, M.: Werner's syndrome: a survey of three
     cases, with review of the literature. Amer. J. Ophthal.
     56:941, 1963.

103. Pomeranz, M. M.: Werner's syndrome – a case report.
     Radiology, 51:521, 1948.

104. Reed, R., Seville, R.H. and Tattersall, R.N.: Werner's
     syndrome. Brit. J. Dermat. 65:165, 1953.

105. Rogers, A.S.: Werner's syndrome. Report of a case with
     unusual complications. J. Florida Med. Ass. 46:436, 1959.

106. Rothmund, A.: Uber Kataract in Verbindung mit einer
     eigentumlichen Hautdegeneration. Arch. f. Ophthal. 14:158,
     1868.

107. Rud, E.: Werner's syndrome in three siblings. Acta Opthal.
     34:255, 1956.

108. Russo, A.: Sindrome genito-sclerodermica e cataratta (Morbo
     di Rothmund). Ann. Ottal. 62:646, 1934.

109. Sainton, P. and Manou, H.: Hyperthyroidisme provoque par la thyroxine synthetique chez un malade atteint d'un syndrome pluriglandulaire avec sclerodermie et cataracte. Bull. Soc. Med. Hop. Paris, 51:1685, 1927.

110. Samols, E. and Bilkus, D.: A comparison of insulin immunoassays. Proc. Exp. Biol. Med. 115:79, 1964.

111. Sannicandro, G.: Sindrome di Rothmund con calcificazioni cutanee e sclerodermia progressiva. Loro rapporti con le lesioni delle paratiroidi. Arch. Ital. Derm. 11:88, 1935.

112. Scarpa, J.B. and Bur, G.E.: Sindrome de Rothmund-Werner: considerations clinicas y etiologicas. Med. Panamer 10:213, 1958.

113. Schott, J. and Dann, S.: Werner's syndrome, a report of two cases. New Engl. J. Med. 240:641, 1949.

114. Schultheisz, E. and Schultheisz, F.: Zwei Falle von Werner-syndrom. Wien. Klin. Wschr. 68:855, 1956.

115. Schwank, R., Stava, Z., Tesar, O. and Dvorak, L.: Pripad Wernerova syndrome (A case of Werner's syndrome). Ceskoslov. Derm. 28:365, 1953.

116. Selye, H., Strebele, R., and Mikulaj, L.: A progeria-like syndrome produced by dihydrotachysterol and its prevention by methyltestosterone and ferric dextran. J. Amer. Geriat. Soc. 11:1, 1963.

117. Setlow, R.B. and Carrier, W.L.: The disappearance of thymine dimers from DNA: an error-correcting mechanism. Proc. Nat. Acad. Sci. U.S. 51:226, 1964.

118. Sheets, R.F.: Werner's syndrome (Progeria of the adult). Amer. Practit. 1:300, 1950.

119. Simon, E.R. and Ways, P.: Incubation hemolysis and red cell metabolism in acanthocytosis. J. Clin. Invest. 43:1311, 1964.

120. Simpson, N.E.: Multifactorial inheritance. A possible hypothesis for diabetes. Diabetes 13:462, 1964.

121. Smith, J.M.: Review lectures on senescence. I. The causes of ageing. Proc. Roy. Soc. (Biol.) 157, 1962.

122. Smith, R.C., Winer, L.H. and Martel, S.: Werner's syndrome--report of two cases. Arch. Derm. 71:197, 1955.

123. Sourreil and Sarrat: Syndrome de Werner. Bull. Soc. Franc. Derm. Syph. 63: 207, 1956.

124. Steinberg, A.G.: Methodology in human genetics. J. Med. Ed. 34:315, 1959.

125. Stojanov, P.K. and Bajdekov, B.: On a limited symptomatology (Bulgarian). Savr. Med. 10:111, 1959.

126. Sulzberger, M.B.: Dyshormonal dermatosis (Werner's syndrome). (Scleroderma, poikiloderma, bilateral juvenile cataract, precocious graying of hair, pluriglandular dysfunction). Arch. Derm. Syph. 36:1256, 1937.

127. Szafran, L: Zacma wzwiazku ze schorzeniami skory (Cataract due to skin diseases). Klinika Oczna (Acta Ophthal. Polonica). 31:267, 1961.

128. Szondy, G.: Werner syndroma (Hungarian). Borgyogy. Vener.
     Szemle 13:94, 1959.

129. Tanner, J.M.: Growth at Adolescence. 2nd Ed., Blackwell
     Scientific Publications, Oxford, 1962, p. 192.

130. Teulires, J. and Chabot, J.: A propos d'un cas de maladie
     de Werner. Bull. Soc. Ophthal. Franc. 4:201, 1950.

131. Thannhauser, S.J.: Werner's syndrome (progeria of the
     adult) and Rothmunds syndrome: two types of closely related
     heredofamilial atrophic dermatosis with juvenile cataracts
     and endocrine features. A critical study with five new
     cases. Ann. Intern. Med. 23:559, 1945.

132. Upton, A.C.: Ionizing radiation and the aging process: a
     review. J. Gerontol. 12:306, 1957.

133. Valero, A. and Gellei, B.: Retinitis pigmentosa,
     hypertension and uraemia in Werner's syndrome. Report of a
     case with necropsy findings. Brit. Med. J. 2:351, 1960.

134. Von Arady, K.: Uber einige seltenere Symptome der
     Sklerodermie. Z. Klin. Med. 106:406, 1927.

135. Vossius, A.: Zwei Falle von Katarakt im Verbindung mit
     Sklerodermie. Z. Augenh. 43:640, 1920.

136. Waxman, S.H., Kelley, V.C., and Motulsky, A.G.: Adrenal
     function studies in Werner's syndrome. Clin. Res. 9:102,
     1961 (Abstract).

137. Werner, O. Uber Katarakt in Verbindung mit Sklerodermie.
     (Doctoral dissertation, Kiel University). Schmidt &
     Klaunig, Kiel, 1904.

138. Wettler, H.: Uber ein Fall von Wernerschem Syndrome.
     Opthalmologica 121:172, 1951.

139. Wilber, I.E.: Werner's syndrome. J. Amer. Med. Wom. Ass.
     15:584, 1960.

140. Wilkins, L.: The influence of the endocrine glands upon
     growth and development, in Textbook of Endocrinology, 3rd
     Ed., ed. by Williams, R.H., W.B., Saunders Company,
     Philadelphia & London, 1962, P. 908.

141. Williams, D.I.: Werner's syndrome. Proc. Roy. Soc. Med.
     42:572, 1949.

142. Winer, N.J.: Hamilton-Schwartz tet and hyperparathyroidism
     in various diseases. Amer. J. Med. Sci. 202:642, 1941.

143. Wolfram, G., Priegnitz, F. and Wagner, H.J.: Zum Werner-
     Syndrome (On Werner's syndrome). Deut. Med. Wschr.
     84:2125, 1959.

144. Worzel, M.H., Newman, J., and Toczek, H. A.: Werner's
     syndrome (A rare and most unusual genodermatosis). J.
     Newark Beth Israel Hosp. 15:40, 1964.

145. Zucker-Franklin, D.: Personal communication.

WERNER SYNDROME: A REVIEW OF RECENT RESEARCH WITH AN ANALYSIS OF
CONNECTIVE TISSUE METABOLISM, GROWTH CONTROL OF CULTURED CELLS, AND
CHROMOSOMAL ABERRATIONS

Darrell Salk

Division of Genetic Pathology, SM-30
University of Washington
Seattle, Washington 98195 USA

ABSTRACT

    Werner syndrome is a rare, autosomal recessive condition
with multiple progeroid features, but it is a phenocopy of aging
rather than accelerated or premature senescence. Somatic
chromosome aberrations occur in multiple tissues in vivo and in
vitro and there is an increased incidence of neoplasia. Thus,
Werner syndrome can be classified in the group of chromosome
instability syndromes. Recent findings provide additional support
for the concept that there is an aberration of connective tissue
metabolism in Werner syndrome, but it is unclear whether this is a
primary or secondary manifestation of the underlying genetic
defect. Abnormal growth characteristics are observed in cultured
skin fibroblast-like cells and this provides another avenue for
current research. Identification of the basic genetic defect in
Werner syndrome might clarify our understanding of the normal aging
process in general, or might elucidate specific aspects such as
the development of neoplasia, atherosclerosis, diabetes, or
osteoporosis.

INTRODUCTION

    Werner syndrome is a rare, autosomal recessive condition in
which young adults display clinical features similar to those
observed in elderly individuals. It is sometimes called "adult

Reprinted from Human Genetics 62:1-15, 1982

progeria" but there are clearly differences between Werner syndrome
and the normal aging process: It is a partial phenocopy rather than
progeria in the sense of precocious or accelerated aging. Recent
evidence indicates that Werner syndrome can be considered a
chromosome instability syndrome similar to xeroderma pigmentosum,
ataxia telangiectasia, Fanconi anemia, and Bloom syndrome. Because
it is inherited in an autosomal recessive fashion, Werner syndrome
is presumably caused by a single gene defect or a small multigene
deletion. It thus provides an opportunity to explore a cascade of
biologic and biochemical events that lead to a partial phenocopy of
aging. Understanding the basic molecular defect in Werner syndrome
may provide insight into the general biology of aging as well as
into the development of specific geriatric diseases.

Historical Background

While working as a medical student in the Ophthalmology Clinic
at Kiel, Otto Werner (1904) published a description of four
siblings with "scleroderma" in association with cataracts.
Oppenheimer and Kugel (1934;1941) drew attention to the condition
in America and reported the first autopsy examination of a case.
Thannhauser (1945) reviewed the reported cases to that date and
made three important contributions: He emphasized that the skin
changes in Werner syndrome were different from those of classical
scleroderma, he provided a list of twelve principal
characteristics, and he included in that listing the tendency of
the condition to occur in siblings.

Epstein and his colleagues (1966) described three new patients
and reviewed 122 other reported cases. This review by Charles
Epstein, George M. Martin, Amelia Schultz and Arno Motulsky stands
as a landmark in Werner syndrome research: The natural history of
the condition was defined and the pathological and histological
changes were extensively documented. Pedigree analysis confirmed
autosomal recessive inheritance and the gene frequency was
estimated. Skin fibroblast-like (FL) cells were cultured for the
first time and noted to grow poorly. These researchers emphasized
the differences between Werner syndrome and natural aging, despite
remarkable clinical similarities, and referred to the condition as
a "caricature" of aging.

Since 1966 interest in Werner syndrome has expanded and there
have been a number of reports of both clinical and in vitro
studies. Japanese researchers have made several important
contributions including the identification of 15 living patients by
M. Goto et al. (1978) and an additional nine patients·by Murata and
Nakashima (1982), an analysis of 42 families that confirmed
autosomal recessive inheritance (Goto et al., 1981), and
identification of a new clinical characteristic of Werner syndrome,
excessive excretion of hyaluronic acid in urine (Tokunaga et al.,

1975; Goto and Murata, 1978; Goto et al., 1978; Murata, 1982).
Italian researchers have recently identified three unrelated
families with at least ten affected members (Rabbiosi and Borroni,
1979; Cerimele et al., 1982). In our own laboratory, we have
analyzed two unusual characteristics of cultured skin FL cells from
Werner syndrome patients: Reduced growth potential (Martin et al.,
1970; Salk et al., 1981a) and somatic chromosome rearrangements
(Hoehn et al., 1975; Salk et al., 1981b). Chromosome aberrations
have recently been confirmed in FL cells and observed in peripheral
blood lymphocytes (Schonberg et al., 1981, 1982; Scappaticci et al.,
1982).

     The purpose of this paper is to review selected studies of
Werner syndrome reported in the fifteen years since Epstein et
al.'s (1966) summary. I will begin with a brief discussion of the
clinical and genetic features of Werner syndrome as described by
Epstein et al. (1966) and updated by others. Then I will discuss
in detail research in three specific areas: Connective tissue
abnormalities, control of growth in cultured skin fibroblasts, and
chromosomal aberrations.

CLINICAL FEATURES

     Thannhauser (1945) listed 12 principal characteristics of
Werner syndrome: 1) Shortness of stature and a characteristic
habitus (thin extremities with stocky trunk); 2) premature greying
of the hair; 3) premature baldness; 4) patches of apparently
stiffened skin, particularly in the face and lower extremities
("scleropoikiloderma"); 5) trophic ulcers of the legs; 6) juvenile
cataracts; 7) hypogonadism; 8) tendency to diabetes; 9)
calcification of blood vessels; 10) osteoporosis; 11) metastatic
calcifications; and 12) tendency to occur in siblings. The skin
changes are interesting because the apparent stiffening is not
scleroderma, but is usually the result of dermal atrophy over areas
in which subcutaneous adipose tissue is depleted. This results in
shiny, smooth skin that is adherent to underlying tissues.

     Several other characteristic features of Werner syndrome have
subsequently been described. Epstein et al. (1966) pointed out that
almost half of the 125 patients they reviewed were said to have
thin, high-pitched, or hoarse voices, and laryngeal abnormalities
were observed in half of the patients studied by laryngoscopy.
These authors also emphasized the increased incidence of neoplasia,
as discussed below. Goto et al. (1978) commented on the presence of
flat feet, hyperreflexia, and excessive urinary excretion of
hyaluronic acid in all 15 of their patients. Murata and Nakashima
(1982) noted, in addition, irregular dental development in 10 of 15
patients examined.

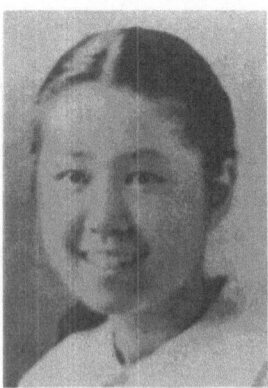 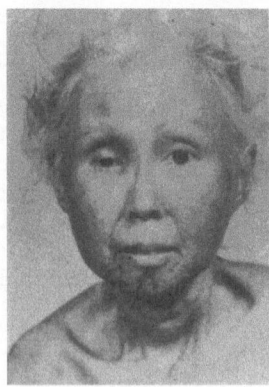 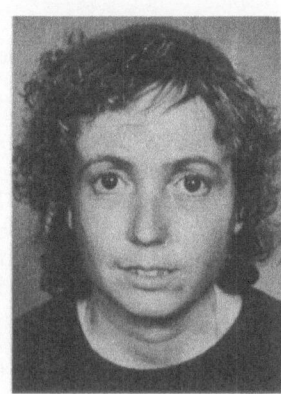

Figure 1: The two photographs on the left show a Japanese-
American woman as a teenager and at 48 years of age (case
1 in Epstein et al., 1966; reproduced with permission of
the author and Williams & Wilkens Co., Baltimore). Her
parents were not known to be related but came from the
same small town in Japan. She had eight siblings, two of
whom were also affected. At 48 years of age she was
short and had thin extremities. The skin of her feet and
legs was thin, taut, and dry, and she had chronic
ulcerations over the malleoli and Achilles tendons. The
senile appearance of her face resulted from the
combination of atrophy of the skin and soft tissues and
graying and loss of hair. The right eye had been
enucleated several years previously after an attack of
acute glaucoma following bilateral cataract extractions
at 27 years of age. She required above-the-knee
amputation at 54 years of age because of chronic foot
ulcers, and died at 57 years of age following a
protracted illness involving urinary tract infection and
bilateral bronchopneumonia.

The photograph on the right is a 29-year-old woman
reported by Gottesman et al. (1980). She shows the
characteristic facial appearance: Round face with thin,
beaked nose and thin lips. She was the tallest girl in
her class during elementary school, but did not grow
during adolescence and gradually became the shortest in
her class. She noted the appearance of grey hairs
starting at 14 years of age and visual symptoms due to
cataracts at about the same time. By age 29 she was
aware of skin changes, primarily thickening of skin on
the lower legs and ankles, and had the characteristic
habitus with thin extremities. Her parents are not known
to be related but their families lived in small
communities in neighboring valleys in Switzerland.
(Photograph courtesy of Dr. Mark Mumenthaler, University
of Berne, Switzerland.)

Among the patients reported by Epstein, the initial diagnosis
of Werner syndrome was made at 38.7 (21-58) years although signs
and symptoms had generally appeared several years earlier. In
retrospect, some features may have been apparent in childhood since
many patients were described as having been small with thin
extremities, and since shortness of stature (a constant feature)
was due to cessation of growth at approximately 13 (10-18) years of
age. The age of appearance of the typical features varied widely
but averaged as follows: Greying of hair, 20 years; skin changes,
25.3 years; loss of hair, 25.8 years; alterations of the voice,
26.6 years; visual symptoms or detection of cataracts, 30 years;
skin ulcers, 30 years; and diabetes, 34.2 years. The average age
at death was 47 (31-63) years; the two principal causes being
malignancy and myocardial or cerebrovascular accidents. Murata and
Nakashima (1982) found similar ages of onset in their review of 177
Japanese cases. Figure 1 shows two women with several of these
features.

A complete review of the symptomatology, pathology, and
clinical studies of Werner syndrome is beyond the scope of this
article; for further details the reader is referred to the
extensive clinical reviews by Epstein et al. (1966), Zucker-Franklin
et al. (1968), Goto et al. (1978), and Murata and Nakashima (1982).
However, four aspects deserve special mention: Neoplasia, the
immune and endocrine systems, and a comparison of the features of
Werner syndrome with the features of normal aging.

Neoplasia

There is an increased incidence of neoplasia in Werner
syndrome. Epstein et al. (1966) emphasized the unusual number of
non-carcinomatous tumors: 13 (10%) of the patients had significant
neoplasms; one patient had two and among the 14 tumors there were
seven malignant sarcomas, three meningiomas, and only four
carcinomas. Goto et al. (1981) reviewed 195 patients reported in
the Japanese literature: They found 11 patients (5.6%) with
malignant tumors, a relatively high incidence in Japan, although
not as high as that reported by Epstein et al. (1966). They also
noted the unusual number of neoplasms of mesenchymal origin and
pointed out that although there were several rare tumors, there
were no cases of prostatic or pancreatic cancer (common among
elderly patients), nor gastric or lung cancer (common in Japan).
These authors also report for the first time a relatively high
incidence of cancer deaths among siblings of patients with Werner
syndrome: 4.2% compared with 0.11% in the general Japanese
population.

Table 1 summarizes the tumors reported in patients with Werner
syndrome. The unusual number of mesenchymal tumors is evident,
including a surprisingly large number of meningiomas. The

TABLE 1. Tumors reported in patients with Werner's syndrome.

Ref*	Age	Sex	Tumor
			MESENCHYMAL
			(Malignant)
1	38	M	Fibroliposarcoma
2	–	–	"
3	31	M	Fibrosarcoma (unspecified origin)
4	+44	M	" (unspecified origin)
5	++46	M	" (mediastinum)
3	61	F	" (unspecified origin)
1	42	F	Hemangiolipoma with occasional mitosis
1	36	F	Leiomyosarcoma (uterus)
3	40	M	" (unspecified origin)
6	+++45	F	Malignant myofibroxanthoma
1	42	F	Melanotic sarcoma
1	>52	F	Nerve sheath sarcoma
1	49	F	Osteogenic sarcoma
7	50	F	"
1	39	F	Spindle cell sarcoma
			MESENCHYMAL
			(Benign)
8	28	M	Meningioma
1	34	F	"
9	39	M	"
4	41	M	"
1	++++42	F	"
4	+44	M	"
1	51	M	"
10	51	F	"
11	56	M	"
3	–	–	Fibroadenoma (breast)
3	–	–	Lymphangioma
3	–	–	Leiomyoma (uterus)
1	42	F	" "
			EPITHELIAL
			(Malignant)
3	53	M	Carcinoma of bladder
1	41	F	Carcinoma of breast
3	46	F	"
1	36	M	Carcinoma of hepatic duct
3	60	M	Carcinoma of larynx
2	–	–	Carcinoma of liver

Ref	Age	Sex	Tumor
1	++++42	F	"
6	+++45	F	Carcinoma of ovary (papillary cystadeno-)
12	48	M	Carcinoma of prostate (undifferentiated)
3	42	F	Carcinoma of thyroid (anaplastic giant cell)
1	39	M	" (papillary)
13	29	M	Carcinoma of skin (basal cell)
13	46	F	" (basal cell)
5	++57	M	" (multiple basal cell)
14	56	M	" (squamous cell)
13	40	M	Carcinoma of stomach
3	49	M	Cholangiocarcinoma
3	37	F	Pseudomyxoma peritonei (ovary)

EPITHELIAL
(Benign)

Ref	Age	Sex	Tumor
4	42	F	Adenoma of the thyroid
3	-	-	6 patients with adenoma of the thyroid
2	-	-	1 patient with microfollicular adenomata of the thyroid
1	-	-	"Several" patients with adenoma of the thyroid or adrenal

OTHER
(Malignant)

Ref	Age	Sex	Tumor
15	24	F	Leukemia (Acute myeloblastic)
6	32	M	" (Acute)
3	36	M	" (Acute myelocytic)
3	40	F	Melanoma

Footnotes
+, ++, +++, ++++ Patients with two tumors
*References are as follows: (1) Epstein et al, 1966; (2) Zucker-Franklin, 1968; (3) Goto et al, 1981; (4) Nakao et al, 1980; (5) Hrabko et al, 1982; (6) Bjornberg, 1976; (7) Rosen et al, 1970; (8) Kobayashi et al, 1980; (9) Tokunaga et al, 1976; (10) Our own unpublished observation of case 2 in Epstein et al, 1966; (11) Hoppe and Koritsch, 1972; (12) Martin et al, 1970; (13) Rabbiosi and Borroni, 1979; (14) Zalla, 1980; (15) Tao et al, 1971.

carcinomas are not particulary unusual but there is a relative
paucity of tumors commonly observed in the general population:
Lung, skin, prostate, colon, and ovary.

Immune System

It has been suggested that abnormalities of the immune system
may be associated with aging, either as cause or effect (Burnet,
1970; Makinodan et al., 1975; Buckley and Roseman, 1976; Yunis et
al, 1976). A number of authors have therefore studied aspects of
the immune system in Werner syndrome. Although there is some
variability, most parameters are reported to be normal, as
summarized in Table 2.

Abnormalities in the B-cell and complement systems were noted
in only one study (Nakao et al., 1980). The percentage of B-cells
that became positive for cytoplasmic immunoglobulin in response to
pokeweed mitogen was reduced in three of four patients, and total
hemolytic complement (CH50) was reduced in three of four patients.
There were occasional reports of elevated immunoglobulin levels,
probably due to intercurrent infections.

With regard to cellular immunity, the percentage of T-
lymphocytes were normal or low normal and the pattern appears to be
similar to that observed with normal aging, including a shift in
the Tμ/Tμ ratio. The interpretation of these findings is
complicated by the fact that many family members studied at the
same time also had low Tμ/Tμ ratios, and it should be noted that no
functional abnormalities have been observed (Gupta, 1981). The
response of lymphocytes to concanavalin-A was slightly reduced in
three of six patients tested, but the response to
phytohemagglutinin was almost uniformly normal. Epstein et al.
(1966) noted that there was lymphoid depletion in all available
autopsy material; however, this might be related to a patient's
chronic or terminal illness, and in any case is a concomitant of
normal aging. One significant difference from normal aging is
that eight of twelve patients examined had naturally occurring
anti-T cell antibodies; other autoantibodies were not observed.

No unusual association of HLA type has been reported in
studies of 19 patients (Goldstein and Singal, 1974; Djawari et al.,
1980; Nakao et al., 1980; Goto et al., 1981). Expression of HLA
antigens on lymphocytes is normal, but is reported to be reduced in
cultured skin fibroblasts from the three patients who were studied
(Goldstein and Singal, 1974; Nakao et al., 1980).

In summary, the phenotypic changes affecting immune function
are complicated and the progeroid manifestations in Werner syndrome
are probably not due to any primary deficiency in immune function.

Table 2.

Studies of the immune system in patients with Werner Syndrome. Results are shown as normal (N), increased or decreased (↑ or ↓), or present or absent (+ or -). The numbers in parenthesis refer to the number of patients with the indicated results/total number of patients tested).

Reference[a]:	1	2	3	4	5	6	7	8	Summary
Humoral immune system									
% B cells:		N(7/7)	N(5/5)		↓(1/1)	N(1/1)	N(1/1)	N(1/1)	N(15/16)
Response to									
PWM[b]:			↓(3/4)						↓(3/4)
SpA[c]:			N(5/5)						N(5/5)
Serum Ig[d]:	N(7/7)		N(5/5)		↑(1/1)	N(1/1)		N(1/1)	N(15/16)
Complement									
CH50[e]:			↓(3/4)						↓(3/4)
C3:			↑(2/4)				N(1/1)		N(3/5)
C4:			↓(2/4)				N(1/1)		N(3/5)
Cellular immune system									
% T cells:	↓(2/6)	N(7/7)	↓(2/5)	N(2/2)	↓(1/1)	N(1/1)	N(1/1)	N(1/1)	N(17/24)
T /T ratio:			↑↓(2/4)	↓(3/4)					↓(4/8)
Response to									
PHA[f]:			N(5/5)		↓(1/1)	N(1/1)		N(1/1)	N(8/9)
Con-A[g]:			↓(2/5)			↓(1/1)			↓(3/6)
MLR[h]:			N(5/5)						N(5/5)
DHSR[i]:	N(15/15)		N(5/5)		-(1/1)	N(1/1)	N(1/1)	N(1/1)	N(23/24)
LMIF[j]:			N(3/3)			N(1/1)			N(4/4)
Phagocytic function									
Phagocytosis:							N(1/1)		N(7/7)
Chemotaxis:			N(4/4)				N(1/1)		N(5/5)
Killing[k]:							↓(1/1)		↓(1/1)
Autoantibodies									
NTA[l]		+(6/7)	+(2/5)						+(8/12)
Other[m]		+(4/7)	N(5/5)			N(1/1)	N(1/1)	N(1/1)	N(12/15)

(Table 2 continued next page)

(Table 2 continued)

Footnotes:

a References are (1) Goto et al., 1978; (2) Goto et al., 1979; (3) Nakao et al., 1980; (4) Gupta, 1981; (5) Salamon et al., 1978; (6) Blohme and Smith, 1979: (7) Djawari et al., 1980; (8) Beadle et al., 1978.

b Pokeweed mitogen

c Staphylococcus aureus protein A – Sepharose 4B

d Serum immunoglobulins

e Hemolytic complement

f Phytogemagglutinin

g Concanavalin-A

h One way mixed lymphocyte response

i Delayed-type hypersensitivity reaction (skin testing)

j Production of leukocyte migration inhibition factor

k Intracellular killing oc Candida albicans

l Naturally occurring anti-T cell antibody

m The autoantibodies and number of patients tested are as follows: antinuclear antibody (ANA) (14), rheumatoid factor (8), anti-DNA (13), anti-thyroid (6), anti-smooth muscle (6), anti-gastric (1), anti-pituitary (1), anti-pancreas (1), anti-mitochondria (1), anti-insulin receptor (1). Four patients in Goto et al., (1979) had low titres f anti-nuclear antibody.

Although there is apparently no associated functional abnormality, the presence of naturally occurring anti-T cell antibody is intriguing and may deserve further exploration.

Endocrine System

Dysfunction of a variety of endocrine glands has been implicated in Werner syndrome by different authors. Epstein et al. (1966) noted the variable results and concluded that the only relatively consistent endocrine abnormalities are those associated with a clinical tendency to diabetes and, in some patients, hypogonadism that cannot generally be defined as either hyper- or hypogonadotropic. The majority of reports of pituitary, thyroid, parathyroid, and adrenal function are normal, although at the time, growth hormone measurement had not been performed. They pointed out that growth hormone was of particular interest because of the characteristic failure of the adolescent growth spurt in Werner syndrome.

Since the review by Epstein et al. (1966), many reports have included endocrine and/or metabolic studies of Werner syndrome patients (Riley et al., 1965; Gibbs, 1967; Zucker-Franklin et al., 1968; Rosen et al., 1970; Fleishmajer and Nedwich, 1973; Alberti et al, 1974; Aram and Fatourechi, 1974; Zackai et al., 1974; Bjornberg, 1976; Beadle et al., 1978; Goto et al., 1978; Nakao et al., 1978; Blohme and Smith, 1979; Rabbiosi and Borroni, 1979; Angel et al., 1980; Corrales Hernandez et al., 1980; Gottesman et al., 1980; Kobayashi et al., 1980; Smith et al., 1980; Hrabko, 1982; Murata and Nakashima, 1982). As in earlier studies, hormone levels have been variable but principally normal. In particular, fasting growth hormone levels have been reported to be normal in all the patients studied, except the one of Blohme and Smith (1979) who used a technique that could not detect low levels (Riley et al., 1965; Alberti et al., 1974; Zackai et al., 1974; Beadle et al., 1978; Nakao et al., 1978; Angel et al., 1980; Corrales Hernandez et al., 1980). Alberti et al. (1974) found no growth hormone response to stimulation with tolbutamide, insulin, or arginine in their patient; however Zackai et al. (1974), Beadle et al. (1978), and Nakao et al. (1978) found normal growth hormone responses to insulin and/or arginine in four patients and a poor response in only one.

The manifestations of diabetes in Werner syndrome are mild and generally can be controlled by diet alone. Fasting blood sugar levels are normal or only slightly elevated, and ketoacidosis and vascular complications are uncommon. There is relative insulin insensitivity, indicated by the ineffectiveness of insulin therapy, the poor response to insulin tolerance tests, and the hyperinsulinism observed in the fasting state and/or in response to glucose tolerance tests or arginine stimulation. An interesting,

although isolated finding was that of Kobayashi et al. (1980) who
observed correction of hyperinsulinism following surgery for a
large meningioma. Serum insulin binding capacity is normal and
anti-insulin antibodies have not been found (Beadle et al., 1978;
Blohme and Smith, 1979).

This pattern of diabetes is similar to the late-onset type and
that observed in obese patients, and to the rare congenital
lipodystrophy (lipoatrophic diabetes). Because of the similarity
with lipoatrophic diabetes, Field and Loube (1960) suggested that
the loss of subcutaneous fat and a relative absence of fat depots
in Werner syndrome were responsible for the diabetic
manifestations.   Zucker-Franklin et al. (1968) pointed out,
however, that lipoatrophy in Werner syndrome is limited to the
extremities, and Epstein et al. (1966) emphasized that the diabetes
was also similar to the more common, age-associated type. Alberti
et al. (1974) suggested that there may be a decreased response of
peripheral insulin receptors; Nakao et al. (1978) extended this
suggestion to an alteration of a diversity of proteins affecting
hormone receptors in general.

Beadle et al. (1978) directly measured insulin receptors in
isolated fat cells from abdominal subcutaneous adipose tissue of a
woman with Werner syndrome. They found that the fat cells were
extremely large and that the density of insulin receptors on the
cells was decreased, but that the affinity of insulin receptors was
normal. Smith et al. (1980) made similar in vitro measurements of
abdominal adipocytes from another patient: They observed
extremely large cells, an increased lipolytic response to
catecholamines, a reduction in the number of insulin receptors to
about 25 percent of normal, and a decreased antilipolytic effect
of insulin. In an interesting reversal of the suggestion that
diabetes in Werner syndrome results from lipoatrophy and a
reduced fat storage capacity (Field and Loube, 1960), Smith et
al. (1980) suggest that "regional adiposity" of abdominal tissue,
with markedly enlarged fat cells, may be responsible for the
diabetes and metabolic alterations in Werner syndrome that are of
the type usually observed in obesity associated with an increase
of total body fat. They propose that lipoatrophy in the
extremities leads to enlargement of the remaining fat cells with
subsequent increased lipolysis, raised plasma free fatty acids,
and reduced glucose metabolism. This might then result in
hyperinsulinism and peripheral insulin resistance. One
difficulty with this proposal is that variable levels of free
fatty acids are reported in Werner syndrome patients, mostly in
the normal range. In addition, any changes in insulin receptor
concentration associated with normal aging have yet to be
explored.

In summary, the endocrine manifestations of Werner syndrome are hypogonadism of uncertain etiology in some patients and a tendency to develop mild diabetes. In view of the observed functional abnormalities, the lack of complications that are usually associated with diabetes mellitus is striking. The relationship between the diabetes observed in Werner syndrome and that observed in obese or elderly patients remains to be elucidated; a variety of cause and effect mechanisms have been proposed. Recent studies of isolated adipocytes provide intriguing clues for further research.

Comparison with Normal Aging

Some clinical features are common to both Werner syndrome and normal aging, such as vascular disease (atherosclerosis, arteriosclerosis, medial calcinosis), greying of the hair, hypermelanosis, lymphoid depletion and thymic atrophy. Other features are similar but occur more severely and to a greater extent in Werner syndrome: Valvular calcification, osteoporosis, testicular atrophy, and atrophy of the skin appendages. Certain features commonly associated with aging occur to a lesser extent or not at all in Werner syndrome: Senile keratosis and other malignant skin lesions, senile elastosis, hyalinization of pancreatic islets, deposition of lipofuscin pigment, and the presence of corpora amylacea in the brain and spinal cord. The absence of clinical or pathological signs of senile dementia is particularly noteworthy (Martin, 1978) although one patient was reported to have "organic brain syndrome without psychosis" (Fleischmajer and Nedwich, 1973) and Murata and Nakashima (1982) comment that mild senile dementia "appeared occasionally" among their 24 patients.

The major contrasts between Werner syndrome and natural aging are related to certain of the signs considered pathognomonic of the former: Cataracts, skin ulcerations, laryngeal pathology, atrophy of the distal extremities, hyaluronic aciduria, and a relatively high incidence of noncarcinomatous neoplasia. (Although cataracts frequently occur in normal aging, the pathologic appearance is different from the posterior cortical and subcapsular opacities observed in Werner syndrome.) The major differences between Werner syndrome and natural aging are outlined in Table 3.

Genetic Features

The inheritance of Werner syndrome is most compatible with being autosomal recessive. This was demonstrated in 53 sibships by an analysis of the proportion of sibs affected using two different techniques: Correction of ascertainment loss by the simple sib method and by the truncate ascertainment method (Epstein et al., 1966). The resulting estimates ($17.9 \pm 2.5\%$ and $26.5 \pm 3.2\%$) are

reasonably close to the 25% expected for an autosomal recessive
condition. Consanguinity rates are increased among affected
families, the sex ratio of affected individuals is nearly 1:1,
and there is no birth order effect. Similar results have been
reported from an analysis of 42 families in Japan (Goto et al.,
1981). No heterozygote manifestations have been identified, with
the possible exception of early greying of the hair (Epstein et
al., 1966) and increased cancer deaths (Goto et al., 1981).

Using data derived from reports throughout the world, Epstein
et al.. (1966) calculated that the homozygote frequency was between
1 and 22 cases per million population. Goto et al. (1981) used
data from Japan and derived a frequency that is the same order of
magnitude: Between 3 and 45 cases per million population. It is
likely that the incidence in Japan is greater than in the United
States because of more frequent consanguinous marriages. These
calculations indicate that there should be between 110 and 2400
recognizable patients (those more than 30 years of age) with
Werner syndrome in the United States. In fact, I am aware of
fewer than five living patients in this country. This
discrepancy is probably due to the lack of awareness of this rare
disorder among primary care physicians.

Connective Tissue

Epstein et al. (1966) noted that many of the changes in
Werner syndrome were suggestive of an impairment in the
development and metabolism of connective tissue. In addition to
such obvious features as skin changes, osteoporosis, and soft
tissue calcifications, they pointed out the relatively high

Table 3. Principal differences between Werner syndrome and
normal aging.

	Werner syndrome	Aging
Inheritance:	Autosomal recessive	Universal; multi-factorial
Short stature:	Primary	Acquired
Laryngeal abnormalities:	Common	Uncommon
Cataracts:	Juvenile	Senile
Soft tissue calcifications:	Common	Uncommon
Osteoporosis:	Peripheral (limbs)	Central (spine)
Hypertension:	Uncommon	Common
Neoplasia:	Many sarcomas, meningiomas	Mostly carcinomas
Central nervous system:	No changes	Senile changes
Hyaluronic aciduria:	Present	Absent

incidence of mesenchymal tumors and the sharply restricted
lifespan of cultured skin fibroblasts. The two major components
of connective tissue are collagen and proteoglycans. Both of
these types of macromolecules show changes with increasing
age (Hall, 1981; Robert, 1981) but recent studies have also
suggested there may be additional, specific aberrations of
connective tissue metabolism in patients with Werner syndrome.

Collagen

Tokunaga et al. (1979) noted increased urinary excretion of
glucosylgalactose in some but not all patients with a variety of
diseases affecting connective tissue: Chondrosarcoma, rheumatoid
arthritis, Werner syndrome, Rothmund-Thomson syndrome, and
Morquio disease. Glucosylgalactose is a disaccharide thought to
be a metabolite of collagen and/or glycoproteins in connective
tissue. This observation of excess excretion in some patients
but not in others suggests that it is a secondary manifestation
related to an individual's overall clinical status rather than to
a specific disease.

Reports of histologic examination of collagen in the skin of
patients with Werner syndrome have ranged from normal to abnormal,
a fact that may reflect differences between studies of tissue from
"scleroderma-like lesions" and from relatively normal-appearing
skin. In their 1966 review, Epstein et al. reported that dermal
collagen had been variously described as hyalinized, thickened,
frayed, or disorganized. Smith et al. (1955) and Ishii and Hosoda
(1975) stated that skin collagen appeared normal, and Rabbiosi and
Borroni (1979) found no hyalinization of dermal collagen in seven
patients in a single family. Tannenbaum (1965) reported normal
histology of abdominal skin but abnormal findings in a
hyperkeratotic region of the foot: Collagen fibrils appeared
curled, wavy, and interlocking, yet individually distinct.
Fleischmajer and Nedwich (1973) studied skin from a scleroderma-
like lesion on the foot and observed normal collagen in the upper
and mid-layers of the dermis, but hyalinization of collagen at
lower levels with thin, poorly defined fibrils blending into the
surrounding ground substance. Beadle et al. (1978) described
basophilic degeneration of collagen and elastic fibers in the
dermis. Gottesman et al. (1980) examined a biopsy of "paper-thin
skin" and reported no noticeable changes of collagen fibrils. In
an unpublished study of autopsy derived skin from a woman with
Werner syndrome (case 3 in Epstein et al., 1966), R. Iozzo of the
University of Washington observed diffuse collagenization
throughout the dermis, in addition to the usual findings of
atrophy of skin appendages, thinning of the epidermis, and
flattened rete ridges (personal communication, 1980).

Chemical analysis of skin from scleroderma-like lesions has revealed an absolute increase in hydroxyproline content, but no difference in hydroxyproline concentration (mg/g dry weight dermis) (Fleishmajer and Nedwich, 1973; Rabbiosi and Borroni, 1979). This is probably due to replacement of subcutaneous fat by connective tissue containing normal collagen, although there is an apparent abnormality of constituent proteoglycans (see below). Alberti et al. (1974) examined a biopsy from skin without lesions and reported increased soluble collagen with polymeric collagen abnormally unstable for the patient's age. Interestingly, Fleischmajer and Nedwich (1973) also noted an increase in soluble collagen.

Analysis of collagen in cultured skin fibroblast-like cells has been inconclusive. Tajima et al. (1978) reported that cultures of skin from Werner syndrome patients accumulate much more hydroxyproline than normal control cultures, and that the kinetics of accumulation differ between Werner cultures derived from areas of dermal atrophy or from areas of relatively normal appearing skin. These results are difficult to interpret, however, because a small number of normal and Werner cultures of relatively different in vitro age were compared. The lifespan of Werner syndrome fibroblast-like cells is markedly reduced (Salk et al., 1981a) and thus Werner syndrome cultures in passages 1-5, as studied by Tajima et al., may already be senescent or at least demonstrate differences in proliferative activity durng the assay period. Basler et al. (1979) showed that senescent cultures of both normal and Werner syndrome fibroblast-like cells accumulate intracellular and extracellular fibrous debris that was interpreted to be incompletely processed collagen precursor molecules. In preliminary studies of procollagen synthesis by cultures of proliferating mid-passage Werner syndrome and normal fibroblast-like cells, we did not observe qualitative or quantitative differences in the electrophoretic pattern of procollagen molecules on polyacrylamide gels (Salk and Bornstein, unpublished results).

Electron microscopy of skin has yielded more consistently abnormal results. Reed et al. (1953) examined collagen extracted from a biopsy of "scleroderma-like" skin and reported apparently normal collagen fibrils coated with amorphorous debris that could be removed by trypsin treatment; in their published electron micrograph the collagen fibrils are of variable diameter. In a biopsy specimen from an area of thin skin from the leg, Gottesman et al. (1980) observed loose bundling of collagen fibrils, abnormal distribution of fibril diameters, and frequent microfibrillar elements among regular fibrils. A. Vogel at the University of Zurich has continued studies of this material and describes normal banding patterns, an increased amount of fiber bending (as observed in some cases of Ehlers-Danlos syndrome),

bimodality of fibril diameters in some regions but perfectly
normal appearing collagen in other areas. In addition, in the
sub-epidermis (0.2-0.5 mm deep) he observes fibroblasts branching
and interdigitating with collagen bundles, an unusual finding in
normal skin (A. Vogel, personal communication, 1981). Other
unpublished ultrastructural studies of autopsy-derived tissue
obtained from a region of relatively normal appearing skin (Case
3 in Epstein et al., 1966) revealed fraying of collagen fibrils
and variable fibril diameters, even within the same fiber (R.
Iozzo, personal communication, 1980).

These varied observations of abnormal collagen in Werner
syndrome suggest some disturbance of collagen metabolism, but the
mechanism remains to be determined. It is possible that these
abnormalities are a secondary manifestation of some other, more
general defect of cellular metabolism.

Proteoglycans

An abnormality in proteoglycan metabolism might explain
several findings in Werner syndrome, including abnormal collagen
fiber formation since proteoglycans and their constituent
glycosaminoglycans (GAGs) form important structural links between
the cellular and intercellular compartment of all tissues (Wight,
1980). These macromolecules also influence or are influenced by
many different cell processes fundamental to morphogenesis and
aging (Mourao and Machado-Santelli, 1978; Schachtschabel and
Wever, 1978; Elliot and Gardner, 1979; Sweet et al., 1979; Oohira
and Nogami, 1980; Wever et al.,1980; Fellini et al., 1981;
Matuoka and Mitsui, 1981a, 1981b; Sluke et al., 1981; Vogel et
al., 1981). There have been several studies of
glycosaminoglycans both in vivo and in vitro in Werner syndrome,
however techniques for evaluation of the complete proteoglycan
molecule have not yet been applied.

Skin from "scleroderma-like lesions" of Werner syndrome
patients contains an increase in the absolute amount of hexosamines
(Fleischmajer and Nedwich, 1973; Rabbiosi and Borroni, 1979). This
probably reflects an increase in the total amount of connective
tissue, which replaces subcutaneous fat. Within the ground
substance itself, however, there is an increased concentration of
hexosamines and a marked increase in dermatan sulfate, whereas the
hydroxyproline (collagen) concentration remains normal
(Fleischmajer and Nedwich, 1973). These observations imply that
there is a specific aberration of the proteoglycan component of
connective tissue. In studies of autopsy-derived skin obtained
from relatively normal appearing regions, we observed a
significant reduction in total GAGs per weight dry tissue in two
patients compared with skin from 14 normal controls ranging in
age from 20 to 70 years (Iozzo, Salk, and Wight, manuscript in

preparation). The decrease in total GAGs was due to reduced
amounts of hyaluronic acid and dermatan sulfate. The difference
between our findings and those of Fleischmajer and Nedwich (1973)
probably is due to differences between the scleroderma-like
lesions on the lower extremities and the relatively atrophic skin
found elsewhere on Werner syndrome patients. It is not yet known
whether an aberration of proteoglycan metabolism is the cause of
generalized dermal atrophy in Werner syndrome or if it is a
secondary manifestation of some other underlying defect.

Tajima et al. (1981) have recently reported studies of GAG
production by cultured skin fibroblasts from Werner syndrome
patients. They noted an increased accumulation of both
hyaluronic acid and sulfated GAGs in intracellular, pericellular,
and extracellular material. They suggest there may be a deficit
in a metabolic pathway that is common to these several fractions,
such as degradation of GAGs. Preliminary studies of Werner
syndrome cultured skin fibroblasts in our laboratory are
generally consistent with the findings of Tajima et al. (1981).
We observe marginal differences in the synthesis of hyaluronic
acid but marked increases in accumulation of sulfated GAGs
(Bryant, Salk, and Wight, unpublished results). These findings
in cultured skin fibroblasts suggest that GAG metabolism is
altered in the skin of Werner syndrome patients and that our
observation of decreased GAG content in Werner syndrome skin may
not be due to decreased synthesis by skin fibroblasts, but rather
to an alteration in GAG turnover.

Abnormal turnover of GAGs is also suggested by the fact that
Werner syndrome patients demonstrate increased urinary excretion of
hyaluronic acid. Tokunaga et al. (1975) studied urine from five
patients with Werner syndrome and noted that although excretion of
total acidic GAGs was within normal limits, the quantity of
hyaluronic acid was increased: 1.7% to 16% of total GAGs compared
with less than 1% for normal subjects. Similar findings were
reported by Goto and Murata (1978) and Goto et al. (1978) who noted
hyaluronic acid content equal to 10-20% of total urinary GAGs in
ten patients. These authors point out that renal tissue is
composed of GAGs rich in hyaluronic acid and suggest that the
urinary GAGs may originate in part from the kidneys, although no
clinical renal dysfunction was evident. Murata (1982) recently
reported more detailed studies of four patients: He observed an
increase in urinary total acidic GAG when expressed on the basis of
body weight. The proportion of hyaluronic acid was elevated 10-
fold compared with normal controls and the proportion of heparan
sulfate was also increased by 20 percent. In addition, the ratio
of chondroitin 4-sulfate to chondroitin 6-sulfate was decreased.
Murata points out that these changes also tend to occur in normal
aging individuals, except for the marked increase in hyaluronic
acid. W.T. Brown and his colleagues have observed excess urinary

excretion of hyaluronic acid in a Puerto Rican woman with Werner
syndrome (personal communication, 1981) bringing the total number
of patients studied to more than thirteen.   Thus, hyaluronic
aciduria appears to be a consistent finding in Werner syndrome
patients and may be useful for diagnosis.   The origin of this
hyaluronic acid is not known, but might represent aberrant turnover
of proteoglycans, the immediate source of urinary excess being
renal tissue.

Control of Growth in Cultured Skin Fibroblasts

Normal human fibroblast-like (FL) cells have a limited
proliferative capacity in vitro.   After being cultured for several
months the cells gradually assume a "senescent" morphology: They
become larger, less regular, and accumulate cytoplasmic fibrils.
Culture growth slows and then ceases after a total of 40-60
population doublings.   The growth potential (or "in vitro
replicative lifespan") of normal human FL cells is inversely
related to the age of the donor (Martin et al., 1970).

By all criteria examined to date, Werner syndrome skin FL
cells are morphologically similar to skin FL cells derived from
normal donors.   Yatscoff et al. (1978) reported identical
electrophoretic patterns of mitochondrial proteins in Werner
syndrome and normal cell cultures, and Subino et al. (1982) reported
similar morphology of their microtubular systems.   Senescent Werner
FL cells appear identical to senescent normal FL cells by both
light and electron microscopy (Basler et al., 1979; Norwood et al.,
1979; Salk et al., 1981f) and they have reduced proteolytic capacity
and increased amino acid efflux, as do senescent normal FL cells
(Goldstein et al., 1976).   Nevertheless, Werner syndrome FL cells
are more difficult to culture than normal cells: They grow more
slowly, assume a senescent morphology more rapidly, and demonstrate
markedly reduced in vitro lifespan (Norwood et al., 1979; Salk et
al, 1981a, 1981f).   The observation of poor growth of Werner
syndrome skin FL cells is a consistent finding: It has been
reported from more than 26 patients from at least eleven
laboratories (Salk, et al., 1981a; Goldstein, 1979; Aso et al.,
1980; Schonberg et al., 1982;   Scappaticci et al., 1982).

We analyzed in detail the growth of 20 independent FL cell
strains from three patients with Werner syndrome and we performed
complementation studies by co-cultivation and cell fusion (Salk et
al., 1981a).   As shown in Table 4, the average population growth
rate of Werner strains during their period of active proliferation
is 55%, and the average replicative lifespan is 27% of the
corresponding values for non-Werner cultures.   Occasional Werner
strains grow as rapidly as the slowest growing normal strains, but
there is no overlap in total replicative lifespans: The longest
Werner strain lifespan is only 75% that of the shortest-lived

normal strain. Exponential growth rates measured by daily in situ cell counts are also reduced in Werner FL cell cultures.

Co-cultivation of normal with Werner syndrome FL cells did not improve the growth of the Werner cells nor reduce the growth of the normal cells. Proliferating hybrid synkaryons of Werner and normal FL cells is difficult to establish because of the poor cloning efficiency and reduced replicative capacity of the parental Werner cells. Using Werner cells from the earliest possible time after explant outgrowth, we have to date isolated only two clones of Werner-normal hybrid cells. We studied these hybrids by measuring ^{3}H-thymidine labeling indices and cumulative population doublings and compared the results with those from proliferating tetraploid (self-fused) normal and diploid (non-fused) Werner clones isolated in the same experiment. Although the data are limited and further studies are needed, it appears that the Werner phenotype (reduced growth potential) was not rescued by fusion with normal cells. These co-cultivation and cell hybridization results suggest that the reduced growth potential of Werner cells is not due to an enzyme defect that can be supplemented by normal enzymes present in another cell. It also appears that Werner cells do not excrete a toxic metabolic by-product or other growth-inhibiting substance because the growth of normal cells is not reduced during co-cultivation.

There is a single report, in Japanese, of reduced activity of serum growth factor in Werner syndrome (Aso et al., 1980). Normal human fetal fibroblasts and marmot epidermal cells were used as indicator cells; their growth in medium containing 10% serum from a 30-year-old male with Werner syndrome was less than in medium containing 10% normal human serum. The significance of this single observation remains to be established.

Examination of the first round of DNA synthesis after fusion of two cell types provides another assay for dominance or recessivity of a cellular phenotype associated with the control of growth. Norwood et al. (1974, 1975) have shown that the phenotype of senescent normal FL cells (reduced DNA synthesis) is dominant in fusions with young, proliferating normal FL cells but is recessive in fusions with HeLa cells. Tanaka et al. (1979, 1980) studied Werner syndrome cells in whole-cell fusions with both normal and HeLa cells and also studied "cybridization" fusions using isolated karyoplasts and cytoplasts. They concluded that Werner syndrome FL cells are essentially similar to senescent normal cells. In our own lab, however, we have observed markedly different behavior of Werner syndrome and normal senescent FL cells: Werner cells were dominant in whole-cell fusions with HeLa cells, significantly reducing DNA synthesis in HeLa nuclei (Norwood et al., 1979). Studies are now in progress to clarify these conflicting results.

Table 4. Population growth rates during the period of active
          growth, and total in vitro replicative lifespan of skin
          fibroblast-like cell strains established from three
          Werner syndrome patients and ten normal individuals (data
          from Salk et al., 1981a).

	No. of Strains	Population growth rate, PD/day* (range)	Lifespan, CPD** (range)
Werner syndrome	20	0.30 (0.21-0.41)	14.6 (3.8-27.8)
Normal	10	0.55 (0.39-0.71)	54.3 (37.0-70.6)

*Population doublings per day
**Cumulative population doublings

Several studies of cultured Werner syndrome FL cells have
demonstrated large heat-labile fractions (14-50%) in three
cytoplasmic enzymes: Glucose-6 phosphate dehydrogenase (G6PD),
6-phosphogluconate dehydrogenase (6-PGD), and hypoxanthine-
guanine phosphoribosyltransferase (HGPRT) (Holliday et al., 1974;
Goldstein and Singal, 1974; Goldstein and Moerman, 1975; Beadle
et al., 1978; Houben et al., 1980). The error catastrophe theory
of aging (Orgel, 1963, 1973) suggests that cell death or
cessation of replication results from an accumulation of self-
perpetuating errors in protein synthesis, and a number of studies
have been performed with cultures of human diploid cells to assay
for the proportion of heat-labile enzymes associated with
increasing in vitro age. Studies with normal cells have yielded
conflicting results (Holliday and Tarrant, 1972; Pendergrass et
al., 1976; Kahn et al., 1977; Shakespeare and Buchanan, 1978),
however the bulk of recent evidence fails to support the error
catastrophe theory as it applies to normal cellular senescence
(Wojtyk and Goldstein, 1980). The significance of increased heat
lability of certain enzymes in Werner syndrome cultures remains
unclear. In all other respects the stability of enzymes in
Werner syndrome cells is similar to those in normal cells:
Lysosomal and mitochondrial enzymes are not modified (Houben et
al., 1980), the fidelity of protein synthesis is normal in both
cell-free and intact cell assay systems (Wojtyk and Goldstein,
1980; Harley et al., 1980), and the thermostability of
erythrocyte G6PD and 6PGD are normal (Brown and Darlington,
1980). It may be that in general the heat lability sometimes
observed in cytoplasmic enzymes results from defects in post-
translational modification (Gershon, 1979; Rothstein, 1979;
Houben et al., 1980) and that Werner syndrome cells manifest a
specific defect in one or more of these systems.

Goldstein and Harley (1979) discuss the relationship between diabetes mellitus, aging, and observations in cultured cells from normal individuals, diabetics, and patients with Hutchinson-Guilford progeria and Werner syndrome. They suggest that a mutant gene affecting a membrane protein common to all cells might explain the association of clinical diabetes mellitus and reduced growth potential of cultured cells. In fact, a variety of aberrations of membrane proteins have been reported in Werner syndrome: FL cells apparently have reduced expression of HLA antigens, although HLA expression in lymphocytes is normal (Goldstein and Singal, 1974; Nakao et al., 1980); "tissue factor" procoagulant activity is increased in Werner FL cells (Goldstein and Niewiarowksi, 1976); some patients demonstrate peripheral resistance to insulin or other hormones (Alberti et al., 1974; Beadle et al., 1978; Nakao et al., 1978; Smith et al., 1980); and Werner FL cells in culture may possibly demonstrate a defect in membrane proteins that regulate amino acid efflux (Goldstein et al., 1976). Goldstein and Singal (1974) point out that the expression of membrane-associated proteins might depend on proper post-translational modifications. Beadle et al., (1978) and Smith et al., (1980) suggest that the insulin receptor concentration is decreased on fat cells in patients with Werner syndrome. The reproducibility and significance of these observations in Werner syndrome remain to be determined and additional studies are indicated, particularly in light of conflicting reports concerning similar measurements of HLA expression, tissue factors, insulin resistance, thermolabile enzymes, and in vitro replicative lifespan in Hutchinson-Guilford progeria (Goldstein and Harley, 1979; Brown, 1980; Brown and Darlington, 1980; Brown et al., 1980).

One can speculate extensively with regard to the possible relationships between aberrant post-translational modification of proteins, reduced growth potential, reduced function of membrane associated proteins, and possible dominant behavior in fusions with HeLa cells. At this time I will only comment that aberrations in connective tissue macromolecules, suggested above, might also result from defective post-translational modification and that these macromolecules may be important, for growth control. Wever et al., (1980) found that treatment of cultured skin FL cells with heparan inhibited cell proliferation and they suggested that heparan sulfate may play a role in the regulation of cell growth. Matuoka and Mitsui (1981b) subsequently demonstrated that cell surface heparan sulfate is involved in density-dependent inhibition of cell proliferation in vitro. Sluke et al. (1981) noted an increase in heparan sulfate in senescent cell cultures. Smith et al., (1982) found that growth factors adherent to cell substrate are mitogenically active in situ, and they suggest that one role of the extracellular matrix is to sequester biologically

active molecules to provide localized, persistent stimulation.
If the extracellular matrix functions poorly in this regard in
Werner syndrome, it might explain both poor growth of cultured
skin FL cells and poor growth of dermal and other tissues in
vivo.

CHROMOSOMAL ABERRATIONS

Variegated Translocation Mosaicism

A variety of non-constitutional, stable chromosome
rearrangements is observed in cultured skin FL cells from
patients with Werner syndrome (Hoehn et al., 1975; Salk et al.,
1981b; Schonberg et al., 1981, 1982; Scappaticci et al., 1982).
These changes range from deletion of a portion of a single
chromosome to multiple translocations involving several
chromosomes in the same cell (Figure 2). Although structurally
abnormal, the number of chromosomes is usually 46 (pseudodiploid)
and the rearrangements can be passed on to daughter cells; thus
clones of cells may be generated that have identical cytogenetic
markers. This pattern of pseudodiploidy with multiple, variable,
stable chromosome rearrangements that are clonal has been called
variegated translocation mosaicism (VTM) (Hoehn et al., 1975).

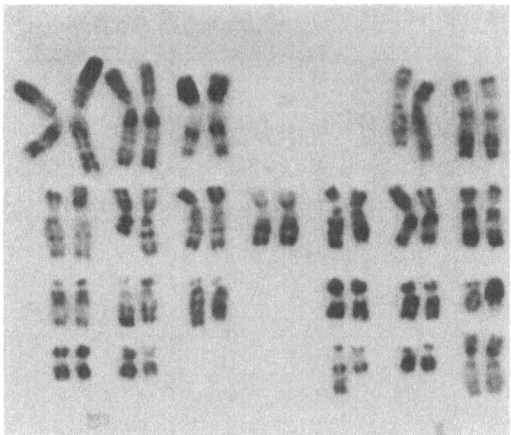

Figure 2: An R-banded karyotype of a Werner syndrome skin
       fibroblast-like cell showing pseudodiploidy with
       structural rearrangements involving five chromosomes:
       46,XX,rea(4),t(6;11)
       (6pter→cen→11qter;11pter→cen→6qter),t(7;21)(7pter→7q3
       1:;21pter→21qter::7q31→7qter),t(10;15)(10pter→10q21::1
       5q14→15qter;15pter→15q14::10q21→10qter). Reproduced
       from Salk et al., (1981b) with permission of the
       publisher, S. Karger AG, Basel.

VTM is occasionally observed in non-Werner FL cell cultures (Hoehn et al., 1975; Littlefield and Mailhes, 1975; Harden et al., 1976), but only rarely to the extent observed in Werner cultures. We found that only eight (8.4%) of 95 non-Werner syndrome FL cell cultures demonstrated VTM: Seven with low-grade VTM (approximately 5% of 300 metaphases), and one with VTM affecting 90-100% of metaphases (Salk et al., 1981b). In Werner syndrome, however, 92% of 1,538 metaphases from 29 independent cultures derived from five patients contained a recognizable, stable structural chromosome rearrangement (Salk et al., 1981b).

As shown in Table 5, the predominant clone in a Werner syndrome FL cell culture may change during its life in vitro. In this example, cells with a deletion of chromosome 11 were predominant in early passages (clone a), whereas cells that contained a translocation, a different deletion, and an unidentifiable marker chromosome were predominant in later passages (clone c). It is likely that this kind of clonal succession also occurs in normal FL cell cultures but is not observed due to lack of multiple cytogenetic markers (Salk et al., 1981d).

Table 5.   Cytogenetic evaluation of 154 R-banded metaphases from sequential passages during the in vitro life of one strain of skin fibroblast-like cells from a patient with Werner syndrome (data from Salk et al., 1981b).

Passages	Normal (46,XY)	Clones (see footnote) a_1	a_2	a_3	a_4	b	c	Misc. unique*
2/3	3	18			13	2		3
4/5	1	19	3	2	11			2
6/7		27			7			
8/9		9					13	1
10/11	1	2			3	1	11	2
TOTAL	5	75	3	2	34	3	24	8

*Miscellaneous unique deletions and/or rearrangements

Clone a_1:   46,XY,del(11)(q23)
a_2:   46,XY,del(11)(q23),inv ins(B)
a_3:   46,XY,del(11)(q23),13q+
a_4:   46,?X,Y,del(11)(q23)
b: 46,XY,t(15;17)(q21;p13)
c: 46,?X,Y,t(2q;6q),del(2)(p16),10p-,-22,+mar

Every chromosome has been observed to be involved in
rearrangements in Werner syndrome, apparently in a random fashion
(Figure 3). However, analysis of specific rearrangement sites
reveals that there are hotspots, or sites where rearrangements are
more frequently observed (Figure 4). The frequency distribution of
rearrangement sites is shown in Table 6. The four sites with nine
or more rearrangement events represent a highly significant
deviation from a random Poisson distribution estimated either from
the size of the zero-event class or from the mean of the non-zero
data. The data in Figures 3 and 4 are adapted from our initial
report (Salk et al., 1981b), and include recent data from our own
and two other laboratories (Salk et al., 1982; Scappaticci et al.,
1982; Schonberg et al., 1982). It is noteworthy that eight new
patients are included and that the addition of these data improves
the resolution of the analysis.

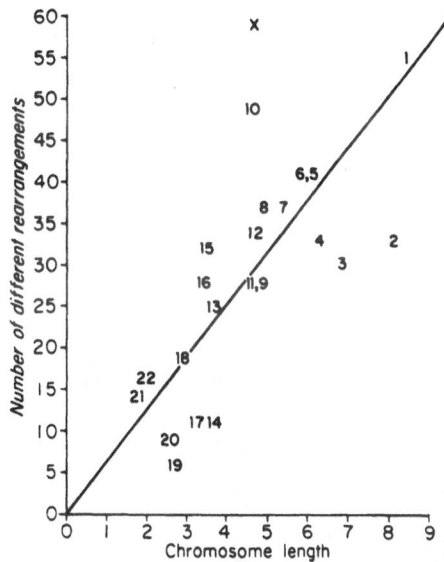

Figure 3: Scattergram showing a correlation between chromosome
          length and the number of times the chromosome is involved
          in different rearrangements in Werner syndrome cells.
          The data of Scappaticci et al. (1982), Schonberg (1982),
          and Salk et al. (1982) have been added to those of Salk
          et al. (1981b), representing a total of 1253 metaphases
          from 11 patients. Each clonal rearrangement was scored
          only once, and the length of the X chromosome has been
          adjusted to account for the number of male metaphases
          included. The regression line was calculated by the
          method of least squares and constrained to go through the
          origin. The slope is 6.34 and the correlation
          coefficient, r, is 0.682.

The frequency distribution shown in Table 6 is consistent with
a model of specific chromosomal hotspots overlying a Poisson-
distributed background of random rearrangement events. The four
sites with nine or more rearrangement events represent only 3% of
the identifiable breakpoints in 1,134 banded metaphases, but they
account for 13% of all definable rearrangements. These four sites
are 1q12, 1q44, 5q12, and 6cen. It is difficult to determine if
any other chromosomal sites are "lesser hotspots." It is possible
that rearrangements occur more frequently at these hotspots or,
alternatively, that there is some selection for cells with
rearrangements at these sites. The site 1q12 has been shown to be
involved with some frequency in structural chromosome
rearrangements in bladder and ovarian cancer (Atkin and Baker,

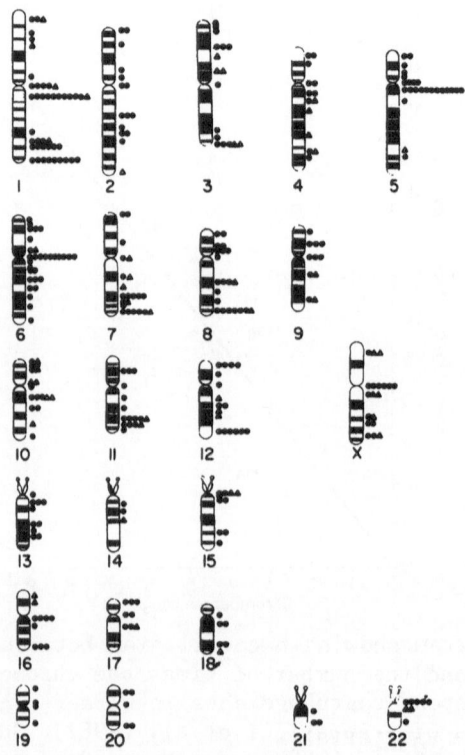

Figure 4: Distribution of identifiable sites involved in
          rearrangements in 1,134 metaphases from 21 skin
          fibroblast-like cell strains from nine patients and from
          peripheral blood lymphocyte cultures from five patients
          with Werner syndrome. Adapted from Salk et al. (1981b)
          with additional data from Salk et al. (1982) (solid
          circles) and Scappaticci et al. (1982) (open triangles).

1978) and in adenovirus 12-infected cells, hematologic disorders, and inborn chromosomal abnormalities (Rowley, 1977); the site 1q44 is frequently involved in breaks in adenovirus 12-infected cells (Rowley, 1977). However, the Werner syndrome hotspots are different from those observed in other non-random chromosomal events (Salk et al., 1981b). It may or may not be relevant that 1q12 is sometimes involved in chromosomal rearrangements in neoplasia, a situation where changes in proliferative capacity may be important (Rowley, 1982).

It is now apparent that the cytogenetic aberration in Werner syndrome is not limited to a single tissue, although the conditions under which expression will occur are not completely understood. The work of Scappaticci et al. (1982), published elsewhere in this issue, is the first observation of stable structural chromosome rearrangements in peripheral blood lymphocytes from patients with Werner syndrome (see Salk et al., 1981b for review).

In another study of banded chromosomes from peripheral blood lymphocytes of one patient, only one cell with a translocation was observed among 25 cells karyotyped in a short-term culture, but multiple clonal chromosome rearrangements were observed in EB-virus transformed lymphoblastoid cell lines (Schonberg et al., 1981; to be published). Preliminary studies of two Werner syndrome

Table 6. Frequency distribution of sites of rearrangement shown in Figure 4, assuming there are 314 identifiable sites on banded metaphase chromosomes.

Number of events	Total number of sites
0	162
1	75
2	39
3	16
4	7
5	5
6	4
7	2
8	0
9	1
10	1
11	1
12	1

lymphoblastoid cell lines in our laboratory revealed normal
chromosome constitution but a high frequency of dicentric
chromosomes in some harvests (Salk et al., 1981b). We have
recently studied a 48-hour lymphocyte culture from a young woman
with Werner syndrome (Figure 1) and observed structural
chromosome rearrangements in six of 14 metaphases (Salk et al.,
1982). Finally, it should be noted that in the original report
of VTM in Werner syndrome there is a description of a clonal
translocation in a strain of putative glial cells derived from
cerebral cortex (Hoehn et al., 1975).

Chromosome Breakage and Other Rearrangements

We were not previously impressed with the amount of chromosome
breakage in comparison with the amount of stable, clonal
rearrangements in our Werner syndrome FL cell cultures, but we did
not do any quantitation (Salk et al., 1981b, 1981c). Similarly,
Schonberg et al. (1982), who quantitated breakage but did not report
parallel control cultures, conclude there is no increase in
chromosome breakage in FL cells, peripheral blood lymphocytes, or
lymphoblystoid cell lines from their two Werner syndrome
patients. However, both Nordenson (1977) and Scappaticci et al.
(1982) report an increase in breakage in Werner syndrome cells
compared with normal controls: 20 to 60-fold (lymphocytes) and
two to four-fold (both lymphocytes and FL cells), respectively.
Nevertheless, even in Nordenson's study the increase is not as
great as that observed in patients with Fanconi anemia.
Nordenson also observed reduced amounts of chromosome breakage
following treatment with the radical scavenging enzymes
superoxide dismutase and catalase, and she suggested that
chromosome instability in Werner syndrome might result from
sensitivity to damage by free oxygen radicals. We were unable to
demonstrate an effect on stable chromosome rearrangements or
growth potential by treating Werner syndrome FL cells either with
the radical scavenging enzymes superoxide dismutase and catalase
or with reduced concentrations of atmospheric oxygen (Salk et
al., 1981c). Marklund et al. (1981) found normal levels of
activity of radical scavenging enzymes in erythrocytes and
lymphocytes from patients with Werner syndrome. Nevertheless,
the findings of Nordenson (1977) and Scappaticci et al. (1982)
suggest that under the right conditions, increased amounts of
chromosomal breakage is manifested by Werner syndrome cells.

Other cytogenetic characteristics of Werner syndrome cells
have been reported to be normal. Scappaticci et al. (1982) observed
premature centromere division of the X-chromosome, a phenomenon
apparently associated with aging (Fitzgerald, 1975; Galloway and
Buckton, 1978). Baseline levels of sister chromatid exchange have
been reported to be normal in Werner syndrome FL cells, peripheral
blood lymphocytes, and lymphoblastoid cell lines (Bartram et al.,

1976; Salk et al., 1981b; Darlington et al., 1981; Schonberg et al., 1982). Mitomycin-C-induced sister chromatid exchange was slightly increased in lymphocytes from one patient with Werner syndrome, but were not significantly elevated in a second patient (Darlington et al., 1981).

In Vivo or In Vitro Phenomenon

Does VTM in Werner syndrome occur in vivo, in vitro, or both? Evolution of clonal chromosome rearrangements (new rearrangements in a previously recognized clone) has been observed in mass cultures of FL cells and this is suggestive, but does not prove, that VTM occurs in vitro (Salk et al., 1981b, 1981d). Schonberg et al (1981, to be published) studied lymphoblastoid cells that were derived using a technique that is felt to establish each line from a single original transformed cell; because of the putative clonal nature of these cell lines and the authors' observation of multiple cytogenetic clones, they concluded that chromosome rearrangements in Werner syndrome can occur in vitro.

Scappaticci et al. (1982) examined Werner syndrome FL cells in the initial outgrowth from skin explants. Their observation of clonal chromosomal rearrangements under these conditions is suggestive, but not compelling evidence that the rearrangements had occurred in vitro: By the time the cells were analyzed they had been in culture for at least 2 to 3 weeks and had undergone an unknown number of divisions in vitro. Stronger evidence for the in vivo occurrence of clonal chromosome rearrangements is the observation of identical rearrangements in two separate blood samples from patient 2 in Scappaticci et al. (1982). There are two examples of rearrangements that were observed in each of two samples taken one year apart: del(11)(q22) and del(17)(q21). It seems unlikely that it would happen twice in one patient, but there is a formal possibility that these two aberrations recurred in vitro by chance, or that the rearrangements are not actually identical. Both aberrations are simple deletions in single cells and it is possible that each "recurrance" actually represents a different cytogenetic event but that the small portions translocated onto other chromosomes were not readily identifiable. The interpretation is made more difficult by four instances of apparently identical rearrangements in unrelated patients or in different tissues from the same patient.

One cytogenetic study of bone marrow from a patient with Werner syndrome has been reported to be normal; however, the morphology of the unbanded bone marrow chromosomes makes interpretation of structural rearrangements difficult (Bertoni and Lostia, 1967).

In recently reported work that is soon to be published in greater detail, we studied FL cell colonies derived from single cells in order to clarify the question of in vitro versus in vivo occurrence of VTM in Werner syndrome (Salk et al., 1981e, 1982). We observed many in vitro structural chromosome changes, including one instance of clonal evolution: Two cells with the same new rearrangement in addition to the basic clonal aberration. We also observed identical clonal chromosome rearrangements in independent cultures derived from a single skin specimen; this demonstrates that the rearrangements were present in multiple cells in the original tissue. Our recent observation of multiple structural chromosome rearrangements in a 48-hour culture of peripheral blood lymphocytes (when essentially all metaphases represent cells in their first division in vitro) provides additional evidence for the in vivo occurrence of chromosome rearrangements. Our findings, in conjunction with those of Scappaticci et al. (1982) and Schonberg et al. (to be published), support the hypothesis that stable structural chromosome rearrangements occur both in vivo and in vitro in Werner syndrome.

VTM and cell growth

The relationship between chromosome aberrations and reduced growth potential in Werner syndrome FL cells is not yet clear. Chromosome instability might be a direct cause of reduced growth: Small losses of genetic material and changes in gene regulation due to position effects could both result from rearrangements that appear to be balanced. However, the chromosomes in Werner syndrome FL cells do not show the high degree of instability demonstrated by cells from patients with Fanconi anemia, ataxia telangiectasia, and Bloom syndrome, and cytogenetic clones have been observed that survive for many weeks in culture despite having multiple rearranged chromosomes (Salk et al., 1981b, 1981d). Schonberg et al. (1981, to be published) suggest that chromosome translocations in Werner syndrome actually provide a proliferative advantage and that this explains the higher proportion of abnormal cells in long-term versus short-term cultures. In support of this, one explanation for the presence of chromosomal hotspots discussed above is that a proliferative advantage is generated by rearrangements at specific sites. However, Schonberg et al.'s observation concerning a difference between long- and short-term cultures is not substantiated by our data or those of Scappaticci et al. (1982) and might also be explained by differences in rearrangement frequency under different culture conditions. As noted previously, the specific conditions for maximal expression of cytogenetic aberrations in Werner syndrome have yet to be established. It is possible that the relationship between chromosome aberrations and reduced growth potential is not one of cause and effect, but rather that they are two distinct manifestations of a single underlying genetic defect.

Chromosome Instability Syndromes

There are four genetic diseases that have classically been referred to as chromosome instability syndromes: Ataxia telangiectasia, Fanconi anemia, Bloom syndrome, and xeroderma pigmentosum (German, 1972). All of these syndromes are autosomal recessive and display chromosome breakage and/or stable chromosome rearrangements either spontaneously or under test conditions when normal cells do not. Abnormal DNA repair has been demonstrated in xeroderma pigmentosum and has been implicated in the other conditions. All of these syndromes also display an increased incidence of neoplasia. The cytogenetic and clinical observations in Werner syndrome justify inclusion of this disease in the general category of autosomal recessive genetic diseases with chromosome instability and an increased incidence of neoplasia. DNA repair and/or survival of Werner syndrome cells appears to be grossly normal following ultraviolet, gamma-, and X-irradiation, but other aspects of DNA replication and repair have yet to be examined (Fujiwara et al., 1977; Higoshikawa and Fujiwara, 1978; Arlett and Harcourt, 1980).

CONCLUSION

Werner syndrome is a rare autosomal recessive condition that displays many features similar to changes that occur during normal aging. It is sometimes referred to as "adult progeria," but it differs from normal aging in several respects. Martin (1978) classifies this condition as a "segmental progeroid syndrome" because it involves major segments of the senescent phenotype rather than being a true acceleration of the aging process. Werner syndrome may also be classified as a chromosome instability syndrome, because it displays multiple stable chromosome rearrangements and, apparently to a lesser extent, chromosome breakage. Chromosome aberrations have been observed in multiple tissues and probably occur both in vivo and in vitro. Like the four classical chromosome instability syndromes, Werner syndrome is associated with an increased incidence of neoplasia.

At the present time there are a number of suggestive observations concerning abnormalities in Werner syndrome both clinically and in cultured cells, but the central underlying problem remains to be elucidated. Patients display abnormalities in connective tissue and recent studies suggest that aberrations of collagen and/or proteoglycans may also be expressed by cells in culture. Skin fibroblast-like cells consistently grow poorly in vitro, a fact that could be related to the dermal atrophy observed in vivo, either as cause or effect. Somatic chromosome aberrations, such as those that occur in Werner syndrome, are

associated with neoplasia and, in some instances, growth
deficiency in the other chromosome instability syndromes.
Abnormalities of DNA repair have been implicated in these other
conditions and deserve further exploration in Werner syndrome.

Werner syndrome apparently results from a single gene
defect, but it remains to be determined whether the aberrant gene
product is a structural protein, an enzyme, or a molecule
involved in gene regulation. The latter two hypotheses are most
consistent with an autosomal recessive pattern of inheritance.
If we can identify the defective gene product in Werner syndrome
it may be possible to trace out the series of biochemical and
physiologic events that lead to the progeroid manifestations and
increased incidence of neoplasia. Although the basic mechanism
underlying Werner syndrome may be different from that underlying
normal aging, the specific events leading to a given
manifestation (such as tumor development, diabetes,
atherosclerosis, or osteoporosis) may not be different. Thus,
understanding Werner syndrome may provide clues for therapeutic
intervention in some of these common geriatric disorders and may
provide insight, or at least open new avenues of research
concerning the basic sequence of events that occur during normal
aging.

Acknowledgements. I thank Ginny Walters, Marguerite Knutsen, and
Sonja Malejew for help with the manuscript and illustrations.
Bruce Walsh assisted with statistical analyses. Thomas Norwood,
Thomas Wight, Hans Ochs and Ed Lipkin reviewed sections of the
manuscript, and P. Johnston, G.B. Finnegan, and Jesse S. provided
many comments and criticisms during all stages of preparation.
Special thanks go to George M. Martin whose abiding interest in
the Werner syndrome and whose encouragement and support over many
years helped to make this work possible. This work was supported
in part by an N.I.A. Clinical Investigator Award (number AG
00144-01) from the National Institute on Aging.

REFERENCES

Alberti KGMM, Young JDH, Hockaday TDR (1974) Werner's syndrome:
    metabolic observations. Proc Roy Soc Med 67:36-38.
Angel M, Cano JF, del Olma JA, Villardell E (1980) Endocrinologic
    aspects of Werner's syndrome. Med Clin (Barc) 74:317-321.
Aram H, Fatourechi V (1974) Werner's syndrome: first reported
    cases in Iran. Cutis 14:215-218.
Arlett CF, Harcourt SA (1980) Survey of radiosensitivity in a
    variety of human cell strains. Cancer Res 40:926-932.

Aso K, Kondo S, Amano M (1980) A case of Werner's syndrome in which lowered activity of a platelet-dependent serum factor for cell growth and reduced growth potential of fibroblasts and epidermal cells were demonstrated. Nippon Hifuka Gakkai Zasshi 90:929-934.

Atkin NB, Baker MC (1978) Abnormal chromosomes and number 1 heterochromatin variants revealed in C-banded preparations from 13 bladder carcinomas. Cytobios 18:101-109.

Bartram CR, Koske-Westphal T, Passarge E (1976) Chromatid exchanges in ataxia telangiectasia, Bloom syndrome, Werner syndrome, and xeroderma pigmentosum. Ann Hum Genet 40:79-86.

Basler JW, David JD, Agris PF (1979) Deteriorating collagen synthesis and cell ultrastructural accompanying senescence of human normal and Werner's syndrome fibroblast cell strains. Exp Cell Res 118:73-84.

Beadle GF, Mackay IR, Whittingham S, Taggert G, Harris AW, Harrison LC (1978) Werner's syndrome, a model of premature aging? J Med 9:377-403.

Bertoni G, Lostia A (1967) Sulla sindrome di Werner (contributo clinico ed istologico). Ottalmologia e Clinica Oculistica 93:1130-1144.

Bjornberg A (1976) Werner's syndrome and malignancy. Acta Derm Venereol (Stockh) 56:149-150.

Blohme G, Smith U (1979) Metabolic studies in a case of Werner's syndrome. Diabete Metab 5:119-124.

Brown WT (1979) Human mutations affecting aging - a review. Mech Ageing Dev 9:325-336.

Brown WT, Darlington GJ (1980) Thermolabile enzymes in progeria and Werner syndrome: evidence contrary to the protein error hypothesis. Am J Hum Genet 32:614-619.

Brown WT, Darlington GJ, Arnold A, Fotino M (1980) Detection of HLA antigens on progeria syndrome fibroblasts. Clin Genet 17:213-219.

Buckley CE, Roseman JM (1976) Immunity and survival. J Am Geriatr Soc 24:241-248.

Burnet FM (1970) An immunological approach to ageing. Lancet 2:358-360.

Cerimele D, Cottoni F, Scappaticci S, Rabbiosi, Borroni G, Sanna E, Zei G, Fraccaro M (1982) High prevalence of Werner's syndrome in Sardinia. Description of six patients and estimate of the gene frequency. Hum Genetics.

Corrales Hernandez JJ, Miralles Garcia JM, Rodriguez Commes JL, Martin Vasallo P, Garcia Diez LC, de Pablo Davila F (1980) New enzymatic and endocrinological aspects in two cases of Werner's syndrome. Med Clin (Barc) 74:355-360.

Darlington, GJ, Dutkowski R, Brown WT (1981) Sister chromatid exchange frequencies in progeria and Werner syndrome patients. Am J Hum Genet 33:762-766.

Djawari D, Lukaschek E, Jecht E (1980) Altered cellular immunity in Werner's syndrome. Dermatologica 161:233-237.

Elliott RJ, Gardner DL (1979) Changes with age in the glycosamino-glycans of human articular cartilage. Ann Rheum Dis 38:371-377.

Epstein CJ, Martin GM, Schultz AL, Motulsky AG (1966) Werner's syndrome: a review of its symptomatology, natural history, pathologic features, genetics and relationship to the natural aging process. Medicine 45:177-221.

Fellini SA, Pacifici M, Holtzer H (1981) Changes in the sulfated proteoglycans synthesized by "aging" chondrocytes. II. Organ cultured vertebral columns. J Biol Chem 256:1038-1043.

Field JB, Loube SD (1960) Observations concerning the diabetes mellitus associated with Werner's syndrome. Metabolism 9:118-124.

Fitzgerald PH (1975) A mechanism of X chromosome aneuploidy in lymphocytes of aging women. Hum Genet 28:153-158.

Fleischmajer R and Nedwich A (1973) Werner's syndrome. Am J Med 54:111-118.

Fujiwara Y, Higashikawa T, Tatsumi M (1977) A retarded rate of DNA replication and normal level of DNA repair in Werner's syndrome fibroblasts in culture. J Cell Physiol 92:365-374.

Galloway SM, Buckton KE (1978) Aneuploidy and ageing: chromosome studies on a random sample of the population using G-banding. Cytogenet Cell Genet 20:78-95.

German J (1972) Genes which increase chromosomal instability in somatic cells and predispose to cancer. Prog Med Genet 8:61-101. Gershon D (1979) Current status of age altered enzymes: alternative mechanisms. Mech Age Devel 9:189-196.

Gershon D (1979) Current status of age altered enzymes: alternatives mechanisms. Mech Ageing Dev 9:189-196.

Gibbs DD (1967) Werner's syndrome ('progeria of the adult'). Proc R Soc Med 60:135-136.

Goldstein S (1979) Studies on age-related diseases in cultured skin fibroblasts. J Invest Dermatol 73:19-23.

Goldstein S, Harley CB (1979) In vitro studies of age-associated diseases. Fed Proc 38:1862-1867.

Goldstein S, Moerman EJ (1976) Defective proteins in normal and abnormal human fibroblasts during aging in vitro. Interdiscipl Topics Geront 10:24-43.

Goldstein S, Moerman EJ (1975) Heat-labile enzymes in Werner's syndrome fibroblasts. Nature 255:159.

Goldstein S, Niewiarowski S (1976) Increased procoagulant activity in cultured fibroblasts from progeria and Werner's syndrome of premature ageing. Nature 260:711-713.

Goldstein S, Singal DP (1974) Alteration of fibroblast gene products in vitro from a subject with Werner's syndrome. Nature 251:719-721.

Goldstein S, Stotland D, Cordeiro RAJ (1976) Decreased proteolysis and increased amino acid efflux in aging human fibroblasts. Mech Ageing Dev 5:221-233.

Goto M, Horiuchi Y, Okumura K, Tada T, Kawata M, Ohmori K (1979) Immunological abnormalities of aging: an analysis of T lymphocyte subpopulations of Werner's syndrome. J Clin Invest 64:695-699.

Goto M, Horiuchi Y, Tanimoto K, Ishii T, Nakashima H. (1978) Werner's syndrome: Analysis of 15 cases with a review of the Japanese literature. J Am Geriatrics Soc 26:341-347.

Goto M, Murata K (1978) Urinary excretion of macromolecular acidic glycosaminoglycans in Werner's syndrome. Clin Chim Acta 85:101-106.

Goto M, Tanimoto K, Horiuchi Y, Sasazuji T (1981) Family analysis of Werner's syndrome: A survey of 42 Japanese families with a review of the literature. Clin Genet 19:8-15.

Gottesman T, Zala L, Vogel A, Mumenthaler M (1980) Das Werner-syndrom. Schweiz med Wochenschr 110:246-250.

Gupta S (1981) Subpopulations of human T lymphocytes. Gerontology 27:181-186.

Hall DA (1981) Gerontology: Collagen Disease. Clin Endocrinol Metab 10:23-55.

Harley CB, Pollard JW, Chamberlain JW, Stanners CP, Goldstein S (1980) Protein synthetic errors do not increase during aging of cultured human fibroblasts. Proc Natl Acad Sci USA 77:1885-1889.

Harnden DG, Benn PA, Oxford JM, Taylor AMR, Webb, TP (1976) Cytogenetically marked clones in human fibroblasts cultured from normal subjects. Somatic Cell Genet 2:55-62.

Higashikawa T, Fujiwara Y (1978) Normal level of unscheduled DNA synthesis in Werner's syndrome fibroblasts in culture. Exp Cell Res 113:438-442.

Hoehn H, Bryant EM, Au K, Norwood TH, Boman H, Martin GM. (1975) Variegated translocation mosaicism in human skin fibroblast cultures. Cyto Genet Cell Genet 15:282-298.

Holliday R, Porterfield JS, Gibbs DD (1974) Premature aging and occurrance of altered enzyme in Werner's syndrome fibroblasts. Nature 248:762-763.

Holliday R, Tarrant GM (1972) Altered enzymes in aging human fibroblasts. Nature 238:26-30.

Hoppe W, Koritsch H-D (1972) Ein weiterer Fall von Meningeom bei einem Patienten mit Werner-Syndrom. Psychiat Neurol Med Psychol (Leipzig) 24:611-617.

Houben A, Houbion A, Remacle J (1980) Lysosomal and mitochondrial heat labile enzymes in Werner's syndrome fibroblasts. Exp Gerontol 15:629-631.

Hrabko RP, Milgrom H, Schwartz RA (1982) Werner's syndrome with associated malignant neoplasms. Arch Dermatol 118:106-108.

Ishii T, Hosoda Y (1975) Werner's syndrome: autopsy report of one case, with a review of pathologic findings reported in the literature. J Am Geriatr Soc 23:145-154.

Kahn A, Guillouzo A, Cottreau D, Marie J, Bourel M, Boivin P, Dreyfus JC (1977) Accuracy of protein synthesis and in vitro aging: Search for altered enzymes in senescent cultured cells from human livers. Gerontology 23:174-184.

Kobayashi S, Gibo H, Sugita K, Komiya I, Yamada T (1980) Werner's syndrome associated with meningioma. Neurosurgery 7:517-520.

Littlefield LG, Mailhes JB (1975) Observations of de novo clones of cytogenetically aberrant cells in primary fibroblast cell strains from phenotypically normal women. Am J Hum Genet 27:190-197.

Makinodan T, Heidrick ML, Nordin AA (1975) Immunodeficiency and autoimmunity in aging. Birth Defects 11:193-198.

Marklund S, Nordensson I, Back O (1981) Normal CuZn superoxide dismutase, catalase and glutathione peroxidase in Werner's syndrome. J Gerontol 36:405-409.

Martin GM (1978) Genetic syndromes in man with potential relevance to the pathobiology of aging. Birth Defects, 14:5-39.

Martin GM, Sprague CA, Epstein CJ (1970) Replicative life-span of cultivated human cells: effects of donor's age, tissue and genotype. Lab Invest 23:86-91.

Matuoka K, Mitsui Y (1981a) Changes in cell-surface glycosamino-glycans in human dipliod fibroblasts during in vitro aging. Mech Ageing Dev 15:153-163.

Matuoka K, Mitsui Y (1981b) Involvement of cell surface heparan sulfate in the density-dependent inhibition of cell prolif-eration. Cell Structure and Function 6:23-33.

Mourao PAS, Machado-Santelli GM (1978) Sulfated glycosaminoglycans of cells grown in culture: dermatan sulfate disappearance in successive fibroblast subcultures. Cell Differ 7:367-374.

Murata K (1982) Urinary acidic glycosaminoglycans in Werner's syndrome. Experientia 38:313-314.

Murata K, Nakashima H (1982) Werner's syndrome: Twenty-four cases with a review of the Japanese medical literature. J Am Geriatr Soc 30:303-308.

Nakao Y, Hattori T, Takasuki K, Kuroda Y, Nakaji T, Fujiwara Y, Kishihara M, Baba Y, Fujita T (1980) Immunological studies on Werner's syndrome. Clin Exp Immunol 42:10-19.

Nakao Y, Kishihara M, Yoshimi H, Inoue Y, Tanaka K, Sakamoto N, Matsukura S, Imura H, Ichihashi M, Fujiwara Y (1978) Werner's syndrome: in vivo and in vitro characteristics as a model of aging. Am J Med 65:919-932.

Nordenson I (1977) Chromosome breaks in Werner's syndrome and their prevention in vitro by radical-scavenging enzymes. Hereditas 87:151-154.

Norwood TH, Hoehn H, Salk D, Martin GM (1979) Cellular aging in Werner's syndrome: a unique phenotype? J Invest Dermatol 73:92-96.

Norwood TH, Pendergrass WR, Martin GM (1975) Reinitiation of DNA synthesis in senescent human fibroblasts upon fusion with cells of unlimited growth potential. J Cell Biol 64:551-556.

Norwood TH, Pendergrass WR, Sprague CA, Martin GM (1974) Dominance of the senescent phenotype in heterokaryons between replicative and postreplicative human fibroblast-like cells. Proc Natl Acad Sci USA 71:2231-2235.

Oohira A, Nogami H (1980) Age-related changes in physical and chemical properties of proteoglycans synthesized by costal and matrix-induced cartilages in the rat. J Biol Chem 255:1346-1350.

Oppenheimer BS, Kugel VH (1934) Werner's syndrome - a heredo-familial disorder with scleroderma, bilateral juvenile cataract, precocious graying of hair and endocrine stigmatization. Trans Assoc Am Physicians 49:358.

Oppenheimer BS, Kugel VH (1941) Werner's syndrome: report of the first necropsy and of findings in a new case. Am J Med Sci 202:629.

Orgel LE (1973) Ageing of clones of mammalian cells. Nature 243:441-445.

Orgel LE (1963) The maintenance of the accuracy of protein synthesis and its relevance to ageing. Proc Natl Acad Sci USA 49:517-521.

Pendergrass WR, Martin GM, Bornstein P (1976) Evidence contrary to the protein error hypothesis for in vitro senescence. J Cell Physiol 87:3-14.

Rabbiosi G, Borroni G (1979) Werner's syndrome: seven cases in one family. Dermatologica 158:355-360.

Reed R, Seville RH, Tattersall RN (1953) Werner's syndrome. Br J Dermatol 65:165-176.

Riley TR, Wieland RG, Markis J, Hamwi CJ (1965) Werner's syndrome. Ann Intern Med 63:285-294.

Robert L (1981) Aging of connective tissues. Experientia 37:1055-1058.

Rosen RS, Cimini R, Coblentz D (1970) Werner's syndrome. Br J Radiol 43:193-198.

Rothstein M (1979) The formation of altered enzymes in aging animals. Mech Ageing Dev 9:197-202.

Rowley JD (1982) Identification of the constant chromosome regions involved in human hematologic malignant disease. Science 216:749-751.

Rowley JD (1977) Nonrandom chromosomal changes in human malignant cells. IN: Sparkes RS, Comings DE, Fox CF (eds) Molecular Human Cytogenetics. Academic Press, New York, pp. 457–472.

Salamon R, Bogdanovic B, Lazovic-Tepavac O, Blazevic A, Macanovic-Bogner K (1978) Werner's syndrome and the cellular immune reactions. Acta Derm Venerol (Stockh) 58:543–544.

Salk D, Bryant E, Au K, Hoehn H, Martin GM (1981a) Systematic growth studies, cocultivation, and cell hybridization studies of Werner syndrome cultured skin fibroblasts. Hum Genet 58:310–316.

Salk D, Au K, Hoehn H, Martin GM (1981b) Cytogenetics of Werner syndrome cultured skin fibroblasts: variegated translocation mosaicism. Cytogenet Cell Genet 30:92–107.

Salk D, Au K, Hoehn H, Martin GM (1981c) Effects of radical scavenging enzymes and reduced oxygen exposure on growth and chromosome abnormalities of Werner syndrome cultured skin fibroblasts. Hum Genet 57:269–275.

Salk D, Au K, Hoehn H, Stenchever MR, Martin GM (1981d) Evidence of clonal attenuation, clonal succession, and clonal expansion in mass cultures of aging Werner's syndrome skin fibroblasts. Cytogenet Cell Genet 30:108–117.

Salk D, Maxwell C, Au K, Hoehn H, Martin GM (1981e) Evolution and clonality of stable chromosome rearrangements in Bloom and Werner syndromes. Am J Hum Genet 33:119A.

Salk D, Carlson C, Martin GM (1981f) Nuclear morphology of senescing and serum starved normal and Werner syndrome cultured skin fibroblasts. Gerontologist 21:89.

Salk D, Au K, Hoehn H, Martin GM (1982) Somatic chromosome rearrangements occur in vivo and in vitro in Werner syndrome (adult progeria). Ms submitted for publication.

Scappaticci S, Cerimele D, Fraccaro M (1982) Clonal structural chromosomal rearrangements in primary fibroblast cultures and in lymphocytes of patients with Werner's syndrome. Hum Genet 62:16–24.

Schachtschabel DO, Wever J (1978) Age-related decline in the synthesis of glycosaminoglycans by cultured human fibroblasts (WI-38). Mech Ageing Dev 8:257–264.

Schonberg S, Henderson E, Niermeijer MF, Bootsma D, German J (1982) Werner's syndrome: preferential proliferation of clones with chromosome translocations. Ms submitted for publication.

Schonberg SA, Henderson E, Niermeijer MF, German J (1981) Werner's syndrome: preferential proliferation of clones with translocations. Am J Hum Genet 33:120A.

Shakespeare V, Buchanan JH (1978) Studies on phosphoglucose isomerase from cultured human fibroblasts: Absence of detectable aging effects on the enzyme. J Cell Physiol 94:105–116.

Sluke G, Schachtschabel DO, Wever J (1981) Age-related changes in
    the distribution pattern of glycosaminoglycans synthesized
    by cultured human diploid fibroblasts (WI-38). Mech Ageing
    Dev 16:19-27.
Smith JC, Singh JP, Lillquist JS, Goon DS, Stiles CD (1982)
    Growth factors adherent to cell substrate are mitogenically
    active in situ. Nature 296:154-156.
Smith RC, Winer LH, Martel S (1955) Werner's syndrome: report of
    two cases. Arch Dermatol 71:197-204.
Smith U, Digirolamo M, Blohme G, Kral JG, Tisell L-E (1980)
    Possible systemic metabolic effects of regional adiposity in
    a patient with Werner's syndrome. Int J Obes 4:153-163.
Subino S, Fiori PL, Lubinu G, Scappaticci S, Cerimele D (1982)
    Immunofluorescence of the tubulin system in human skin
    fibroblasts in Werner's syndrome, Kaposi sarcoma, and
    psoriasis. Arch Dermatol Res 272:143-145.
Sweet MBE, Thonar EJMA, Marsh J (1979) Age-related changes in
    proteoglycan structure. Arch Biochem Biophys 198:439-448.
Tajima T, Iijima K, Watanabe T (1978) Collagen synthesis of
    cultured fibroblast from Werner's syndrome of premature
    aging. Experientia 34:1459-1460.
Tajima T, Watanabe T, Iijima K, Ohshika Y, Yamaguchi H (1981) The
    increase of glycosaminoglycans synthesis and accumulation on
    the cell surface of cultured skin fibroblasts in Werner's
    syndrome. Exp Pathol 20:221-229.
Tanaka K, Nakazawa T, Okada Y, Kumahara Y (1979) Increase in DNA
    synthesis in Werner's syndrome cells by hybridization with
    normal human diploid and HeLa cells. Exp Cell Res 123:261-
    267.
Tanaka K, Nakazawa T, Okada Y, Kumahara Y (1980) Roles of nuclear
    and cytoplasmic environments in the retarded DNA synthesis
    in Werner syndrome cells. Exp Cell Res 127:185-190.
Tanenbaum MH (1965) Werner's syndrome: progeria of the adult.
    Arch Intern Med 116:499-504.
Tao LC, Stecker E, Gardner HA (1971) Werner's syndrome and acute
    myeloid leukemia. Can Med Assoc J 105:952-954.
Thannhauser SJ (1945) Werner's syndrome (progeria of the adult)
    and Rothmund's syndrome: two types of closely related
    heredo-familial atrophic dermatosis with juvenile cataracts
    and endocrine features. A critical study with five new
    cases. Ann Intern Med 23:559.
Tokunaga M, Futami T, Wakamatsu E, Endo M, Yosizawa Z (1975)
    Werner's syndrome as "hyaluronuria." Clin Chim Acta 62:89-
    96.
Tokunaga M, Mori S, Sato K, Nakamura K, Wakamatsu E (1976)
    Postmortem study of a case of Werner's syndrome. J Am
    Geriatr Soc 24:407-411.

Tokunaga M, Wakamatsu E, Yosizawa Z (1979) Excretion of glucose-
    containing oligosaccharides in urines of orthopedic
    patients. Tohoku J Exp Med 128:71-79.
Vogel KG, Kendall VF, Sapien R (1981) Glycosaminoglycan synthesis
    and composition in human fibroblasts during in vitro
    cellular aging (IMR-90). J Cell Physiol 107:271-281.
Wight TN (1980) Vessel proteoglycans and thrombogenesis. Prog
    Hemost Thromb 5:1-39.
Werner O (1904) Uber Katarakt in Verbindung mit Sklerodermie
    (doctoral dissertation, Kiel University). Schmidt and
    Klauning, Kiel.
Wever J, Schachtschabel DO, Sluke G, Wever G (1980) Effect of
    short- or long-term treatment with exogenous glycosamino-
    glycans on growth and glycosaminoglycan synthesis of human
    fibroblasts (WI-38) in culture. Mech Ageing Dev 14:89-99.
Wojtyk RI, Goldstein S (1980) Fidelity of protein synthesis does
    not decline during aging of cultured human fibroblasts. J
    Cell Physiol 103:299-303.
Yatscoff RW, Goldstein S, Freeman KB (1978) Conservation of genes
    coding for proteins synthesized in human mitochondria.
    Somatic Cell Genet 4:633-645.
Yunis EJ, Fernandes G, Greenberg LJ (1976) Tumor immunology,
    autoimmunity and aging. J Am Geriatr Soc 24:258-263.
Zackai AH, Weber D, Noth R (1974) Cardiac findings in Werner's
    syndrome. Geriatrics 29:141-148.
Zalla JA (1980) Werner's syndrome. Cutis 25:275-278.
Zucker-Franklin D, Rifkin H, Jacobson HG (1968) Werner's
    Syndrome: an analysis of ten cases. Geriatrics 23:123-135.

KEYNOTE ADDRESS:
GENETICS AND AGING; THE WERNER SYNDROME AS A
SEGMENTAL PROGEROID SYNDROME

George M. Martin

Departments of Pathology and Genetics
University of Washington
Seattle, Washington 98195 USA

ABSTRACT

The maximum lifespan potential is a constitutional feature of
speciation and must be subject to polygenic controls acting both in
the domain of development and in the domain of the maintenance of
macromolecular integrity. The enormous genetic hererogeneity that
characterizes our own species, the complexities of numerous nature-
nurture interactions, and the quantitative and qualitative
variations of the senescent phenotype that are observed suggest
that precise patterns of aging in each of us may be unique.
Patterns of aging may also differ sharply among species (for
example, semelparous vs. multiparous mammals).

Some potential common denominators, however, allow one to
identify progeroid syndromes in man that could lead to the
elucidation of important pathways of gene action. (The suffix "-
oid" means "like"; it does not mean identity.) Unimodal progeroid
syndromes (eg., familial dementia of the Alzheimer type, an
autosomal dominant) can help us understand the pathogenesis of a
particular aspect of the senescent phenotype of man. Segmental
progeroid syndromes (eg. the Werner syndrome, an autosomal
recessive) may be relevant to multiple aspects of the senescent
phenotype.

Some results of research on the Werner syndrome may be
interpreted as support for "peripheral" as opposed to "central"
theories of aging; they are consistent with the view that gene
action in the domain of development (adolescence, in this instance)

can set the stage for patterns of aging in the adult; they point to
the importance of mesenchymal cell populations in the pathogenesis
of age-related disorders; finally, they underscore the role of
chromosomal instability, especially in the pathogenesis of
neoplasia.

INTRODUCTION

    All phenotypes result from an interaction of nature with
nuture, but all of us participating in this conference have the
conviction, I'm sure, that the most productive route to
understanding the biology and pathobiology of aging (including the
major age-related diseases of human beings) will come from a
dissection of the genetical aspects.

    In this review, I shall briefly summarize the rationale
behind this belief, some genetic approaches to the problem, and how
the so-called progeroid syndromes of man, and especially the
Werner Syndrome, can help in these endeavors.

The Maximum Lifespan Potential is a Constitutional Feature of
Speciation

    The principal rationale for the genetic approach to the study
of aging is the well-established species-specific variation in
maximum lifespan potential (MLSP) (Comfort, 1979). Among mammals,
the range of MLSP is about 40-50 fold (Altman and Dittmer, 1962).
Thus, when genetic variations are such as to lead to the evolution
of a new species, a characteristic lifespan is typically among the
new constitutional features of its phenotype.

Lifespan Must be Subject to Highly Polygenic Controls

    A corollary of the above conclusion is that it is almost
certainly the case that comparatively large numbers of genes are
involved in modulating the rates at which aging (and, presumably,
of age-related diseses) develop, since it is reasonable to assume
that changes in the expression of numerous genes are involved in
speciation.

    Three attempts have been made to estimate the numbers of genes
that might be involved in the aging of Homo sapiens. All of them,
including my own attempt (Martin, 1978) are based upon questionable
assumptions, however, so that a sound quantitative answer to that
important question is still not available.

    The first such attempts, carried out independently by the late
George Sacher (1975) and by Richard Cutler (1975), involved an

essentially identical strategy, based upon the evidence of a
strong, direct correlation of MLSP with brain weight and the
availability of data on the cranial capacities of the fossil
remains of homonid precursors of man. Such evidence pointed to a
comparatively rapid rate of evolution of increasing lifespan during
the rather short time period that lead to the emergence of Homo
sapiens. Extrapolating from estimates of rates of amino acid
substitutions in protein (and, therefore, rates of nucleotide base
substitution), they concluded that circa 200 genes may have been
associated with the increment of MLSP leading to the establishment
of our species. It may the case, however, that chromosomal
rearrangements are more significant in evolution than point
mutations (Wilson et al., 1977). A single chromosomal
rearrangement could potentially regulate the expression of hundreds
or thousands of genes. Thus, the hopeful notion that comparatively
"few" genes are involved in aging (Cutler, 1975) lacks strong
support. (A geneticist would consider any system controlled by
even a few dozen genes to be highly complex.)

My own efforts focussed upon an enumeration of genetic loci of
man, allelic variation or mutation at which resulted in modulations
of the rates of development of various aspects of the senescent
phenotype, as crudely described by human biologists, pathologists
and clinicians. For the most part, these genetic variations
exhibit abiotrophic effects in that degenerative and/or
proliferative events may not be expressed for many years following
birth. The conclusion was that up to around 7% of the genome might
be involved in modulating various aspects of the phenotype, although
I speculated that perhaps only 1% of those might be regularly of
importance in regulating features of aging. In any case, it seems
unlikely that only a few genes control the aging process. It is
therefore more prudent to refer to "aging processes" rather than to
"the aging process."

Two Broad Domains of Gene Action

How might the putative "aging genes" or "longevity assurance
genes" (Cutler, 1976) function? One convenient classification is
to consider two broad sub-sets: those that act in the domain of
development and those that act in the domain of the maintenance of
macromolecular integrity. To use the metaphor of a factory
designed to synthesize proteins, one set of genes could function in
the basic design and construction of the structure, including
specifications of the number of functioning units (cells) of
various types and their dynamics of growth, replacement and
interaction. Another set would specify the system of quality
control at various levels of synthesis, custom modifications,
packaging, shipping and field testing.

Two General Investigative Approaches

The "medical genetics" approach employed in the attempt,
mentioned above, to estimate the proportion of the genome of
potential relevance to the pathobiology of aging (Martin, 1978) is
an example of how gerontologists can utilize spontaneous genetic
variation to study aspects of their science. Our present major
preoccupation—the Werner syndrome—falls in this category. For
completeness, one should mention the other general investigative
approach—namely, the experimental induction of genetic variation
of relevance to aging and age-related disease. An excellent recent
example is provided by the work of Johnson and Wood (1982), in
which recombinant inbred lines of two varieties of the nematode,
Caenorhabditis elegans, revealed wide variances in lifespan,
including lines with lifespans substantially in excess of the
parental organisms; hybrids between those parentals had not
revealed any heterosis effect. Thus, the way is open to a formal
biochemical genetic analysis of genes leading to enhanced
lifespans. Such genes are likely to be of greater relevance to
basic mechanisms of aging than those that cause the progeroid
syndromes that will be shortly discussed.

But would the discovery of such genes necessarily give
universal truths concerning the biology of aging, such that they
could be applied to any species? It seems reasonable that a
proportion of them might apply, but one must be cautious. For
example, until recently, it was believed that all mammalian species
had multiparous modes of reproduction, post-reproductive aging and
functional decline unfolding relatively slowly after multiple
rounds of reproduction, with death occurring after variable, but
comparatively long, periods of time after the cessation of
reproduction. Several examples of semelparity are now known for
marsupial, insectivorous, male "mice" (and perhaps, in some
instances, females). The males die more or less synchronously,
shortly after a single, seasonal, intensive round of repeated
copulations. Death is preceded by an apparently neuroendocrine-
mediated diffuse testicular atrophy and fibrosis (reviewed by
Diamond, 1982). The pathobiology of aging in animals exhibiting
such "big-bang" reproduction may differ in fundamental ways from
the apparently less precisely programmed aging of most mammalian
species.

Genetic Variation in Homo sapiens: Is There Such a Thing as a
Standard Pattern of Aging in Man?

Our species is characterized by an extraordinary degree of
genetic heterogeneity. For example, in 1978, at a time when our
knowledge of the extent of allelic variation at the HLA complex was
far from exhausted, Bodmer and Bodmer (1978) had calculated that
the known genetic variation already could account for 300,000,000

genetically distinctive individuals! Since there is evidence that
allelic variation at the homologous gene cluster in Mus musculus
domesticus is associated with significant differences in the 90th
percentile survivorship of experimental cohorts (Smith and Walford,
1978), it may well be the case that comparable allelic variation in
man may be important determinants of individually unique patterns
of aging. Pathologists who do many autopsies of geriatric subjects
are well aware of the rich variety of quantitatively and
qualitatively distinctive patterns of morphologic findings (Martin,
1979). It is notable that even ubiquitous age-related findings,
such as atherosclerosis, exhibit an increase in variance with age
(Martin, et al., 1975a). Thus, it is safe to assume that
particular nature-nurture interactions in each of us results in
mosaic patterns of aging that, if they could be analyzed in great
detail, would give results that never occurred before in the
history of man, or indeed, are ever likely to occur again.
Nevertheless, there are some apparent common denominators and one
can use these to ask questions about genes that affect aspects of
the phenotype.

Progeroid Syndromes in Man

Since the time of Virchow, pathologists have been devoted to
the suffix "-oid." This expresses their reservations that, although
what is being described is like something else, it does not
necessarily follow that it is the same entity. Virchow, for
example, coined the term "amyloid" (like starch)," because organs
containing those substances gave a positive chemical reaction for
starch. We now know, of course, that amyloids are proteins, not
carbohydrates.

Further research will reveal to what extent the various
"progeroid" syndromes ("like premature senility") are indeed
helpful as model systems for aspects of the senescent phenotype or
as probes for the pathogenesis of important age-related diseases.
There are four general possibilities: 1) It may be that the
responsible genes are part of a sub-set that regularly function in
modulating the rates of aging of virtually all mammals or of
virtually all human subjects. 2) The gene action may exhibit such
properties except that only a single cell type or a few cell types
are affected. 3) The responsible genes are not those that are
ordinarily active in modulating rates of development of the
senescent phenotype but nevertheless can mimic, with varying
degress of fidelity, virtually all aspects of the phenotype. 4)
The responsible genes are not those that are ordinarily active in
modulating rates of development of the senescent phenotype but
nevertheless mimic, with varying degress of fidelity, the aging of
only a single cell type or a single class of cells. It is my bias
that the majority of such genes will prove to be examples of
category number 4, giving rather unfaithful, partial accelerations

of senescence. Even so, the identification of such genes and the
discovery of their biochemical modes of action will be of enormous
importance since the molecular understanding of any unusual pathway
can provide us with a means of discovering the usual pathway.
Moreover, as we have emphasized in the preceding section, all of
us probably have our fair share of private, unusual pathways!

Unimodal Progeroid Syndromes

     This term was introduced to describe the concept that there
are genetic disorders of man that affect, predominantly, a single
aspect of the senescent phenotype (Martin, 1982). An excellent and
exceedingly important example is familial dementia of the Alzheimer
type. There have now been described a number of pedigress in which
the disorder appears to be inherited as an autosomal dominant
(Martin, 1981). The histopathologic hallmarks of that disorder are
confined to the central nervous system, have been found to
accumulate as a function of age in the general population
(Murimatsu et al., 1975) and are quantitatively related to the
extent of clinical dementia (Blessed et al., 1968). In about 4% of
the population over the age of 65, the process appears to be
greatly accelerated, leading to clinically "severe dementia;" the
prevalence of "mild dementia" is about 11% (Katzman. 1976).

     Other examples of unimodal progeroid syndromes include xeroderma
pigmentosum (premature aging of skin), familial hypercholesterolemia
(premature atherosclerosis) and type III amyloidosis (premature
cardiac amyloidosis) (Martin, 1982).

Segmental Progeroid Syndromes

     Genetic syndromes of man in which multiple aspects (or
segments) of the senescent phenotype appear to be involved have
been referred to as "segmental progeroid syndromes" (Martin, 1978).
The Werner syndrome, of course, is the classical example.
Nevertheless, there are very important aspects of the senescent
phenotype that are not observed in the Werner syndrome—for
example, aging in the central nervous system.

     Other examples of segmental progeroid syndromes include the
Down syndrome, the Cockayne syndrome, the Hutchinson-Gilford
syndrome and Ataxia telangiectasia (Martin, 1978).

What Have We Learned so Far from the Study of the Werner Syndrome?"

     Some gerontologists believe that the time of onset of declines
in structure and function of somatic cells is determined by a
"clock" or a "pacemaker" in the central nervous system and is
mediated by neuroendocrine substances (Martin, 1980). The
distinguished gerontologist and psychologist, James E. Birren, has

referred to such gerontologists as "centralists" to differentiate them from those who believe that primary changes occur in various peripheral tissues and that these are independent of the central nervous system ("peripheralists")(Birren, personal communication). If we can presume that such age-related changes in peripheral somatic tissues set the stage, in human subjects, for such common age-related disorders as atherosclerosis, arteriolosclerosis, medial calcinosis, osteoporosis, diabetes mellitus, occular cataracts, neoplasms, regional fibrosis, and atrophy of skin, subcutaneous fat and gonads, then the mutation associated with the Werner syndrome provides evidence in support of the "peripheralists." Two lines of evidence support (but do not prove) this assertion. Firstly, there is the well-documented observation that cultured mesenchymal cells from such subjects exhibit accelerated in vitro aging (Martin et al, 1970). They also exhibit an increased propensity to undergo chromosomal mutations (Hoehn et al., 1975; Salk et al., 1981a), which, according to the work of the late Howard Curtis and others (Crowley and Curtis, 1963; Curtis et al., 1966; Curtis and Miller, 1971; Brooks et al., 1973) may constitute a basic parameter of cellular aging. Our information as to the extent to which chromosomal aberrations accompany in vitro aging is incomplete. Aneuploidy, polyploidy, breaks and translocations have been found late in the natural history of the cultures and have been interpreted as secondary events (Saksela and Moorhead, 1963; Thompson and Holliday, 1975). Because of the complexities of clonal selection, clonal attenuation and clonal succession in such cultures, however (Martin et al., 1974; Salk et al., 1981b), the extent and significance of such cytogenetic pathology may have been underestimated. It should be pointed out, parenthetically, that the finding of such cytogenetic lesions would not rule out cell differentiation theories of clonal attenuation (Martin et al., 1974; Martin et al., 1975b). Consider, for example, the extreme cytogenetic lesion that accompanies mammalian erythropoesis -- the elimination of the entire nucleus! However, even if one accepts the limited replicative lifespan of cultivated somatic cells as a valid model of at least some aspects of aging (a notion that continues to be rejected by such gerontologists as Robert Kohn) (Kohn, 1982), there would still remain the formal possibility that neuroendocrine events actually <u>initiate</u> heritable alterations in the somatic cells of patients with the Werner syndrome that then lead to the phenotype of limited replicative lifespan in vitro.

A second line of evidence in support of the "peripheralists" is that there have been no generally accepted, consistent, significant alterations in the neuroendocrine system of subjects with the Werner syndrome. However, since one does not really know what neuroendocrine parameters to examine in detail, such negative evidence is not particularly compelling.

One might also argue that the Werner syndrome provides some support for the idea that inappropriate gene action in the domain of development (specifically, failure of the physiological growth spurt associated with adolescence) can lead to premature onset and increased severity of a large number of age-related disorders in later adult life. One possibility is that there is a failure of a genetically defective pool of stem cells to undergo an appropriate degree of clonal amplification and differentiation in response to the new hormonal environment of adolescence. Studies of the pathology of the Werner syndrome (Epstein et al., 1966), which will be reviewed at this conference, and the cell culture investigations mentioned above, would implicate mesenchymal cells as the principal target cell population. Hayflick and Moorhead (1961) may therefore have made a very wise decision in focussing on cultivated fibroblast-like cells as a model for the study of cellular aging!

A final point (among many that might be made) is that the Werner syndrome appears to be of major importance to the understanding of the pathogenesis of neoplasia. It can now be added to a small list of inborn errors that can be considered to be chromosomal instability syndromes and which lead to greatly increased risks of diverse neoplasms. These include the Bloom syndrome, Ataxia-telangiectasia and Fanconi's anemia (German, 1983). In the Werner syndrome, the increased propensity of somatic cells to undergo such events as reciprocal translocations, inversions and deletions presumably lead (via effects on expression and dosage of genes involved in mitotic cell cycle control and differentiation) to an acceleration of one or more of the multiple steps of tumor initiation and tumor progression. Such events are now being intensively scrutinized at the molecular level.

Since the Werner syndrome is inherited as an autosomal recessive, we can assume that the molecular lesion results in an enzyme deficiency. The challenge before us is to discover this enzyme (or family of enzymes, if a sub-unit of multimeric proteins) and to determine both its role in normal physiology and its role in the pathogenesis of the Werner syndrome, ordinary aging, and various specific age-related disorders.

REFERENCES

Altman, P.L. and Dittmer, D.S. (1962), Lifespans: mammals. In
    Growth. Biological Handbook, Fed. Am. Soc. Exp. Biol.,
    Washington, D.C., pp. 445-450.
Blessed, G., Tomlinson, B.E. and Roth, M.L. (1968), The association
    between quantitative measures of dementia and of senile change
    in the cerebral grey matter of elderly subjects, Brit. J.
    Psychiat., 113:797.

Bodmer, W.F. and Bodmer, J.G. (1978), Evolution and function of the HLA system, Brit. Med. Bull. 34:309.

Brooks, A.L., Mead, D.K. and Peters, R.F. (1973), Effect of aging on frequency of metaphase chromosome aberrations in liver of Chinese hamster, J. Gerontol. 28:452.

Comfort, A. (1979), The Biology of Senescence, Elsevier, New York.

Crowley, C. and Curtis, H.J. (1963), The development of somatic mutations in mice with age, Proc. Natl. Acad. Sci. USA 49:626.

Curtis, H.J., Leith, J. and Tilley, J. (1966), Chromosomal aberrations in liver cells of dogs of different ages, J. Gerontol. 21:268.

Curtis, H.J. and Miller, K. (1971), Chromosomal aberrations in liver cells of guinea pigs, J Gerontol. 26:292.

Cutler, R.G. (1975). Evolution of human longevity and the genetic complexity governing aging rate. Proc. Natl. Acad. Sci. M.S. 72:4664.

Cutler, R.G. (1976). On the nature of aging and life maintenance processes, in Interdisciplinary Topics in Gerontology, (ed. by R.G. Cutler), Vol. 9, Karger, Basel, p. 83.

Diamond, J.M. (1982). Big-bang reproduction and ageing in male marsupial mice, Nature, 298:115.

Epstein, C.J., Martin, G.M., Schultz, A.L., and Motulsky, A.G. (1966), Werner's syndrome. A review of its symptomology, natural history, pathologic features, genetics and relationship to the natural aging process, Medicine, 45:177.

German, J. (ed.)(1983), Chromosome Mutation and Neoplasia, Alan R. Liss, New York.

Hayflick, L. and Moorhead, P.S. (1961), The serial cultivation of human diploid cell strains, Exp. Cell. Res. 25:585.

Hoehn, H., Bryant, E.M., Au, K., Norwood, T.H., Borman, H. and Martin, G.M. (1975), Variegated translocation mosaicism in human skin fibroblast cultures, Cytogenet. Cell Genet. 15:282.

Johnson, T.E. and Wood, W.B. (1982), Genetic analysis of life span in the nematode, Caenorhabditis elegans, Proc. Natl. Acad. Sci. U.S.A., 79:6603.

Katzman, R. (1976), The prevalence and malignancy of Alzheimer Disease, Arch. Neurol. 33:217.

Kohn, R.R. (1982), Evidence against cellular aging theories, in Testing the Theories of Aging (ed. by R.C. Adelman and G.S. Roth), CRC Press, Boca Raton, Fla., pp. 221-231.

Martin, G.M., Sprague, C.A. and Epstein, C.J. (1970), Replicative life-span of cultivated human cells: Effect of donor's age, tissue and genotype, Lab. Invest. 23:86.

Martin, G.M., Sprague, C.A., Norwood, T.H. and Pendergrass, W. (1974), Clonal selection attenuation and differentiation in an in-vitro model of hyperplasia, Amer. J. Path, 74:137.

Martin, G.M., Ogburn, C.E. and Sprague, C.A., (1975a), Senescence and vascular disease, in Explorations in Aging (ed. by V.J. Cristofalo, J. Roberts and R.L. Adelman), Plenum Press, New York, Adv. Exp. Med. Biol. 61:163.

Smith, G.S. and Walford, R.L. (1978). Influence of the H-2 and H-1
    histocompatibility systems upon the lifespan and spontaneous
    cancer incidences in congenic mice, in Genetic Effects on
    Aging (ed. by D. Bergsma and D.E. Harrison), Original Article
    Series, Vol. 14, No. 7, Alan R. Liss, New York, pp. 281-312.
Wilson, A.C., White, T.J., Carlson, S.S. and Cherry, L.M. (1977).
    Molecular evolution and cytogenetic evolution. In Molecular
    Human Cytogenetics, ICN-UCLA Symposium on Molecular and Cell
    Biology, Vol. 7, Academic Press, New York, pp. 375-393.

CLINICAL, ENDOCRINE AND METABOLIC ASPECTS OF THE WERNER SYNDROME
COMPARED WITH THOSE OF NORMAL AGING

Hiroo Imura*, Yoshinobu Nakao**, Hideshi Kuzuya *,
Motozumi Okamoto*, Mikiko Okamoto* and Kazunori Yamada*

 * Department of Medicine, Kyoto University Faculty of
   Medicine, Sakyo-ku, Kyoto 606
** Department of Medicine, Kobe University School of
   Medicine, Chuoku, Kobe 650, Japan

ABSTRACT

    Data on the clinical features of the Werner syndrome in 102
patients in Japan were collected by sending questionnaires to
major hospitals and analyzed. The male-to-female ratio was 3 to
2 and the incidences of consanguinity and familial occurrence
were 51% and 39.4%, respectively. These patients were divided
into 3 subgroups; group 1, 2, and 3 lacked short stature,
cataract, and hypogonadism, respectively. Each group had
somewhat different clinical features.

    Endocrine and metabolic abnormalities in the Werner syndrome
patients were compared with those in normal aged subjects.
Impaired plasma growth-hormone responses to insulin and arginine
were more common and impaired plasma thyrotropin responses to TRH
were less common in the Werner syndrome patients than in aged
subjects. Plasma LH and FSH levels were higher in most patients
than those in age- and sex-matched controls; also, their serum
testosterone concentrations were lower than those in age-matched
controls and testicular biopsy revealed more marked atrophy than
in aged subjects. Serum triiodothyronine levels tended to be
lower than in age-matched controls. Oral glucose tolerance test
revealed diabetic glucose tolerance in 55% and impaired glucose
tolerance in 22%, although fasting blood glucose levels were
elevated only in 20%. Plasma insulin response to glucose was
more exaggerated in those with the Werner syndrome than in normal
aged subjects. The euglycemic glucose clamp method revealed

171

lower glucose disposal rates and insulin sensitivity indices in the Werner syndrome than in normal subjects of similar age. The number of erythrocyte insulin-binding sites was normal in the Werner syndrome patients. These results suggest a postreceptor defect in insulin resistance in the Werner syndrome.

INTRODUCTION

The Werner syndrome has drawn much attention as a model of at least some aspects of normal aging, because of the similarity of its characteristic features to those of normal aged subjects. Since the Werner syndrome is inherited in an autosomal recessive fashion, it is presumably caused by a single gene defect and may serve as a tool to explore the mechanism of aging. However, there also seem to be some dissimilarities between the Werner syndrome and normal aging, and thus the phenotypic differences between the two conditions require investigation.

This article deals with the clinical and biochemical features of Japanese patients with the Werner syndrome, and some endocrine and metabolic tests performed in our laboratory.

CLINICAL FEATURES OF THE WERNER SYNDROME IN JAPAN

By sending questionnaires to major hospitals in Japan, we have collected the data of 102 patients with the Werner syndrome: 61 males and 41 females (male-to-female ratio approximately 3:2). In the review of Epstein et al. (1966), the male to female ratio was 70 to 64. In our studies, a history of consanguineous marriage was recorded in 50 of 98 cases (51.0%) and the occurrence in siblings was found in 39 of 99 cases (39.4%). Studies of familial cases suggested autosomal recessive inheritance, although there are many sporadic cases in whom the mode of inheritance could not be determined because of the lack of data concerning atypical cases or stillbirth.

Age at onset as judged by the occurrence of one of the major clinical manifestations of the Werner syndrome is shown in Table 1. Ten-to-nineteen years was the age at which the onset most frequently occurred, followed by 20-29 years.

Table 2 shows the clinical features in these 102 patients. As a whole, the major clinical manifestations were cataract (95.1%); skin manifestations such as hyperkeratosis (88.1%), atrophy (85.1%), sclerotic changes (83.1%) and ulceration (41.8%); loss (76.0%) and/or graying (81.0%) of hair; and a change of voice (79.0%). Although a little less frequent, short stature, low body weight, and genital atrophy were also important

Table 1

Werner's syndrome in Japan

No. of Cases		102
Sex: Male		59.8 %
Female		40.2 %
Family History:	Consanguity	51.0
	Familial occurrence	39.4
Age of onset:	Below 10	10.7
	10 - 19	51.6
	20 - 29	22.5
	30 - 39	11.8
	Over 40	1.1

symptoms. Other symptoms included bone or connective-tissue abnormalities, such as deformity, osteoporosis, and soft-tissue calcification. Goto et al. (1978) reported 15 cases and postulated both flat foot and hyperreflexia as additional important clinical manifestations in the Werner syndrome.

Although the Werner syndrome is considered to be an abnormality of one major gene, there are many atypical or abortive cases and the combination of clinical manifestations is not uniform, even in typical cases. To analyze the heterogeneity of the clinical manifestations, we divided the majority of the patients into 3 groups: Group 1 were of normal body height; Group 2 had no sign of cataract; Group 3 had normal or almost normal sexual function. As shown in Table 2, onset tended to be late in patients in Group 1, bone changes and hypogonadism were infrequent, and frequency of skin manifestations was high. Group 2 patients were usually of short stature and less frequently had skin or hair changes and bone abnormalities; onset of the disease tended to be early. Group 3 patients had a history of onset after puberty and a less frequent association of short stature, skin ulcer, hair abnormality, and osteoporosis. In spite of such difference in clinical manifestations, there were no differences in the incidence of consanguinious marriage and familial occurrence among three groups.

Table 2

Clinical features and subtypes of Werner's syndrome

		Total	Group 1	Group 2	Group 3
Number of patients		102	22	6	23
Heredity—Consanguinity		51.0%	50.0%	50.0%	56.0%
	Familial occurrence	39.4	31.8	33.3	40.0
Body size	Short stature	75.7	0	83.3	48.0
	Low body weight	74.7	54.5	50.0	48.0
Age of onset	0–10	10.7	0	33.3	12.0
	10–19	51.6	36.3	33.3	26.0
	20–29	22.5	27.2	33.3	36.0
	30–39	11.8	36.3	0	20.0
	40+	1.1	0	0	4.0
Skin	Sclerosis	83.1	90.9	33.3	76.0
	Hyperkeratosis	88.1	90.9	83.3	72.0
	Atrophy	85.1	95.4	66.6	72.0
	Ulceration	41.8	36.3	16.6	16.0
Hair	Graying	81.0	95.4	50.0	68.0
	Alopecia	76.0	63.6	33.3	56.0
Eye	Cataract	95.1	95.4	0	68.0
Larynx	Change of voice	79.0	86.3	50.0	64.0
Bone and Connective Tissue					
	Osteoporosis	61.4	50.0	50.0	40.0
	Bone deformity	44.7	31.8	83.3	36.0
	Calcification	32.1	18.1	50.0	32.0
Gonads	Hypogonadism	70.3	54.5	50.0	0
Complications					
	Diabetes	61.3	54.5	33.3	52.3
	Neoplasms	13.8	0	36.6	8.0
	Liver dysfunction	35.4	27.2	33.3	43.0

The Werner syndrome is known to be associated with the dysfunction of a variety of organs. In our series, mild liver dysfunction was noted in 35.4%, suggesting the presence of a fatty liver. EEG abnormalities were recorded in 28.0% and neurological abnormalities in 14.5%. Some patients showed brain atrophy when tested by computed tomography but the incidence of this is unclear. Renal function was impaired in 12.2%. Sclerosis of retinal arteries was noted in 26.3%. Frequent association of mesodermal neoplasia with the Werner syndrome have been repeatedly pointed out since the report of Epstein et al. (1966). In our group, 13.8% of patients were associated with malignancies that included 3 cases of meningioma, 2 cases each of fibrosarcoma, malignant melanoma, and thyroid tumors, and 4 cases of miscellaneous tumors.

ENDOCRINE ABNORMALITIES IN THE WERNER SYNDROME

One of the characteristic abnormalities in the Werner syndrome is in endocrine function. Table 3 shows the results of pituitary function tests in the Werner syndrome in comparison with those in aged subjects. Plasma growth hormone response to insulin-induced hypoglycemia and to argine was impaired in patients with the Werner syndrome far more frequently than in normal aged subjects. A similar decreased response of plasma growth hormone has been reported (Alberti et al., 1974; Miyamoto et al., 1977; Nakao et al., 1978). These observations are of considerable interest, since the adolescent growth spurt, which is probably attributable to the combined action of growth hormone and androgens, is usually absent in the Werner syndrome. However, such impaired response of plasma growth hormone to hypoglycemia and arginine does not necessarily imply growth-hormone deficiency, because the propranolol-insulin stimulation test, a more potent provocative test, elicited a normal response in 4 of the 5 patients studied. The reason for an impaired response of growth hormone to insulin-induced hypoglycemia and arginine is not clear, but some abnormalities can be assumed in the central nervous system that involves the regulation of growth-hormone secretion.

In contrast to the growth-hormone findings, plasma prolactin responses in the Werner syndrome patients to thyrotropin-releasing hormone (TRH) were not significantly different from those in aged subjects. However, plasma thyrotropin response to TRH tended to be higher in patients with the Werner syndrome than normal octogenarians. A progressive decrease in thyrotropin response to TRH with age has been reported by several investigators (Snyder and Utiger, 1972); the reason for this decrease is still unknown. Miyamoto et al. (1977) reported that

Table 3

Pituitary function tests in patients with
the Werner syndrome and aged subjects

	Werner syndrome impairment	Aged subjects impairment
Plasma GH responses to:		
Insulin-induced hypoglycemia	73.7%	10.0%[*]
Arginine	42.1	8.5 [*]
Propranolol-insulin	20.0	---
Plasma PRL responses to TRH	12.5	18[*]
Plasma TSH responses to TRH	10.7	24.2[**]
Plasma cortisol or ACTH responses to:		
ACTH	0	0[*]
Metyrapone	0	0[*]

   * over 60 years old
  ** over 80 years old

plasma thyrotropin response to TRH was somewhat exaggerated in
the Werner syndrome. In the present series, however, most of the
patients studied showed normal thyrotropin response to TRH,
coinciding with normal serum T_4 concentrations, as will be
discussed later. Plasma cortisol responses to ACTH and plasma
ACTH responses to metyrapone were all within normal limits both
in patients with the Werner syndrome and in normal aged subjects.

Plasma luteinizing hormone (LH) levels change with age in
both males and females. There is considerable individual
variation, but in normal females an abrupt rise is observed after
age 50, whereas a gradual increase after 60 years of age is noted
in males (Fig. 1). Most of the patients with the Werner syndrome
showed higher basal LH levels than did the sex- and age-matched
controls. Similar changes were observed in plasma follicle
stimulating hormone (FSH) levels, increasing abruptly after age
50 in females and gradually after age 60 in males (Fig. 2). Most
of the patients with the Werner syndrome showed high basal plasma
FSH levels, even below age 50.

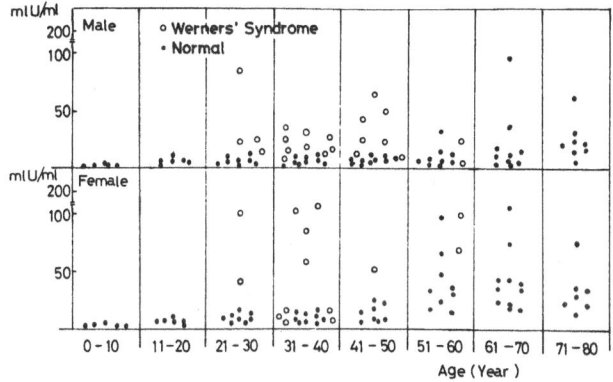

Fig. 1:   Plasma LH levels in normal subjects of various ages and patients with the Werner syndrome.

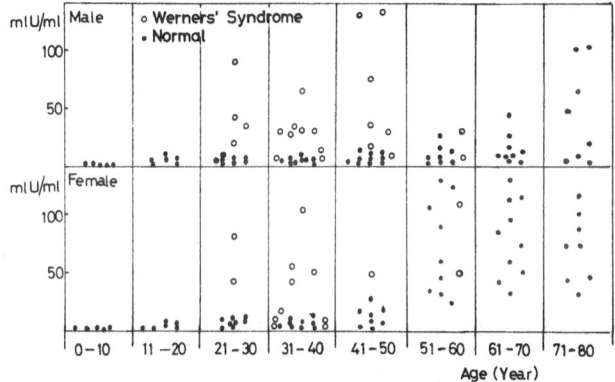

Fig. 2:   Plasma FSH levels in normal subjects of various ages and patients with the Werner syndrome.

Plasma LH and FSH responses to luteinizing hormone-releasing hormone (LHRH) were exaggerated in 20 of 28 Japanese patients in comparison with those in normal young adults. Fig. 3 shows results in 5 cases in our laboratory. There were considerable individual differences but, in general, the responses to LHRH were comparable to or greater than those in aged male subjects.

Serum testosterone levels in normal males tend gradually to decrease with age after maturity, although there are marked individual variations. In our studies 7 of 9 patients with the Werner syndrome showed lower values than those in age-matched controls. Low serum testosterone levels associated with elevated plasma LH levels in Werner's syndrome suggest the primary failure

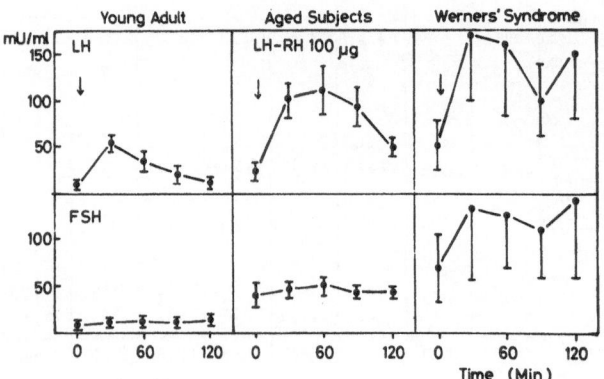

Fig. 3:   Plasma LH and FSH responses to 100 µg of LHRH in normal
           young and elderly male subjects and patients with the
           Werner syndrome.

of Leydig's cell function. This was confirmed by the human
chorionic gonadotropin (hCG) loading test. Repeated hCG
injections for 3 days are associated with a marked increase of
serum testosterone in young adults and a low or equivocal
increase in aged subjects. Three Werner's syndrome patients
studied by us showed no significant increase.

     Testicular biopsy performed in three patients revealed
moderate-to-severe atrophy; diminished spermatogenic activity and
thickening of the tubular wall were seen. These results agree
with previous observations (Epstein et al., 1966; Ishii and
Hosoda, 1975). Such histological changes of the testes in the
Werner syndrome are essentially the same as those in aged
subjects, although they were more severe in some patients with
the Werner syndrome.

     Serum thyroxine levels did not change significantly with
age, whereas serum levels of triiodothyronine (T_3), an active
thyroid hormone, gradually decrease with age, with a linear
regression line as shown in Fig. 4 (Nishikawa et al., 1981).
There was no significant sex difference in serum T_3 levels.
Patients with the Werner syndrome had normal serum T_4 levels in
our series as already reported by Epstein et al. (1966).
However, these patients tended to have serum T_3 levels lower than
those of age-matched controls and the mean level in 9 patients
was almost comparable to that of the seventh decade. The reason
for the decrease of serum T_3 levels is unknown, but it might be
caused by a decrease in the demand for T_3 in the Werner syndrome,
as in aged subjects.

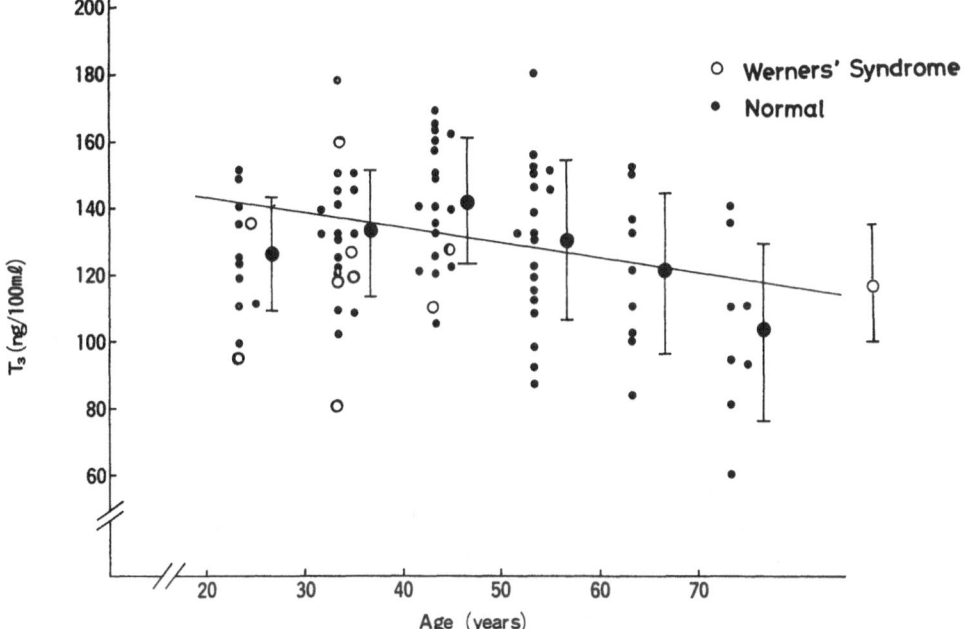

Fig. 4:   Serum triiodothyronine (T_3) levels in normal subjects
          of various ages and patients with the Werner syndrome.
          The mean ($\pm$SE) T_3 levels in the Werner syndrome is
          shown on the right side by an open circle.

METABOLIC ABNORMALITIES IN THE WERNER SYNDROME

    One of the characteristic abnormalities in the Werner
syndrome is decreased glucose tolerance or diabetes mellitus,
which has been reviewed repeatedly (Irwin and Ward, 1953; Field
and Loube, 1960; Epstein et al., 1966). Epstein et al. (1966)
reported that diabetes was recognized in 55 of 125 cases (44.4%)
in the medical literature, although only 5 cases had significant
symptoms such as polyuria, polydipsia, pruritus, and weight loss.
The percentage is much higher if abnormal glucose tolerance
curves are considered. In fact, Field and Loube (1960) reported
that 21 of 32 cases reported in the literature had diabetic
glucose tolerance curves. Among our collected cases, 49 patients
had the oral glucose tolerance test: when the criteria proposed
by WHO was used, 27 (55%) of them fell into the category of
diabetes mellitus and 11 (22%) into the category of impaired
glucose tolerance. Only 11 patients showed normal glucose
tolerance curves. Fasting blood glucose concentrations were
elevated more than 120 mg/dl only in 10 patients, suggesting that

the impairment of glucose tolerance is generally mild in the Werner syndrome.

A decrease in glucose tolerance with age in normal subjects has been repeatedly reported by many investigators. Wingerd and Duffy (1977) performed oral glucose tolerance test in 2248 women between 18 and 61 years of age and concluded that blood glucose levels at 1 hour and 2 hours after oral glucose loading increase 10 mg/dl and 5 mg/dl, respectively, per decade. In our studies, however, the impairment of glucose tolerance in aged subjects was milder than that in the Werner syndrome (Fig. 5).

Plasma insulin response to the oral glucose tolerance test was exaggerated in the Werner syndrome in all three groups of glucose tolerance, even in the diabetic glucose tolerance group. Of the 27 patients in this group, plasma insulin was measured in 19. Plasma insulin levels at 30 minutes after glucose challenge ranged from 6 to 330 μU/ml and the peak values ranged from 12 to 463 μU/ml. Although there was a tendency toward delayed responses, definitely decreased responses of plasma insulin (peak values below 30 μU/ml) were noted only in 2 of the 19 patients studied. None of the patients studied was obese. These results are in contrast to our previous results in non-obese, not-insulin

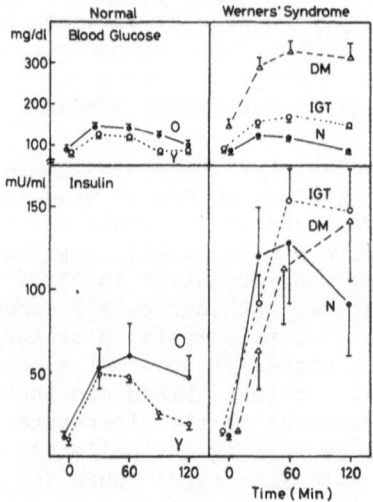

Fig. 5:   Responses of blood glucose and plasma insulin in normal
            young (Y) and elderly (O) subjects and patients with
            the Werner syndrome (right frame). The patients were
            divided into groups of normal glucose tolerance (N),
            impaired glucose tolerance (IGT) and diabetes mellitus
            (DM).

dependent diabetic patients, in whom plasma insulin response was
usually decreased (Imura et al., 1977). Results of plasma
insulin response to oral glucose loading in aged subjects are
variable, although many investigators report slightly exaggerated
responses (Davidson, 1979). In our studies, plasma insulin
response was slightly greater in aged subjects than in young
adults. However, the peak insulin values in aged subjects were
lower than those in the Werner syndrome. It appears, therefore,
that the exaggerated plasma insulin response to glucose is a
characteristic feature in the Werner syndrome.

Several factors can be considered to explain decreased
glucose tolerance in aged subjects and in patients with the
Werner syndrome. Decreased insulin secretion is not a cause of
glucose intolerance as discussed above. Decreased dietary intake
(starvation diabetes) and physical inactivity are also possible
causes of glucose intolerance, but these factors are probably not
important in our cases, since they were eating a fairly normal
amount of foods and were physically active. The third
possibility is a decrease in lean body mass, which stores dietary
carbohydrate. It is well known that lean body mass decreases
with age, as does the disappearance rate of glucose administered
intravenously: the two factors correlate to some extent but the
correlation is of low magnitude, suggesting other factors may be
important (Davidson, 1979). Although not estimated accurately,
the lean body mass is decreased in the Werner syndrome, possibly
more than in elderly subjects; this might explain, in part, the
decreased glucose tolerance in the Werner syndrome.

Another, and probably the most likely possibility is insulin
antagonism. To test insulin sensitivity, we have applied the
euglycemic glucose clamp technique (DeFronzo, 1979) in normal

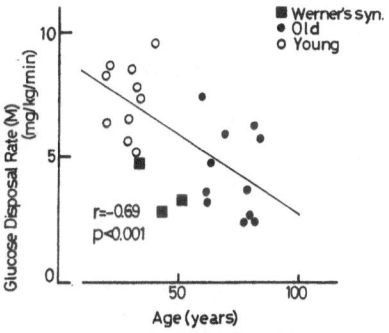

Fig. 6:   Glucose disposal rate estimated by euglycemic clamp
technique plotted against age, in young and elderly
subjects and patients with the Werner syndrome.

subjects and patients with the Werner syndrome. As shown in Fig.
6, the glucose disposal rate measured by this technique decreases
linearly with age. Two of three patients with the Werner
syndrome showed a low glucose disposal rate. Steady-state plasma
insulin concentrations were higher in the Werner syndrome and in
aged subjects than in young controls, suggesting decreased
insulin clearance in the first two groups. Therefore, the
insulin sensitivity indices, as calculated by dividing the
glucose disposal rate by the steady-state plasma insulin
concentration, are low in aged subjects and even lower in the
Werner syndrome (Fig. 7). DeFronzo (1979) also observed
decreases in glucose disposal rate and insulin sensitivity index
in aged subjects using the euglycemic clamp method.

What causes tissue insensitivity to insulin in aged subjects
and patients with the Werner syndrome? To explore this question,
we studied 125I-insulin binding to cultured fibroblasts obtained
from two patients with the Werner syndrome. 125I-insulin binding
per cell tended to be higher in the Werner syndrome, possibly
because of the increased size of fibroblasts in culture. These
results contradict previous reports that insulin receptors in
isolated fat cells are decreased in the Werner syndrome (Beadle
et al., 1978; Smith et al., 1980). The reason for such a
discrepancy might be explained by tissue differences, because
both studies used fat cells that were quite large. Our
observations strongly suggest that the major defect in insulin
action in aged subjects and in the Werner syndrome is in the
post-receptor step.

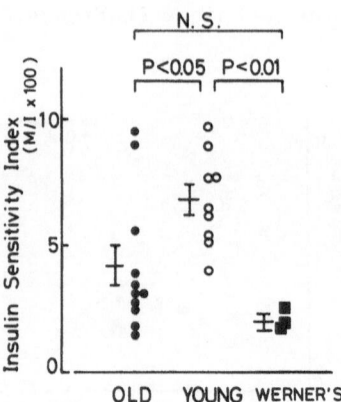

Fig. 7:   Insulin sensitivity indices calculated by dividing
           glucose disposal rate by steady state insulin
           concentrations in normal subjects and patients with the
           Werner syndrome.

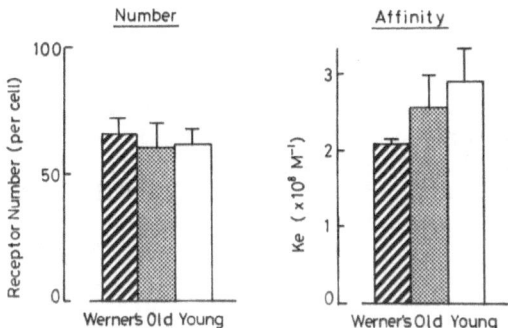

Fig. 8:   The number and affinity of insulin-binding sites on
           erythrocytes obtained from normal young and elderly
           subjects and patients with the Werner syndrome.

DISCUSSION

In our present studies, we have collected data on 102
patients with the Werner syndrome in Japan. The incidences of
the various symptoms were not greatly different from those given
in the previous review (Goto et al., 1978). One point worth
mentioning is the relatively low incidence of arteriosclerosis in
our series and in the literature in Japan (Goto et al., 1978),
whereas Epstein et al. (1966) stressed arteriosclerosis as a
prominent feature of the Werner syndrome. This difference may be
explained by different environmental factors. Such lower
incidence of arteriosclerosis is different from that in normal
aging. Hypertension is known to be also less frequent in the
Werner syndrome. On the contrary, skin change, especially
ulceration, and atrophy of muscle and adipose tissue are more
prominent in the Werner syndrome. The high incidence of
neoplasms of mesodermal origin was confirmed in our present
series.

Although the Werner syndrome may be a disease entity caused
by a single gene mutation, we were able to divide our patients
into 3 subgroups. Each subgroup had somewhat different clinical
features (Table 2). However, the significance of the phenotypic
heterogeneity of the Werner syndrome is not known and must await
further clarification. Another aim of the present study was to
compare the endocrine and metabolic aspects of the Werner
syndrome with those of normal aged subjects. Table 4 summarizes
the major differences. Impaired growth hormone responses to
insulin and arginine are relatively common in the Werner
syndrome. On the other hand, the plasma thyrotropin response to
TRH is somewhat decreased in aged subjects. Primary testicular

atrophy as revealed by the measurement of serum testosterone, plasma LH and FSH and also by testicular biopsy is more prominent in the Werner syndrome than in normal aged subjects. Another important difference is severe insulin insensitivity in the Werner syndrome. This is partly explained by a decrease of lean body mass, but mainly is due to tissue resistance to insulin. The basic mechanisms causing primary testicular atrophy and insulin resistance are still unknown and require further study.

Table 4

Comparison of endocrine and metabolic aspects of
the Werner syndrome with those of aging

	Werner syndrome	Aging
Impaired GH responses to various stimuli	Common	Uncommon
Decreased TSH response to TRH	Uncommon	Not uncommon
Testicular atrophy	Severe	Mild
Plasma insulin response to oral glucose loading	Exaggerated	Almost normal
Insulin insensitivity	Severe	Less severe

REFERENCES

Alberti, K.G.M.M., Young, J.D.H., and Hockaday, T.D.R. (1974), Werner's syndrome: metabolic observations, Proc. Roy. Soc. Med., 67:36.
Beadle, G.F., Mackay, I.R., Whittingham, S., Taggert, G., Harris, A.W., and Harrison, L.C. (1978), Werner's syndrome, a model of premature aging? J. Med., 9:377.
Davidson, M.B. (1979), The effect of aging on carbohydrate metabolism: A review of English literature and a practical approach to the diagnosis of diabetes mellitus in the elderly, Metabolism, 28:688.
DeFronzo, R.A. (1979), Glucose intolerance and aging. Evidence for tissue insensitivity to insulin, Diabetes, 28:1095.
Epstein, C.J., Martin, G.M., Schultz, A.L., and Motulsky, A.G. (1966), Werner's syndrome. A review of its symptomatology,

natural history, pathologic features, genetics and
relationship to the natural process, Medicine, 45:177.

Field, J.B. and Loube, S.D. (1960), Observations concerning the
diabetes mellitus associated with Werner's syndrome,
Metabolism, 9:118.

Goto, M., Horiuchi, Y., Tanimoto, K., Ishii, T. and Nakashima, H.
(1978), Werner's syndrome: Analysis of 15 cases with a
review of the Japanese literature, J. Am. Geriat. Soc.,
16:341.

Imura, H., Ikeda, M. and Seino, Y. (1977), Significance of the
measurement of plasma insulin and glucagon in the diagnosis
of diabetes mellitus, Jpn. J. Med., 16:55.

Irwin, G.W. and Ward, P.B. (1953), Werner's syndrome -- with a
report of two cases, Am. J. Med., 15:266.

Ishii, T. and Hosoda, Y. (1975), Werner's syndrome: Autopsy
report of one case, with a review of pathologic findings
reported in the literature, J. Am. Geriat. Soc., 13:145.

Miyamoto, M., Ueda, M., Nakabayashi, H., Uchida, K., Saito, Z.,
Takeda, R. and Tomari, Y. (1977), Werner's syndrome, Jpn. J.
Geriat., 14:178.

Nakao, Y., Kishihara, M., Yoshimi, H., Inoue, Y., Tanaka, K.,
Sakamoto, N., Matsukura, S., Imura, H., Ichihashi, M. and
Fujiwara, Y. (1978), Werner's syndrome. In vivo and in vitro
characteristics as a model of aging, Am. J. Med., 65:919.

Nishikawa, M., Inada, M., Naito, K., Ishii, H., Tanaka, K.,
Mashio, Y. and Imura, H. (1981), Age-related changes of serum
3,3'-diiodothyronine, 3'5'-diiodothyronine and 3,5-
diiodothyronine concentrations in man, J. Clin. Endocrinol.
Metab., 52:517.

Smith, U., Digiorolamo, M., Blohme, G., Kral, J. and Tisell, L-E
(1980), Possible systemic metabolic effects of regional
adiposity in a patient with Werner's syndrome, Int. J. Obesity,
4:153.

Snyder, P.J. and Utiger, R.D. (1972), Response to thyrotropin
releasing hormone in man, J. Clin. Endocrinol. Metab. 34:380.

Wingerd, J. and Duffy, T.J. (1977), Oral contraceptive use and
other factors in the standard glucose tolerance test, Diabetes,
26:1024

PATHOLOGY OF THE WERNER SYNDROME

Toshiharu Ishii[1], Yasuhiro Hosoda[1], Yoshiro Hamada[2], Sadaaki Nakagawa[3], Goro Asano[4], and Yoshimune Horibe[5]

Departments of Pathology[1,3,4,5] and Dermatology[2], Keio University School of Medicine[1], Shinjukuku Tokyo 160, Japan; also Numazu Municipal Hospital[2], Kawasaki Medical School[3], Nippon Medical School[4], and Nagoya Fujita Gakuen Medical School[5]

INTRODUCTION

Anatomic-pathological observation remains one of the fundamental approaches to the understanding of multiple system disease of unknown etiology. In this paper, we review the results of such anatomic investigations of necropsies of subjects with the Werner syndrome, including five cases (all Japanese subjects) that we have personally autopsied, one of which (Case 5) has not been previously reported.

NECROPSIED CASES OF JAPANESE PATIENTS WITH THE WERNER SYNDROME

Case 1 (Hamada, 1966). The patient was a 51-year-old childless, married male furniture manufacturer.

Chief complaints: nasal bleeding and cardiac arrhythmias.

Family history: No consanguinity. The father had died in a motor vehicle accident, the mother of pneumonia. The patient was the fourth of six siblings. His elder brother, who had died of pulmonary tuberculosis, was said to have been constitutionally small (both for height and weight). He had suffered from bilateral ocular cataracts since his adolescence and apparently had premature graying of the hair and was somewhat bald. The other siblings appeared to be normal.

187

Past history: The patient had noticed progressive emaciation and hoarseness since he was 18 years old. His hair began to drop out and turn grey and the skin of his lower lips became taut from about age 28. At age 30, ocular cataracts were noted, and he sustained a fracture of the knee joint. Intractable skin ulcers of the right lateral malleolus developed at age 36, and of the left heel at age 44, both persisting until his death.

Present illness: He was admitted to the Numazu Municipal Hospital on 20 Oct., 1969, at the age of 50. His body height was 150 cm and body weight, 20 kg. His intelligence was normal and his countenance looked senile. Skeletal muscle, subcutaneous adipose tissue, and genital organs were atrophic. Axillary and pubic hair were both sparse. The skin showed generalized sclerosis, which was bilaterally pronounced on the forearms, lower limbs and dorsal areas of the feet. The skin overlying the elbow and knee joints showed hyperkeratosis with atrophy and telangiectasia. On admission, pulmonary tuberculosis was diagnosed because of an abnormal chest X-ray and elevated erythrocyte sedimentation rate. Treatment with streptomycin was initiated. Nasal bleeding, present at the time of admission, was no longer observed. In the area of the intractable skin ulcer of the feet, the bone was exposed and osteomyelitis was diagnosed from cultures of Staphlococci and from X-ray findings. The osteomyelitis was resistant to antibiotic therapy. Positive laboratory findings were as follows: anemia (RBC 329 x 10^4/mm^3, haemoglobin 75% of normal); proteinuria (+) and glycosuria (++); unstable glucose tolerance test (the results fluctuated between those of normal and diabetics); serum calcium 7.3 mEq/l and basal metabolic rate +21%.

A diagnosis of the Werner syndrome was made. The results of a skin biopsy were consistent with this clinical diagnosis. The patient became dyspneic, cardiac arrhythmias persisted, and he became febrile (39.6° C). He died of pneumonia on 13 Oct., 1970 at the age of 51.

Necropsy findings: The skin showed a marked generalized atrophy, especially on forearms, legs and feet (Fig. 1). The skin of the right malleolus and heel was ulcerated, with partial exposure of the underlying bone. Hyperkeratotic scales were seen on both elbow joints and telangiectasia was noted on both patellar regions. The skin of the back revealed both epidermal atrophy and hyperatosis. The epidermis showed atrophy of the rete ridge and slight hyperpigmentation. In the dermis, sweat gland atrophy and intimal thickening of the small arteries were seen. The heart weighed 300 g and did not reveal significant change histologically. The brain, weighing 1190 g, appeared atrophic, but otherwise was unremarkable. The aorta and other arteries showed somewhat advanced sclerotic changes for his age.

The left lung weighed 350 g and the right, 720 g. In the right
upper pulmonary lobe, focal fibrosis was seen, associated with
scattered old calcified tuberculous nodules. In the surrounding
tissues, there was broncho-pneumonia. The liver, weighing 750 g,
was atrophic. Histologically, there was centrilobular congestion
and slight degree of fatty alteration. Fresh fibrin thrombi were
present in the arterioles in the portal triad. The kidneys, each
weighing 100 g, were congested and several retention cysts were
noted. Arteriosclerosis was noted in the renal arterial system.
The spleen, weighing 40 g, was congested and fibrous. The
endocrine organs were not weighed. The thyroid and parathyroid
appeared to be atrophic, however. Except for arteriosclerosis,
no qualitative alterations were noted in the pituitary, adrenal
and pancreatic tissues. The testes were extremely atrophic,
spermatogenesis being completely absent. About half the
testicular tissue consisted of Leydig's cells. The prostate
appeared to be hypoplastic (Fig. 2).

Case 2 (Nakagawa et al., 1974): 44-year-old male farmer.

Chief complaint: Left upper-arm tumor.

Family history: The patient was a product of a
consanguineous marriage. One of the mother's siblings had had
an opthalmological disease since adolescence. The patient was
the fifth among five siblings; the fourth, a female, was
schizophrenic. The patient was married and had two apparently
normal children.

Past history: A short stature had been noted since his
elementary school years and he had ceased to grow at adolescence.
At about that time his skin had gradually become taut. He had
also complained of tremor and tachycardia when he was 16 years
old, and had undergone an hemithyroidectomy. (The diagnosis at
that time was not certain). Ocular cataracts were removed from
the left eye at age 27 and from the right eye at age 30. A tumor
of the left upper arm was noted at age 40. He was admitted to
the Kawasaki Medical School Hospital for resection of this tumor.

Present illness: Upon admission his body height was 148 cm
and body weight 43 kg. His hair was black, but extremely sparse.
His countenance looked senile. The skin of the limbs, especially
the legs, was remarkably sclerotic and tense. In addition, the
skin way hyperkeratotic on the hand and foot, and an ulcer had
formed on the outer area of the right foot. A diagnosis of the
Werner syndrome was made. The tumor was located in the brachial
biceps muscle and was histologically identified as a
leiomyosarcoma. Laboratory findings were unremarkable except for
an elevated basal metabolic rate (+41.7%). He was discharged
after a wide resection of the tumor, but multiple subsequent

hospitalizations were required because of recurrence and metastasis of the tumor. He died of widespread metastatic disease at age 44.

Necropsy findings: While the lengths of the trunk and the limbs were proportional, the limbs were extremely slender. The skin of the trunk showed slight atrophy (Fig. 3). Hyperkeratosis was noted in the regions of the hand and foot (Fig. 4). An intractable skin ulcer had formed on the lateral side of the right foot. Both axillary and pubic hair were sparse. Histologically, the epidermis was slightly hyperkeratotic, with shortening of the rete ridge and with hyperpigmentation. The dermis was thick and fibrotic. The skin appendages were atrophic. The recurring tumor of the left upper arm had invaded the surrounding muscular tissues. Metastatic tumors were observed in both lungs and pleurae, and in a left pulmonary hilar lymph node. The left lung was atelectatic, apparently because of the numerous metastatic nodules. Histologically, these lesions proved to be leiomyosarcoma (Fig. 5). The lungs also showed congestion, edema and broncho-pneumonia. The heart, weighing 170 g, showed brown atrophy with lipofuscin deposits in myocytes. No other changes were noted. No remarkable findings were observed in the brain, which weighed 1010 g. The kidneys were congested and weighed 150 g (left) and 140 g (right). The interlobular and arcuate arteries were arteriosclerotic. The glomeruli were normal. The spleen, weighing 80 g, showed congestion and slight fibrosis of the splenic sinuses with hemosiderin deposition in moderate degrees. A follicular adenoma was noted in the thyroid; it was well demarcated with a distinct capsule. The rest of the thyroid tissue was histologically normal (Fig. 6). The adrenals, weighing 4.6 g (left) and 4.5 g (right), showed cortical atrophy. Their structures appeared normal. The pancreas, weighing 50 g, although small, was normal in shape. Both acinar tissues and Langerhans islets were histologically unremarkable. The testes, weighing 6.6 g (left) and 5.5 g (right) appeared to be atrophic. Microscopically, the seminiferous epithelium was underdeveloped and spermatogenesis was not observed. Most of the seminiferous tubules were atretic and hyalinized. The Leydig's cells appeared to be hyperplastic (Fig. 7). The trabeculae of the bone appeared to be markedly atrophic (Fig. 8) and the bone marrow revealed a depression in haematopoiesis. No significant alterations were noted in the skeletal muscle.

Case 3 (Asano et al., 1970): A 49-year-old male real estate dealer.

Chief complaints: Upper bowel pain and thirst.

Family history: The patient was the product of a consanguineous marriage. The father had died of a cancer of the

stomach. The patient was one of 10 siblings. One of the elder
brothers had also died of cancer of the stomach; medical history
for the others was unremarkable. The patient's marital status
was not clear.

Past history: He had rheumatic fever when 10 years old, but
had recovered. He had suffered from a cataract in the right eye
since age 38 and in the left eye since age 40. He contracted
pulmonary tuberculosis at age 42. When he was 49 years old,
gastric ulcers and diabetes mellitus were diagnosed after an
investigation for complaints of lateral abdominal pain and
thirst. Because of a worsening of the abdominal pain, he was
admitted to the Nippon Medical School Hospital in April, 1970.

Present illness: Upon admission, body height was 155 cm and
body weight was 35.5 kg. His limbs were slender and his jaw was
hypognathic. The scalp showed alopecia. His countenance had a
bird-like appearance. The skin and skeletal muscles were
generally atrophic. The soles of his feet were flat and
ulcerated. By May, he complained of nausea, vomiting, hoarseness
and dysphagia. A diagnosis of scleroderma was made. In June,
generalized jaundice appeared. At about that time, diabetes
mellitus was confirmed through laboratory examinations and the
diagnosis was changed from scleroderma to the Werner syndrome.
The icterus progressed, consciousness became dulled and the
patient died in July, 1970 at the age of 49.

Necropsy findings: The skin, especially in the lower limbs,
was atrophic, glossy and scaly. Telangiectasia was also noted on
the skin of the legs. The epidermis of the lower limbs was
atrophic, with hyperkeratosis and flattened dermal papillae. The
dermis was markedly fibrotic. Capillaries were remarkably
distended in the most superficial portions of the dermis. In the
subcutaneous portions of the right forearm, an oval-shaped nodule
was found that measured 1.5 cm in diameter. Histologically it
was proven to be a vascular leiomyoma (Fig. 10). The heart,
weighing 200 g, showed brown atrophy grossly and lipofuscin
pigment in myocytes histologically. The aorta showed
atherosclerosis to a moderate-to-marked extent (Fig. 11) and the
arterial tree was, in general, highly sclerotic in the various
organs. The lung, weighing 260 g (left) and 390 g (right) was
entirely congested and edematous. An old calcified tuberculous
nodule was noted in the left upper lobe. Broncho-pneumonia was
seen bilaterally in the lower lobes and there was an abscess in
the right lower lobe. Microscopically, foci of metastatic
adenocarcinoma were found scattered throughout the lungs. In one
hepatic lobe, a fist-sized tumorous lesion was seen.
Microscopically, this tumor was diagnosed as a cholangioma (Fig.
12). The adjacent hepatic tissue was stuffed with bile. The
tumor had spread throughout the whole abdominal cavity, and the

abdomen was in a state of carcinomatous peritonitis with abundant
ascites. No particular change was otherwise seen in the liver.
The kidneys, each weighing 140 g, were grossly swollen.
Microscopically, the renal tubular epithelium appeared hydropic
and the lumens often contained bile pigments. These findings
were compatible with a diagnosis of cholemic nephrosis. In the
arterial tree, sclerotic changes extended to the arterioles. The
spleen, weighing 60 g, showed a remarkable degree of hemosiderin
deposition. The splenic artery was highly sclerotic. In the
brain, weighing 1200 g, cerebral infarcts were noted in the
frontal lobe and bilaterally in the lenticular nuclei. These
infarcts were 1 cm each in diameter. Histologically, these
lesions showed liquefaction. The basilar and middle cerebral
arteries were markedly atherosclerotic. The pituitary was not
thought to be abnormal. The thyroid, weighing 5.4 g, was
markedly atrophic, with interstitial fibrosis. The size of the
parathyroid glands was within normal limits and histologically,
the acidophilic cells were proportionally decreased. The
adrenals were distinctly atrophic, particularly the cortices.
The pancreas, weighing 46 g, was grossly atrophic.
Histologically, an adenocarcinoma was noted to invade the
peripancreatic adipose tissue and the interlobular interstitium,
associated with which there was fibrosis and a lymphocytic
infiltration. The pancreatic acini were ectatic, possibly as a
result of cholemic nephrosis. No significant changes were seen
in the islets of Langerhans. The testes together weighed 8 g and
were markedly atrophic. The seminiferous tubules were atreitic.
The testicular stroma was partly replaced with a proliferation of
Leydig's cells (Fig. 13). An acute peptic ulcer was noted in the
stomach; the ulceration involved submucosal tissues. Vertebral
bone appeared normal. No skeletal muscle alterations were
observed.

Case 4 (Ishii and Hosoda, 1975): 29-year-old male clerk.

Chief complaints: Dyspnea, nausea and fatigability.

Family history: The patient was a product of a
consanguineous marriage. Both parents were normal. The patient
had two siblings. The elder brother died of renal failure, but
there was no history of ocular cataract, loss of hair or
sclerodema-like skin changes.

Past history: Patient noticed hoarseness at the age of 14,
and a solar skin sclerosis appeared at 16. He ceased to grow and
hair began to drop off and turn gray at 18. He complained of a
loss of visual acuity at 19, and an operation for a cataract of
the left eye was performed at age 21. Post-operatively, he had
suffered from sympathetic ophthalmia, and the left eye had to be
extirpated. Another operation for a cataract of the right eye

was performed at age 22. Thereafter, his condition remained
generally stationary for some period. However, headaches and
nasal bleeding began when he was 28, and hypertension was noted
(200/140 mm/Hg). He was admitted to Keio University Hospital at
that time with a diagnosis of the Werner syndrome.

Present illness: Upon admission, hypertension and renal
failure were noted. He was treated with diuretics and
cardiotonics and was discharged. He had to be readmitted,
however, because of dyspnea, nausea and fatigability shortly
thereafter (March 1971) at age 29. Upon admission, body height
was 161 cm and body weight 41 kg. Blood pressure was 220/120
mm/Hg and pulse was 110/min. There was evidence of anemia,
radial artery arteriosclerosis, alopecia, a cardiac systolic
murmer, moist rales in the lung, lower limb edema, scleroderma-
like atrophy of the skin of the limbs and bilateral hyper reflex
of the Achilles tendon. He died of cardiac failure in July,
1971.

Necropsy findings: The height was 161 cm and the weight 41
kg. Marked emaciation and severe edema of the limbs were
evident. The scalp was completely bald except for the bilateral
parietal regions. The skin was atrophic on the right side of the
abdominal wall and on the anterior surface of the lower limbs.
Axillary and pubic hair were sparse. In the skin of the upper
thigh, there was thinning of the epidermis, slight
hyperpigmentation of the basal layer and shortening of the
papillae. The dermis was slightly fibrotic, but the collagen
fibers had not changed significantly. The heart, weighing 450 g,
showed left ventricular hypertrophy. Histologically there was
also evidence of myocardial hypertrophy. The aorta was highly
atherosclerotic, considering the patient's age. No specific
findings were noted on the brain, except for cerebral
arteriosclerosis. The kidneys were atrophic, weighing 84 g
(left) and 77 g (right). Marked arteriosclerosis and
arteriolosclerosis, atrophy of the tubules and loss of glomeruli
were observed. In some glomeruli, focal of diffuse glomerular
epithelial proliferation, fibrinoid necrosis and serum
infiltration could be seen. These findings suggested that
malignant nephrosclerosis had developed (Fig. 14, 15). The
liver, weighing 810 g, showed no significant changes expect for
arteriosclerosis within the portal triad. The spleen, weighing
42 g, was congested, and the splenic artery and arterioles were
highly sclerotic. The thyroid, weighing 8 g, was markedly
atrophic. Microscopically, interstitial fibrosis was observed.
The parathyroids were normal in size; histologically, chief cells
predominated with a relative decrease in acidophilic cells. The
adrenals weighed 6 g each; microscopically, nodular aggregates of
cortical cells were observed. In the peri-adrenal adipose
tissue, the small arteries were sclerotic. The small pancreas

weighed 52 g; histologically, there was a slight fatty
infiltration; no significant changes were noted in the islets of
Langerhans. The thymus was completely involuted. The testes,
weighing 8 g (left) and 9 g (right), were atrophic. Although
spermatogenesis was preserved, the number of mature sperm was
reduced. In the interstitium, Leydig's cells were hyperplastic
and deposits of lipofuscin were scattered throughout. The
prostate was atrophic, and the interstitium was histologically
fibrotic. Mönckeberg arteriosclerosis was also seen in the
prostate. The vertebral bones showed atrophy of the trabeculae
without dilatation of the Haversian canals. The skeletal muscles
showed no significant histological changes.

Case 5: 56-year-old female housewife.

Chief complaints: Fever and drowsiness.

Family history: No consanguinity. The patient's father died
at age 91 and mother at age 82. There were no remarkable clinical
findings in the other four siblings.

Past history: At the age of 43, the patient had sustained a
stroke which left her with a left hemiparesis. At that time a
local physician made a diagnosis of Werner syndrome because of
her countenance, constitution and skin appearance.

Present illness: By the end of November 1979, she
complained of right-sided hemiparesis, dysarthria, gait
disturbance and headache. She also had a high fever (39.5° C).
These symptoms prompted admission to the Nagoya Fujita Gakuen
Medical School Hospital. Upon admission, she was 130 cm in
height and weighed 26 kg. Almost immediately following
admission, she became comatose. Babinski, Chaddock and
Schaffer's reflexes were bilaterally positive. High fever
persisted thereafter and pneumonia was diagnosed from chest X-
rays. Despite antibiotics and hydrocortisol therapy, she died of
pneumonia on 10 Dec., 1979. The laboratory findings during her
hospitalization were: RBC 231-408 x 10^4/mm^3, Hct 22.8-41.0, WBC
12,500-41,300/mm^3 and blood sugar level 170-323 mg/dl.

Necrospsy findings: The scalp hair was entirely grey and
cataracts were present in the eyes. The skin showed generalized
atrophy, especially in the limbs and at the finger tips.
Histologically, the skin of the upper thighs and abdominal wall
showed epidermal atrophy with slight hyperkeratosis. The dermis
was slightly thickened with a slight increase in collagen fibers.
Skin appendages were also atrophic. The heart, weighing 140 g,
showed brown atrophy. Microscopically, lipofuscin pigments were
somewhat increased, but no other alterations were noted except
for coronary artery atherosclerosis (Fig. 16). The aorta was

atherosclerotic, especially in the abdominal portion. The brain,
weighing 910 g, was atrophic, although the gross weight, the
depth of the sulci, and the width of the gyri were proportional.
At the cut surfaces, the thickness of the cortex and medulla was
also proportional. The cerebral arteries showed moderate-to-
marked atherosclerosis. Old infarcts were seen in the right
basal nuclei and in the right posterior lobe; the diameter of
each was 2.5 cm (Fig. 17, Fig. 18). Histologically, both were
old lesions, with liquefaction, reticular degeneration and a
massive infiltration of gitter cells. The left lung, weighing
300 g, was congestive and edematous. Broncho-pneumonia and
abscess formation were noted in the left lower lobe. The right
lung (485 g) showed only broncho-pneumonia. In the pulmonary
artery, a fresh fibrin thromboembolism was noted. The liver,
weighing 630 g, the kidneys, weighing 90 g (left) and 65 g
(right), and the spleen, weighing 40 g, were all atrophic.
Arteriosclerosis and congestion were noted in these organs.
Hemosiderin and calcium were dispersed throughout the splenic
parenchyma and present in Gandy-Gamna's nodules. The thyroid (10
g) and adrenal glands (left, 3g; right, 2.5 g) appeared to be
atrophic. The pancreas was also grossly atrophic.
Microscopically, these endocrine organs appeared to be
unremarkable, although sclerotic arteries and arterioles were
noted. The uterus was atrophic, the cervical canal being
atretic. In the ovary, corpora albinicantia had formed. The
vertebral bones showed slight trabecular atrophy. Haematopoiesis
was slightly depressed.

PATHOLOGICAL LESIONS IN THE WERNER SYNDROME

     Up to 20 necropsied cases of Werner syndrome have been
described in the literature (Oppenheimer and Kugel, 1941; Boyd
and Grant, 1950; Perloff and Phelps, 1958; Valero and Gellei,
1960; Jacobson et al., 1960; Hamada, 1966; Laugier et al., 1967;
Zucker-Franklin et al., 1968; Asano et al., 1970; Pavlik and
Korp, 1971; Nakagawa et al., 1974; Ishii et al., 1975; Tokunaga
et al., 1976), including the 5 cases in the present manuscript.
We will attempt to summarize the descriptions of the histological
findings for each organ (Table I).

Skin: In the limbs where the skin is taut and tense, the
epidermis was thin because of atrophy of the rete ridges, and was
often associated with hyperkeratosis, hyperpigmentation and
telangiectasia. The dermis showed fibrosis, which frequently led
to hyalinization, a process that results in atrophy of the
pilosebaceous and sweat glands. These changes often extended
also to the palm and the sole, in which case hyperkeratosis was
usually accentuated, sometimes with clavus formation. In
addition, the skin was sometimes ulcerated in the lower limb, and

especially at the lateral malleolus, olecranon and heel where the
bone mass is superficially protuberant.

Heart: Myocardial hypertrophy has been frequently described.
Judging from their clinical history, most of those with
myocardial hypertrophy had a hypertensive pathogenesis. In
contrast, the obvious brown atrophy noted in some cases was seen
without any causative complication (Boyd et al., 1950).
Excluding the two hearts with hypertension hypertrophy, the
average weight of the three Japanese hearts with brown atrophy
was 180 g. Considering the microplanchnic state in the Werner
syndrome and clinical information on blood pressure, the brown
atrophy itself appears to be the natural cardiac state of this
syndrome. Myocardial infarcts, fibrosis and calcification have
been exclusively reported in the Western literature (Oppenheimer
et al., 1941; Boyd et. al., 1950; Rogers, 1958). These changes
may be sequelae of coronary atherosclerosis as the counterpart of
generalized atherosclerosis.

Aorta and other arteries: Atherosclerosis was pronounced in
almost every case. Coronory (Perloff et al., 1958; Rogers,
1958; Jacobson et al., 1960), renal and carotid arteriosclerosis
(Perloff et al., 1958), were specified, and renal artery
thrombosis was also referred to (Valero et al., 1960).
Otherwise, generalized atherosclerosis has been repeatedly
described. In the Japanese cases, also, atherosclerosis was seen
in the aorta, especially in the abdominal portion, and
arteriosclerosis in the various organs in moderate-to-marked
degree. Mönckeberg-type arteriosclerosis with calcified media
has been rarely mentioned (Oppenheimer et al., 1941), but it was
shown also in Case 4 of this paper.

Brain: It is noteworthy that among the Japanese cases,
myocardial infarction never occurred. Instead, there were two
cases of cerebral infarction. It is generally accepted that, in
the Japanese, cerebral atherosclerosis occurs not only earlier
but more severely than in Americans (Resch et al., 1969).
Preferential occurrence of cerebral infarction among the Japanese
patients with the Werner syndrome may be related to such a
background. This issue has further significance from the fact
that the occurrence of cerebral infarction has not yet been
described among the 14 Western-necropsied cases of this syndrome.
There were no particular findings in the brain other than such
sporadic occurrences of infarction. Remarkable cerebral aging
changes were seldom identified.

Endocrine organs:

A.   Pituitary. Atrophy with normal cell composition has been
reported (Asano et al., 1970; Rogers, 1958; Jacobson et al.,

Table I

Pathological Findings in the Werner Syndrome

Skin (12 out of 12 necropsies in which the skin was referred to)

    epidermal atrophy
    dermal fibrosis and/or hyalinisation
    atrophy of the appendages
    reduction of subcutaneous adipose tissue

Heart

    left and/or biventricular myocardial hypertrophy (8 of 20)
    myocardial ischaemic lesions (2 of 20)
    myocardial calcification (described in one case)
    brown atrophy (4 of 20)

Vascular system

    athero- and/or arteriosclerosis (4 of 20)
    Mönckeberg-type arteriosclerosis (described/found in 2 cases)
    arteriolosclerosis (described or found in 5 cases)

Endocrine organs

    pituitary gland atrophy (4 of 16 cases)
    thyroid atrophy (7 of 15) and adenomas (described in 3 cases)
    adrenal atrophy (5 of 11) and adenomas (described in 2 cases)
    pancreatic atrophy (3 of 13)

Genital organs

    testicular atrophy (9 of 15 cases)
    uterine atrophy (3 of 5)
    prostatic atrophy (4 of 7)
    prostatic hypertrophy (1 of 7)

Malignancies (5 of 20 necropsies)

    liver cell carcinoma, thyroid adenocarcinoma, cholangioma,
    fibrosarcoma, leiomyosarcoma

1960). In particular, Perloff et al. (1958) made a histometrical study and found the pituitary gland to be normal. Pinhead-sized chromophobe adenoma (Valero et al., 1960) or basophilic cell hyperplasia (Tokunaga et al., 1976) have also been reported, but the findings had no clinical significance because of the absence of pituitary symptoms in these patients.

B.   Thyroid. The thyroid gland was generally atrophic. Multiple adenomata occurred in two cases (Oppenheimer et al., 1941; Laugier et al., 1967) and papillary adenocarcinoma (Valero et al., 1960) in one case. In addition, follicular adenoma occurred in the Japanese Case 3. From the point of view of a general pathologist, it seems tumorous lesions occur frequently. In other words, at least 4 such lesions occurred out of 20 cases.

C.   Parathyroid. The chief cells were proportionally increased in the Japanese Case 4, and a similar finding was also described in one Western case (Oppenheimer et al., 1941). In contrast, there was an increase of acidophilic cells in the Japanese Case 3. No symptoms of parathyroidal dysfunction were seen in these cases, and parathyroidal function was found to be normal in endocrinological studies (Schott and Dann, 1949). There was little of significance in the parathyroid morphology.

D.   Adrenal. The adrenal gland was consistently atrophic in most of the necropsied cases. Nodular hyperplasia was reported in one Western case (Valero et al., 1960) and was seen in the Japanese Cases 4 and 5. Adenoma had also formed in two cases (Boyd et al., 1950; Rogers, 1958). However, these conditions would not appear to have been significant, judging from the clinical information. In addition, adrenal dysfunction has not been mentioned in the necropsied cases.

E.   Pancreas. The pancreas tended to be grossly atrophic. No qualitative changes have so far been shown in the islets of Langerhans. The islets tended to be slightly reduced in the Japanese Cases 2 and 3, but no qualitative degeneration was seen in them, even in association with diabetes. It is generally accepted that diabetics having the Werner syndrome are resistant to insulin. Also, it has recently been suggested that diabetes mellitus in the aged could result from the lean body mass (Dudl and Ensinck, 1977). Small body mass in the Werner syndrome might be related to such a mechanism. We have come across no evidence in the literature of diabetic glomerulosclerosis among the necropsied cases.

In summary, the endocrine organs in the Werner syndrome were generally atrophic, but there was no single pathological finding that can explain the widespread manifestations of the Werner syndrome. The atrophic tendency in the endocrines should be

considered together with the microsplanchnic tendency in the
Werner syndrome, i.e., there is an overall tendency of the whole
body to be underdeveloped.

Genital organs: In the male patients, there is good evidence for
atrophy of the testes (Oppenheimer et al., 1941; Perloff et al.,
1958; Valero et al., 1960; Jacobson et al., 1960).
Hypospermatogenesis (Perloff et al., 1958; Valero et al., 1960)
and aspermatogenesis (Oppenheimer et al., 1941; Boyd et al.,
1950) have both been described. A similar tendency was
consistently shown in the four Japanese male patients. The
female patient also had an atrophic tendency. Although female
necropsied cases are few (Rogers, 1958; Laugier et al., 1967;
Pavlik et al., 1971), this tendency to atrophy is distinct in the
reports (Laugier et al., 1967, Pavlik et al., 1971) and in our
Japanese Case 5. In males, the prostate was usually atrophic
(Oppenheimer et al., 1941; Boyd et al., 1950), as in the Japanese
Cases 1 and 4. The prostate usually shows hypertrophy with
advancing age, so it is noteworthy that the prostate in the
Werner syndrome tends to be atrophic, and this atrophic tendency
of the Werner syndrome may be interpreted as a local expression
of the general constitution in the Werner syndrome.

Bone: It has been well documented that osteoporosis occurs in
almost every patient. Osteoporosis may occur systemically, but
it is especially severe in the limb bones. At the same time, the
soft tissue in the extremities is calcified (Jacobson et al.,
1960). Histologically, we were able to observe the osteoporotic
tendency also in the vertebral bone in most of the Japanese
cases. When we examined the peripheral bones, osteoporosis was
observed in every case.

Liver, Kidney, and Spleen: In these organs, no specific lesion
was seen other than those associated with the secondary
pathological condition.

ORGANS RESPONSIBLE FOR PATHOLOGICAL LESIONS IN THE WERNER SYNDROME

Histological alterations were concentrically distributed in
the skin, arteries and bone in the Werner syndrome, apart from
the external manifestation of short stature, grey hair, hair loss
and cataracts, and there were no other pathologically appreciable
lesions in the parenchymal and endocrine organs. The lesions
seen in the parenchymal organs of the liver, kidneys, spleen,
heart and lungs were always ascribed to the secondary changes
resulting from the main pathological state of each patient.
Other than the small size and occasional infarcts, no significant
findings were seen in the brain. Lesions, such as Alzheimer's
neurofibrillar change, Marinesco bodies, torpedo cells and Lewy

bodies were not observed. The endocrine and genital organs
simply reduce their gross weight, retaining their normal
histological structure. This atrophy may occur in parallel with
the generalized atrophy. It can thus be concluded that the
pathognomonic findings are characteristically concentrated within
the mesenchymal tissues of the skin, arteries, bone and ocular
lens in the Werner syndrome.

Skin lesions are most severe in the limbs, especially the
lower limb, and are often associated with intractable ulceration
of the tissue overlying protuberant portions of the bone mass of
the leg or foot. Remarkable histological changes include
epidermal atrophy, often with hyperkeratosis and
hyperpigmentation, and dermal fibrosis. Fibrosis is not only
limited to the upper dermis, but extends to the deeper layers.
The skin appendages are usually atrophic, possibly as a result of
dermal fibrosis. These findings resemble the skin changes of
scleroderma at the sclerotic and atrophic phases, although the
skin always lacks inflammatory-cell infiltration and edema in
the Werner syndrome.

Considering the various visceral and systemic lesions of
scleroderma, we conclude that the histogenesis of the skin
lesions of the Werner syndrome is distinct. Scleroderma might
best be categorized as an immunologically-determined degenerative
disorder. The lesions of the Werner syndrome also appear to be
different from that of normal aging of the skin. The collagen
changes of aging skin are characterized as elastotic
degeneration, the aberrations originating in connective tissue
fibers (collagen and elastin) of the dermis, especially in skin
exposed to sunlight. Such degenerations of collagens and elastic
fibers are not observed in the Werner syndrome. Instead, one
sees fibrosis, with increased deposits of collagen.
Mucopolysaccharides should also be considered in the pathogenesis
of the fibrosis. The materials we collected, however, were all
fixed in formalin, and therefore precise interpretations of
staining for mucopolysaccharides is not possible; nevertheless,
the special stains we have carried out do not reveal any drastic
accumulations of such substances.

Because of the observation of dermal fibrosis, we examined
the extent of collagen production of fibroblast-like cell
cultures from the skin of the thigh of patients with the Werner
syndrome and controls (Fig. 19). The cultures were maintained in
Eagle's Minimum Essential Medium with 10% bovine fetal serum.
The cultures were harvested when subconfluent. Figure 19
summarizes the results when collagen production is expressed as
total hydroxyproline in the medium. No significant differences
were found between the Werner syndrome and controls. Although it
had previously been suggested that the Werner syndrome skin

fibroblasts produce an increased amount of collagens (Tajima et al., 1978), that conclusion was based upon only a single case. In that case, moreover, only fibroblasts from the skin of the thigh showed an increased production of collagen; cultures from the skin of the abdominal wall of the same patient gave normal results. Further studies should consider other biochemical constituents, such as hyaluronic acid, the urinary secretion of which has been reported to be elevated among patients with the Werner syndrome (Tokunaga et al., 1975).

Arteries, both in our examined Japanese cases and in the reported cases from Western countries, seem to show an accelerated progression of generalized atherosclerosis. This atherosclerosis is qualitatively similar to that of ordinary senile atherosclerosis. No abnormal substance was seen to have accumulated in any component of the atherosclerosis.

In connection with our interest in the atherosclerosis of the Werner syndrome, we conducted a pathoepidemiological study of the risk factors of atherosclerosis among 1239 ordinary Japanese (unpublished). Table II summarizes "critical threshold levels" of certain risk factors on the basis of multivariate analysis, in which the grades of aortic and coronary atherosclerosis have been analyzed. When we compare this result with our previous study of 15 living patients with the Werner syndrome (Goto et al., 1978), the mean serum cholesterol level in patients with the Werner syndrome (207 mg) is somewhat elevated. Similar increased cholesterol levels were reported from the U.S.; the figures were 322 mg in the Werner syndrome and 245 mg in the normal (Zucker-Franklin et al., 1968). We can thus conclude that atherosclerosis in Werner's syndrome results, in part, from a hyper-cholesterolemic state. It has been fully established that cholesterol is a distinct risk factor of myocardial infarction; and its risk increases in parallel with the cholesterol level (Dawber et al., 1980). Myocardial infarction in the Werner syndrome, however, exclusively occurred in the Western necropsied cases; it never occurred in the Japanese ones.

Although cholesterol is high in the Japanese patients with this syndrome, the Japanese level is far lower than the American level. The difference in the occurrence of myocardial infarction in this syndrome may be based upon the difference in cholesterol levels.

Mönckeberg arteriosclerosis is another vascular sign of aging. This type of arteriosclerosis is usually interpreted as the sequela of medial degeneration, possibly the result of insufficient vascular perfusion from the adventitial side, resulting from the medial hypertrophy of aging. It may be a sequela of metastatic calcification. We do not know which mechanism is responsible for the occurrence of such

Table II

"Critical Threshold Levels" for Atherosclerosis*

Artery	Systolic blood pressure	Total cholesterol
Thoracic aorta	140 mm/Hg	180 mg/dl
Abdominal aorta	140	180
LAD coronary artery	140	180
LCX coronary artery	140	180
RCA coronary artery	140	180

LAD = left anterior descending
LCX = left circumflex
RCA = right circumflex

* 1239 cases (mean patient age 48.7 years)

arteriosclerosis; however, it may be worthwhile to record this condition, as it occurred in 2 cases.

Bone lesions have not often been mentioned in previously necropsied cases, although osteoporosis has been described in some cases. Osteoporosis is chiefly distributed in the bones of the limbs. We did not examine the bones of the limbs histologically; however, the osteoporotic tendency was consistently observed in the vertebrae of the Japanese necropsied cases. The bone matrix did not show any qualitative changes other than trabecular atrophy.

We should thus turn our attention to the connective tissues of skin, artery, bone and ocular lens, changes in each of which constitute the principal pathology of the Werner syndrome. It is instructive to compare the pathology of the Werner syndrome with that observed in very aged human subjects. We made a pathological study of centenarians in 1978 (Ishii and Sternby, 1978a,b,c). Among the representative pathological findings were reduced body height and weight, atherosclerosis and osteoporosis, all comparable to that in the Werner syndrome. In contrast, amyloid deposition, pulmonary emphysema, and formation of colonic diverticulae were exclusively seen in centenarians. These lesions thus preferentially occur in the normal aged. Scleroderma-like skin changes, however, never occurred in the centenarians.

Bearing in mind the role of the connective tissue in the Werner syndrome, we studied amyloid deposition in the normal aged and in the Werner syndrome. Senile amyloid deposition is thought to comprise immunoamyloid and amyloid protein AL. Senile amyloid deposition is believed to originate from the repeated immunological stimuli experienced during the long life of the aged (Ishii et al., 1983). The Werner syndrome is associated, on the other hand, with immunological deterioration (Goto et al., 1979). This condition may be expected to evoke amyloid deposition chronologically earlier than the normal state. Although we used Congo red staining, amyloid deposition could not be detected in 4 of our cases of the Werner syndrome, not even when we included cases associated with tuberculosis (49- and 51-year-old male patients). This discrepancy may be part of the segmental manifestation of the aging phenomenon in the Werner syndrome.

Among the reported Western cases associated with malignancies, sarcomas predominate. When we make comparisons with the cancers in the control Japanese aged population (Ishii et al., 1979), this sarcoma-prone tendency is also obvious in the Japanese patients with the Werner syndrome. Sarcomas have been reported in 11 out of 16 cases of malignancy in the Western patients and 8 out of 10 in the Japanese (Kizukuri et al., 1980). In the Western patients, the sarcomas are of several varieties; however, it is noteworthy that in the Japanese, 5 malignant melanomas have been reported out of 8 sarcomas. This sarcoma-prone tendency also highlights the importance of the connective tissue in the Werner syndrome. It is suggested that even the core characters of the Werner syndrome, being a hereditary disease, is modified through ethnic or environmental factors.

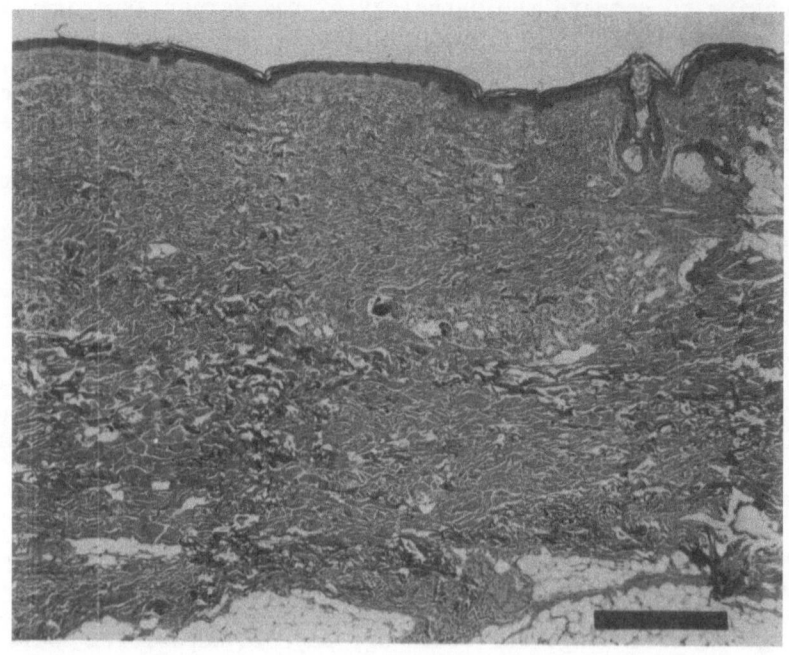

Fig. 1. Skin. HE. The scale bar indicates 500 microns.

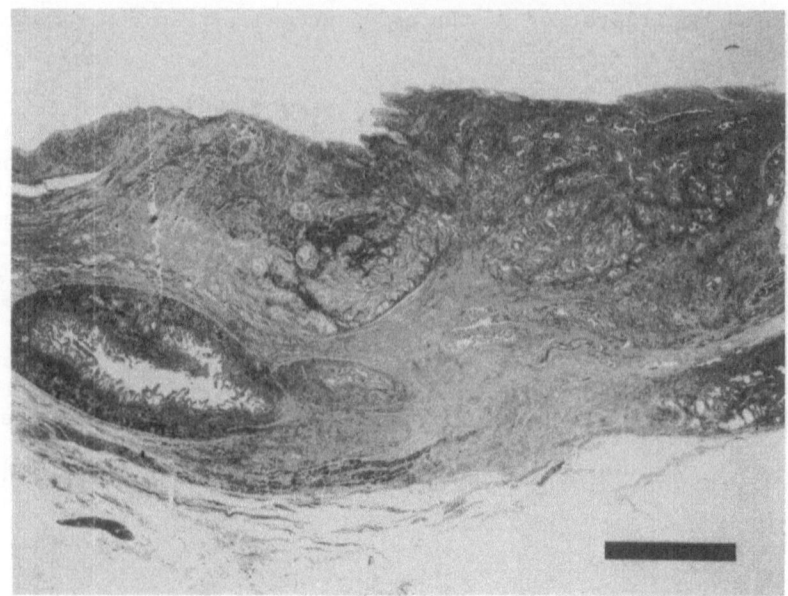

Fig. 2. Prostate. Mallory's stain. The scale bar indicates
         3080 microns.

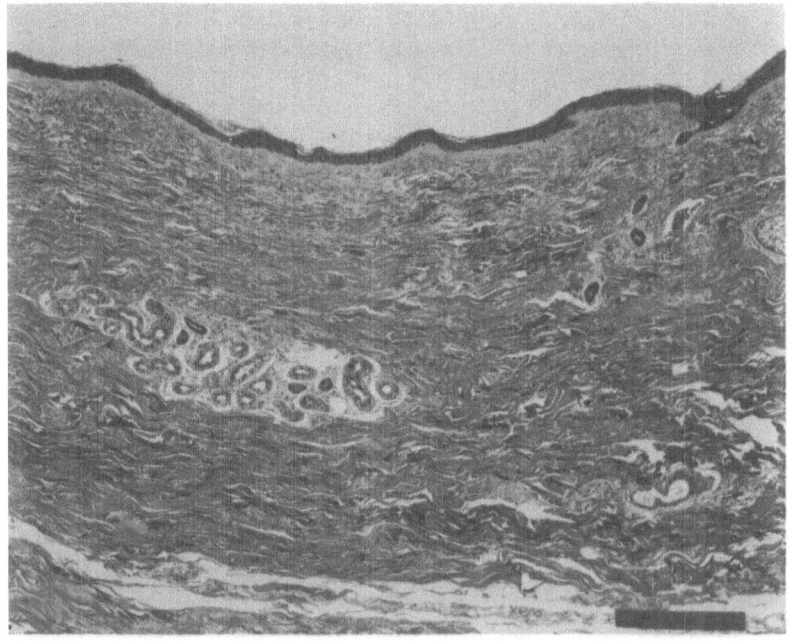

Fig. 3. Skin. HE. The scale bar indicates 310 microns.

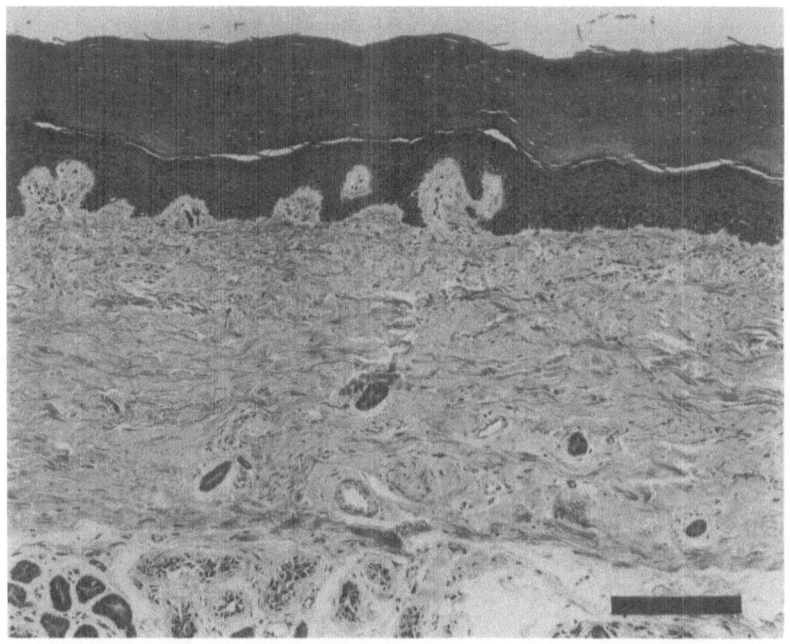

Fig. 4. Skin. HE. The scale bar indicates 200 microns.

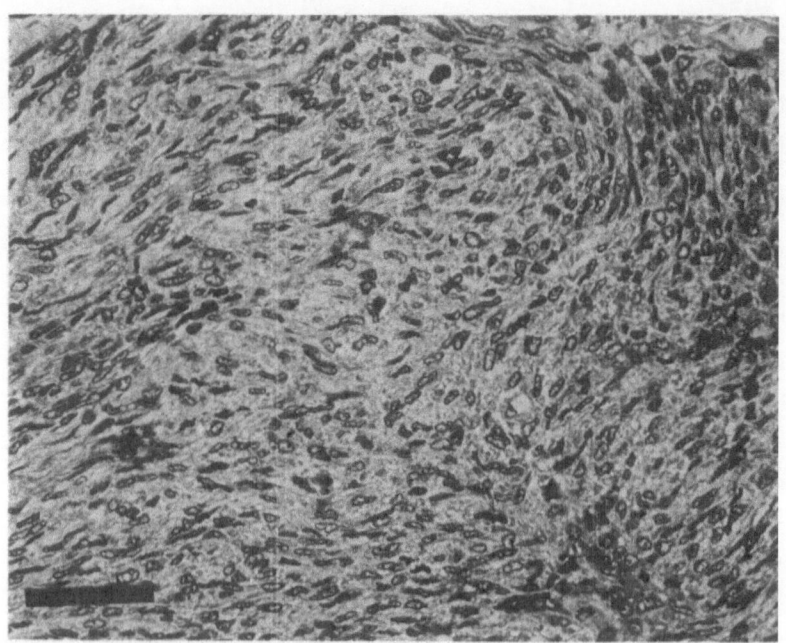

Fig. 5.   Leiomyosarcoma of the left upper tumor. HE. The scale
          bar indicates 200 microns.

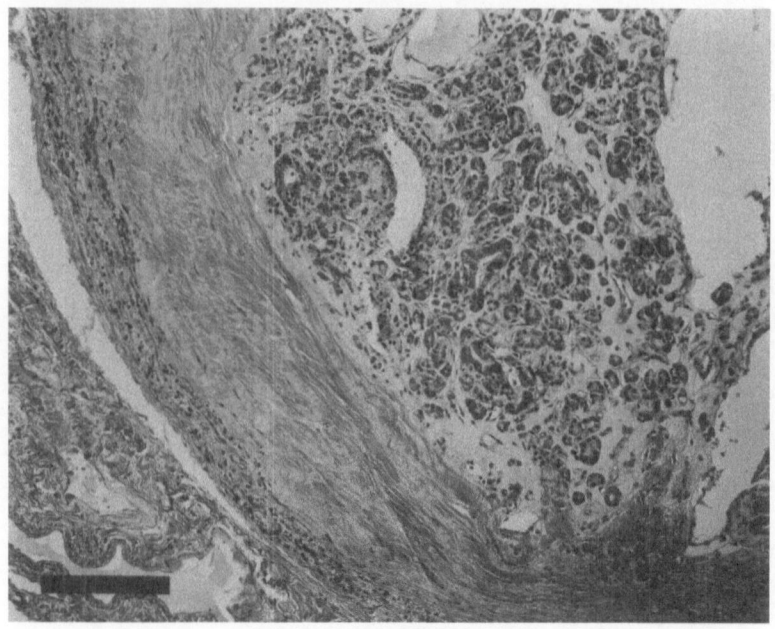

Fig. 6.   Follicular adenoma of the thyroid. HE. The scale bar
          indicates 200 microns.

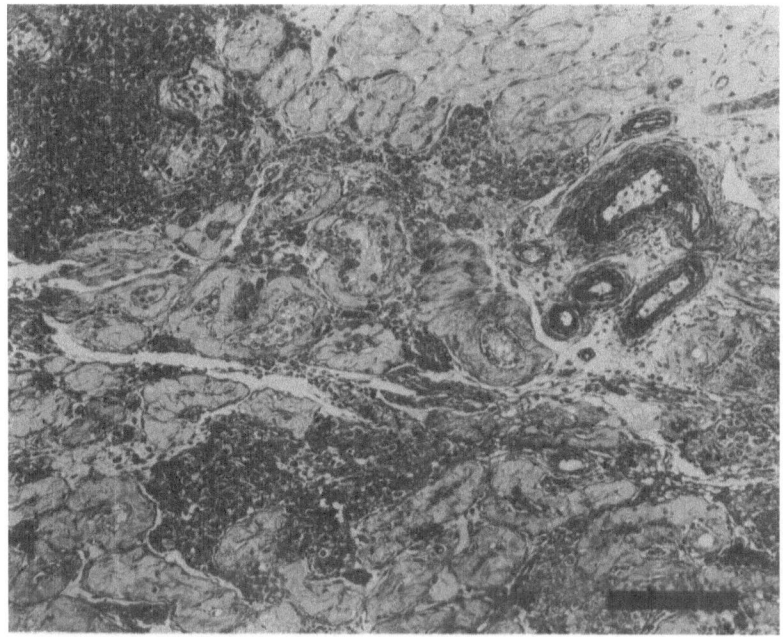

Fig. 7. Testis. HE. The scale bar indicates 200 microns.

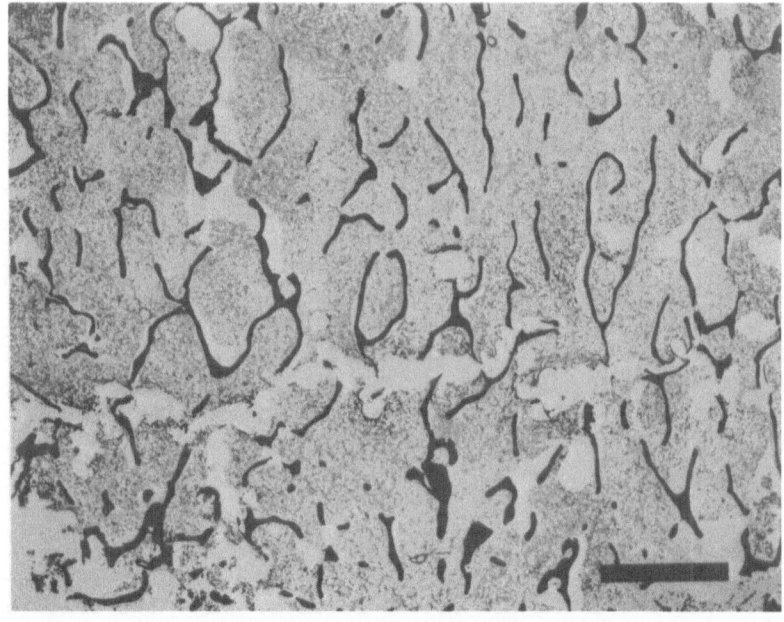

Fig. 8. Vertebral bone. Elastic van-Gieson's stain. The scale
bar indicates 3080 microns.

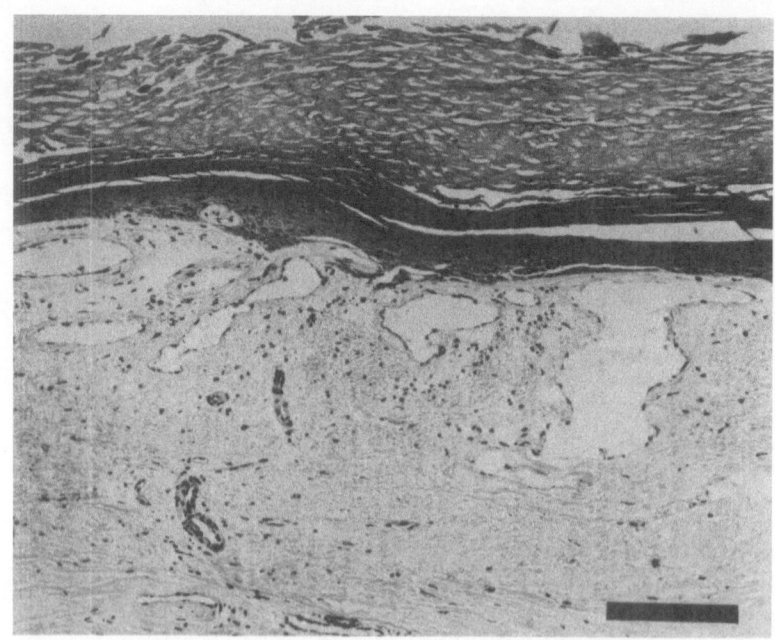

Fig. 9. Skin. HE. The scale bar indicates 200 microns.

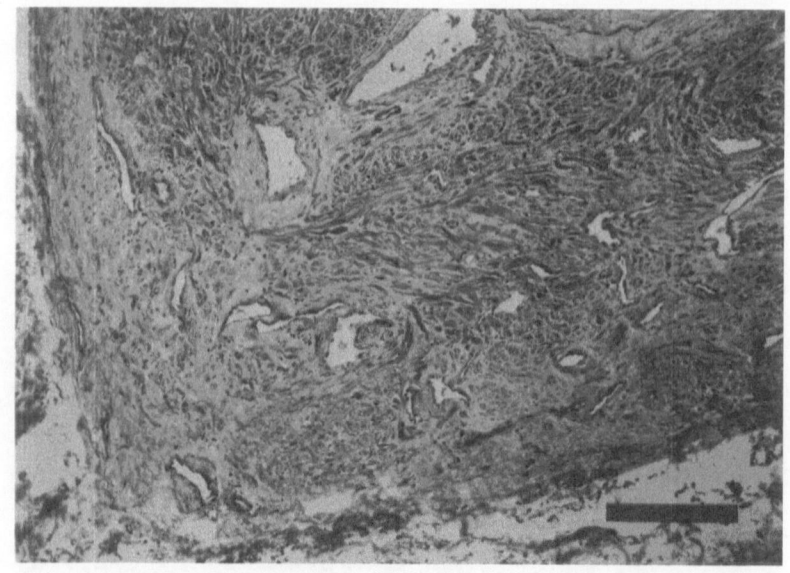

Fig. 10. Vascular leiomyoma of the forearm. HE. The scale bar
          indicates 200 microns.

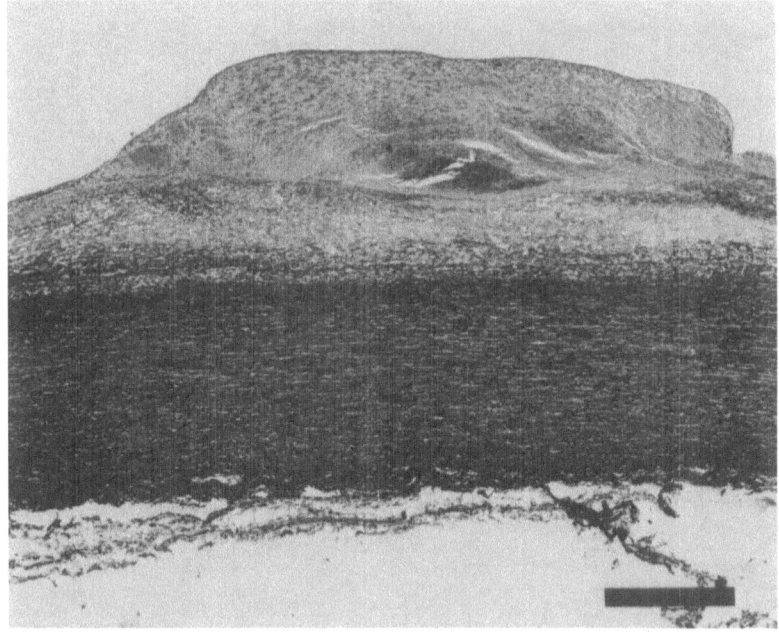

Fig. 11. Aorta. HE. The scale bar indicates 870 microns.

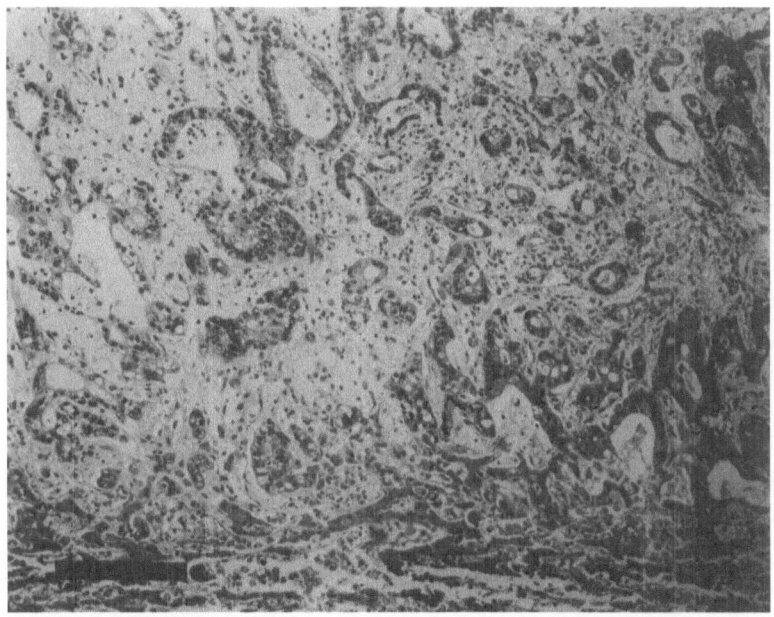

Fig. 12. Cholangioma. HE. The scale bar indicates 200 microns.

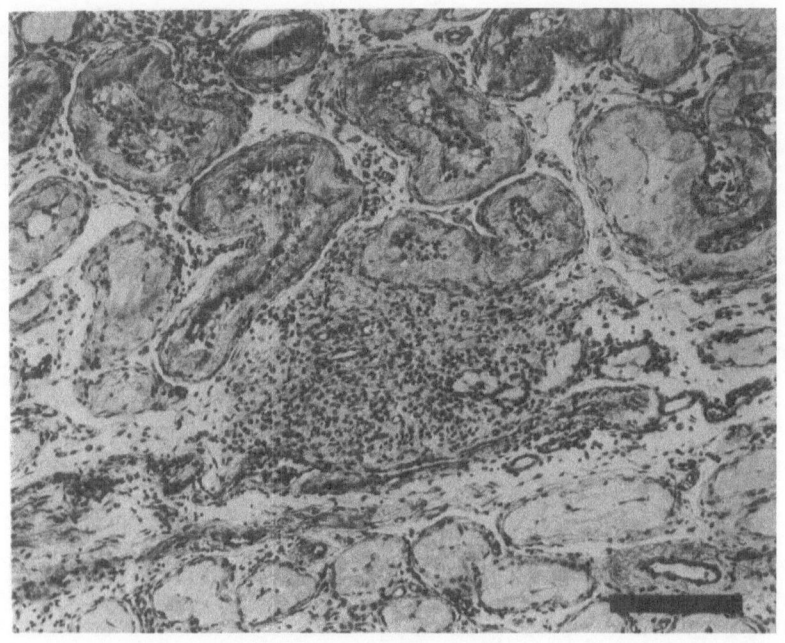

Fig. 13. Testis. HE. The scale bar indicates 200 microns.

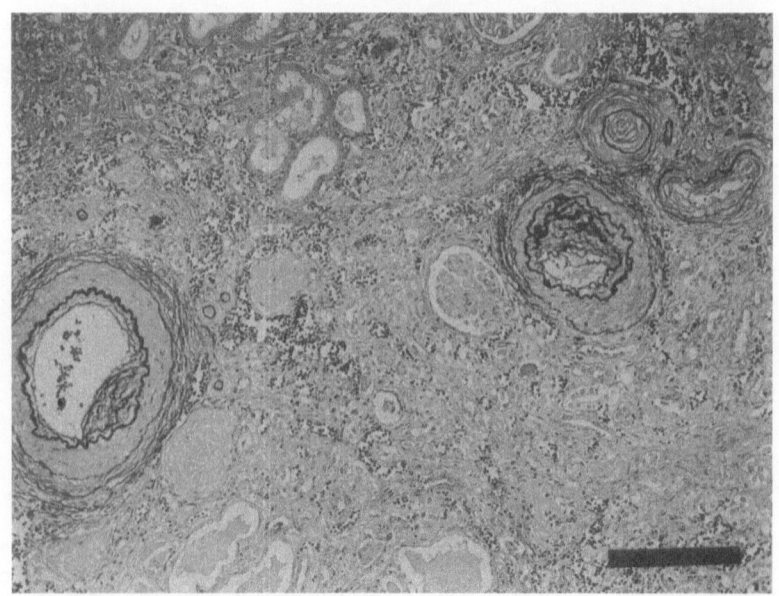

Fig. 14. Kidney. Elastic van-Gieson's stain. The scale bar
          indicates 200 microns.

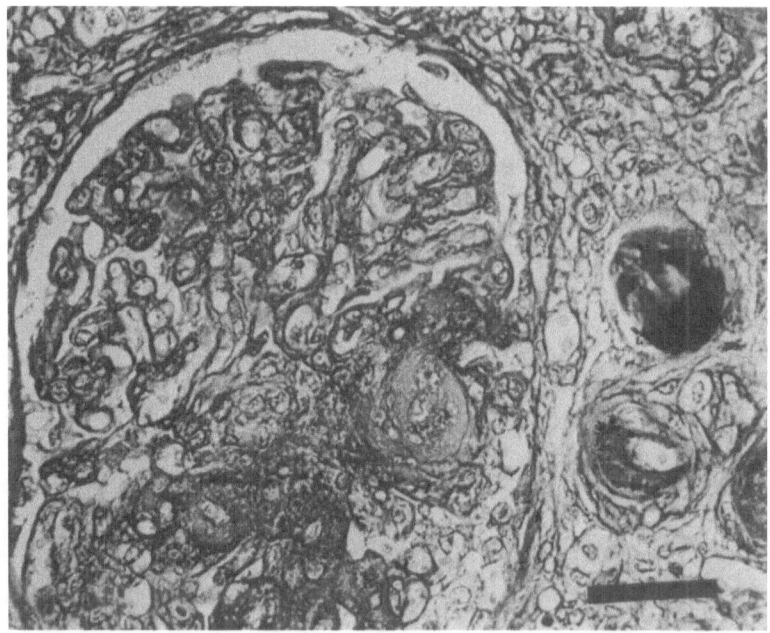

Fig. 15. Kidney. Mallory's stain. The scale bar indicates 50
microns.

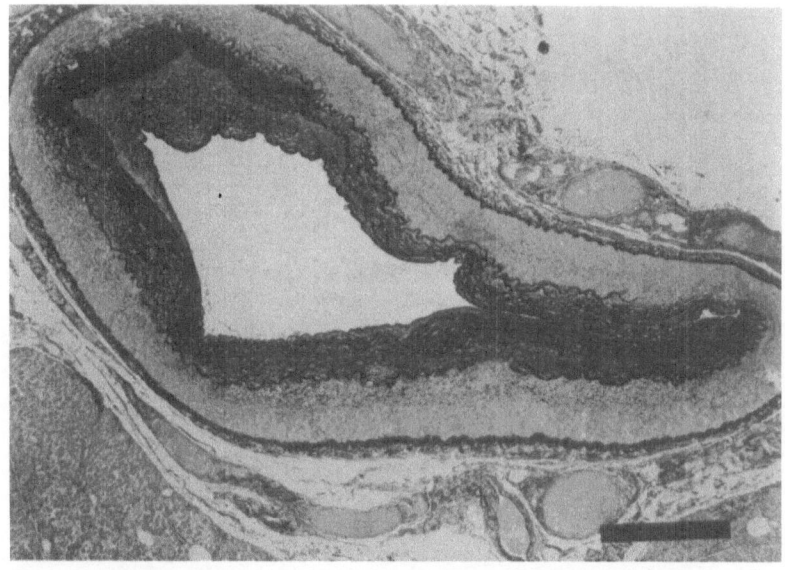

Fig. 16. Coronary artery. Elastic van-Gieson's stain. The
scale bar indicates 500 microns.

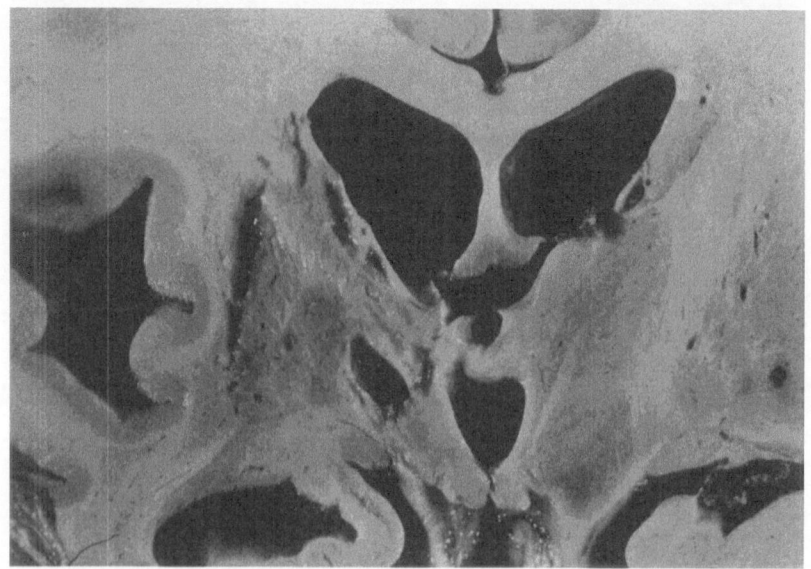

Fig. 17. Old cerebral infarction in the right basal ganglia.

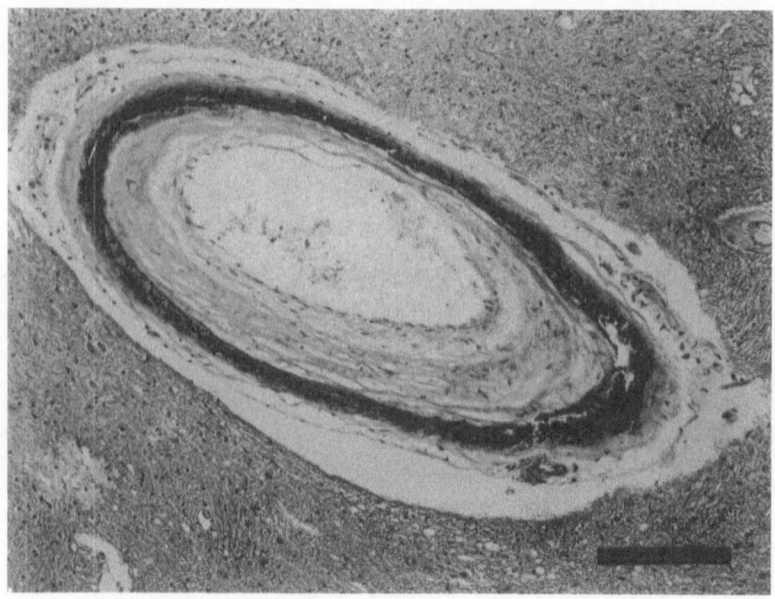

Fig. 18. Cerebral arteriosclerosis neighboring the infarction.
          HE. The scale bar indicates 200 microns.

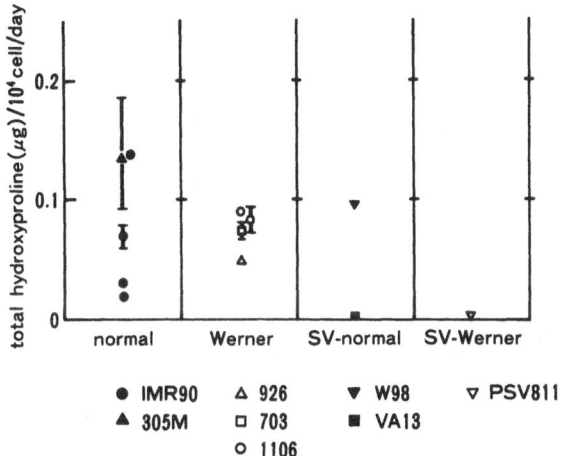

Fig. 19. Collagen production efficiency in the Werner syndrome and normal subjects.

REFERENCES

Asano, G., Aihara, K., Ito, T. and Yamate, N., 1970, An autopsy case of Werner's syndrome, Nippon Ika Daig. Z., 37:162.

Boyd, M.W.J. and Grant, A.P., 1950, Werner's syndrome (progeria of the adult): Further pathological and biochemical observation, Brit. Med. J., 2:920.

Dawber, T, 1980, The Framingham Study, Harvard University Press, Boston.

Dudl, R.J. and Ensinck, J.W., 1977, Insulin and glucagon relationships during aging in man, Metabolism, 26:33.

Goto, M., Horiuchi, Y., Okumura, K. and Tada, T., 1979, Immunological abnormalities of aging. An analysis of T lymphocyte subpopulation of Werner's syndrome, J. Clin. Invest., 64:695.

Goto, M., Horiuchi, Y., Tanimoto, K., Ishii, T. and Nakashima, H., 1978, Werner's syndrome: Analysis of 15 cases with a review of the Japanese literature, J. Am. Geriatrics Soc., 26:341.

Hamada, Y., 1966, Werner's syndrome: Report of a case with portmortem findings. Dermatologica et Urologica (Tokyo) 20:1321.

Ishii, T. and Hosoda, Y., 1975, Werner's syndrome: Autopsy report of one case, with a review of pathologic findings reported in the literature, J. Am. Geriatrics Soc., 23:145.

Ishii, T., Hosoda, Y., Ikegami, N. and Shimada, H., 1984, Senile amyloid deposition, J. Path. 139:1.

Ishii, T., Maeda, K., Nakamura, K. and Hosoda, Y., 1979, Cancer in the aged: An autopsy study of 940 cancer patients, J. Am. Geriatrics Soc., 27:307.

Ishii, T. and Sternby, N.H., 1978a, Pathology of centenarians. I. The cardiovascular system and the lungs, J. Am. Geriatrics Soc., 26:108.

Ishii, T. and Sternby, N.H., 1978b, Pathology of centenarians. II. Urogenital and digestive systems, J. Am. Geriatrics Soc., 26:391.

Ishii, T. and Sternby, N.H., 1978c, Pathology of centenarians. III. Osseous system, malignant lesions and causes of death, J. Am. Geriatrics Soc., 26:529.

Jacobson, H.G., Rifkin, H. and Zucker-Franklin, D., 1960, Werner's syndrome. A clinicoroentgen entity, Radiology. 74:373.

Kizukuri, T., Katoh, M., Uesugi, T. and Jimbow, K., 1980, Werner's syndrome with malignant melanoma, Nippon Hifuka Gakkai Zasshi, 90:677.

Laugier, P., Ellena, V., Risold, J.C., Bulte, C., Oppermann, A. and Pageaut, G., 1967, Syndrome de Werner: Constatations necropsiques, Bull. Soc. Franc. Derm. Syph., 74:38.

Nakagawa, S., Shinohara, K., Kojima, H., Ishikawa, F. and Murakami, T., 1974, An autopsy case of Werner's syndrome associated with leiomyosarcoma, Jap. J. Clin. Med., 32:859.

Oppenheimer, B.S. and Kugel, V.H., 1941, Werner's syndrome: Report of first necropsy and of findings in new cases, J. Am. Med. Sci., 202:629.

Pavlik, F. and Korp, W., 1971, Werner-syndrom, Wien Med. Wschr., 121:87.

Perloff, J.K. and Phelps, E.T., 1958, A review of Werner's syndrome with a report of the second autopsied case, Ann. Intern. Med., 48:1205.

Resch, J.A., Okabe, N., Loewenson, R.B., Kimoto, K., Katsuki, S. and Baker, A.B., 1969, Pattern of vessel involvement in cerebral atherosclerosis, J. Atheroscl. Res., 9:239.

Rogers, A.S., 1958, Werner's syndrome, J. Florida Med. Assn., 46:436.

Schott, J. and Dann, S., 1949, Werner's syndrome: A report of 2 cases, New Engl. J. Med., 240:641.

Tajima, T., Iijima, K. and Watanabe, T., 1978, Collagen synthesis of cultured fibroblast from Werner's syndrome of premature aging, Experientia, 34:1459.

Tokunaga, M., Futami, T. and Wakamatsu, E., 1975, Werner's syndrome as 'hyaluronuria,' Clin. Chim. Acta, 62:89.

Tokunaga, M., Mori, S., Sato, K., Nakamura, K. and Wakamatsu, E., 1976, Postmortem study of a case of Werner's syndrome, J. Am. Geriatrics Soc., 24:407.

Valero, A. and Gellei, B., 1960, Retinitis pigmentosa, hypertension and uremia in Werner's syndrome, Brit. Med. J., 2:351.

Zucker-Franklin, D., Rifkin, H. and Jacobson, H.G., 1968, Werner's Syndrome: An analysis of ten cases, Geriatrics, 23:123.

NEUROPATHOLOGY OF THE WERNER SYNDROME

S.M. Sumi

University of Washington
Department of Pathology
Seattle, Washington

INTRODUCTION

In his original report, Werner (1) described four siblings who had in common shortness of stature, senile appearance, early graying of the hair and appearance of cataracts, skin changes and early cessation of menstruation. Subsequent authors added premature balding, tendency to diabetes mellitus and calcification of blood vessels to this picture. Although patients with this syndrome appear to exhibit premature aging, evidence for this is difficult to document (2), and this is particularly true with regard to the central nervous system.

The clinical hallmark of the aging brain is considered to be the appearance of dementia, a general deterioration of intellect. Pathologically, this is characterized by the appearance of senile plaques and neurofibrillary degeneration of the cerebral cortical neurons. These changes, both clinical and pathological, in "old age" are quite common but far from universal, and their appearance before this time is abnormal annd may be considered to indicate premature aging. More common, and less pathological evidence of aging, is the accumulation of corpora amylacea in the subpial regions of the central nervous system and accumulation of lipofuscin granules in the various neuronal cell bodies. What is the evidence for premature cerebral aging in the Werner syndrome?

When considering this question one must remember that there are few detailed descriptions of the nervous system in Werner's syndrome. However, as Martin (3) pointed out the absence of

clinical or pathological signs of dementia in most reports is
particularly noteworthy. However, Fleischmajor and Nedwich (4)
reported one patient with "organic brain syndrome without
psychosis," while Rabbiosi and Berroni (5) found mental
retardation in three of seven siblings but gave no further
details. Murata and Nakashima (6) stated that "premature
senility was present in all 24 patients" they reviewed. These
reports appear to be exceptions both in that there was even any
reference to the nervous system and in their reports of
intellectual abnormality.

Neuropathologically, it appears to be universally agreed
that senile plaques and neurofibrillary tangles, the hallmarks of
Alzheimer's disease, are not found in the Werner syndrome (7).
Most of the attention has been focussed on lipofuscin
accumulation in neurons with particular attention to whether they
may be abnormal in quality or quantity. Again, the consensus is
that there is no abnormality in either respect. In the related
condition of progeria (8,9) no such abnormalities in lipofuscin
were found. In fact, even in Alzheimer's disease, there is
question whether there is any increase in the amount of
lipofuscin beyond what might be expected with the age of the
patient (10,11).

Case Reports

We present our findings in two of three sisters of Japanese
descent who died of the Werner syndrome.

Clinical Summary: The first patient was 57 years old at the time
of her death (Case 1 in Epstein, et al., 1966). She was very
short in stature, had cataracts diagnosed at the age of 22, her
hair had turned gray in her 20s and she had had menopausal
symptoms since 33 years of age. She also developed adult onset
diabetes mellitus. She had thin hyperpigmented skin and she
lacked secondary sexual characteristics.

Her sister died at 51 years of age of myocardial infarction
(Case 2 in Epstein, et al., 1966). She was also of short stature
and her hair began to turn gray when she was in high school. By
age 24 she developed senile cataracts which were removed the
following year. She underwent menopause in her 20s. She had
bilateral leg amputations because of chronic ulcers and
osteomyelitis.

Both sisters were considered to be intellectually normal.

Neuropathological Findings: The brain was grossly normal in
appearance but in both it was generally small, weighing 800 gm in
the first and 900 gm in the second. Microscopically, no senile

plaques or neurofibrillary tangles were found in either of the
brains. As in the previously reported cases of progeria, the
amount of lipofuscin in the various neurons did not appear to be
excessive.

The only finding in these brains which had not been
previously recorded was the presence of small, round eosinophilic
inclusions in the nuclei of the neurons in the substantia nigra.
These were rather small, being no larger than the nucleoli at
their largest. One or more of these bodies were present, but
usually no more than two or three occurred in any one nucleus.
They had all the features of Marinesco bodies.

Marinesco (12) described such eosinophilic nuclear
inclusions in melanin-containing neurons of the substantia nigra
and thelocus caeruleus and reported that they occurred in all age
groups and that they appeared to increase in number with age.
Yuen and Baxter (13), in the only systematic survey of Marinesco
bodies in a series of routine autopsies, found them in the
substantia nigra in the majority (125) of 160 patients over the
age of 21 years. There was no correlation between the presence
of these bodies and the type of terminal illness. Although found
in all age groups, they were more numerous in the older patients,
the largest numbers being found in those 55 and older. They
concluded that Marinesco bodies were not of pathological
significance and possibly reflected an aging or involutional
change in the pigmented neurons.

The fact that Marinesco bodies have not been reported in
previous cases of the Werner syndrome and progeria probably is
only a reflection of the care with which the brains had been
examined.

It would appear that there is really no compelling evidence,
either clinically or pathologically, that the brain is a site of
premature aging in the Werner syndrome.

REFERENCES

1. O. Werner, Uber Katarka in Verbindung mit Skeerodermie
   (Doctoral Dissertation, Kiel University), Schmidt und
   Klaunig, Kiel, (1904).
2. C.J. Epstein, G.M. Martin, A.L. Schultz, and A.G. Motulsky,
   Werner's Syndrome, Medicine. 45:177-221 (1966).
3. G.M. Martin, Genetic syndromes in man with potential
   relevance to the pathobiology of aging, Birth Defects.
   14:5-39 (1978).
4. R. Fleischmajor, and A. Nedwich, Werner's syndrome, Am J
   Med. 54:11-118 (1978).

5. G. Rabbiosi, G. Borroni, Werner's syndrome: Seven cases in
    one family, Dermatologica. 158:355-360 (1979).
6. K. Murata, H. Nakashima, Werner's syndrome: Twenty-four
    cases with a review of the Japanese medical literature, J
    Am Geriat Soc. 30:303-308 (1982).
7. D. Salk, Werner's syndrome, Hum Genet. 327:1-15 (1982).
8. A.M. Spence, M.M. Herman, Critical re-examination of the
    premature aging concept in progeria: A light and electron
    microscopic study, Mech Age Develop. 2:211-227 (1973).
9. C.D. West, A quantitative study of lipofuscin accumulation
    with age in normals and individuals with Down's syndrome,
    phenylketonuria, progeria and transneuronal atrophy, J Comp
    Neurol. 186:109-116 (1979).
10. D.M.A. Mann, K.G.A. Sinclair, The quantitative assessment of
    lipofuscin pigment, cytoplasmic RNA and nucleolar volume in
    senile dementia, Neuropath Appl Neurobiol. 4:129-135
    (1978).
11. J.H. Dowson, Neronal lipofuscin accumulation in aging and
    Alzheimer dementia: A pathogenic mechanism, Brit J
    Psychiat. 140:142-148 (1982).
12. G. Marinesco, Sur la presence des corpuscules acidophiles
    paranucleolaires dans les cellules du locus coeruleus, C R
    Acad Sci. 135:1000 (1902).
13. P. Yuen, D.W. Baxter, The morphology of Marinesco bodies
    (paranucleolar corpuscles) in the melanin-pigmented nuclei
    of the brainstem, J Neurol Neurosurg Psychiat. 26:178-183
    (1963).

WERNER'S SYNDROME AND AGING: A REAPPRAISAL

Charles J. Epstein

Departments of Pediatrics and of Biochemistry and
Biophysics; University of California, San Francisco
San Francisco, California   94143 USA

ABSTRACT

   Although a clear distinction between the Werner syndrome and
premature aging was made in our review published in 1966, repeated
allusions in the literature indicate either an ambivalence about
this relationship or a belief that the two conditions are fundamentally related to one another. Therefore, the criteria for
premature aging originally used have been reexamined and found to
be still acceptable. Evaluation of the features of the Werner
syndrome in the light of these criteria once again indicates that
there is no substantial evidence to support and considerable
evidence to oppose equating the Werner syndrome with aging. This
conclusion applies not only to the Werner syndrome in toto, but
also to those aspects of the syndrome considered to qualify it as a
segmental progeroid syndrome and to its characteristic cellular
abnormalities (severely limited in vitro proliferation and
variegated translocation mosaicism). The Werner syndrome should
not, therefore, be forced into the mold of premature aging but
should be studied on its own merits as a condition which may
provide us with clues to the pathogenesis of many important
problems.

INTRODUCTION

   In our review of the Werner syndrome published in 1966
(Epstein et al., 1966), we discussed in some detail the
relationship between the Werner syndrome and aging and came to the
following conclusion:

The Werner syndrome is certainly not merely a process of precocious (earlier onset) or accelerated (more rapid progression) aging. There are too many differences in the degree and nature of the various features of the two entities to allow them to be closely identified with each other. The Werner syndrome may be better considered a "caricature" of aging, exaggerating, although not necessarily by the same mechanisms, some of the clinical and pathologic features which connote aging. If one takes the view that both the Werner syndrome and aging represent the results of generalized metabolic processes, or aberrations thereof, and that the various tissues of the human organism have only a limited number of reactions to such processes, then the overlap between the two entities is not surprising. . . Many of the similarities may be fortuitous, with the convergence of the various pathological processes occuring only at the level of the various affected end organs. However, other similarities may denote a more fundamental identity, with common biochemical and physiological mechanisms actually being involved. Therefore, even if the Werner syndrome and aging are considered to be distinct entities, an analysis of those features that they have in common could conceivably be useful in achieving an understanding of both.

At the time it was written, I believed that this was a strong statement of our belief that, despite the superficial similarities based mainly on overall appearances, the Werner syndrome and aging did not represent the same process and, therefore, that the Werner syndrome was not in fact either identical to or a model of accelerated or precocious aging. The possibility that there might be some common features at the pathogenetic level was left open, although just barely. However, in the sixteen years that have elapsed since the appearance of the review from which I have quoted, numerous articles have appeared which contain statements that appear to disagree with our original conclusions, either directly or by inference. A few examples will be quoted, in chronological order of appearance:

". . . cells from Werner's patients have at least one biochemical defect in common with senescent fibroblasts derived from a normal individual, and this strengthens the view that the early death of Werner's cells in culture is really due to premature ageing, and makes it more likely that there is a direct relationship between in vivo and in vitro aging." (Holliday et al., 1974)

". . . Werner's syndrome, a hereditary disease of premature aging . . ." ". . . these observations taken together with the decreased replication potential that occurs during normal

aging and the more severe growth limitation observed in
Werner's and progeria firoblasts, strengthens the view that
the rate of fibroblast aging in vitro is directly related to
the rate of aging in vivo." (Goldstein and Moerman, 1975)

". . . there seems to be no difference between the changes in
Werner's syndrome and the senile changes which usually occur
in the aged." (Ishii and Hosada, 1975)

". . . Hutchinson-Gilford progeria syndrome (HGPS) and
Werner's syndrome (WS), typical inherited premature aging
diseases. . ." (Fujiwara et al., 1977)

"Human Genetic Disorders that Feature Premature Onset and
Accelerated Progression of Biological Aging." (Goldstein,
1978)

". . . Werner's syndrome is considered to be an excellent
human model for 'aging'. . ."
". . . An important link between Werner's syndrome and natural
human aging." (Goto et al., 1978)

". . . possibly the syndrome is a model of genetically
determined changes which partially resemble normal aging
phenomena." (Nakao et al., 1978)

"A very rare disease, it (progeria) is thought by many to
represent a model for precocious aging...Werner's syndrome is
similar to progeria in many ways, although its salient
manifestations occur in later years...If Werner's syndrome and
progeria are examples of accelerated aging. . ." (Hayflick,
1981)

Some of these statements are being quoted out of context (and
for this I apologize), and the authors may have qualified or even
contradicted them elsewhere in the articles. Nevertheless, they do
serve to point out that at the minimum there is an ambivalence
about the relationship of the Werner syndrome to aging and an
unwillingness to affirm that the two entities are fundamentally
unrelated; in some instances, the statements appear to reflect the
conclusion that the two conditions are fundamentaly related to one
another.

Because of this less than universal acceptance of what
appeared to me to be an obvious truth, I felt that it would be
appropriate, in the context of this meeting, to review the bases of
our original conclusion and to determine whether our reasoning was
faulty then and/or whether new information has appeared which
seriously contradicts that conclusion.

For some reason, radiobiologists appear to be the most
scrupulous about developing criteria for assessing precocious and
accelerated aging, and in our original discussion we quoted the
criteria advanced by Casarett (1964) which were based on earlier
criteria set forth by Comfort (1959). As presented in somewhat
abbreviated form in our review, Casarett's criteria for premature
aging were:

1) An earlier increase in mortality, without alteration of
   the shape of the mortality curve.

2) Proportional advancement in time of all diseases or
   causes of death, without alteration of degree, sequence,
   or absolute incidence, and without induction of disease.

3) Proportional advancement in time of all morphological and
   physiological manifestations of the aging process.

Review of the gerontological literature indicates that these
criteria have not changed since 1964. They were used by Walburg
(1975) in his review of the relationship of radiation-induced life-
shortening and premature aging and were again restated by Comfort
in 1979. It is of interest that Walburg (1975), in applying these
criteria to the effects of radiation, concluded, previous
assertions notwithstanding, that

> . . . almost none of the characteristic lesions associated
> with senescence that have been studied adequately reflects a
> radiation effect analogous to premature aging. In fact, most
> of the age-related changes show no effect of radiation at all,
> and many of those that do (for example, graying of hair,
> sterility, cataract formation) do not appear to be due to
> similar mechanisms.

The parallelism of many of the manifestations of radiation
induced senescence with those of the Werner syndrome is obvious and
again serves to caution us against using a relatively small number
of highly visible characteristics as the basis for making judge-
ments.

In assessing the applicability of the Casarett criteria, the
easiest is, of course, the first--the time of death, and it has
long been recognized that patients with the Werner syndrome appear
to die early. Unfortunately, relatively little new data on this
point have appeared since our original review in which we
calculated the average age of death as 47 years. Moreover, the
data as they now exist are not in a form which permits us to
construct a mortality curve (of the Gompertz type) by which to
determine whether the shape of the curve has remained unaltered (as
required for precocious aging) or reflects the change

characteristic of an increased rate constant, alpha (as required for accelerated aging). We have neither the required information for calculating the probability of death from the Werner syndrome as a function of age nor the necessary control data, although both might ultimately be obtained by the analysis of the large pedigrees now under investigation in Japan and elsewhere.

The second criterion of Casarett refers to pathology, both in the form of disease and as causes of death. Insofar as the causes of death are concerned, the data were and still are insufficient to determine whether these causes are advanced in time "without alteration of degree, sequence, or absolute incidence." A great many more cases will have to be studied, with appropriate controls, before the question can be answered. However, considerably more information is available about diseases in patients with the Werner syndrome, and even a cursory examination of the data indicates that the Werner syndrome by its very definition does not meet the criterion just stated. Thus, consideration of those findings which can be considered as similar, but different in degree (calcification of valve rings and leaflets, hyalinization of seminiferous tubules, atrophy of skin appendages, and osteoporosis) violates the requirement of non-alteration of degree, while those aspects considered as characteristic of the Werner syndrome (cataracts, ulcerations and atrophy of extremities, laryngeal atrophy, high proportion of sarcomas and connective tissue tumors, and soft tissue calcification) violate the requirement of unchanged absolute incidence and the additional requirement of non-induction of new disease.

Finally, the third criterion of Casarett requires that all morphological and physiological manifestations of the aging process be proportionally advanced in time. In this regard, attention in the Werner syndrome has been paid principally to morphological characteristics--for example, graying of the hair, hypermelanosis, lymphoid depletion and thymic atrophy, and even atherosclerosis (if for the sake of discussion we list it as a morphological change rather than as a disease), but aside from the graying and possibly the atherosclerosis the evidence that these changes are advanced in time is not compelling. Furthermore, virtually nothing at all has been studied with regard to those physiological changes which might be considered as correlated with aging. Such changes have been intensively studied in aging individuals, particularly in association with attempts to devise methods for defining biological age. They include factors such as skin elasticity, systolic blood pressure, vital capacity, hand grip strength, reaction time, vibratory sense, and visual and auditory acuity (Hollingsworth et al., 1965; Shock, 1981), and Comfort (1979) has provided an even more extensive list of possible criteria. Based primarily on animal data, Ludwig and Smoke (1980) have attempted to define quantifiable criteria for biological age which are both morphological and

physiological: thickness of the glomerular basement membrane,
density of neuronal cells, chromosomal aberrations, thymic weight,
lipofuscin accumulation in the Purkinje cell layer of the
cerebellum, reactive astrocytes in the hippocampus, thermal
contractibility of tail tendon, physiological capacitance in the
stressed organism, spleen cell response to T-cell mitogens,
thyroxin degradation rate, and cell doubling potential of skin
fibroblasts.

Although the theoretical bases of these two approaches differ,
both agree in avoiding the use of frankly pathological or disease
related changes. They focus on changes presumed to result from
whatever processes cause or determine aging (referred to by some as
primary aging [Hofecker et al., 1980]), and which might predispose
to but are distinguished from disease. Unfortunately, any attempts
to apply these considerations to the Werner syndrome are doomed to
failure, since the relevant data just do not exist. Even Ludwig
and Smoke (1980), in asserting that the Werner syndrome represents
an extreme discrepancy between biological and chronological age, do
so without any real basis in fact. It is worth noting, however,
that some of the categories of features just mentioned have been
looked at in the Werner syndrome--collagen and connective tissue, the
endocrine system, immune responses, and cell proliferation--and in
no instance can it be concluded that the changes are the same as
obtained in natural aging (see Salk, 1982, for review of recent
data). Therefore, if we generate a "score-card" for how the Werner
syndrome meets Casarett's criteria for premature aging, it will
look as follows:

	Criterion	Score for the Werner Syndrome
1.	Shape of mortality curve	Unknown
2.	Advances in time of	
	causes of death	Unknown
	diseases	Unlike aging
3.	Advances in time of	
	morphological changes	Unknown
	physiological changes	Unknown

Overall, the data are insufficient to support the conclusion
that the Werner syndrome represents premature aging, and when they
are sufficient they contradict it.

The foregoing discussion might be considered as "overkill",
since few if any investigators appear to be willing to argue, in
the face of the evidence just cited, that the Werner syndrome is
identical with premature aging. Nevertheless, some, perhaps many,
do still appear to hold to the notion that at least some of the
features of the Werner syndrome are identical with those of aging.
In advancing this view, Martin (1978) coined the term "segmental

progeroid syndrome" to refer to conditions manifesting a limited number of pathophysiological and cellular features regarded as criteria of aging. The implication of this designation is that the particular features considered as a part of the syndrome do (or may) in fact represent true aging phenomena. By the scoring system used, the Werner syndrome was considered to manifest twelve of these features, including "potential relevance to the 'intrinsic mutagenesis' hypothesis of aging," increased frequency of non-constitutional chromosomal aberrations, increased susceptibility to one or more types of neoplasms of relevance to aging, possibility of a defect in a stem cell population or in the kinetics of stem-cell proliferation, premature graying or loss of hair or both, diabetes mellitus, hypogonadism, degenerative vascular disease, osteoporosis, cataracts, regional fibrosis and variation in amounts and/or distribution of adipose tissue.

I find the concept of segmental progeroid syndromes a difficult one to accept, both in terms of the criteria used for assigning genetic conditions to this category and of the implied assumption that there may be a mechanistic relationship underlying the features present in one of these syndromes and in natural aging. The criteria chosen for evaluation are very mixed indeed, and their significance to aging is not always obvious. Furthermore, I would submit that if we are willing to entertain the concept of segmental progeria, then those features included in the progeroid syndrome should follow Casarett's criteria as best they can, and it is for this reason that I devoted so much time to their consideration. In particular, the proposed features should obey the second and third criteria which would require that the diseases, morphological alterations, and physiological changes characterizing the progeroid syndrome should again resemble those features of natural aging in terms of their degree, sequence, and incidence. Review of even those potentially acceptable features supporting inclusion of the Werner syndrome in the list of segmental progeroid syndromes indicates that these criteria cannot be met for the reasons already outlined earlier. Once again we are looking at the specific effects of a specific disease process, and not at accelerated aging--even in part.

The two most striking laboratory features of the Werner syndrome are the severely limited in vitro replication of cultured skin fibroblasts (Martin et al., 1970) and the development of clonal structural chromosome rearrangements--the so-called variegated translocation mosaicism (Salk et al., 1981). The latter is clearly not a manifestation of natural aging and constitutes one more of the unique features of the Werner syndrome. Similarly, despite attempts to argue to the contrary, the extreme shortening of in vitro cell survival is well beyond the limits observed in fibroblasts obtained from even the most aged individuals. Rather than being regarded merely as advanced in vitro cellular senescence, it must be considered, in my opinion, as a pathological consequence of the underlying defect in the Werner syndrome.

If, as this reappraisal indicates, the Werner syndrome still cannot be considered a form of accelerated aging, in whole or in part, is there any value in studying it over and above that derived from understanding one more rare disease? In the concluding paragraph of our 1966 review we suggested that there is, and that conclusion remains as valid today as it was then:

> The elucidation of the primary defect of the Werner syndrome and tracing of its adverse ramifications thus remains a tantalizing challenge. In one hereditary disorder are combined two major diseases of modern man—vascular disease and neoplasia, as well as others of widespread importance— diabetes, cataracts, and osteoporosis. The solution of the puzzle of Werner's syndrome may, therefore, provide us with clues to the pathogenesis of many diverse problems.

In 1965, we (Epstein et al., 1965) referred to the Werner syndrome as a "caricature of aging, a genetic model for the study of degenerative diseases," and I still believe that is what it is. Forcing the Werner syndrome into the mold of premature aging does nothing to enhance its value as a subject for study and, by requiring us to make tenuous and often unsubstantiated associations, serves only to detract from the outcome of our investigations. Let us study the condition on its own merits— there will still be many valuable and fascinating things to be learned.

REFERENCES

Casarett, G.W., 1964, Similarities and contrasts between radiation and time pathology. Advan. Gerontol. Res., 1:109-163.

Comfort, A., 1959, Natural ageing and the effects of radiation. Radiat. Res. (Suppl.), 1:216-234.

Comfort, A., 1979, "The Biology of Senescence," 3rd ed., Elsevier, New York.

Epstein, C.J., Martin, G.M., and Motulsky, A.G., 1965, Werner's syndrome: Caricature of aging, a genetic model for the study of degenerative diseases. Trans. Assoc. Amer. Phys., 78:73-81.

Epstein, C.J., Martin, G.M., Schultz, A.L. and Motulsky, A.G., 1966, Werner's syndrome. A review of its symptomatology, natural history, pathologic features, genetics and relationship to the natural aging process. Medicine, 45:177-221.

Fujiwara, Y., Higashikawa, T., and Tatsumi, M., 1977, A retarded rate of DNA replication and normal level of DNA repair in Werner's syndrome fibroblasts in culture. J. Cell. Physiol., 92:365-374.

Goldstein, S., 1978, Human genetic disorders that feature premature onset and accelerated progression of biological aging, In "The Genetics of Aging", E. L. Schneider, ed., Plenum Press, New York.

Goldstein, S. and Moerman, E.J., 1975, Heat-labile enzymes in Werner's syndrome fibroblasts. Nature, 255:159.

Goto, M., Horiuchi, Y., Tanimoto, K., Ishii, T., and Nakashima, H., 1978, Werner's syndrome: analysis of 15 cases with a review of the Japanese literature. J. Amer. Geriatrics Soc., 26:341-347.

Hayflick, L., 1981, The biology of human aging. Plastic Reconstru. Surg., 67:536-550.

Hofecker, G., Skalicky, M., Kment, A., and Niedermuller, H., 1980, Models of the biological age of the rat. I. A factor model of age parameters. Mech. Ageing Develop., 14:345-359.

Holliday, R., Porterfield, J.S., and Gibbs, D.D., 1974, Premature aging and occurrence of altered enzyme in Werner's syndrome fibroblasts. Nature, 248:762-763.

Hollingsworth, J.W., Hashizumi, A., and Jablon, S., 1965, Correlations between tests of aging in Hiroshima subjects—an attempt to define "physiological age." Yale J. Biol. Med. 38:11-26.

Ishii, T. and Hosoda, Y., 1975, Werner's syndrome: autopsy report of one case, with a review of pathologic findings reported in the literature. J. Amer. Geriatrics Soc., 23:145-154.

Ludwig, F.C. and Smoke, M.F., 1980, The measurement of biological age. Exp. Aging Res., 6:497-522.

Martin, G.M., 1978, Genetic syndromes in man with potential relevance to the pathobiology of aging. Birth Defects Orig. Art. Series 14(1):5-39.

Martin, G.M. Sprague, C.A., and Epstein, C.J., 1970, Replicative lifespan of cultivated human cells: effects of donor's age, tissue and genotype. Lab. Invest., 23:86-91.

Nakao, Y., Kishihara, M., Yoshimi, H., Inoue, Y., Tanaka, K., Sakamoto, N., Matsukura, S., Imura, H., Ichihashi, M., and Fujiwara, Y., 1978, Werner's syndrome. In vivo and in vitro characteristics as a model of aging. Amer. J. Med., 65:919-932.

Salk, D., 1982, Werner's syndrome: a review of recent research with an analysis of connective tissue metabolism, growth control of cultured cells, and chromosomal aberrations. Hum. Genet., 62:1-15.

Salk, D., Au, K., Hoehn, H., and Martin, G.M., 1981, Cytogenetics
    of Werner's syndrome cultured skin fibroblasts: variegated
    translocation mosaicism. <u>Cytogenet. Cell Genet.</u>,
    30:92-107.
Shock, N.W., 1981, Indices of functional age, <u>In</u> "Aging: A
    Challenge to Science and Society. Vol. 1, Biology," D. Danon,
    N.W., Shock and M. Marois, eds., Oxford University Press,
    Oxford.
Walburg, H.E., Jr., 1975, Radiation-induced life shortening and
    premature aging. <u>Advan. Radiat. Biol.</u>, 5:145-179.

A COMPARISON OF ADULT AND CHILDHOOD PROGERIAS: WERNER SYNDROME AND HUTCHINSON-GILFORD PROGERIA SYNDROME

W. Ted Brown, Fred J. Kieras, George E. Houck, Jr.,
Regina Dutkowski, and Edmund C. Jenkins

The New York State Institute for Basic Research in
Developmental Disabilities, Staten Island, New York and
Cornell University Medical College, New York, New York

INTRODUCTION

The Werner syndrome, also known as progeria of the adult,
and the childhood Hutchinson-Gilford Progeria Syndrome (hereafter
Progeria), both serve as genetic disease models of human aging
(Brown, 1979). A comparison of their similarities and
differences may be useful in order to gain insight into the
nature of the genetic mutations underlying these conditions.
Their modes of inheritance indicate the involvement of a single
gene. This implies that some specific genes may lead to a
phenotype of greatly accelerated senescence and that such genes
may have direct effects on the rate of aging. Determining the
basic mechanisms involved in producing their phenotypes may point
the way to an understanding of important pathogenetic aspects
underlying the aging process.

Down syndrome (trisomy 21) individuals may show more
features of accelerated senescence than either Werner syndrome or
Progeria (Martin, 1977), however, Down's individuals are
recognizable by physical abnormalities at birth and show
developmental delays from early infancy. The abnormalities and
growth delay in Progeria are not usually apparent at birth, but
progressively develop usually beginning in the first year of
life. Likewise the recognizable phenotype of the Werner syndrome
is not often apparent until the individuals are in their mid-
teens to their twenties, and diagnosis is not usually made until
they are in their thirties.

229

Here, we review and compare the clinical, genetic, and laboratory features of the Werner syndrome and Progeria in order to help assess their role as disease models of accelerated aging.

CLINICAL FEATURES OF THE WERNER SYNDROME AND PROGERIA

The Werner syndrome (Epstein et al., 1966) has a number of clinical features which appear to resemble Progeria (Debusk, 1972), but a number of striking differences as well. The general similarities and differences between the Werner syndrome, Progeria and aging are summarized in Table 1. The widespread atherosclerosis of the Werner syndrome is also seen in Progeria. Calcification of the heart valves (in the Werner syndrome) is usually more marked and more severe than in Progeria and aging. The graying and whitening of the hair is striking in the Werner syndrome and usually occurs in the teenage years. Total alopecia is rare, but hair loss and thinning of the hair occurs over most of the body. In Progeria, loss of scalp hair usually begins to occur with the first year of life. A pattern of total alopecia, with perhaps a few sparse hairs remaining, is common by the age

Table 1

Features	Werner Syndrome	Progeria	Aging
1 Atherosclerosis	present	present	present
2 Graying of Hair	present	present	present
3 Loss of Hair	present	present	present
4 Aged Appearing Skin	present	present	present
5 Hypermelanosis Skin	present	present	present
6 Skin Calcification	present	absent	absent
7 Ankle Ulcerations	present	absent	absent
8 Hyperkeratosis	present	absent	absent
9 Short Stature	present	present	variable
10 Osteoporosis	present	present	present
11 Coxa Valga	absent	present	absent
12 Facial Disproportion	absent	present	absent
13 High Pitched Voice	present	present	variable
14 Thymic Atrophy	present	variable	present
15 Hypogonadism	present	present	variable
16 Diabetes	variable	rare	variable
17 Cortical Atrophy	present	absent	variable
18 Dementia	variable	absent	variable
19 Cataracts	present	absent	present
20 Neoplasms	frequent	absent	frequent

of 3 to 6. Male pattern baldness is common with normal aging,
but total alopecia is not usual and is very rare in females. The
skin changes in the Werner syndrome and Progeria appear similar,
but they are different than in normal aging. In both Werner and
Progeria there is a loss of subcutaneous tissue which is
particularly marked in the extremities. Widespread "metastatic"
calcification of subcutaneous tissue is noted in the Werner
syndrome, but not seen in Progeria or normal aging.
Hyperkeratosis of the soles of the feet and ankle ulcerations are
particularly striking in the Werner syndrome but usually absent
in Progeria and normal aging. Osteoporosis as seen in normal
aging also occurs in the Werner syndrome and Progeria. However,
it has differences; in the Werner syndrome, it usually has a
peripheral distribution, while in Progeria it has a dysplastic
character with osteolysis of the distal clavicles and fibrous
tissue replacement. Coxa valga and aseptic necrosis of the head
of the femur are seen in Progeria. Hip dislocations are common
and a marked delay in bone fracture healing is frequent. The
face in the Werner syndrome tends to be rounded but fairly normal
in appearance. In Progeria the face is strikingly unusual.
Although the head circumference is of a normal proportion for
height, there is mandibular hypoplasia which produces a severe
facial disproportion and gives a somewhat alien appearance.
Laryngeal atrophy produces a high pitched voice in both Progeria
and the Werner syndrome. This is also seen in normal aging but
to a lesser degree. Thymic atrophy has been reported to occur in
both the Werner syndrome and normal aging. This is not usually
seen in Progeria and thymic enlargement has occasionally been
noted. Hypogonadism occurs in both the Werner syndrome and
Progeria. Diabetes mellitis of a peripheral insulin resistance
type is common in the Werner syndrome. It has been noted to
occur late in the course in several cases of Progeria but is
generally rare. Cortical atrophy has been noted at autopsy in
several Werner syndrome cases, perhaps secondary to the severe
atherosclerosis. No changes of senile dementia of the Alzheimer
type have been reported in the Werner syndrome or Progeria.
Cataracts of a subcapsular type are usual in the Werner syndrome,
but are different than the senile type seen in normal aging.
They are lacking in Progeria. Neoplasms, particularly sarcomas,
are frequent in the Werner syndrome. Only one case of a neoplasm
in a Progeric patient has been reported. The average weight of
patients with Progeria is approximately 25-30 lbs. A few
patients with Progeria have weighed on the order of 40-60 lbs.,
and have lesser degrees of atherosclerosis. This suggests that
atypical forms of Progeria with partial expression can occur.
Werner syndrome patients generally weigh 70-90 lbs., and a
failure of adolescent growth spurt is commonly seen. Thus, at a
superficial level at least, many similarities exist between the
Werner syndrome, Progeria and aging. This may reflect similar
underlying mechanisms at a genetic level.

GENETIC FEATURES

The mode of inheritance of the Werner syndrome is clearly autosomal recessive, and as is the case for rare recessives, there exists increased consanguinity among the affected families. Epstein et al. (1966) estimated a rate of between 19 to 36% consanguinity among a predominantly caucasian population, whereas Goto et al. (1981) found a rate of 70% in Japan. From these estimates, using the Dahlberg formula, Epstein et al. estimated the homozygote incidence in the U.S. to be from 1 to 22 cases per million population. Similarly, Goto et al. (1981) estimated the Japanese incidence to be from 3 to 50 per million population. In addition to an increased consanguinity, the proportions of affected sibs is expected to be 25% for a recessive mode of inheritance. In the U.S. study (Epstein et al., 1966) the proportion of affected sibs was estimated by two different methods with the results that approximately 25% of sibs were found to be affected. The Japanese study (Goto et al., 1981) also allowed or led to a 25% frequency estimate.

The mode of inheritance of Progeria appears to be that of a sporadic autosomal dominant mutation. Support reasoning for this derives from three different lines of evidence.

First, the consanguinity rate is lower than would be expected for a recessive as rare as Progeria. Debusk (1972) mentions that consanguinity was present in 3 out of 19 families in which it was specifically sought and was absent or not sought in 41 additional families for an estimated rate of 5-16%. Rautenstrouch and Snigula (1977) report a rate of 6% among cases in which it could be determined. Using the Dahlberg formula, assessing a birth incidence of Progeria to be 1 per 8 million and a population consanguinity frequency of either 0.5, 1 or 3% leads to estimates of expected consanguinity of 47, 64, and 85% in Progeric families. Thus, the observed consanguinity frequency in Progeria is much lower than would be expected for a rare recessive. Although the reported incidence of Progeria is about 1 in 8 million births (Debusk, 1972), true incidence may be somewhat higher as not all cases are reported. Perhaps 1 in 4 million is a reasonable estimate. In the U.S., we have seen 10 Progeric patients. Of these, only 4 had not yet been previously reported including the two youngest cases. In none of their families was there any history of consanguinity. Even if Progeria were to have a 1 in a million incidence, this would still lead to a prediction using the Dahlberg formula of an expected consanguinity frequency of from 24 to 66%. This is much higher than the low frequency which is seen in Progeria.

Second, a paternal age effect has been observed in Progeria which is highly suggestive of sporadic dominant mutations. Jones et al. (1975) found that among 18 cases the father was older than the mother by an average of 4.4 years which was a significant difference and similar to that seen in seven other disorders with new mutations for which autosomal dominant inheritance had been established (Basal Cell Nevus syndrome, Waardenburg syndrome, Crouzon syndrome, Cleido-cranial dysostosis, Oculo-dental-digital syndrome, Treatcher-Collins syndrome, and multiple exostoses) and for 4 disorders in which older paternal age in the setting of new mutation had been previously indicated (Achondroplasia, Apert syndrome, Fibrodysplasia ossiticons progressiva, and Marfan syndrome).

Third, for a recessive condition, the proportion of affected sibs should be about 25%, whereas for Progeria it is clearly much less with the majority of cases being sporadic. For example, the case of identical Progeric twins reported from Brazil had 14 normal sibs. As noted by McKusick (1976), for new dominant mutations, one may occasionally expect the mutation to occur in a germ line leading to somatic mosaicism and several new cases within one family. This has been reported (Gabr et al., 1960; Rava, 1967; Erecinski, 1961; Franklyn, 1976; Rautenstrauch and Snigula, 1977). An alternative but less attractive hypothesis is that while the majority of cases may represent sporadic dominant mutations, a few cases may be the result of recessively inherited mutations.

We have examined 10 living cases of Progeria in the U.S. The data on their paternal-maternal ages and sibling frequency is summarized in Table 2. The fathers were older than the mothers by an average of 6.0 years, whereas about 2.8 years difference is expected (Jones et al., 1975). Thus, a paternal age effect was observed in these 10 cases which can be added to strengthen the paternal age affect previously reported in 18 Progeric cases (Jones et al., 1975). Among these 10, no family had more than one affected child. The number of unaffected sibs was 26. One would expect there to be 25% or 6 to 7 sibs affected if a recessive mode of inheritance were to apply to these 10 Progeria families.

LABORATORY STUDIES OF WERNER SYNDROME AND PROGERIA

Laboratory studies which we conducted involved an attempt to identify a genetic or metabolic marker for these diseases. Such a marker might help define the nature of the underlying defects in these diseases. We have not found a specific DNA repair capacity defect in cultured Progeric cells (Brown et al., 1980a). We found sister chromatid exchange frequencies to be normal in Pregeria and the WS patients (Darlington et al., 1981). We found no increase in

Table 2. Paternal Age Effect and Number of Normal Sibs in 10 U.S.
          Progeric Sibships

Case		Age	Normal Sibs	Mother's Age at Birth	Father's Age at Birth
1	TS	14	3	26	26
2	MC	27	6	40	46
3	PS	5	2	24	23
4	AG	12	6	24	49
5	LC	2	2	35	42
6	BM	16	1	27	27
7	KC	12	2	24	24
8	SK	6	1	33	47
9	FM	13	2	28	25
10	BS	10	2	26	38
			26	28.7 (+5.5)	34.7 (+10.7)

thermolabile components of the erythrocytic enzymes, glucose-6-
phosphate dehydrogenase and 6-phosphogluconate dehydrogenase, in
patients with Progeria and the Werner syndrome (Brown and
Darlington, 1980b). We found no abnormality in HLA antigen
expression in Progeric fibroblasts (Brown et al., 1980c). We
interpret these findings to indicate that widespread errors in
protein synthesis are unlikely to underlie these diseases.

     As summarized elsewhere in this volume, two of the more
notable abnormalities in laboratory studies of the Werner
syndrome are likely to involve chromosomal abnormalities and
glycosaminoglycan abnormalities. Here we would like to present
results recently obtained in our laboratory on these
abnormalities in WS and Progeric patients.

Patients

     A 37-year-old female (NV) was diagnosed as having the Werner
syndrome. She was born in Puerto Rico and developed gray-white
hair at the age of 12. Diabetes mellitus developed at age 30
requiring insulin therapy. Bilateral femoral-popliteal bypass
surgery was performed at age 32 for circulatory insufficiency.
Bilateral cataract extractions were performed at age 36. At age
37, non-healing ankle ulcers led to a below-the-knee amputation
of the left leg. She was 4 feet, 10 inches tall and weighed 90
lbs. She had hyperpigmentation spots on the skin and an aged
appearance. She had eight normal siblings and one 23-year-old
brother with short stature who had developed gray hair. Parental
consanguinity was not known to be present.

A 37-year-old white male (JS) was diagnosed as having the
Werner syndrome. A summary of his medical history, kindly
supplied by Dr. Reed Pyretz, Johns Hopkins Hospital, included the
following: cataracts requiring extirpation occurred at ages 30
and 31. Dyspnea on exertion and angina developed at age 32. At
age 37, arteriography showed 50 to 90% obstruction of the
coronary arteries. Stature was short with a height of 5 feet 3
inches. His weight was 135 lbs. Proximal and distal
interphalangeal joints showed bony hypertrophy. Brachydactyly
was present. Alopecia was present, but not diabetes, ankle
ulcerations, or sclerodermatous skin changes. Family history was
negative for consanguinity and 2 siblings were normal.

Chromosomal Studies

Heparinized whole blood from patient NV and from three
normal female volunteers was grown for 96 hours in either medium
RPMI 1640 or TC 199 with 19% undialized fetal calf serum, and
phytohemagglutinin P. Unbanded chromosomes were prepared as
previously described (Darlington et al., 1980). Slides were
coded and blindly scored for frequency of gaps, chromatid, and
chromosome breaks, exchange figures, and fragments. The results
are shown in Table 3.

There was a 3-4 fold higher number of gaps and chromatid
breaks in WS blood grown in TC 199 as compared to the control
bloods grown in TC 199. Bloods grown in RPMI 1640 showed less or

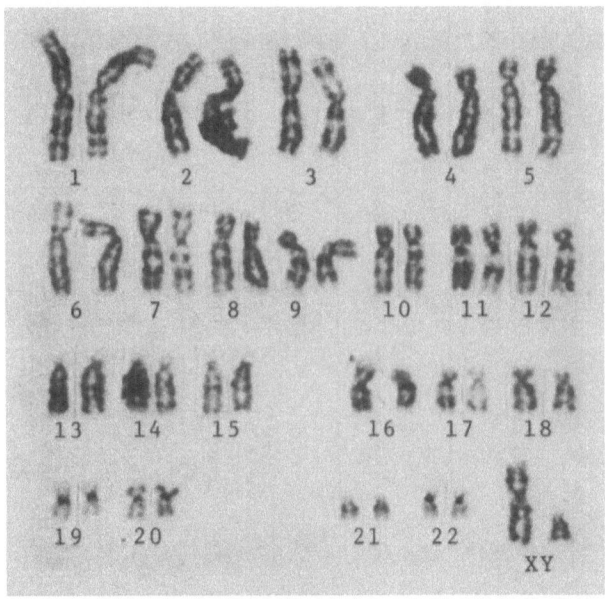

Figure 1.

Table 3

Table 3. Chromosome Aberrations in Werner Syndrome Peripheral Blood
          Comparison of Two Media — RPMI 1640 vs TC199

Subject	Media	Gaps	Chromatid	Chromosome	Exchange Figures	Fragments	Total	Cells Analyzed
Werner (NV)	RPMI	17	10	3	1	1	32	100
	TC199	39	20	7	2	1	69	100
Control #1	RPMI	6	11	5	0	0	22	100
	TC199	13	8	3	0	3	17	100
Control #2	RPMI	2	7	4	0	0	13	100
	TC199	9	5	4	0	3	21	100
Control #3	RPMI	10	7	4	0	0	21	100
	TC199	5	7	5	0	5	22	95

no comparable differences. This may be analogous to induction of
fragile sites seen when bloods from fragile X syndrome
individuals are grown in TC 199 medium which is relatively folate
deficient but not in RPMI 1640 which is relatively folate
enriched. Thus we have confirmed a finding of increased
chromosomal aberrations as reported by Nordenson (1977) in WS
blood, which appears to be dependent upon the medium in which the
cells are grown.

A punch skin biopsy was obtained from Werner patient JS and
explanted into 25 cm^2 plastic T flasks (Falcon). It was
incubated at pH 7.2 in RPMI 1640 (GIBCO), 16% fetal bovine serum,
1 mM glutamine, 1,000 u/ml at 37° C. After 3 weeks, the skin
fibroblasts were subcultured with 0.25% trypsin (GIBCO). The
subcultures were harvested for Giemsa-banded chromosomal analysis
within one week (second passage).

A total of 21 metaphases with 46 chromosomes were karyotyped
photographically. Nine cells from one of the flasks had a normal
46,XY karyotype. Eleven metaphases from another second passage
culture were also normal. Example is shown in Fig. 1.
One cell of the 21 cells exhibited a possible del(7)(q11). The
chromosome 7 may have broken in that cell. An unidentifiable
fragment or distorted chromosome with bands that were not clear
was also present. This material could have been the 7q11 to ter
portion of broken chromosome 7. The 7q11 break point did not
correspond to any of the break points that have been identified
by Salk (1981b, 1982) and Scappaticci (1982) in a total of 1134
fibroblast metaphases from WS individuals. Other than this
cell, there was no evidence of deletion or translocation of any
other chromosomes in the 21 metaphases.

Our normal observations may be due to individual differences
in patients diagnosed as having the Werner syndrome.
Alternatively, the present normal results may have been due to
the cell culture conditions including the age of the cells or the
type of medium. This was apparently the 15th Werner syndrome
individual whose fibroblasts were analyzed for variegated
translocation mosaics (VTM), including those reported by Hoehn et
al. (1975), Norwood et al. (1979), Salk et al. (1981, 1982),
Schonberg et al. (1981, 1982) and Scappaticci (1982) in
fibroblasts, peripheral blood lymphocytes, and long-term
lymphoblastoid cell cultures. Salk (1982) has noted one type of
chromosomal abnormality in early passage cells and completely
different types in later passage cells from the same individual.
We cultured cells in RPMI 1640 while those of Hoehn et al.
(1975), Norwood et al. (1979), and Salk et al. (1981, 1982) were
in Dulbecco-Vogt medium. Littlefield and Maihles (1975) observed
occasional VTMs in non-Werner fibroblasts where RPMI 1640 was the
basal medium used.

Studies of Hyaluronic Acid

We have analyzed hyaluronic acid (HA) in urine samples
obtained from three Progeric patients and from one WS patient.
The samples were diluted with water to salt concentrations of
0.3M or less and filtered to remove insoluble material. The
samples were brought to a cetylpyridinium chloride (CPC)
concentration of 0.4% (w/v) and the glycosaminoglycans (GAGs)
precipitated overnight at 4°C. The precipitated GAGs were
collected by centrifugation at 4°C and washed 3 times with
absolute ethanol containing 1% potassium acetate to remove excess
CPC. The crude GAGs were treated overnight with 0.5 mg of
proteinase K at 37°C in 0.1 M Tris HCl, pH 7.5. The digests were
dialyzed against distilled water, concentrated, and the GAGs
precipitated by addition of 4 volumes of absolute ethanol
containing 1% potassium acetate. The GAGs were collected by
centrifugation at 10,000 g for 15 min at 4°C, dried in vacuuo,
and redissolved in water. These were for further analysis.

Electrophoresis was performed on SEPRAPHORE III cellulose
acetate strips (5.7 x 14.4 cm). The electrolytes used were 0.1 N
HCl at 10 ma for 40 min or 0.3 M Cd(OAc)$_2$, pH 4.1, at 5 ma for 3
hrs. Strips were stained in 0.1% (w/v) Alcian Blue in 0.1% (v/v)
acetic acid to locate GAG and destained in 0.1% (v/v) acetic
acid. Hexosamine analysis after hydrolysis in 4N HCl for 8 hrs
at 100°C was performed by the procedure of Elson and Morgan
(1933). Uronic acid was determined using glucuronic acid (GlcUA)
as standard by the method described in Damle et al. (1979). GAGs
were fractionated on an anion exchange resin BioRad AG1X2, (200-
400 mesh) as described by Schiller et al. (1961) using increasing
concentrations of NaCl. Hyaluronidase was assayed in fibroblast
extracts by the method of Orkin et al. (1982). Beta-N-acetyl
hexosaminidase and beta-glucuronidase were assayed as described
by LeRoy et al. (1972) and Hall et al. (1973). GAG samples were
digested with chondroitinase ABC or with bacterial hyaluronidase
as described in Damle et al. (1979).

The GAG preparations from the 4 patients were analyzed for
uronic acid and hexosamine and the molar ratios of these
components are presented in Table 4.

In pure GAG this ratio is very close to 1. The deviations
from unity in these preparations indicate that some components
other than GAGs may be present.

All of the samples were analyzed by electrophoresis in 0.1 N
HCl. In this solvent the distance migrated is proportional to
the sulfate content of the GAGs. HA migrates only slightly from
the origin while heparin migrates the greatest distance. The

Werner syndrome and Progeria samples showed bands coincident with HA suggesting that these patients had more than normal amounts of HA in their urines. Adequate amounts of urinary GAGs were available from the Werner syndrome (NV) patient and from the Progeria patient (TS) and these were subjected to further study to characterize and quantitate the urinary HA.

Table 4. Uronic and Hexosamine Molar Ratio in Urinary GAGs From Werner syndrome and Progeria

Patient	Uronic Acid: Hesosamine (Molar Ratio)
Progeria	
P.S.	0.91
L.C.	0.88
T.S.	0.80
Werner syndrome	
N.V.	1.16

A known amount of GAG was applied to a column of AG1X2 (anion exchange resin) and eluted with water, 0.5 M NaCl (HA enriched fraction) -and 4 M NaCl (sulfated GAG fraction). The salts were removed by dialysis, the samples concentrated, and further analyses performed.

Total recovery of uronic acid in the Werner Syndrome (NV) was 73%, while with the Progeria sample (TS) it was 93%. All samples were subjected to electrophoresis in 0.1 N HCl. In both patients a band coincident with HA was found in the 0.5 M NaCl fraction and this accounted for most of the Alcian Blue staining material in this fraction. The water and 4 M NaCl fractions did not contain HA.

The fractions from the anion exchange were then digested with Streptococcal hyaluronidase (specific for HA) and analyzed by electrophoresis in 0.1 N HCl and in 0.3 M $Cd(OAc)_2$. Essentially, all of the material in 0.5 M fraction was removed by this treatment while the other fractions remained unchanged. This indicates that almost all of the GAG in the 0.5 M NaCl fraction is HA and allows us to quantitate the urinary HA in these patients after correcting for recovery of Uronic Acid from the column.

Table 5. Reactionation of Urinary GAG on AG1x2

NaCl Concentration	% Total Uronic Acid in Fraction	
	Werner Syndrome (NV)	Progeria (TS)
H_2O Wash	26	0
0.5 M NaCl	19	17
4.0 M NaCl	55	83

Two years previously, four 24-hour urine samples were kindly analyzed for us by Dr. Jack Distler, University of Michigan, for the presence of HA using a method previously described (Jourdian et al., 1979). The first sample was a baseline collection. Three months later while the patient (NV) was hospitalized another 24-hour collection was obtained. Then the patient received approximately 100 units of an injectable form of hyaluronidase, Wydase (Wyeth Laboratories), given subcutaneously every 2 hours for 36 hours. During this time, two additional 24 hour urine collections were obtained. The results shown in Table 6 indicated a baseline level of about 20% HA which dropped to less than 1% during the injections. It is known that injected hyaluronidase rapidly appears in the urine of rabbits (Morton Lipshutz, Wyeth Laboratories, Personal Communication), so it may be reasonable to assume that in this case the HA in the urine could be degraded by the excreted hyaluronidase. Alternatively, the injected enzyme could be acting in the extracellular space to act upon the HA present there. If Werner patients lack a normal level of hyaluronidase, this approach might offer a mode of therapy.

Our results confirm and extend the earlier findings of increased HA in the urine of WS patients by Goto et al. (1981). We have also established that HA is increased in the urine of a Progeria patient which confirms an early report of Tokunaga et al. (1978).

Enzyme Activities in Extracts of Cultured Fibroblasts

Because of increased excretion of HA in the urine of these patients, a possible metabolic defect may be in the deficient

Table 6. Urinary Hyaluronic Acid (HA) in Werner syndrome

Sample	Conditions	HA as % GAG
1	Baseline 3 mo.	20.8
2	Pretreatment	20.2
3	Hyaluronidase	0.4
4	Hyaluronidase	0.2
5	Post-treatment 1 yr	15.0
6	Later Baseline 2 yr	19.0

24 hr urine collections, samples 2, 3, and 4 were collected sequentially, Hyaluronidase used was Wydase (Wyeth) 30 U. injected S.C. every 2 hrs. Patient - N.V., Control Values less than 1%.

degradation of HA. Three enzymes which may be involved in the degradation of HA are hyaluronidase, β-glucuronidase, and β-N-Acetyl glucosaminidase. These 3 enzymes were assayed in extracts of control (normal) fibroblasts and fibroblasts from Progeria and Werner syndrome. Within experimental limits, the values of hyaluronidase and β-glucuronidase in patients' cells were normal. However, in Progeria fibroblasts the β-N-acetyl glucosaminidase level was 12% of the normal value. This might account for increased levels of HA in the urine of the patients, but further experiments must be performed to confirm this result and to rule out other possibilities.

CONCLUSIONS

The basic defect in either the Werner syndrome or Progeria is unknown. It has been suggested (McKusick, 1983) that dominant type mutations may in general be of a different type which involve structural molecules rather than the mutations seen in recessive diseases which often involve a lack of an enzymatic activity. However, some genetic diseases are known with both dominant and recessive forms. For example, the Erhlos-Danlos syndrome of loose jointedness and stretchable skin, is now recognized as being due a number of subtypes with several autosomal dominant types, and several recessive types (McKusick, 1983). A mutation involving the collagen molecule directly appears to account for some of the dominant forms, while deficiency of post translational modifying enzymes that affect collagen cross linkage appear to account for some of the recessively inherited forms.

A similar situation involving some key gene product could apply to the Werner syndrome and Progeria. Thus, although the Werner syndrome is due to an autosomal recessive mutation and Progeria likely represents a sporadic dominant mutation, there may be a similar genetic pathology in the two diseases. A mutation of a structural molecule or a deficiency of a modifying enzyme might lead to a somewhat similar phenotype apparently affecting a similar aspect of the aging process. It would appear that mesenchymal and connective tissues are severely affected in both diseases. It is intriguing that elevated levels of hyaluronic acid have been seen in both conditions. This may reflect some common pathogenic mechanism in the extracellular connective tissue compartment. Further research may clarify the basis for these abnormalities in the Werner syndrome and Progeria, and provide insight into their molecular basis. These two distinct yet similar genetic experiments of nature may provide an understanding of a metabolic factor which apparently affects the aging process.

ACKNOWLEDGEMENTS

We wish to thank Talitha Curtis and Bruce Kastin for technical assistance, Gretchen Darlington for helpful discussions during the course of this work, the Sunshine Foundation, for clinical assistance, and the Bedminster Foundation for financial support.

REFERENCES

Brown, W.T., 1979, Human mutations affecting aging -- a review, Mechanisms of Aging and Development, 9:325.

Brown, W.T., Ford, J., and Gersey, E.L., 1980a, Variation of DNA repair in Progeria Cells unrelated to growth conditions, Biochemical and Biophysical Research Communications, 97:347.

Brown, W.T., Darlington, G.J., 1980b, Thermolabile in progeria and Werner Syndrome: Evidence contrary to the protein error hypothesis, Am. J. Hum. Genet., 32:614.

Brown, W.T., Darlington, G.J., Fotino, M., and Arnold, A., 1980c, Detection of HLA antigens on progeria fibroblasts, Clinical Genetics, 17:213.

Damle, S.P., Kieras, F.J., Tzeng, W.-K., and Gregory, J.D., 1979, Isolation and characterization of proteochondroitin sulfate from pig skin, J. Biol. Chem., 254:1614.

Darlington, G.J., Dutkowski, R., Brown, W.T., 1981, Sister chromatid exchange frequencies in progeria and Werner syndrome patients, Am. J. Hum. Genet., 33:762.

DeBusk, F.L., 1972, The Hutchinson-Gilford progeria syndrome, J. Pediat., 697.

Elson, L.A., and Morgan, W.T.J., 1933, A colorimetric method for the determination of glucosamine and chondrosamine, Biochem. J., 27:1824.

Epstein, C.J., Martin, G.M., Schultz, A.L., Motulsky, A., 1966, Werner's syndrome: a review of its symptomatology, natural history, pathological features, genetics and relationship to the natural aging process, Medicine, 45:177.

Erecinski, K., Bittel-Dobryzynska, N., Mostowiec, S., 1961, Zespol progerii u dwoch braci, Pol. Tyrg, Lek., 16:806.

Franklin, P.P., 1976, Progeria in siblings, Clin. Radiol., 27:327.

Gabr, M., Hashem, M., Fahmi, A., Safouh, M., 1960, Progeria, a pathologic study, J. Pediat., 57:70.

Goto, M., Tanimoto, K., Horuichi, Y., Sasuzuji, T., 1981, Family analysis of Werner's syndrome: A survey of 42 Japanese families with a review of the literature, Clin. Genet., 19:8.

Hall, C.W., Cantz, M., Neufeld, E.F., 1973, A beta-glucuronidase deficiency mucopolysaccharidosis: Studies in cultured fibroblasts, Arch. Biochem. Biophys., 155:32.

Hoehn, H., Bryant, E.M., Au, K., Norwood, T.H., Boman, H., Martin, G.M., 1975, Variegated translocation mosaicism in human skin fibroblast cultures, Cyto. Cell Genet., 15:282.

Jones, K.L., Smith, P.W., Harvey, M.A.S., Hall, B.D., Quan, L., 1975, Older paternal age and fresh gene mutation: Data on additional disorders, J. Pediat., 86:84.

Littlefield, L.G., Mailhes, J.B., 1975, Observations of de novo clones of cytogenetically aberrant cells in primary fibroblast cell strains from phenotypically normal women, Am. J. Hum. Genet., 27:190.

Martin, G.M., 1977, Genetic syndromes in man with potential relevance to the pathobiology of aging, Birth Defects Orig. Article Series, Genetics of Aging, 14:5.

McKusick, V.A., 1983, "Mendelian inheritance in man, catalogs of autosomal dominant, autosomal recessive and X-linked phenotypes," 7th Edn., Johns Hopkins Univ. Press, Baltimore.

Norwood, T.H., Hoehn, H., Salk, D., Martin, G.M., 1979, Cellular aging in Werner's syndrome: a unique phenotype? J. Invest. Derm., 73:92.

Nordenson, I., 1977, Chromosome breaks in Werner's syndrome and their prevention in vitro by radical-scavenging enzymes, Hereditas, 87:151.

Okada, S., Veath, M.L., Lerry, J., O'Brien, J.S., 1971, Ganglioside GM_2 storage diseases: Hexosaminidase deficiencies in cultured fibroblasts, Amer. J. Hum. Genet., 23:55.

Orkin, R.W., Underhill, C.B., Toole, B.P., 1982, Hyaluronate degradation in 3T3 and Simian virus-transformed 3T3 cells, J. Biol. Chem., 257:5821.

Rautenstruauch, T. and Snigula, F., 1977, Progeria: A cell
    culture study and clinical report of familial incidence,
    Europ. J. Pediat., 124:101.
Rava, G., 1967, Su un nucleo familiare di progeria, Minerva Med.,
    58:1502.
Salk, D., Au, K., Hoehn, H., Martin, G.M., 1981, Cytogenetics of
    Werner's syndrome cultured skin fibroblasts: variegated
    translocation mosaicism, Cytogenet. Cell Genet., 30:92.
Salk, D., 1982, Werner Syndrome: A review of recent research with
    an analysis of connective tissue metabolism, growth control
    of cultured cells, and chromosomal aberrations, Hum. Genet.,
    62:1.
Scappaticci, S., Cerimele, D., Fraccaro, M., 1982, Clonal
    structural chromosomal rearrangements in primary fibroblast
    cultures and in lymphocytes of patients with Werner's
    syndrome, Hum. Genet., 62:16.
Schiller, S., Slover, G.A., Dorfman, A., 1961, A method for the
    separation of acid mucopolysaccharides: Its application to
    the isolation of heparin from the skin of rats, J. Biol.
    Chem., 236:983.
Schonberg, S., Henderson, E., Niermeijer, M.F., Bootsma, D.,
    German, J., 1982, Werner's syndrome: preferential
    proliferation of clones with chromosome translocations, MS
    submitted for publication.
Schonberg, S.A., Henderson, E., Niermeijer, M.F., German, J.,
    1981, Werner's syndrome: preferential proliferation of
    clones with translocations, Am., J. Hum. Genet., 33:120A.
Tokunaga, M., Wakamatsu, E., Sato, K., Satake, S., Aoyama, K.,
    Saito, K., Sugawara, M., Yosizawa, Z., 1978, Hyaluronuria in
    a case of progeria (Hutchinson-Gilford Syndrome)., J. Amer.
    Geriatrics Soc., 26:296.
Varadi, D.P., Cifonelli, J.A., Dorfman, A., 1967, The acid
    mucopolysaccharides in normal urine, Biochim, Biophys. Acta,
    141:103.

CLINICAL, DEMOGRAPHIC, AND GENETIC ASPECTS

OF THE WERNER SYNDROME IN JAPAN

Makoto Goto, Fujio Takeuchi, Kiyoaki Tanimoto,
and Terumasa Miyamoto

Department of Internal Medicine and Physical Therapy
Faculty of Medicine, University of Tokyo, 7-3-1, Hongo
Bunkyo-ku, Tokyo 113, Japan

ABSTRACT

A total of 196 typical patients with the Werner syndrome, a
caricature of aging, was studied to define the details of the
clinical manifestations, demography and genetic aspects in Japan.

Most of the previously reported clinical characteristics and
the autosomal recessive inheritance of this syndrome were
confirmed, but no significant linkage was revealed between
specific HLA type and the Werner syndrome. The frequency of the
Werner syndrome in Japan was estimated using two methods which
indicated approximately 300 cases among 100 million people.

INTRODUCTION

The Werner syndrome was originally described by Otto Werner
in 1904 in his doctoral thesis "On cataract in combination with
scleroderma" (Werner, 1904).

Since then about 400 cases have been reported all over the
world, thus justifying the eponym, "the Werner syndrome." The
disease characteristics have recently been defined on the basis
of review articles written by Oppenheimer and Kugel (1934),
Thannhauser (1945), Epstein et al. (1966), Goto et al. (1978,
1981) and Salk et al. (1982) as follows: a distinctive habitus
(short stature with a stocky trunk and slender extremities),

scleroderma-like skin changes frequently associated with chronic ulcerations over the ankles and heels, accelerated conditions of a variety of age-associated clinical manifestations (alopecia, greying of the hair, cataracts, arteriosclerosis, neoplasia, and osteoporosis) and endocrinological abnormalities (diabetes mellitus and hypogonadism). A high incidence of consanguinity of parents was also reported.

Because of its several similarities to natural aging, the Werner syndrome has been considered to be an excellent model of accelerated aging, or a caricature of aging; however, it is somewhat different from natural aging (Epstein et al., 1966; Salk, 1982). About half of the 400 cases were reported in Japan and the incidence seemed high partly because of a higher rate of consanguineous marriages in rural areas of Japan (Goto et al., 1981).

This paper describes the symptomatology, chronology, demography, and genetics of the Werner syndrome in Japan in more detail than did in the previous papers (Goto et al., 1978, 1981). It is based on 196 carefully selected patients described in the Japanese literature during the 63 years from 1917 to 1979.

HISTORICAL BACKGROUND OF THE WERNER SYNDROME IN JAPAN

In Japan, the Werner syndrome was first described in 1917 by Dr. R. Ishida, an ophthalmologist. Before 1960, all of the 33 cases reported were reported by either opthalmologists or dermatologists because of the high incidence of cataracts and scleroderma in this syndrome. Since 1961, both internists and orthopedic surgeons have begun to pay attention to the Werner syndrome and have reported 34 cases in a decade. Doctors

Table 1. Case reporting of the Werner syndrome in Japan for 63 years (1917-1979).

Reported by	Time period in which reported			
	1917-1960	1961-1970	1971-1979	Total
Internists	0	14	80	94
Ophthalmologists	23	3	6	32
Dermatologists and Urologists	10	8	13	31
Orthopedic surgeons	0	9	20	29
Otorhinolaryngologists	0	0	4	4
Psychiatrists	0	0	3	3
Geneticists	0	0	3	3

from a variety of departments have been aware of this rare
syndrome since 1971 and 129 cases had been reported up to 1979
(Table 1).

In 1975, Tokunaga et al. discovered an excessive excretion
of urinary hyaluronic acid in patients with the Werner syndrome
and coined the term "hyaluronuria," an observation which was
later confirmed by Goto and Murata (1978). Thus, the Werner
syndrome is characterized by two unique laboratory features in
addition to the typical clinical manifestations: hyaluronuria
and the short lifespan of cultured fibroblasts (Martin et al.,
1970).

In 1981, Goto et al. summarized 195 cases of WS that had
been reported previously in the Japanese literature. Their
review described the largest series of patients with the Werner
syndrome.

SYMPTOMATOLOGY

Since there are no generally accepted criteria for the
diagnosis of the Werner syndrome, a tentative list of diagnostic
criteria has been proposed (Goto et al., 1981). There are
several characteristic signs and symptoms in the Werner syndrome:

a) Characteristic habitus and stature. Short stature and
light body weight, slender extremities with a stock trunk, and a
beak-shaped nose.

b) Scleroderma-like skin changes. Atrophic skin and
muscle, circumscribed hyperkeratosis, telangiectasia, tight skin
over the bones of the feet, skin ulcers, and metastatic
calcification.

c) Signs and symptoms of premature senescence. Bird-like
appearance, alopecia, greying of the hair, skin
hyperpigmentation, hoarseness, diffuse arteriosclerosis, juvenile
bilateral cataracts, and osteoporosis.

d) Endocrinological abnormalities. Diabetes mellitus and
hypogonadism.

e) Miscellaneous manifestations. Mental disorders and
malignant tumors.

f) Consanguineous marriage of parents.

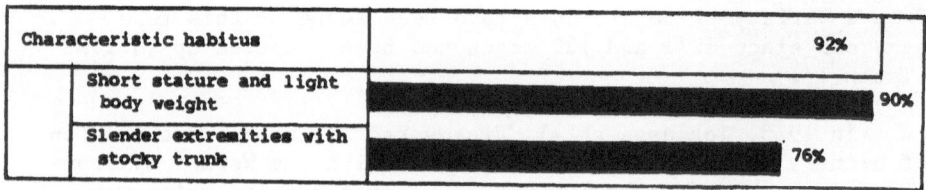

Figure 1

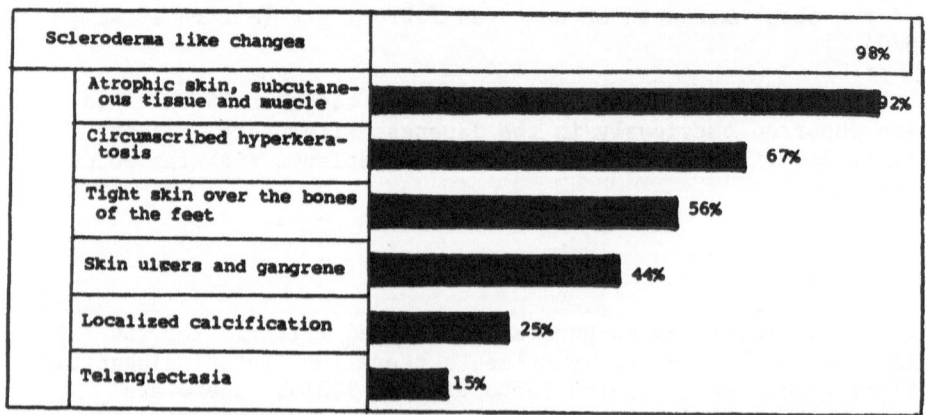

Figure 2

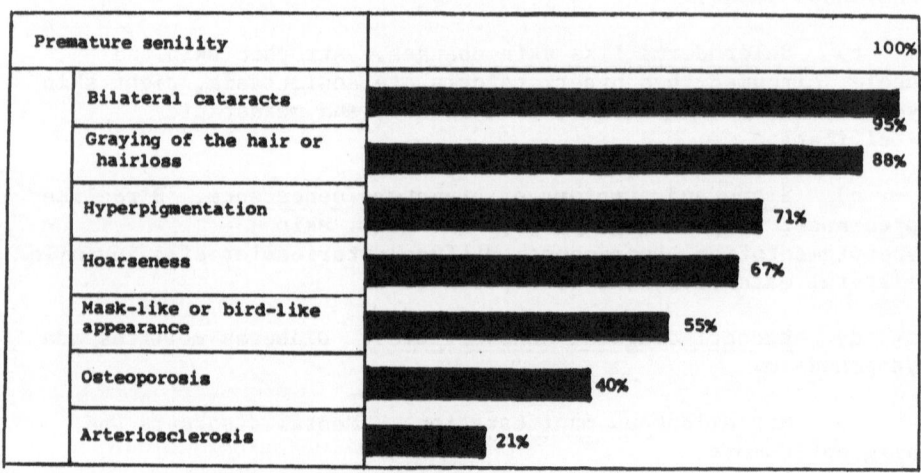

Figure 3

Figures 1, 2 and 3. Characteristic signs and symptoms in
    the Werner syndrome.

In this paper, 196 patients having at least three of the
four major signs and symptoms described above (a-d) were selected
for further investigation as having the Werner syndrome.

Characteristic habitus and stature (92% of Japanese cases, Fig. 1)

The Werner syndrome was sometimes diagnosed by its
characteristic habitus and stature. Short stature (90% of
Japanese cases), which resulted from a failure of the adolescent
growth spurt, was a common finding in the Werner syndrome.
Heights ranged from 122 cm to 161 cm (average 141.5 cm) and
weights from 19 kg to 52 kg (average 35.7 kg) for both sexes.
The patients were usually normal at birth and in childhood.
Their growth stopped shortly after adolescence (14-20 years of
age), but the parts of the body were almost proportional in size.
Slender extremities and a stocky trunk (Cushingoid habitus) were
observed in most patients (76%), although there was no sign of
striae cutis. Atrophy of peripheral subcutaneous and muscular
tissues was a constant feature and creatinuria (greater than 100
mg/day) was also described in 5.1% of the cases.

Scleroderma-like skin changes (98% of Japanese cases, Fig. 2)

Scleroderma-like appearance of the skin was as follows:
atrophic skin, subcutaneous tissue and muscle (92% of Japanese
cases), circumscribed hyperkeratosis especially on the soles of
the feet (67%), atrophic or deformed nails (45%), telangiectasia
on the cheeks and anterior chest (15%), tight skin over the bones
of the feet (56%), skin ulcers and gangrene in the legs (44%),
and localized soft-tissue calcification over the Achilles
tendons, knees, and elbows (25%).

Because of the several similar skin changes in the Werner
syndrome and progressive systemic sclerosis, patients with the
Werner syndrome were occasionally misdiagnosed. However, unlike
progressive systemic sclerosis, the Werner syndrome was not
characterized by Raynaud's phenomenon, esophageal dilation, lung
fibrosis, or sicca syndrome. On the other hand, patients with
progressive systemic sclerosis rarely had juvenile bilateral
cataracts, osteoporosis, diabetes mellitus, or hypogonadism, but
on rare occasions, they developed hoarseness as a result of
cricoarytenoid joint disease (Grossman et al., 1961). Chronic
ulceration over pressure points in the feet sometimes resulted in
gangrene and in amputation, despite the use of hyaluronidase
dressings (Tokunaga et al., 1975) or fresh blood transfusions.

Flat feet, with the occasional complication of hallux valgus
(5.1%), and painful corns may be acquired because of sclerotic
skin and weakness of the foot tendons.

<u>Signs</u> <u>and</u> <u>symptoms</u> <u>of</u> <u>premature</u> <u>senescence</u> (100% of Japanese cases, Fig. 3).

All the patients had an accelerated form of at least one of the age-associated clinical manifestations such as greying of the hair, alopecia, skin hyperpigmentation, hoarseness, diffuse arteriosclerosis, juvenile bilateral cataracts, and osteoporosis.

The patients showed almost identical facial characteristics; a bird-like or mask-like appearance (55%), grey hair or alopecia (88%), juvenile bilateral cataracts (95%), atrophic auricles, atrophy of the skin and subcutaneous tissue over the neck (Fig. 4).

Juvenile bilaterial cataracts (polaris posterior type) were reported in almost all the patients (usually with a history of onset at about age 30) and were not related to the presence of diabetes mellitus.

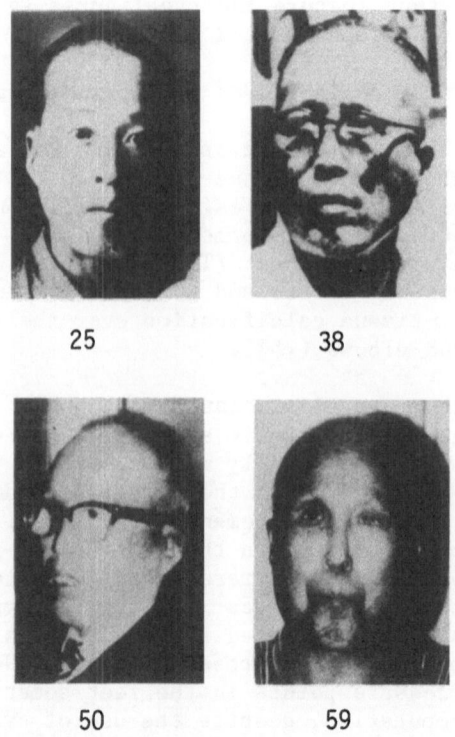

Figure 4.   Chronological change of the facial expression of a patient with the Werner syndrome (numbers indicate the patient's age).

Several common features found in natural aging such as diminished auditory acuity (1.5%), presbyopia, prostatic hypertrophy, Parkinsonism, and senile dementia were rarely reported in the patients with the Werner syndrome.

Endocrinological abnormalities (79% of Japanese cases, Fig. 5)

Several endocrinological dysfunctions including abnormal glucose tolerance (46%) and hypogonadism (77%) were frequently associated with the Werner syndrome. Most diabetic patients with either chemical (subclinical) diabetes (28%) or overt (clinical) diabetes (18%) were controlled by diet alone or small doses of sulfonylurea or biguanide. However, 19% of overt diabetic patients required over 200 units of insulin for control of hyperglycemia and one patient had a history of ketoacidosis. The mean serum level of insulin was 21.2 u V/ml with a range of 2 to 38 u V/ml (normal: 5 to 15 u V/ml). As shown in Fig. 6, serum insulin levels during a 100g oral glucose tolerance test remained unchanged in most cases, suggesting that inappropriate insulin levels may contribute to the diminished glucose tolerance in the Werner syndrome. The parents of all these diabetic patients made first-cousin marriages.

Male hypogonadism was reported in 49% of the patients, with 60% showing a hypergonadotrophic type with high urinary levels of gonadotropin, aspermatogenesis and an increase of Sertoli cells; 9% having a hypogonadotropic type with an increase of Leydig cells, and 31% showing an unknown type. Gynecomastia was observed in 22% of the hypergonadotropic hypogonadism patients. Amenorrhea, early onset of menopause and sterility were occasionally reported among the female patients. The plasma levels of several sex hormones are presented in Table 2, and indicate an imbalance of sex hormones in most cases.

Thyroid function was evaluated by standard methods, including the basal metabolic rate (BMR), 24-hour thyroidal[131]I uptake, and the serum level of protein-bound iodine. Most of these measurements indicated normal thyroid function, but 6% of the cases showed a low BMR and 8%, an elevated BMR. Three patients had a thyroid adenoma, one had hyperthyroidism and one had myxedema.

The serum levels of parathyroid hormone, thyroid-stimulating hormone and growth hormone were within the normal range.

Miscellaneous (Fig. 5)

Neurological and psychological abnormalities were reported in some cases. Nine percent had a low IQ, 3% had paranoia schizophrenia and 3% had grand mal-type epilepsy. In all of

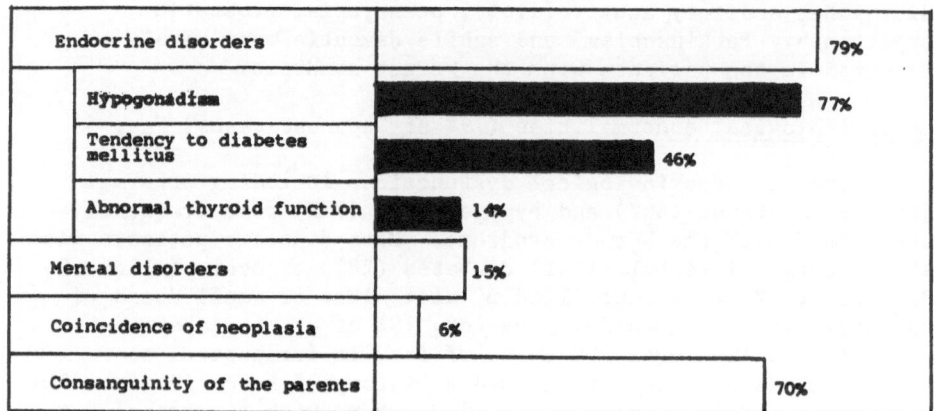

Figure 5.   Characteristic signs and symptoms in the Werner
            syndrome.

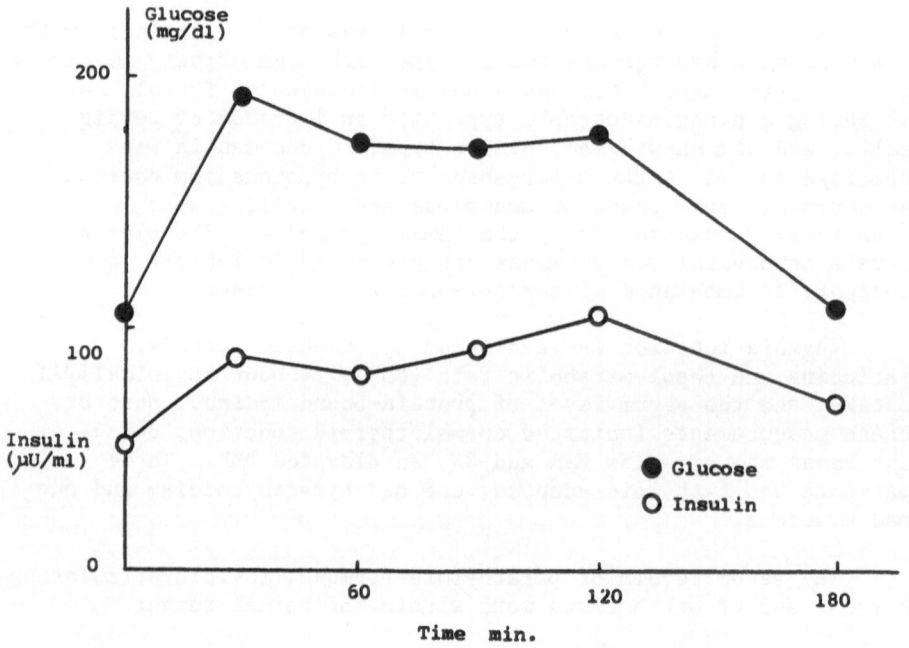

Figure 6.   Serum insulin and glucose levels during an oral
            glucose tolerance test in the patient with the Werner
            syndrome.

Table 2. Sex hormone levels in the plasma from the patients with the Werner syndrome.

Cases	Age	Sex	Estrone (pg/ml)	Estradiol (pg/ml)	Estriol (pg/ml)	Testosterone (ng/ml)	Dehydroepiandrosterone-sulfate (pg/ml)
1	20	M	10.0	27.7	5.0	4.05	341
2	32	F	22.1	62.8	9.45	0.36	332
3	34	F	50.5	78.2	7.34	2.41	299
4	35	M	68.3	21.2	5.0	2.16	491
5	40	M	112.0	28.6	5.0	4.86	1464
6	50	F	67.1	10.4	5.0	1.48	50
7	52	M	55.0	35.7	5.0	3.16	119
8	55	M	71.7	10.0	5.0	3.14	419
9	59	M	10.0	45.4	5.0	4.37	333
Normal	20-63	M	5.0-40.0	10.0-41.0	0-15.0	4.17-12.0	400-1500
Premenopausal	20-41	F	30.0-100.0	20.0-121.0	5.0-40.0	0.15-0.89	400-1500
Postmenopausal	45-60	F	44.0-98.0	13.0-16.0	5.0-16.0	0.15-0.89	400-1500

these cases, the parents of the patients were first cousins. In
contrast to natural aging, hyperreflexia was often observed in
the patients with the Werner syndrome; however, the specific
pathological abnormality of the neuromuscular system was not
presented.

Of the 196 patients, 11 had malignant tumors (5.6%); i.e.,
one cholangioma (40-year-old male), one melanoma (40-year-old
female), one cystic bladder carcinoma (53-year-old male), one
laryngeal cancer (60-year-old male), one anaplastic carcinoma of
the thyroid (42-year-old female), one psedomyxoma peritonei of
ovarian origins (37-year-old female), one leiomyosarcoma (40-
year-old male), two fibrosarcomas (31-year-old male and 61-year-
old female), one acute myelocytic leukemia (36-year-old male) and
one breast cancer (46-year-old female).

A relatively high incidence of malignant tumors among family
members of probands with the Werner syndrome was also described
(Goto et al., 1981). The patients also showed benign tumors,
including six adenomas of the thyroid, one myoma of the uterus,
one lymphangioma, one meningioma, and one fibroadenoma of the
breast. In this series, the preponderance of tumors with a
mesenchymal original should be emphasized.

Other laboratory findings included mild liver dysfunction
(8%) and hyperlipidemia (11%) with high serum levels of both
cholesterol and triglycerides, often in the setting of diabetes
mellitus.

The serum level of uric acid fluctuated with hyperuricemia
was sometimes observed, in agreement with the observation by
Zucker-Franklin et al. (1968). Two patients with the Werner
syndrome had a gouty attack that was controlled by colchicine.
An analysis of several serum enzyme levels related to uric acid
metabolism is presented in Table 3.

Excessive urinary excretion of hyaluronic acid had been
observed in the Werner syndrome and so far "hyaluronuria" has
been reported in 12 out of 14 cases tested (86%). Mild renal
dysfunction (abnormal urinary concentration, abnormal response to
PSP test, and proteinuria) was frequently observed, but there was
so far no clear-cut relationship between the renal function and
hyperuricemia or hyaluronuria (Goto et al., 1978). Immunological
data will be presented in another chapter.

Table 3. Serum enzyme levels related to uric acid metabolism in the Werner syndrome.

Enzymes	Normal	Case 1	Case 2	Case 3	Case 4
PRPPS* (n mol/mg protein/h)	40 + 18	56.6	49.2	39.9	49.0
HGRPT † (n mol/mg protein/h)	75 + 24	70.4	62.0	77.4	98.8
APRT ‡ (n mol/mg protein/h)	25 + 10	40.0	23.4	20.3	25.2
ADA § (m unit/mg protein)	0.9+0.5	0.71	0.76	0.93	1.44
PNP ¶	15 + 7	9.7	7.5	34.3	101.6

*Phosphoribosyl-1-pyrophosphate synthetase
†Hypoxanthine guanine phosphoribosyl transferase
‡Adenine phosphoribosyl transferase
§Adenosine deaminase
¶Purine nucleoside phosphorylase

Consanguineous marriage of the parents (70% of Japanese cases, Fig. 5).

Seventy percent of the patients were the product of a consanguineous marriage, of which 73% were between first cousins.

CHRONOLOGY

The mean age at which patients were first diagnosed as having the Werner syndrome was 36.7 years (range of 15 to 70 years) (Fig. 7). However, the mean age at which patients or their families recognized several characteristic manifestations of the Werner syndrome was 20 years (range 2 to 40 years).

The earliest sign was greying of the hair or alopecia at a mean age of 20.3 years, followed in order by voice changes (hoarseness) (22.5 years), skin changes (24 years), cataracts (29.6 years), diabetes mellitus (31.7 years) and skin ulcers (34.7 years) (Table 4).

Fifty-five percent of the patients were first recognized as having the Werner syndrome because of their having cataracts,

greying of the hair, or alopecia; 18 per cent were recognized
because of their characteristic stature and habitus; 25 percent
because of changes in their skin or voice.

Data relating to the age and cause of death were available
for only 10 of the cases. The average lifespan of patients with
the Werner syndrome in Japan was 43.5 years (range 29 to 70
years).

Seven patients died of malignant tumors (31–46 years), one
of myocardial infarction (70-year-old male), one of renal failure
(29-year-old male), and one of pneumonitis (51-year-old male).

DEMOGRAPHY

As shown in Fig. 8, the number of patients was plotted by
prefecture according to the patient's registered address or birth
place. This reporting has been carried out in almost all the
prefectures in Japan. Patient aggregates were detected in
several areas. Tokyo district had 29 cases, Osaka district 27
cases, the North Kanto 18 cases, the Hokuriku area 16 cases, the
South Kyushu district 9 cases, and Tohoku area 24 cases.

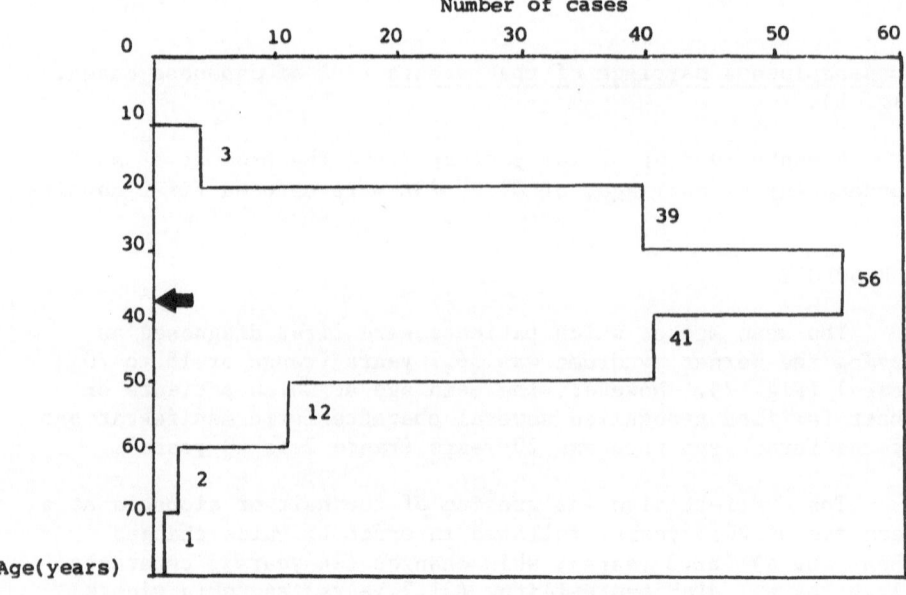

Figure 7.   Distributions of the ages of diagnosis of patients
      with the Werner syndrome. The mean age was indicated as an
      arrow.

Table 4. Ages of diagnosis of the Werner syndrome

	Average age	Earliest Age
Diagnosis	36.7	17.0
Symptoms		
Greying of hair or alopecia	20.3	6.0
Voice change	22.5	11.0
Skin change	24.0	7.0
Cataracts	29.6	8.0
Diabetes mellitus	31.7	15.0
Skin ulcers	34.7	7.0

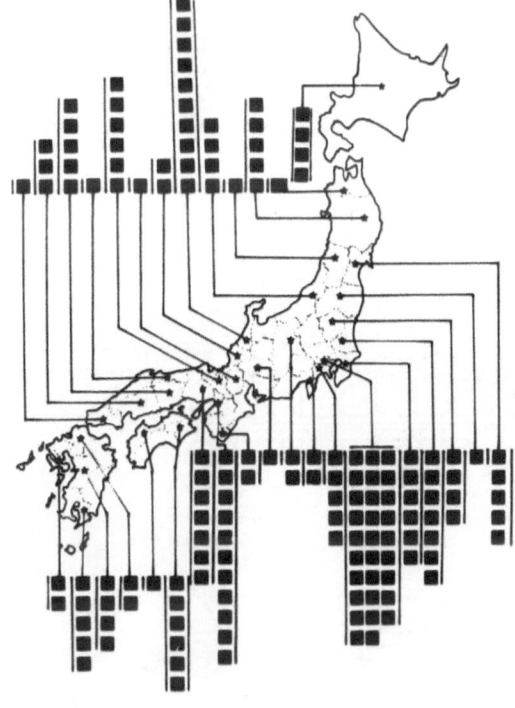

UNKNOWN —30

Figure 8. Case reporting of the Werner syndrome Japanese cases
    by prefecture.

PEDIGREE CHARTS AND GENETICS

A total of 196 individuals with the Werner syndrome
fulfilled the tentative diagnostic criteria. The diagnoses were
partly based on family records: 42 pedigree charts with 80
syndrome patients were collected from Japanese medical journals.
Several representative pedigree charts are presented in Figure 9.

The sex ratio was 92 males to 96 females (8 were unknown
sex) and according to Morton's segregation analysis under
incomplete ascertainment (Morton, 1959), it appears that an
autosomal recessive gene is responsible for this disease (Goto et
al., 1981).

Further, it is of interest that there was a report of a
family with three patients having both WS and xeroderma
pigmentosum (autosomal recessive inheritance).

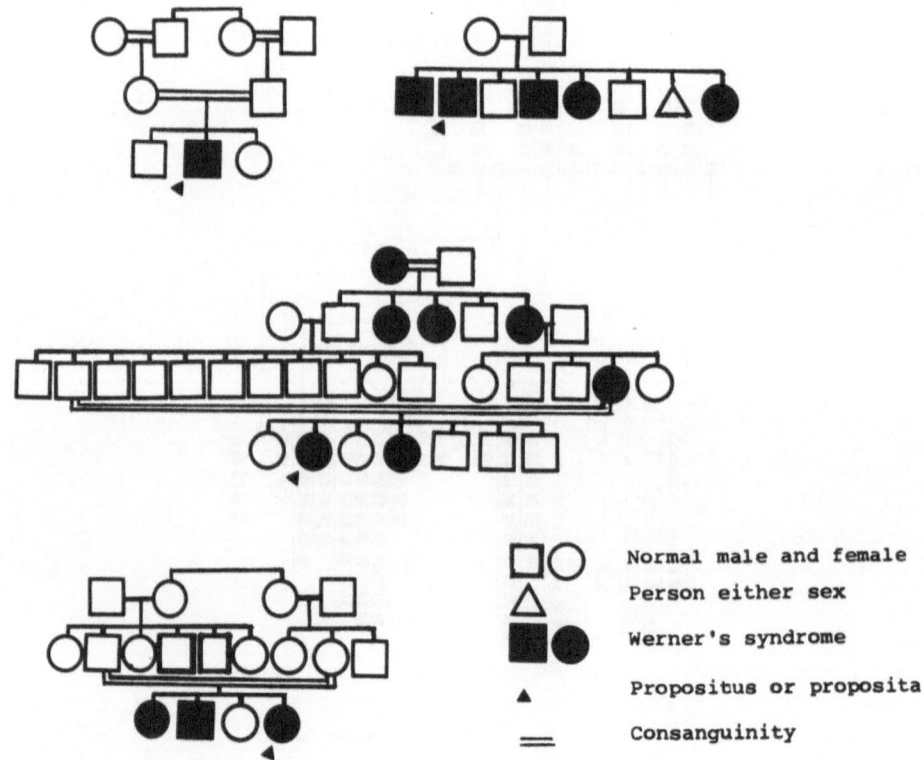

Figure 9. Representative pedigree charts and key to symbols

FREQUENCY OF THE WERNER SYNDROME IN JAPAN

The frequency of the Werner syndrome in Japan was estimated by two methods (Goto et al., 1981). Firstly, the incidence of the Werner syndrome in several prefectures from 1977 to 1979 was estimated according to a survey of relatively closed communities. Five patients were found in a population of 1,700,000, four in 1,600,000, and seven in 2,170,000. These patients may represent more than 50% of the cases in these areas, giving a prevalence of 1:300,000 to 1:400,000. Secondly, the homozygote frequency was estimated according to Dahlberg's formula (1950). Using Dahlberg's formula, the theoretical number of homozygote individuals with the Werner syndrome in Japan was calculated to be between 1,000 and 5,000 on the basis of a total Japanese population of about 110,000,000.

In actuality, 162 living cases have been reported since 1961 in Japan. On the basis of these cases, the estimated prevalence of living WS patients in Japan was 1:500,000, a figure which approximates the theoretical value calculated above.

Chromosomal Analysis

Chromosomal examination was made in 20 patients and revealed two abnormal cases. One had a mosaic-type Klinefelter syndrome (46,XY/47, XXY) and the other, an "abnormal" pattern.

Table 5. HLA type of the Werner syndrome

Case	HLA-A		HLA-B	
1	9	–	5	w40
2	10	–	5	w40
3	2	–	40	–
4	9	33	12	–
5	10	–	w15	w17
6	9	11	w16	–
7	9	–	5	w40
8	9	31	51	–
9	2	10	w54	–
10	9	–	5	w54
11	2	–	40	51
12	2	11	15	51
13	24	–	5	44
14	2	–	27	40
15	w24	26	w52	w60
16	w24	26	w52	w60

HLA Typing

Peripheral blood lymphocytes from patients with the Werner syndrome were typed for HLA-A and -B antigens, by the standard serological method (Sasazuki, et al., 1976), using the 7th Histocompatibility Workshop sera and loca sera obtained in Japan. HLA phenotypes of the patients are summarized in Table 5. No significant association was found between any HLA specificities and the Werner syndrome.

REFERENCES

Dahlberg, G., 1950, Methods for population genetics, Am. J. Biol. 25:90–104.

Epstein, C.J., Martin, G.M., Schultz, A.L., Motulsky, A.G., 1966, Werner's syndrome: A review of its symptomatology, natural history, pathologic features, genetics and relationship to the natural aging process, Medicine, 45:177–221.

Goto, M., Urata, K., 1978, Urinary excretion of macromolecular acidic glycosaminoglycans in Werner's syndrome, Clin. Chim. Acta, 85:101–106.

Goto, M., Horiuchi, Y., Tanimoto, K., Ishii, T., Nakashima, H., 1978, Werner's syndrome: Analysis of 15 cases with a review of the Japanese literature, J. Am. Geriatr. Soc., 26:341–347.

Goto, M., Tanimoto, K., Horiuchi, Y., Sasazuki, 1981, Family analysis of Werner's syndrome: A survey of 42 Japanese families with a review of the literature, Clin. Genet. 19:8–15.

Grossman, A., Martin, J.R., Root, H.S., 1961, Rheumatoid arthritis of the crico-arytenoid joint. Laryrngoscope, 71, 530–544.

Ishida, R., 1917, A case of cataract in combination with scleroderma, Jap. J. Opthalmol., 21:1025–1029.

Martin, G.M., Sprague, C.A., Epstein, C.J., 1970, Replicative lifespan of cultivated human cells: Effects of donor's age, tissue and genotype, Lab. Invest., 23:86–91.

Morton, N.E., 1959, Genetic tests under incomplete ascertainment, Am. J. Hum. Genet., 11:1–16.

Oppenheimer, B.S., Kugel, V.H., 1941, Werner's syndrome: Report of the first necropsy and of findings in a new case, Am. J. Med. Soc., 202:629–642.

Salk, D., 1982, Werner's syndrome: A review of recent research with an analysis of connective tissue metabolism, growth control of cultured cells, and chromosomal aberrations, Hum. Genet., 62:1–15.

Sasazuki, T., McMichael, A., Radvawy, R., Payne, R., McDevitt, H.O., 1976, Use of high dose of x-irradiation in the MLC reaction, Tissue Antigens, 7:91–96.

Thannhauser, S.J., 1945, Werner's syndrome (progeria of the
    adult) and Rothmund's syndrome: Two types of closely
    related heredo-familial atrophic dermatosis with juvenile
    cataracts and endocrine features. A critical study with
    five new cases, Ann. Intern. Med., 23:559-626.
Tokunaga, M., Futami, T., Wakamatsu, E., Endo, M., Yosizawa, Z,
    1945, Werner's syndrome as "hyaluronuria," Clin. Chim.
    Acta., 62:89-96.
Werner, C.W.D., 1904, "Uber Katarakt in Verbingung mit
    Sklerodermie (doctoral dissertation, Kiel University),
    Schmidt and Klauning, Kiel.
Zucker-Franklin, D., Rifkin, H., Jacobson, H.G., 1968, Werner's
    syndrome: An analysis of ten cases, Geriatrics, 23:123-135.

IMMUNOLOGICAL ASPECTS OF WERNER'S SYNDROME:

AN ANALYSIS OF 17 PATIENTS

Makoto Goto, Kiyoaki Tanimoto, and Terumasa Miyamoto

Department of Internal Medicine and Physical Therapy
Faculty of Medicine
University of Tokyo
Tokyo, Japan

INTRODUCTION

The Werner syndrome, a caricature of aging, is characterized
by a variety of clinical manifestations associated with natural
aging. In brief, the Werner syndrome is a rare genetically
determined disease inherited as an autosomal recessive trait.
Patients manifest failure of the adolescent growth spurt, graying
of hair in the teens, juvenile bilateral cataracts, mild diabetes
mellitus, arteriosclerosis, and scleroderma-like skin changes.
The average lifespan is 47 years (Goto et al., 1978, 1981). A
high incidence of neoplasia of mesenchymal origin was also
reported.

A striking shortening of lifespan and slow elongation rate
of the DNA chains of cultured fibroblasts have been demonstrated
(Martin et al., 1970; Fujiwara et al., 1977). The increased
proportion of heat-labile enzymes (Goldstein and Moerman, 1975;
Holliday et al., 1977) as well as the excessive excretion of
urinary hyaluronic acid (Goto and Murata, 1978) have also been
documented, all of which probably relate to the pathogenesis of
this rare syndrome.

Recently, both gerontologists and immunologists have paid a
great deal of attention to the immunologic disturbances
associated with natural aging, either as cause or effect
(Makinodan et al., 1975; Buckley and Roseman, 1976; Yunis et al.,
1976). These include production of multiple autoantibodies,

increaseed susceptibility to infectious agents and frequent
neoplastic proliferation in aged individuals. Thus the Werner
syndrome has several characteristics that are akin to natural
aging and to progressive systemic sclerosis (sclerodema), a
connective-tissue disease with several immunological
abnormalities. Mild renal dysfunction is frequently observed
(Goto et al., 1978), but extensive immunological analysis of
the Werner syndrome has never been reported.

        This communication, based on our recent experiments,
describes the results of the analysis of the cell subsets in the
peripheral blood lymphocytes and of the autoantibodies frequently
detected in autoimmune diseases.

ANALYSIS OF CELL SUBSETS

Peripheral Blood Lymphocytes

        The absolute number of peripheral blood lymphocytes was
counted on the blood smear from 26 patients with the Werner

Table 1

Absolute number of peripheral blood lymphocytes

Werner's syndrome*   Healthy controls

No. of lymphocytes/mm^3 (mean SD)	Age group (yrs)	No. of lymphocytes/mm^3 (mean SD)
3124 ± 908 (n=3)	10--19	2093 ± 719 (n=5)
2471 ± 1213 (n=4)	20--29	2217 ± 912 (n=7)
2191 ± 566 (n=5)	30--39	2308 ± 956 (n=8)
2128 ± 363 (n=7)	40--49	2081 ± 877 (n=8)
2023 ± 473 (n=4)	50--59	2002 ± 837 (n=8)
1849 ± 148 (n=3)	60--69	1781 ± 881 (n=6)

*Absolute number of peripheral blood lymphocytes was obtained
from our 16 cases of the Werner syndrome and from additional 10
cases in the literature.

syndrome (WS), including 10 cases in the Japanese literature. Thirty-nine age-matched healthy controls were also examined. As shown in Table 1, the absolute number of peripheral blood lymphocytes declined with age in WS patients and healthy controls.

T Cells (E-rosette Forming Cells)

Peripheral blood lymphocytes were collected from heparinized whole blood by centrifugation over a Ficoll-Hypaque density gradient (Boyum, 1968). Lymphocytes were washed three times in RPMI 1640 containing 10% heat-inactivated fetal bovine serum (FBS) and antibiotics.

Sheep red blood cells (SRBC) were washed three times with phosphate-buffered saline (PBS) and treated with neuraminidase as described by Weiner et al. (1973).

Equal volumes of the SRBC (2×10^8/ml) and 7×10^6/ml of lymphocytes were mixed and incubated at 37°C for 15 min. After centrifugation at 400 rpm for 5 min, the reaction mixtures were kept at 0° C for 60 min. and then were suspended gently. Lymphocytes surrounded by more than four SRBC on the surface were counted under the microscope as positive rosette-forming cells, and their percentages were calculated out of a total of 200 lymphocytes.

Among healthy individuals the percentage of T cells (20-65 years) ranged from 51.0 to 73.8; 3 of 8 patients examined showed a reduced decreased percentage of T cells (Table 2). Of interest, the percentage of E-rosette-forming cells declined drastically with advancing age among WS syndrome patients.

B-cells (EAC-rosette Forming Cells)

Sensitized SRBC (EA) were prepared in the conventional manner, except for the use of IgM rabbit anti-SRBC isolated by Sephadex G-200 gel filtration. EA were mixed with appropriately diluted human complement in which natural antibody to SRBC had been absorbed in advance. After a 10-min. incubation at 37°C, the reaction was stopped by the addition of 0.1M ethylenediamine tetra acetate (EDTA), and the cells (EAC) were washed three times with 0.15 M geletan veronal buffer containing 0.03mM Ca^{2+}, 0.01mM Mg^{2+}, and 0.01M EDTA.

For rosette formation, equal volumes of 2×10^8/ml EA and 7×10^8/ml lymphocytes were incubated at 37°C for 15 min. After centrifugation at 400 rpm for 5 min., the pellets were gently resuspended and EA-rosette-forming cells were calculated in the

same manner as were E-rosette-forming cells (Morito et al.,
1978).

The percentage of B cells remained unchanged with aging (20-
65 years) among healthy individuals (n=65) and only one patient
showed a slightly elevated percentage of B cells with a highly
decreased percentage of T cells (Table 2).

B cells (surface immunoglobulin (Ig)-positive cells) were
also detected by staining with fluoresceinated rabbit anti-human
Ig by the method described by Blakeslee and Baines (1976). One
out of 7 patients showed a slightly elevated percentage of B
cells (control 20-35%) (Goto et al., 1979).

Table 2

Case	Age (yrs)	% of lymphocyte subpopulations	
		T(E-rosetting)*	B(EAC-rosetting)*
1	17	80.0	21.4
2	29	59.4	28.9
3	40	59.4	32.5
4	41	53.0	nd
5	43·	55.3	29.7
6	48	46.2	38.0
7	59	30.0	48.0
8	61	30.0	nd
Control (n=65)	20-65	51.0-73.8	17.0-42.0

*T and B lymphocyte subpopulations in patients with Werner's
syndrome. T cells were rosetted with sheep RBC for E-rosette
formation. B cells were rosetted with complement-treated
sensitized sheep RBC (EAC-rosette formation).

The percentage of T cells was low in some patients with WS, but the percentage of B cells was essentially unchanged with age in both healthy controls and WS patients.

Further Characterization of T-cell Subpopulations

Two antibodies against surface markers of T-cell subpopulations, i.e. antilymphocyte antibodies (ALA) that are naturally found in patients with systemic lupus erythematosus (SLE) (Okudaira et al., 1979) and antibodies reactive to human brain-associated T-cell antigen (anti-BAT) (Golub, 1972; Stratton and Byfield, 1977; Dalchan and Fabre, 1979) were used to stain a nylon wool column purified T cells (> 98% T cells).

Rabbit anti-BAT was obtained by immunizing rabbits twice with the human brain homogenate in Freund's complete adjuvant. The collected sera were absorbed extensively with human erythrocytes, bone marrow, and B-cell-type chronic lymphocytic leukemia cells to remove hemagglutinating activity and anti-B cell activity (Goto et al., 1979).

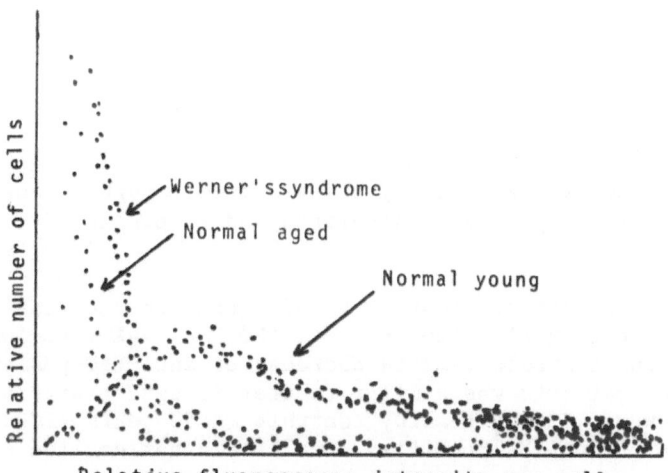

Fig. 1. Fluorescence distribution of peripheral-blood T cells stained with anti-BAT. T cells from a young WS patient (30 years), a normal young donor (30 years), and a normal aged donor (96 years) were incubated with anti-BAT for 30 min at 4°C, and incubated for an additional 30 min at 4°C with fluoresceinated goat anti-rabbit Ig. The cells were analyzed with FACS. Distributions are based on cumulative analysis of 10,000 viable cells.

For the routine fluorescence-activated cell sorter (FACS) analysis of peripheral blood lymphocytes, the nylon wool column-purified lymphocytes were incubated with anti-BAT at 4°C for 30 min. Normal rabbit serum with human peripheral blood lymphocytes absorbed were used as a negative control stain.

After three washes, the cells were stained with fluoresceinated goat anti-rabbit Ig at 4°C for 30 min. Analysis of the flourescence profile of stained cells was performed according to the method described by Herzenberg et al. (1976). Normal lymphocytes from young (20-36 years) and aged individuals (90-96 years) were stained with same reagents and analyzed under the identical conditions to make comparisons. The analytical pattern was recorded by photographing the oscilloscope. To express the fluorescence distribution of lymphocytes, control lymphocytes from healthy young individuals were stained with reagents and run in the FACS with a suitable gain, which gave a heterogeneous pattern on the oscilloscope of continuous fluorescence distribution from very dull to bright (Fig. 1).

A point of fluorescence intensity was set, at which the whole area was divided in half and the analysis of the samples was performed under the defined condition. The percentage of bright and dull populations was calculated by measuring the area divided by this point. When the cells from WS patients or healthy aged individuals over 90 years were analyzed under the same conditions, the fluorescence profile demonstrated a drastic decrease in the brightly stained population when compared with those of healthy young controls.

The ratio of the brightly stained T-cell populations to the total T cells analyzed was calculated and is presented in Table 3.

All seven patients tested showed a drastic decrease in cells which stained brightly with anti-BAT ($20.3 \pm 7.4\%$ v.s. 50% in healthy young controls). This decrease of anti-BAT-positive cells in WS patients was similar to that in aged controls over 90 years. However, among healthy controls (< 90 years olds) the percentage of anti-BAT-positive T cells did not decline with age.

The same preparation of T cells was stained with IgM antilymphocyte antibodies from patients with SLE and analyzed under conditions similar to that of anti-BAT. As presented in Table 3, 5 out of 7 WS patients and the healthy aged individuals showed a decrease in the brightly stained cell populations when compared with the healthy young controls. The antibodies used here were not monoclonal and they may have been heterogenous in their specificities.

The isotype of most ALA, which are analogous to natural thymocytotoxic antibodies in New Zealand Black mice, was shown to be IgM (Messner et al., 1975; Winfield et al., 1975), but the specificities of ALA against human T-Cell subsets have not been established (Okudaira et al., 1979). The ALA in patients with SLE were reactive with suppressor T cells, K cells, natural killer cells, and so on (Winfield et al., 1975; Kippel et al., 1979; Goto et al., 1980). The anti-BAT antibodies were also heterogenous and were reactive to human T-cell subpopulations, including those responsive to concanavalin A (Golub, 1972; Stratton and Byfield, 1977; Dalchan and Fabre, 1979).

The present studies were carried out at a time when monoclonal antibodies were not available, but this type of investigation is needed for further characterization of the cellular changes in aged individuals and patients with WS.

Mitogen Stimulation of Lymphocytes

Since the proportion of the various cell subsets in the patients with WS differed from that of normal control, the mitogenic response of T cells in 4 patients with WS was studied by using two T cell mitogens; phytohemagglutinin (PHA) and concanavalin A (Con A).

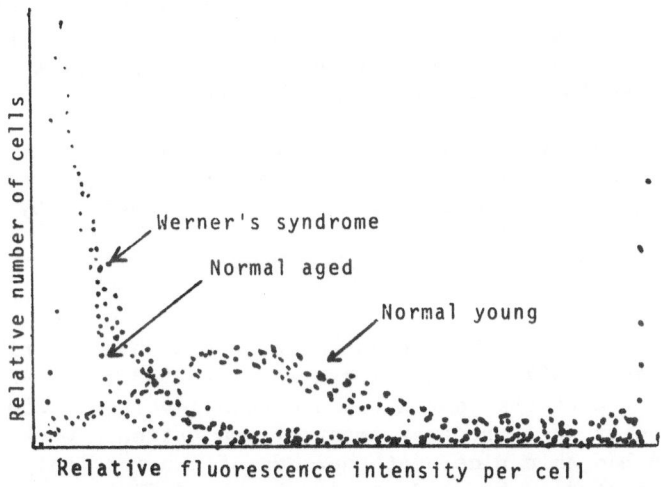

Fig. 2. Fluorescence distribution of peripheral-blood T cells stained with ALA.

Table 3

Case	Age	Anti-BAT⁺T cells	ALA⁺T cells
	(yrs)	(%)	(%)
1	17	20	38
2	29	10	26
3	30	10	33
4	31	30	32
5	40	21	40
6	45	22	52
7	59	29	51
Control	20-36	50	50
	90-96	6-11	14-18

*T-cell subpopulations reactive with anti-BAT and ALA in patients with the Werner syndrome. Percentages of anti-BAT and ALA-positive T cells are given by dividing brightly stained T cells by total T cells.

Peripheral blood lymphocytes (1 x 10^6/ml) in RPMI 1640-10% FBS medium were cultured for 3 days in the presence of optimal doses of PHA or Con A in humidified air + 5%CO_2. Cells were pulsed with ^{3}H-thymidine for 17 h before harvest.

PHA response was normal in 4 patients tested, but two patients had a lower Con A response than that of age-sex matched controls. This tendency was similar to that reported by Nakao et al. (1980).

Serum CH50

Serum CH50 levels were measured by the method described by Kabat and Mayer (1971). Normal ranges were 29.3 to 43.9U/ml. Six out of 12 patients tested had elevated levels of CH50, irrespective of age; however, most of the patients with high CH50 levels had skin ulcers at the time of examination. None of the patients studied had a decreased level of CH50.

Quantitation of Immune Complexes

Circulating immune complexes were detected by two methods; Raji-cell radioimmunoassay and human red blood cell radioimmunoassay. The Raji cell radioimmunoassay was performed as described by Theofilopoulos et al. (1976). Raji cells (2 x 10^6) in 200 ul 1% bovine serum albumin and Eagle's minimal essential medium (BSA-MEM) were left to react with 25 ul of a 1:4 dilition of test serum for 45 min at 37°C. The cells were washed three times with 1% BSA-MEM and then exposed to approximately 2.5 ug goat anti-human IgG labeled with ^{125}I in 30 ul 1% BSA containing ^{125}I-BSA for 30 min at 4°C. The cells were washed once in 1% BSA-MEM, and the radioactivity in the cell pallet was determined in a gamma scintlistron counter. The uptake of ^{125}I-goat antihuman IgG was calculated after correcting for nonspecific binding of ^{125}I-BSA and referring to a standard curve of the uptake of antibody by cells incubated with aggregated human gamma globulin in normal human serum. The amount of complexes in the test serum was expressed as ug of aggregated human gammaglobulin equivalent per ml of serum. The red blood cell radioimmunoassay was originally developed by Aikawa et al. (1979). Briefly, 50ul 4% preincubated human red blood cells were mixed with equal amount of ^{125}I-labelled rabbit human IgG and incubated at 37°C for 60 min. After three washings, equal volumes (250ul) of human red blood cells, normal human sera, and the heat-inactivated sample were mixed and incubated at 37°C for 15 min.

The human red blood cell suspensions were washed three times with gelatin veronal buffer containing 0.5% bovine serum albumin (BSA). Radioactivity incorporated by the human red blood cells was measured in a gamma scintillation counter. Circulating immune complex levels in 12 patients examined were within normal limits (less than 10ug IgG equivalent/ml).

Serum Level of Immunoglobulings

The titers of serum immunoglobulings (IgG, IgM, and IgA) in 16 patients with the Werner syndrome were examined by immunodiffusion. As indicated in Table 4, the IgG level was elevated in 4 patients, IgM in one, and IgA in 3.

In Vitro Immunoglobulin Synthesis

Ig synthesis in vitro was studied in the presence of pokeweed mitogen (PWM) by the method described previously (Okudaira et al., 1980).

In brief, one million lymphocytes in RPMI-10% were cultured in the presence or absence of 10ug/ml of PWM at 37 °C in a humidified 5% CO_2 atmosphere for 7 days. The supernatants were collected by centrifugation at 400g for 10 min and the levels of IgG and IgM were measured.

Human IgG was isolated from Cohn Fraction II by DEAE cellulose column chromatography and labeled with $125I$ by the chloramine-T method (MaConahey and Dixon, 1966). Human IgM preparations were purified from the euglobulin fraction of the serum from a patient with Waldenstrom's macroglobulinemia by Sephadex G 200 gel filtration and radiolabeled in the same manner as IgG preparations. One hundred microliters of the supernatant was added to equal volumes of 10-20 ng/ml $125I$-labeled human IgG and 1:3,000 diluted rabbit anti-human IgG, and incubated at 4 C for 48 H. Then, 100ul of 1:6 diluted goat anti-rabbit IgG and 100ul of 1:150 diluted normal rabbit serum were added to the mixtures and incubated at 4°C for an additional 24 h. The mixtures were centrifuged at 4,000 x g for 30 min and the supernatants were separated from the precipates. The radioactivities of the supernatants and precipitates were counted in a gamma scintillation counter. The percent radioactivity of the precipitates in relation to that of both the supernatants and the precipitates was calculated. IgG concentrations were calculated on the basis of a standard curve using purified IgG.

The levels of IgM in the culture supernatants were measured in the same manner as were IgG levels, except for the use of $125I$-labeled human IgM preparations and rabbit anti-human IgM.

Two patients out of 6 tested showed decreased IgG and IgM synthesis (Table 4). No patient showed increased Ig synthesis in the absence of PWM, which may indicate that spontaneous polyclonal B-cell activation (Dixon et al., 1978) is not an important phenomenon in the Werner syndrome.

Detection of Autoantibodies

It has been reported that autoantibodies can be detected in healthy aged individuals (Hooper et al., 1972), patients with scleroderma (Rothfield and Rodnan, 1965), and patients with some endocrinologic diseases, such as diagetes mellitus and hypogonadism (Kahn et al., 1976; Isojima et al., 1972).

Since the Werner syndrome is characterized by age-associated signs, scleroderma-like skin changes, and endocrinologic abnormalities, the sera in 17 Werner's syndrome patients were analyzed for the presence of several autoantibodies.

Anti-lymphocyte Antibodies (ALA)

ALA, formerly termed NTA (naturally occurring thymocytotoxic

antibody), have been detected in a variety of conditions
including SLE, rheumatiod arthritis, scleroderma, juvenile
rheumatiod arthritis, Sjogren's syndrome, viral infection and
natural aging (Mittal et al., 1970; Mottironi and Terasaki, 1970;
Okudaira et al., 1979, Ooi et al., 1974; Strelkauskas et al.,
1978; Terasaki et al., 1970).

Kreisler detected ALA in a wide variety of disease
conditions including allergy, pregnancy, amyloidosis, myasthenia,
myeloma, and tuberculosis (1971). The isotype of most ALA was
found to be IgM, but some ALA were shown to be IgG (Kawata et
al., 1980).

As described above, some T cell populations reactive to ALA
decreased in the Werner syndrome and it is conceivable that
autoantibodies reactive to lymphocytes may exist in the
circulation of WS patients.

Peripheral blood lymphocytes from healthy young individuals
were incubated with anti-F(ab)$_2$'-precoated dishes at 37°C for 60
min to remove B cells. T cells (> 90%; 1 x 10^6/0.1ml) were
incubated with the patient's serum at 4°C for 30 min to detect
ALA. The cells were then stained with fluoresceinated
isothiocyanate rabbit anti-human IgG or IgM and analyzed by the
fluorescence-activated cell sorter.

Analysis of the fluorescence profile of stained cells was
basically the same as described above. A representative
fluorescence profile is presented in Figs. 3 and 4. IgM-type ALA
was detected in 13 out of 15 serum samples from WS patients
(Table 5). Of interest, 6 out of 13 serum samples showed IgG-
type ALA, however, the titer of the ALA was quite low and no sera
stained more than 20% of the T cells, even at a dilution of 1:1.

The ALA detected in the sera from WS patients were
heterogenous and the titer was so low that extensive
characterization of the antibody was difficult and remained to be
determined.

Anti-nuclear Antibody (ANA)

Detection of ANA was carried out by the indirect
immunofluorescent technique described by Tan (1967) and Weitzman
and Walker (1977).

As shown in Table 5, the titer of ANA was very low and only
a speckled pattern of ANA (5 out of 16) was detected. The
technique used here was the classical screen test. At present,
ANA are recognized as the collective of a variety of
autoantibodies to DNA, histones, non-histone nuclear proteins,

Table 4

Case synthesis	Age	Serum immunoglobulins			Immunoglobulin	
		IgG	IgM	IgA (mg/dl)	IgG	IgM (ng/ml)
1	15	1422	134	289	nd	
2	20	2050	140	416	540	670
3	28	1800	92	468	340	530
4	30	1050	185	335	nd	
5	33	1120	160	120	2100	2500
6	34	1990	90	160	nd	
7	35	1040	80	140	2300	2050
8	40	1008	91	128	nd	
9	40	1750	85	150	nd	
10	41	1500	160	190	nd	
11	45	1500	205	370	nd	
12	45	1080	80	358	nd	
13	48	2140	294	458	1890	1160
14	48	1600	248	352	nd	
15	50	1920	228	370	nd	
16	59	1460	133	240	nd	
17	61	1660	92	495	2020	1950
Control	20-60	800-1800	80-250	90-450	900-3000	700-4000

*Serum immunoglobulin levels and immunoglobulin synthesis in vitro in the Werner syndrome. Immunoglobulin synthesis was assayed by culturing peripheral blood lymphocyte in the presence of PWM (10ug/ml). The levels of IgG and IgM were measured in the supernatants by radioimmunoassay.

RNA-protein complexes and so on (Tan, 1982). To further characterize the ANA in the sera from the Werner syndrome patients, anti-DNA antibodies and anti-centromere antibodies were detected.

Anti-DNA Antibodies

Radioimmunoassays for anti-double-stranded DNA and anti-single-stranded DNA in IgG class were done by using the same method already described (Aotsuka et al., 1979).

Briefly, each serum sample was appropriately diluted, and 2ul was added to polystyrene tubes coated with double- or single-stranded DNA as well as to uncoated control tubes. After incubation at 37°C for 120 min, the tubes were washed three times and then ^{125}I-labeled rabbit anti-IgG was added to the tubes. The tubes were incubated overnight at room temperature and washed again three times. The radioactivity retained in the tubes was counted in an automatic gamma scintillation counter. The titers of anti-double and single-stranded DNA antibodies were determined

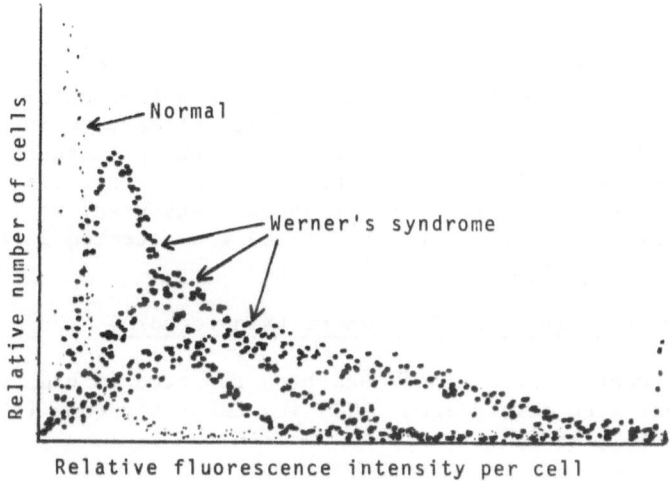

Fig. 3. Fluorescence distribution of peripheral-blood T cells labelled with the sera from WS patients and normal donors (20-96 years) and of fluoresceinated rabbit anti-human IgM.

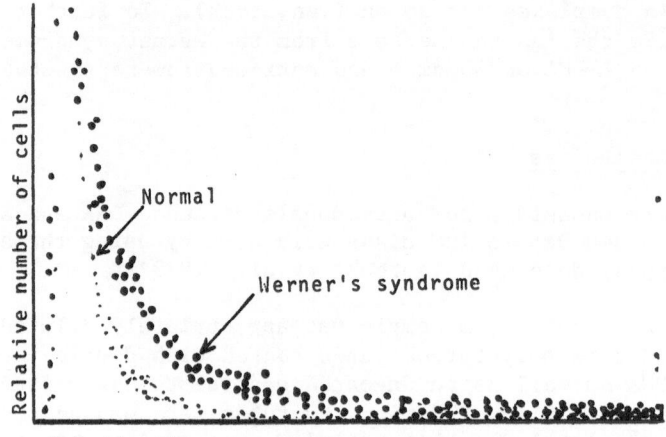

Fig. 4.   Fluorescence distribution of peripheral-blood T cells
labelled with the sera from a WS patient (40 years) and a
normal donor (35 years) and of fluoresceinated rabbit anti-
human IgG.

from their radioactivity counts and expressed as ug/ml, using a
standard curve. As shown in Table 6, both anti-double- and anti-
single-stranded DNA antibodies in the IgG class were increased in
the circulation of WS patients compared with age-matched control
levels and similar to those in the aged group. However, when a
less sensitive Millipore filter technique was used, no
significant DNA binding activity (< 5%) was detected in any serum
from WS patients (Casales et al., 1963).

Detection of Antibody to Centromere (Kinetochore)

     Anti-centromere antibody has been reported in high incidence
in patients with scleroderma (30%) and CREST syndrome (88%)
(Moroi et al., 1980).

     Because of the scleroderma-like skin changes, sera from 16
WS patients were examined by Dr. Moroi for the presence of
anticentromere antibodies. The indirect immunofluorescent
antibody technique was used to determine the nuclear staining
patterns produced by the sera under study (Moroi et al., 1980).

TABLE 5

Case	Age (yrs)	ANA	ALA IgM	IgG
1	15	−	+	+
2	20	speckled 1:10	+	−
3	29	−	+	nd
4	30	−	−	nd
5	33	−	−	−
6	35	nd	+	−
7	40	speckled 1:20	+	+
8	40	−	nd	nd
9	40	speckled 1:10	+	+
10	41	−	+	−
11	45	−	+	−
12	45	−	nd	nd
13	48	speckled 1:20	+	nd
14	48	−	+	+
15	50	−	+	+
16	59	speckled 1:20	+	−
17	61	−	+	+

*Demonstration of antibodies in the sera from Werner's syndrome patients. Antinuclear antibodies (ANA) were detected by indirect immunofluorescence technique. Antilymphocyte antibodies (ALA) were detected by FACS.

The substrate used here was Wil II cells. The slides of Wil II
cells were placed in a dry oven at 37°C for 29 min, fixed for 19
min in peroxidate/lysine/paraformaldehyde fixative at 4°C, and
washed in balanced salt solution for 5 min. Slides were not
allowed to dry but were used immediately for anticentromere
antibody testing.

Anticentromere antibodies were not detected in any of the 16
sera tested, however, the serum from a 59-year-old male patient
showed nucleolar staining, which has been frequently found in the
sera from scleroderma patients (45%) (Bernstein et al., 1982).

Anti-Insulin-Receptor Antibody

In 1975, Kahn et al., demonstrated that one of the syndromes
of insulin-resistant diabetes mellitus results from insulin-
receptor antibodies.

Recently anti-insulin-receptor antibodies were also found in
the sera from patients with scleroderma (Weinstein et al., 1980).
Insulin-resistant diabetes mellitus was reported in several cases
in the Werner syndrome.

Dr. Kasuga at NIH examined the sera from 3 WS patients for
the presence of an anti-insulin-receptor antibody, using insulin-
binding and immunoprecipitation assays. Two out of 3 patients
showed a normal glucose tolerance test reaction and no signs of
insulin resistance.

The standard competition binding assay consisted of
incubating solubilized human plancental membranes with a tracer
concentration of ^{125}I-insulin and increasing concentrations of
unlabelled insulin in a total volume of 200ul in 0.1M sodium
phosphate buffer at 22°C for 60 min. The reaction was terminated
by cooling to 4°C; the ^{125}I-insulin bound to the receptor, but
not free ^{125}I-insulin, was precipitated with polyethylene glycol
in carrier gamma-globulin. Specific binding was determined by
subtracting the radioactivity that remained bound in the presence
of 10^{-6}M unlabelled insulin.

The immunoprecipitation assay consisted of three steps: 1)
the solubilized receptor was incubated with tracer ^{125}I-insulin
at 22°C for 60 min; 2) serum containing receptor antibodies was
added and the incubation was allowed to proceed at 22°C for a
further 60 min; 3) the incubation mixture was cooled to 4°C and
immunoprecipitation was affected by the addition of a slight
excess of second antibody (goat anti-human IgG) for 4h at 4° C.
The immune complexes were then precipitated by centrifugation and
the pellet was washed once with Triton buffer and the
radioactivity was counted in a gamma counter. The concentration

Table 6

Donor	Anti-ssDNA (ug/ml)	Anti-dsDNA (ug/ml)
Werner's syndrome (N=16) (15-61 yrs)	5.52 ± 1.40	4.59 ± 0.11
Healthy control (n=30) (15-61 yrs)	1.16 ± 0.30	1.21 ± 0.27
(61-98 yrs) (n=15)	5.47 ± 0.98	3.01 ± 0.63

*Anti-DNA antibodies in IgG class in patients with the Werner syndrome. Both anti-single-stranded DNA antibodies and anti-double-stranded DNA antibodies were measured by solid-phase radioimmunoassay.

of second antibody required for optimum immunoprecipitation curves with several dilutions of sera in the presence of trition.

By using these two methods, no anti-insulin receptor antibody was detected in sera from 3 patients.

Beadle et al. (1978) reported the marked decrease of insulin-binding to receptors on thhe patients' fat cells and concluded that the insulin receptor concentration, at least on fat cells, decreased in the Werner syndrome.

Sperm-Immobilizing Antibodies

The sperm-immobilizing antibodies to human spermatozoa as well as to sperm-coating antigens that are present in seminal plasma were found in the sera of some sterile women (Isojima, 1972).

Analysis of sperm immobilizaion was carried out by Dr. Koyama at Hyogo Medical College by the method previously described (Isojima, 1972).

Sera from 4 female patients were selected.

A volume of 250ul of heat-inactivated serum, 50ul of

complement solution, and 35ul of human sperm suspension (60 x 106 /ml) were mixed in a small test tube and incubated at 32°C for 60 min. As a control, 250ul of heat-inactivated serum without sperm-immobilizing activity, 50ul of complement, and 25ul of sperm suspension were mixed and incubated in the same way as the specimen of serum. After 60 min of incubation, one drop of sperm suspension from the small test tube was placed on a slide, and the number of motile spermatozoa among 50 spermatozoa were counted in one microscopic field. The percentage of motile spermatozoa among the 200 spermatozoa examined was calculated (T %). This percentage was also calculated for the control (C%). The sperm-immobilization value (< 2 in normal sera) was calculated as C/T.

The sperm immobilization value for all four sera was less than 2. Other antibodies frequently found in endocrinological diseases such anti-microsomal antibody and anti-thyroglobulin antibody were not detected in 5 patients tested.

Discussion and Conclusion

Several antibodies including antinuclear antibodies, anti-lymphocyte antibodies and anti-DNA antibodies were detected in low titers in the sera from WS patients by using sensitive techniques.

The role of these antibodies in the pathogenesis of the Werner syndrome remains unclear and to be further determined.

Decreases of some T cell subpopulations reactive to the anti-lymphocyte antibodies or the anti-brain associated T cell antigen antibodies were quite pronounced, however further studies concerning lymphocyte functions in Werner's syndrome are needed.

Summary

Several immmunological assessments of the Werner syndrome are described, including detection of antibodies frequently found in autoimmune diseases and analysis of age-related changes of cell subpopulations.

By using sensitive techniques such as fluorescence-activated cell sorting and solid-phase radioimmunoassay, anti-lymphocyte antibodies and anti-DNA antibodies were frequently detected in the sera from patients with the Werner syndrome. Anti-nuclear antibodies were also detected in a conventional manner; however, the titers of these antibodies were very low. Examination of cell populations revealed marked decreases in the T cell subsets reactive to both antilymphocytic antibodies and anti-brain associated T cell antigen antibodies.

Acknowledgement. The authors are grateful to Dr. Alan Cohen for valuable discussion and for preparing our manuscript.

References

Ablin R. J., Baird W. M., 1971, Lymphocytotoxic antibodies in prostatic cancer, JAMA., 216:2015.

Aikawa T., Mitamura T., Tanimoto K., Horiuchi Y., 1979, Detection of circulating immune complexes by using human red blood cells, J Lab Clin Sci., 94:902.

Aotsuka S., Okawa M., Ikebe K., Yokohari R., 1979, Measurement of anti-double stranded DNA antibodies in major immunoglobulin classes, J Immunol Methods., 28:149.

Beadle G. F., Mackay L. R., Whittingham S., Taggart G., Hanis A. W., Harrison L. C., 1978, Werner's syndrome, A model of premature aging?, J Med., 9:377.

Bernstein R. M., Steigerwald J. C., Tan E. M., 1982, Association of antinuclear and antinucleolar antibodies in progressive sclerosis, Clin Exp Immunol., 48:43.

Blakeslee D., Baines M., 1976, Immunofluorescence using dichlorotriazinyl-aminofluorescein, J Immunol Methods., 13:305.

Bluestein H. G., Zvaifler N. J., 1976, Brain-reactive lymphocytotoxic antibodies in the serum of patients with systemic lupus erythematosus, J Clin Invest., 57:507.

Boyum A., 1968, Isolation of monuclear cells and granulocytes from human blood, Scand J Clin Lab Invest., 21:77.

Buckley C. E., Roseman J. M., 1976, Immunity and survival, J Am Geriatr Soc., 24:241.

Casales S. P., Friou G. J., Teague P. O., 1963. Specific nuclear reaction pattern of DNA antibody in lupus srythematosus sera, J Lab Clin Med., 62:625.

Dalchan R., Fabre J. W., 1979, Tissue distribution of brain-thymus shared antigens recognized by anti-brain xenosera in the rat, dog and man, Clin Exp Immunol., 35:425.

DeHoratius R. J., Henderson C., Strickland R. G., 1976, Lumphocytotoxins in acute and chronic hepatitis, characterization and relationship to changes in circulating T lymphocytes, Clin Exp Immunol., 26:21.

Dixon F. J., Theofilopoylos A. N., Wilson C. B., 1978, Etiology and pathogenisis of a spontaneous lupus-like syndrome i mice, Artjrotos Rheum., 21:64S.

Fujiwara Y., Higashikawa T., Tatsumi M., 1977, A retarded rate of DNA replication and normal level of DNA repair in Werner's syndrome fibroblasts in culture, J Cell physiol., 92:365.

Golub E. S., 1972, The distribution of brain-associated O antigen cross-reactive with mouse in the brain of other species, J Immunol., 109:168.

Goldstein S., Moerman E. J., 1975, Heat-labile enzymes in
    Werner's syndrome fibroblasts, Nature., 255:159.
Goto M., Murata K., 1978, Urinary excretion of macromolecular
    acidic glycosaminoglycans in Werner's syndrome, Clin Chim
    Acta., 62:89.
Goto M., Horiuchi Y., Tanimoto K., Ishii T., Nakashima H., 1978,
    Werner's syndrome: Analysis of 15 cases with a review of te
    Japanese literature, J Am Geriatr., 26:341.
Goto M., Horiuchi Y., Okumura K., Tada T., Kawata M., Ohmori K.,
    1979, Immunological abnormalities of aging: An analysis of
    T lymphocyte subpopulations of Werner's syndrome, J Clin
    Invest., 64:695.
Goto M., Tanimoto K., Horiuchi Y., 1980, Natural cell mediated
    cytotoxicity in systemic lupus erythematosus. Supression by
    antilymphocyte antibody, Arthritis Rheum., 23:1274.
Goto M., Tanimoto K., Aotsuka S., Okawa M., Yokohari R., 1982,
    Age-related changes in auto- and natural antibody in the
    Werner's syndrome, Am J Med., 72:607.
Harrison I. C., Flier J. S., Roth J., Karlsson F. A., Hohn C. R.,
    1979, Immunoprecipitation of the insulin receptor: A
    sensitive assay for receptor antibodies and specific
    technique for receptor purification, J Clin Endocrinol
    Metab>, 48:59.
Herzenberg L. A., Sweat R. G., Herzenberg L. A., 1976,
    Fluorescence-activated cell sorting, Sci Amer., 234:108.
Holliday R., Poterfield J. S., Gibbs D. D., 1974, Premature aging
    and occurrence of altered enzyme in Werner's syndrome
    fibroblasts, Nature., 248:762.
Hooper B., Whitingham S., Mathews J. D., Mackay I. R., Curnow D.
    H., 1972. Autoimmunity in rural community, Clin Exp
    Immunol., 12:79.
Isojima S., Tsuchiya K., Koyama K., Tauchi G., Naha O., Adachi
    H., 1972, Further studies on sperm-immobilizing antibody
    found in sera of unexplained cases of sterility in women, Am
    J Obstet Gynecol., 112:198.
Kahn C. R., Flier J. S., Bar R. S., Archer J. A., Gorden P.,
    Maning M. M., Roth J., 1978, The syndromes of insulin
    resistance and acanthosis nigricans, N Engl J Med., 294:739.
Klippel J. H., Bluestein H. G., Zvaifler N. M., 1979, Lymphocyte
    reactivity of antisera to cryoproteins in systemis lupus
    erythematosus, Clin Immunol Immunopath., 12:52.
Koike T., Kobayashi S., Yoshiki T., Itoh T., Shirai T., 1979,
    Differential sensitivity of functional aubsets of T cells to
    the cytotoxicity of natural T-lymphotoxic antibody of
    systemic lupus erythematosus, Arthritis Rheum, 22:123.
Korsmeyer S., Strickland R. G., Wilson I. D., Williams R. C.,
    1974, Serum lymphocytotoxic and lymphocytophilic antibody
    activity in inflammatory bowel disease, Gastroenterology.,
    67:578.

Kreisler M., Naito S., Terasaki P. I., 1971, Cytotoxins in
    diseases, Transplantation Proc., 3:112.
Mikinodan T., Heidrick M. L., Nordin H. A., 1975,
    Immunodeficiency and autoimmunity in aging, Birth Defects.,
    11:193.
Martin G. M., Sprague C. A., Epstein C. H., 1970, Replicative
    lifespan of cultured human cells: effects of donor's age,
    tissue, and genotype, Lab Invest., 23:89.
McConahey P. I., Dixon F. J., 1966, A model of trace iodination
    of proteins for immunologic studies, Int Arch Allergy Appl
    Immunol., 29:185.
Messner R. P., Kennedy M. S., Jelinak J. G., 1975, Antilymphocyte
    antibodies in SLE. Effect on lymphocyte surface
    characteristics, Arthritis Rheum., 18:201.
Mittal K. K., Rossen R. D., Sharp J. T., Lipsky M. D., Butler W.
    T., 1970, Lymphocyte cytotoxic antibodies in systemic lupus
    erythematosus, Nature., 225:1255.
Morito T., Tanimoto K., Horiuchi Y., Juji T., 1978, Fc-rosette
    inhibition by pregnant women's sera and by rabbit anti- 2-
    microglobulin, Int Arch Allergy Appl Immunol., 56:247.
Morol Y., Gritzler C. P. M. J., Steigerwald H., Tan E. M., 1980,
    Auto-antibody to centromere (kinetochore) in scleroderma
    sera, Proc Natl Acad Sci USA., 77:1627.
Mottironi V. D., Terasaki P. I., 1970, Histocompatibility
    testing, Copenhagen, Munksgaard, 231.
Nakao Y., Hattori T., Takatsuki K., Kuroda Y., Nakaji T.,
    Fujiwara Y., Kishihara M., Baba Y., Fujita T., 1980,
    Immunological studies on Werner's syndrome, Clin Exp
    Immunol., 42:10.
Okudaira K., Nakai H., Hayakawa T., Kashiwado T., Tanimoto K.,
    Horiuchi Y., Juju T., 1979, Detection of antilymphocyte
    antibody with two-color method in systemic lupus
    erythematosus and its heterogenous specificities against
    human T cell subsets, J Clin Invest., 64:1213.
Okudaira K., Tanimoto K., Nakamura T., Horiuchi Y., 1980,
    Spontaneously enhanced in vitro immunoglobulin synthesis by
    B cells in systemic lupus erythematosus, Clin Immunol
    Immunopath., 16:267.
Ooi B. S., Orlina A. R., Masaitis L., First M. R., Dallak V. E.,
    Ooi Y. M., 1974, Lymphocytotoxin in aging, Transplantation.,
    18:190.
Pathfield N. D., Rodnan G. P., 1968, Serum antinuclear antibodies
    in systemic sclerosis (Scleroderma), Arthritis Rheum.,
    11:607.
Stratton J. A., Byfield P. E., 1977, Reactions of anti-human
    brain serum with human lymphocyte subpopulations, Cell
    Immuno., 28:1.

Strelkauskas A. J., Schauf V., Wilson B. S., Chess L., Schlossman
    S. F., 1978, Isolation and characterization of naturally
    occurring subclasses of human peripheral blood T cells with
    regulatory functions, J Immunol., 120:1278.
Tan E. M., 1967, Relationship of nuclear staining patterns with
    precipitating antibodies systemic lupus erythematosus, J Lab
    Clin Med., 70:800.
Tan E. M., 1982, Autoantibodies to nuclear antigens (AMA). Their
    immunobiology and medicine, Adv Immunol., 33:167.
Terasaki P. I., Mottironi V. D., Barnett E. V., 1970, Cytotoxins
    in disease. Autocytotoxins in lupus, N Engl J Med.,
    283:724.
Theofilopoulos A. N., Wilson C. B., Dixon F. J., 1977, The Rafi
    cell radioimmune assay for detecting immune complexes in
    human sera, J Clin Invest., 57:169.
Weiner M. S., Bianco C., Nussenzweig V., 1973, Enhanced binding
    of neuraminidose-treated sheep erythrocyte human T
    lymphocytes, Blood., 42:939.
Weinstein P. S., High K. A., Dercole A. J., Jeanette J. C., 1980,
    Insulin resistance due to receptor antibodies: A comparison
    of progressive systemic sclerosis, Arthritis Rheum., 23:101.
Weitzman R. J., Walker S. E., 1977, Relation of titered
    peripheral pattern ANA to anti-DNA and disease activity in
    systemic lupus erythematosus, Ann Rheum Dis., 36:44.
Winfield J. B., Winchester R. J., Werner P., Fu M., Kunkel H. G.,
    1975, Nature of cold-reactive antibodies to lymphocyte
    surface determinants in systemic lupus erythematosus,
    Arthritis Rheum., 18:1.
Yunis E. J., Fernandes G., Greenberg L. O., 1976, Tumor
    immunology, autoimmunity and aging, J Am Geriatr Soc.,
    24:258.

CLINICAL AND METABOLIC STUDIES ON WERNER'S SYNDROME:

WITH SPECIAL REFERENCE TO DISORDERS OF LIPID AND LIVER FUNCTION

Katsumi Murata and Hiroaki Nakashima

Department of Medicine and Physical Therapy
University of Tokyo School of Medicine, Tokyo
Third Department of Medicine
Kagoshima University School of Medicine
Kagoshima, Japan

Supported in part by Grants-in-aid from the Ministry of Education,
Science and Culture of Japan and grants from the Life Science
Section of the Institute of Physical and Chemical Research and
from Adult Disease Clinic Memorial Foundation, Tokyo

INTRODUCTION

Werner's syndrome was first described by Werner (1904) as a
mesodermal disorder clinically characterized by multifarious facets
of premature senility. Numerous papers on Werner's syndrome have
since been written (Oppenheimer and Kugel 1934; Thannhauser 1945;
Irwin and Ward 1953; Epstein et al., 1966). However, reports of a
disorder of lipid metabolism and liver dysfunction were limited
(Zucker-Franklin et al., 1968). The occurrence of Werner's syndrome
is relatively higher in Japan (Murata and Nakashima, 1982). To
date, numerous clinical reports on this syndrome are to be found in
the literature, but some of them are either incomplete or
occasionally overlap. Only by cautious selection from among the
publications in the medical literature, excluding incorrect cases,
is it possible to reveal the clear-cut clinical features of this
syndrome.

The present paper describes the conspicuous clinical
characteristics of 24 cases of Werner's syndrome. The typical
clinical symptoms of this syndrome were compared with 172 cases
reported in the Japanese literature, after careful exclusion of
fragmentary or overlapping cases. During this investigation,
special attention was paid to disorders of lipid metabolism and

liver function in patients with Werner's syndrome, because they have
not been precisely described in previous papers (Murata, 1983).

LITERATURE REVIEW

The clinical features of Werner's syndrome are unique and
appear as either A general or a local manifestation. The high
frequency of consanguineous marriages was recognized in 19 of our 24
cases (79%), and 68% in the Japanese cases, among whom the male-
female ratio was nearly 1:1. The conspicuous clinical
manifestations that the WS patients have in common with the Japanese
cases are as follows. The average height in 18 male patients with
Werner's syndrome was 151.1 cm, in 6 female patients 131.7 cm, and
the average weight in male patients was 38.8 kg, in female patients
32.5 kg. All the patients were characterized by short stature,
light body weight, sparse hair, slim extremities with a fat trunk, a
high-pitched or hoarse voice, a bird-like face with receding jaw,
juvenile bilateral cataracts, scleroderma-like skin, and
hyperkeratosis. We also noted the frequent presence of the
following unrecorded signs: flat feet, hyperreflexibility,
irregularly arranged teeth, and thin, sparse, and colour-faded hair.

Premature senility in Werner's syndrome, which is interpreted
as a connective-tissue disorder related to aging, appeared so
frequently that it accounted for all the patients of the present
study and 99% in the literature. The facial expression was quite
similar in all Werner's patients. The bird-like appearance of the
face was due to the atrophy of the subcutaneous tissue in the neck
during the early stage of Werner's syndrome. Sparse grey hair or
loss of hair, or both, was not only confined to the scalp but also
affected the eyebrows and eyelashes (Fig. 1). "Sparse, thin and
light" hair is quite commonly encountered in Japan. This is in
contrast to dark coarse hair of the patient with Sanfillipo's
syndrome. The hair signs of Werner's syndrome begin at the age of
13-26. The eyes occasionally appear protuberant because of either
the loss of circumorbital connective tissue or the deposition of
postorbital lipid. In all the patients, juvenile bilateral
cataracts were conspicuous from the age of 13-27 years. In 10 of
the 24 patients, the dentition had grown irregularly and in some had
to be replaced artifically. Atrophy with hyperpigmentation of the
skin was frequently observed in skin exposed to sun, such as the
face and distal extremities. The voice became high-pitched or
hoarse at the age of 14-25. On X-ray examination, severe
osteoporosis was detected in all of our cases, especially after the
4th decade. In several, the lower extremities were most severely
affected. Generalized arteriosclerosis was found not only in the
aorta (Fig. 2) but also in the small arteries (Fig. 3).
Calcification of the soft connective tissue occurred in 12 cases,
most frequently localized in the Achilles tendon (Fig. 4), followed
by the knee and elbow tendons (Fig. 5).

The scleroderma-like appearance was common in the legs of all the Werner's patients. Atrophy of subcutaneous and muscular tissues was usually observed in the limbs. Circumscribed hyperkeratosis was found in all Werner's patients. This sign of "flat feet" was a conspicuous characteristic and was found in 20 of the 24 cases of Werner's syndrome. Attention to flat feet as well as

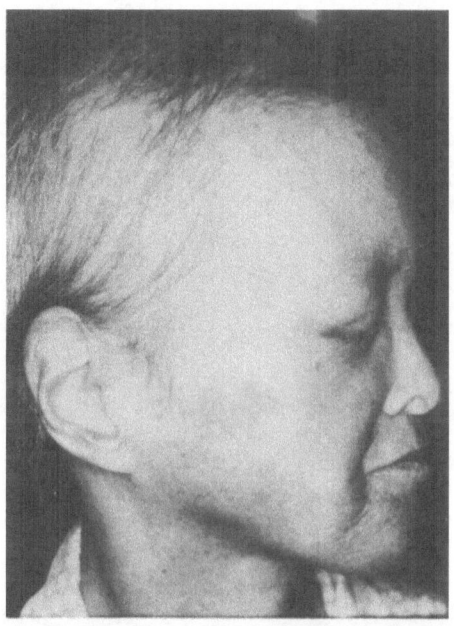

Fig. 1:   Thin, sparse, and colour-faded black hair was observed in a patient (50 year-old female) of Werner's syndrome. Note irregular pigmentation on her face.

hyperreflexibility was first paid in reports of the initial seven cases (Goto and Murata, 1977). Weakness of the tendon construction and translocation of the bones in the feet would cause flat feet (Fig. 6).

Ulceration of the skin of the legs or feet was surrounded by pigmented or depigmented tight and hard skin and was observed quite often over the age of 36. Severe ulceration was difficult to reverse and occasionally was the cause of amputation. In the early stage, xanthoma was occasionally observed of skin of neck, chest, and legs (Fig. 7), indicating lipid disturbance in Werner's syndrome.

A dysfunction of glucose tolerance or a tendency towards diabetes mellitus, or both, were detected 67% in the WS cases

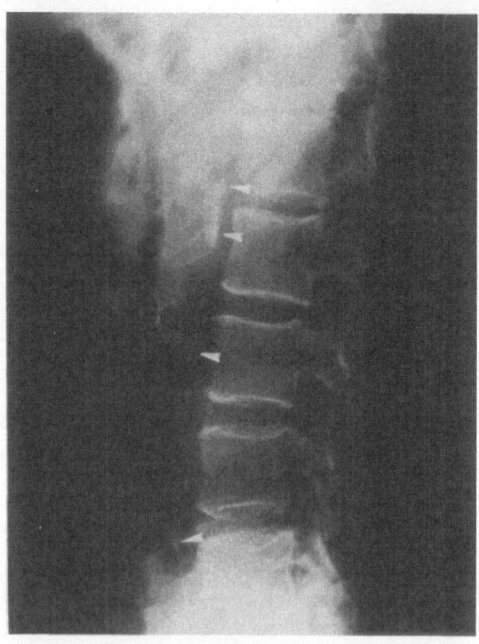

Fig. 2:   Calcification of the abdominal aorta of a patient with
          Werner's syndrome (54 year-old male).

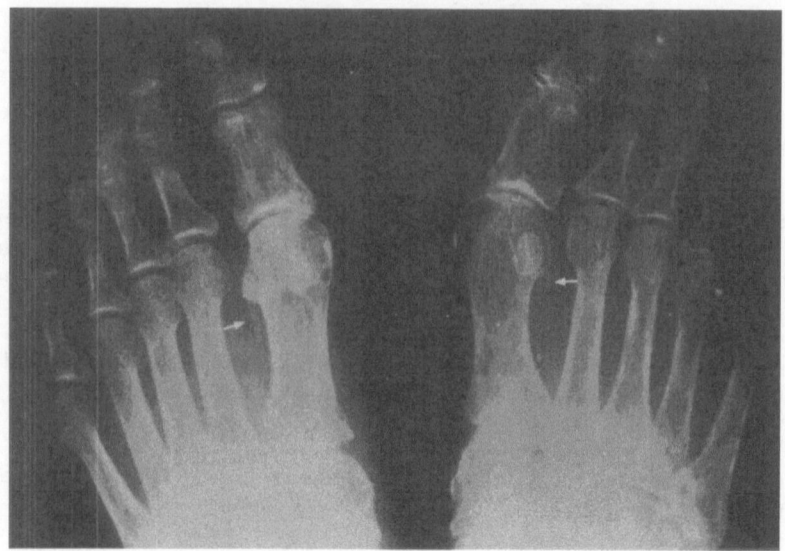

Fig. 3:   Osteoporotic changes of the toe bones and calcification of
          metatarsal arteries indicated in the arrow.

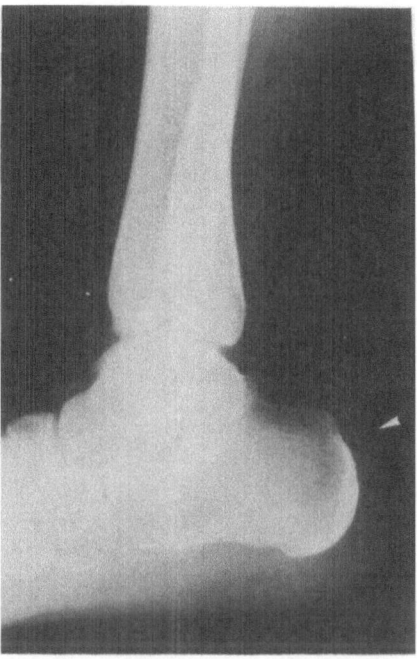

Fig. 4:   Calcification of the Achilles tendon of a patient with
           Werner's syndrome (Case 3). Note the flat feet and the
           corresponding location of the talo-crural joint.

and 61% in the Japanese literature. The fasting blood sugar level
was within normal range in two-thirds of the WS patients in this
study. The others showed various responses to the glucose
tolerance test and suffered from the delayed type of diabetes
mellitus, being progressively resistant to insulin treatment.
Secondary sexual underdevelopment occured in 15 cases (63%) and
hypogonadism in 17 cases (21%) of the all Werner's patients. No
striking abnormalities showed up in the hormonal data of any of the
WS patients. Routine immunological analysis showed a slight
increase in one of the immunoglobulins but its type was not
identified.

     Serum biochemical data obtained from the present cases of
Werner's syndrome included certain deviations of liver function and
lipid levels. The average level of serum cholesterol was 208 mg/100
ml and that of triglycerides 185 mg/100 ml. The averaged urea
nitrogen level was 18.4 mg/100 ml and ranged from 0.6 mg/100 ml to
23.0 mg/100 ml. Mild liver dysfunctions were also observed. The
average level of alanine aminotransferase was 33.6 units, ranging
from 13 units to 48 units, but excessive amounts over normal ranges
(69-90 units) were occasionally found in 10 cases. The amount of

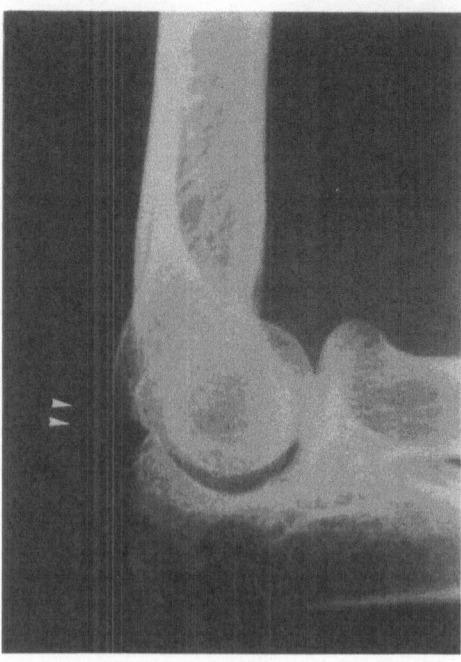

Fig. 5: Calcification of the tendon at the elbow joint in a
         patient with Werner's syndrome (Case 2).

asparatate aminotransferase averaged 36.1 units and increased as
high as from 61-143 units in nine cases. The elevated amounts of
aminotransferase were common in the three WS cases with
hyperlipidemia. Serum lactic dehydrogenase averaged 311 units,
ranging from 140 units to 410 units. Serum alkaline phosphatase
was almost all within normal range. No hyperuricemia was observed,
even in the hyperlipidemic cases.

     A high frequency of hyperreflexia of the patella was observed
in almost all the patients, followed by hyperreflexia in the
Achilles, biceps, and triceps tendons. The phenomenon was first
observed by us as a disorder of nerve system. In addition to
hyperreflexibility, flat feet were also noted at various ages (15-
61 years) in our 8-year serial study (Murata and Nakashima). Since
then, we confirmed by careful examination that both signs occur
quite frequently in patients with Werner's syndrome. Hyperreflexia
should be interpreted, in part, as a pyramidal sign and also as
hardness of the tendon. The intelligence quotient of Werner's
patients remained normal or was rather higher than 100. Some
patients were well educated and worked actively at the high
positions in society. Psychogenic disturbance was observed
occasionally as an expression of mild senile dementia.

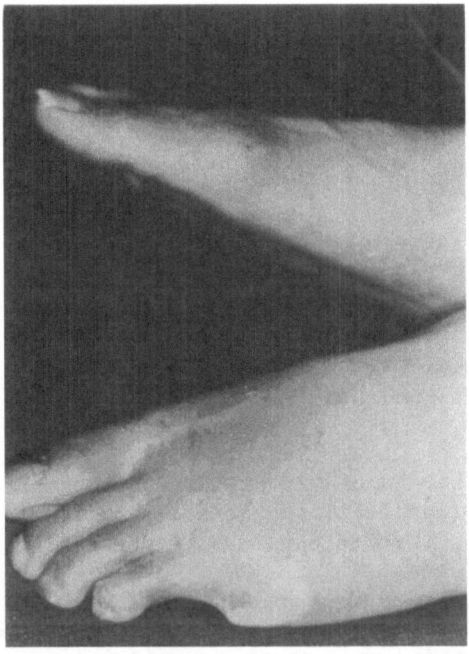

Fig. 6:   Flat feet and autoamputation at the right fifth toe of a
          male patient with Werner's syndrome at age 54.

     Generalized arteriosclerosis had been detected in the
cardiovascular system of WS patients (Zackai and Noth, 1974).   On
electrocardiography, ST-segment depression and inverted T waves were
observed in 11 out of 21 of the WS patients, and may have been due
to coronary arteriosclerosis. Hypertension combined with
arteriosclerosis, was observed in 4 cases, kidney dysfunction in
nine. The individual signs were proteinuria in 7 cases, abnormally
delayed excretion of phenolsulfonphtalein in 3, increased
concentration of urine in 3, elevated urea nitrogen in 1 and
persistent microhematuria in 1. Hypertension and uremia were
reported by Valero and Gellei (1960). Pneumonia (Fig. 8) seemed to
be a major cause of death among WS patients.

THREE CASES OF WERNER'S SYNDROME WITH HYPERLIPEMIA AND LIVER
DYSFUNCTION

Case 1: 43-year-old housewife:

     Weight, 43.5 kg; height, 150
cm. Werner's syndrome was also found in her youngest sister (case
2) among seven brothers and sisters. At the age of 18, she noticed

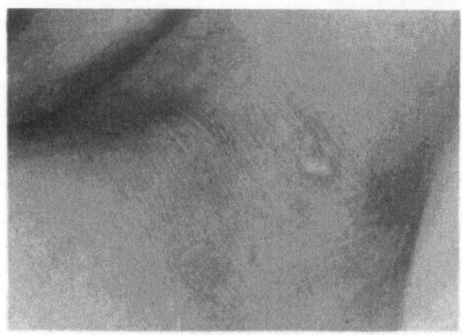

Fig. 7:   Xanthoma of the left foot of a 34-year-old female with
          Werner's syndrome.

sparse hair. At the age of 22, Hallux valgus started. She married
at 24 years of age and had 3 spontaneous abortions. At the age 26,
bilateral cataracts were recognized. Hypertension started at the
age of 37.

     Her face was bird-like with a receding jaw. Her hair was thin,
sparse and colour-faded and her skin was dried and dark with
pigmentation. Her slimmed extremities and fatty abdomen were
remarkable. Her extremities where exposed to the sun were darkly
pigmentated. Digital angiitis was noticed on all fingers.
Teleangiectasia was detected in the ears. Her teeth were all
artificially replaced. All tendon reflexes especially in the
extremities were increased. Her Achilles tendon was calcified and
her feet were flat. Blood pressure was 188/90 mmHg. An
electrocardiogram was normal.

     Laboratory data showed hyperlipemia (Tables 1 and 2). Blood
cell counts were within normal limits. Serum total protein was
relatively elevated than the normal, reflecting a higher proportion
of B-globulin. Thymol turbidity was as high as 6.9 units. Serum
transaminases were consistently higher than the normal. The level
of asparatate aminotransferase averaged 38.3 units, ranging from 39
to 47 units, while that of alanine amino-transferase was 36.2 units,
ranging from 30 to 46 units. The enhanced levels of transaminases
have consistently been detected for the last 5 years. The value of
x-GPT was slightly increased. Responses to the blood sugar
tolerance test and insulin levels were both within normal ranges.
Somewhat higher levels of serum calcium and IgA were observed.
Daily excretion of urinary 17-KS and 17-HCS tended to be elevated.

     The most conspicuous change was detected in serum lipid
components of the patients of Werner's syndrome. The average
triglyceride level was as high as 1173 mg/100 ml, ranging from 878

Table 1. Laboratory data of liver dysfunction in three hyperlipemic cases of the Werner syndrome

	Case 1	Case 2	Case 3
Blood cells			
Red blood cell count ($10^4/mm^3$)	425	414	485
Hemoglobin (g/100 ml)	13.4	12.5	15.1
Hematocrit (%)	38.5	37.5	39.0
Platelet count ($10^4/mm^3$)	21.5	22.1	25.1
White blood cell count ($10^3/mm^3$)	5.0	6.2	7.5
Serum analysis			
Total protein (g/100 ml)	8.94 (5) / 8.0 – 9.4	8.54 (5) / 8.3 – 9.2	8.37 (7) / 7.8 – 8.4
A/G ratio	1.27	1.38	1.42
Albumin (%)	55.9 (4) / 52.2 – 62.9	58.2 (4) / 58.0 – 58.3	58.7 (4) / 56.0 – 62.0
α_1-globulin (%)	2.5 (4) / 2.1 – 2.8	3.0 / 2.7 – 3.3	2.1
α_2-globulin (%)	9.1 (4) / 8.6 – 9.7	8.7 / 7.0 – 10.3	9.0
β-globulin (%)	13.5 (4) / 11.4 – 16.0	14.0 / 13.9 – 14.0	12.1
γ-globulin (%)	19.0 (4) / 12.0 – 22.8	16.1 / 14.2 – 18.3	18.1
Fibrinogen (mg/100 ml)	280	250	290

(continued)

Table 1. (Continued)

Serum analysis (cont.)	Case 1	Case 2	Case 3
Total bilirubin (mg/100 ml)	0.15 - 0.27	0.27 - 0.41	1.06 (10) / 0.80 - 1.60
Direct bilirubin (mg/100 ml)	0.08 - 0.17	0.10 - 0.19	0.14 / 0.10 - 0.20
Indirect bilirubin (mg/100 ml)	0.06 - 0.10	0.12 - 0.22	0.92 / 0.70 - 1.50
Thymol turbidity test (units)	6.9 (6) / 6.5 - 10.8	5.4 (5) / 4.0 - 7.4	3.1
Zinc sulfate test (units)	9.8 (6) / 8.6 - 11.1	4.6 (7) / 3.3 - 8.9	10.5
Biochemical analysis			
Alkaline phosphatase (K.A. units)	4.4 (6) / 4.8 - 5.3	5.4 (7) / 4.7 - 6.8	7.4 (10) / 5.7 - 9.6
Asparate-amino transaminase (units)	38.3 (4) / 39 - 47	38.2 (4) / 34 - 46	35.2 (6) / 19 - 85
Alanine amino-transaminase (units)	36.2 (5) / 30 - 46	36.2 (5) / 28 - 54	56.3 (6) / 28 - 131
Lactic dehydrogenase: total (units/l)	201 (5) / 190 - 227	230 (4) / 204 - 228	144 (13) / 131 - 340
Isozyme I (%)	18	18	ND
II (%)	41	38	
III (%)	24	22	
IV (%)	5	6	
V (%)	12	16	
Cholinesterase (Δ pH)	1.52 (5) / 1.4 - 1.6	1.4 - 1.6	ND

	Case 1	Case 2	Case 3
Biochemical analysis (cont.)			
Leucine aminopeptidase (units)	153 (5) 142 - 165	128 - 248	ND
γ-glutamyl transpeptidase (units)	33.2 (6) 23 - 40	76.3 55 - 99	32.4 (10) 8 - 41
Serum amylase (Somogi units)	102	100	ND
Creatine phosphokinase (mU/ml)	10	17	ND
Urea nitrogen (mg/100 ml)	8.7	11.7	10 - 16
Creatinine (mg/100 ml)	0.6	0.7	0.6 - 0.8
Uric acid (mg/100 ml)	3.3	3.7	6.1 5.0 - 7.3
Serum electrolytes			
Sodium (mEq/L)	143	140	140-144
Potassium (mEq/L)	4.4	4.5	3.6 - 4.6
Chloride (mEq/L)	96	99	96 - 103
Calcium (mEq/L)	4.8 - 5.1	4.7 - 5.1	4.7 - 5.6
Phosphorus (mg/100 ml)	3.0	2.7	3.2 - 3.6
Magnesium (mEq/L)	1.9	1.8	ND
Iron (μg/100 ml)	83	91	45 - 99
Copper (μg/100 ml)	134	134	ND

Table 2. Endocrinological, immunological and serum lipid data

Endocrine findings

	Case 1	Case 2	Case 3
Trisorb (ng/100 ml)	99	119	88
Tetrasorb (µg/100 ml)	6.3	6.9	6.0
Thyroid stimulating hormone (µU/ml)	3.0 - 3.1	3.1 - 3.1	3.0
Insulin (µ units/ml)	15.8	13.9	11.9
Glucose (mg/100 ml)	90	97	$\frac{123\ (8)}{93\ -\ 125}$
Serum aldosterone (pg/ml)	57.5	65.8	ND
Urinary aldosterone (µg/day)	0.9	1.5	ND
Urinary 17KS (mg/day)	10.3	9.6	9.0
Urinary 170HCS (mg/day)	6.3	7.5	4.0

Glucose tolerance test and insulin level

	Case 1		Case 2		Case 3	
	Glucose (mg/100 ml)	Insulin (µ units/ml)	Glucose (mg/100 ml)	Insulin (µ units/ml)	Glucose (mg/100 ml)	Insulin (µ units/ml)
Before	86	15.8	90	13.9	169	ND
30'	124	47.4	155	105.9	286	
60'	148	86.9	150	118.9	337	

Glucose tolerance test and insulin level (cont.)

	Case 1		Case 2		Case 3	
	Glucose (mg/100 ml)	Insulin (u units/ml)	Glucose (mg/100 ml)	Insulin (u units/ml)	Glucose (mg/100 ml)	Insulin (u units/ml)
90'	150	135.2	139	153.3	324	
120'	128	97.7	89	61.3	255	
180'	57	15.8	76	14.4	187	

Immunological findings

	Case 1	Case 2	Case 3
CH$_{50}$ (unit/ml)	35.6	44.5	37.8
Anti-DNA-binding activity (%)	12	11	9
Ig G (mg/100 ml)	1600	970	2100
Ig A (mg/100 ml)	450 - 480	310	460
Ig M (mg/100 ml)	110	140	140
Ig D (mg/100 ml)	< 3.0	5.5	4.0
Ig E (I units/ml)	62	77	125
C-reactive protein	-	-	-
RA test	-	-	-
Anti-polyADPR activity (%)	15	12	11

(continued)

Table 2. (Continued)

Urinalysis	Case 1 Continuous microhematuria	Case 2 Within normal limits	Case 3 Glucose
Urinary glycosaminoglycans	Hyaluronic acid (+)	Hyaluronic acid (+)	Hyaluronic acid (+)
Serum lipid components			
Total cholesterol (mg/100ml)	$\frac{264\ (6)}{219-317}$	$\frac{237\ (6)}{194-319}$	$\frac{286\ (4)}{212-326}$
Triglyceride (mg/100 ml)	$\frac{1173\ (6)}{878-1538}$	$\frac{1101\ (6)}{736-1562}$	$\frac{468\ (4)}{363->1000}$
β-lipoprotein (mg/100 ml)	$\frac{1180\ (6)}{926-1507}$	$\frac{1077\ (6)}{806-1477}$	ND
Phospholipid (mg/100 ml)	310	284	294
HDL-cholesterol (mg/100 ml)	$\frac{36.8\ (5)}{22-45}$	$\frac{31.0\ (5)}{21-34}$	35.0
LDL (mg/100 ml)	528	509	435
VLDL (mg/100 ml)	551	1218	505
α-lipoprotein (%)	25	24	27
Pre β-lipoprotein (%)	36		34
β-lipoprotein	39	76	39
Lipoprotein lipase activity	4.42	3.14	5.60

The numbers in parenthesis indicate the determination numbers of each case.
Underlined numbers indicate out of the normal ranges. ND = not determined

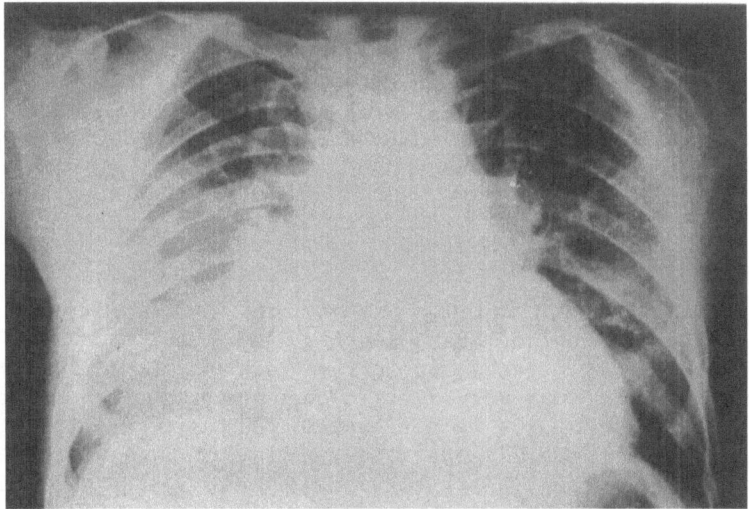

Fig. 8:   Clear radiograph shows pneumonic change in the lower part
           of the right lung and enlargement of the heart in a 53-
           year-old patient with Werner's syndrome.

mg/100 to 1538 mg/100 ml.   The levels of both total cholesterol and
phospholipid were somewhat higher than normal.   Average HDL-
cholesterol was as low as 36.8 mg/100 ml, ranging from 22 mg/100 ml
to 45 mg/100 ml: the normal range in Japanense women is 55 mg/100
ml - 75 mg/100 ml (Nakazawa and Murata, 1980).

Case 2:   35-year-old housewife.

Weight, 45.3 kg; height, 150 cm.   She was the youngest sister of
Case 1.   She was healthy in childhood and married at the age of 27.
She noticed that she had a fat trunk, and thin extremities with
dried and pigmented skin.   At the age of 34, bilateral cataracts
started.   Her face had typically bird-like features, with a fat neck
and receding jaw.   She had thin and sparse hair.   Her voice was high
pitched, her feet flat.   On X-ray examination, Achilles and elbow-
tendon calcification was detected (Fig. 5).   Almost all tendon
reflexes in the extremities, especially the patella tendon reflex,
were increased.   Her usual blood pressure was almost within normal
range but it increased occasionally to the maximum value of 180/100
mmHg.   She had a healthy 5-year-old boy.

     Laboratory examination revealed persistent hyperlipidemia as
in her elder sister (Table 1 and 2).   Serum total protein and β-
globulin were somewhat increased.   Hormonal examinations revealed
that the values were nearly normal.   The levels of serum x-GPT,
thymol turbidity, and transaminases were somewhat higher than the
normal.

Conspicuous disorders of serum lipid fractions were detected
as follows: the average level of serum triglyceride was as high as
1101 mg/100 ml, ranging from 736 mg/100 ml to 1562 mg/100 ml. The
average level of serum B-lipoprotein was also increased to 1077
mg/100 ml, ranging from 806 mg/100 ml to 1477 mg/100 ml. The
values of serum cholesterol and phospholipid were slightly
increased. The average high-density lipoprotein cholesterol was as
low as 31.0 mg/100 ml, ranging from 27 mg/100 ml to 34 mg/100ml.

Case 3: 19-year-old man.

Body weight, 50 kg; height, 155 cm. He was healthy until the
age of 14, when he noticed hoarseness and bilateral cataracts. The
latter were recently treated surgically. His pigmented skin was
dried and hard, his feet were flat. Tendon reflexes at the patella,
heel and other extremities were elevated. His hair was thin and
sparse and the black colour was faded. Calcification was detected
in the Achilles tendon by X-ray examination (Fig. 4). Thus, nearly
all the symptoms of Werner's syndrome were presented. Blood
pressure was normal.

On laboratory examination, hypertriglycemia was also present.
The average level of triglyceridemia was 468 mg/100 ml, ranging from
363 mg/100 ml to over 100 mg/100 ml. The levels of total
cholesterol and phospholipid were somewhat above the normal. HDL-
cholesterol was as low as 35 mg/100 ml.

The values of serum transaminases were slightly elevated. The
level of fasting blood sugar was 112 mg/100 ml to 145 mg/100 ml and
slight glycosuria was occasionally noticed and they were decreased
towards normal values after dietary and medical treatment.

Thus, in these three cases out of 24 Werner's diseases,
hypertriglycemia was found to be the most conspicuous change of
serum lipid metabolism. Serum cholesterol and phospholipid were
somewhat elevated above the normal. The low level of serum HDL-
cholesterol seemed also to be characteristic in these patients.
The levels of serum very-low-density lipoprotein were higher than
normal. Serum pre-B-lipoprotein and B-lipoprotein increased more
than a-lipoprotein. These findings substantiated the predominance
of hypertriglyceride in the three cases of Werner's syndrome.

Serum lipoprotein lipase activity (LPL) was examined by
injecting heparin, (Novo heparin) at a dose of 125 units/kg of body
weight, to reduce serum triglyceride and to increase serum
nonesterified fatty acid (NEFA) in the two sister cases and one
female case (Fig. 9). The level of serum triglyceride decreased
approximately 20-30% of the initial level at 10 and 15 min after the
injection of heparin and more than 50% at 60 min and 120 min. This
was the same in the third case. Thus, the administration of heparin

increased the LPL activity of hypertriglyceridemia in three cases of Werner's syndrome. The reduction of hypertriglyceridemia by heparin injection resulted in the degradation of it to (NEFA). Serum NEFA level was elevated several fold at 5 min after heparin injection and

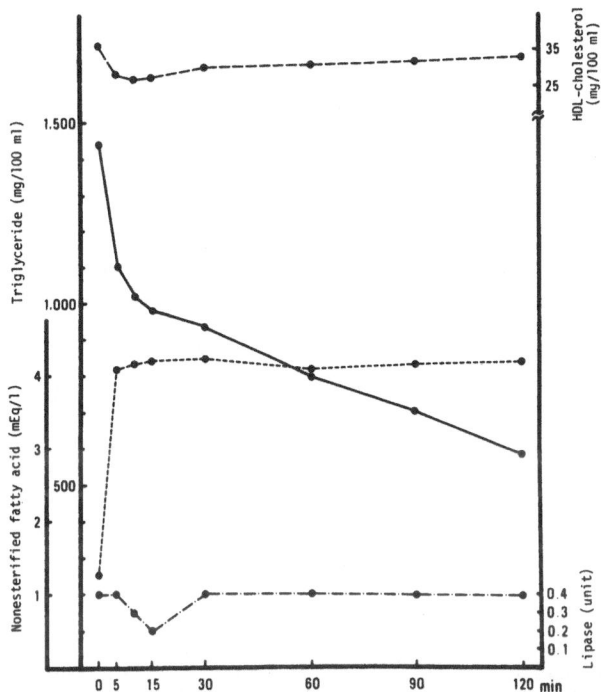

Fig. 9: Changes of plasma triglyceride and nonesterified fatty acid levels after intravenous injection of heparin (125 units/kg of body weight) in a patient with Werner's syndrome (Case 2). Note the immediate increase of nonesterified fatty acid after heparin injection and the succeeding decrease of triglycerides that continued for 120 min.

the enhanced NEFA level remained almost unchanged until 120 min. The LPL activity determined by heparin injection for the two sister cases of Werner's syndrome was less than that of diabetic patients with hypertriglyceridemia. Serum HDL-cholesterol and lipase activity decreased slightly immediately after the injection and the values returned towards the initial level.

DISCUSSION

These data indicate that (1) the obesity in the trunk and slimmed extremities as well as the xanthoma and atherosclerosis of the patients with Werner's syndrome are related to the lipid disturbance; (2) the tendency towards diabetes mellitus in the disease causes hyperlipidemia, hypertriglyceridemia in particular; and (3) the continual liver function disorder results in the lipid dysfunction.

In a clinical examination, we have studied 24 cases of Werner's syndrome that clinically coincide with those described by Epstein et al. (1966). In the serial study of Werner's syndrome, the hyperreflexibility of tendons in the extremities, flat feet and irregular tooth arrangement were frequently observed among the other usual symptoms reported previously (Epstein et al., 1966). These newly added signs were noticed at the early period of the serial field investigation and afterwards the high frequency of these three signs was confirmed. In addition, the signs of thin, sparse, and colour-faded hair could be seen in the patient of Werner's syndrome. Since these three signs can be detected so easily, they could help to diagnose Werner's syndrome. Hyperreflexibility may be due to either irritable phenomenon of the pyramidal tract or a certain constructive reaction of hard tendons. Flat feet are possibly due to the heavy body weight of fatty trunk relative to the slim legs and the poor development of foot's connective tissue. The irregular arrangement of the teeth would be a disorder of exodermal tissue with hereditary diseases. Sparse, thin, and colour-faded hair seemed to be observed more frequently in young WS patients. Therefore, the sign would be helpful as the initial sign of Werner's syndrome.

Conspicuous clinical manifestations of Werner's syndrome are summarized as follows. A high incidence of short stature, low body weight, slim limbs and fatty trunk, thin, sparse, and colour-faded hair, bilateral cataracts, and hardness of skin in the extremities was observed over 80% of the total cases. Calcification of soft tissue, atherosclerosis, and the trend towards diabetes mellitus were in low incidence.

Serum lipid levels as well as the serum data of liver function in Werner's syndrome have usually been reported to be within normal limits. In fact, not much attention has previously been paid to the disturbances of lipid metabolism and liver function. On examining the medical reports of patients with Werner's, it is apparent that a slight increase of serum lipids has only sporadically been reported. No paper has mentioned hyperlipidemia as described in this study. In addition, not much information has been available regarding liver function, although hepatomegaly was mentioned by Oppenheimer and Kugel (1941). A disorder of lipid metabolism such as extremity-elevated triglyceridemia as well as liver dysfunction would be interpreted as a facet of multiple defects of gene expression in Werner's syndrome. The elder sisters of the two sister cases did not exhibit any feature of Werner's syndrome but their serum lipid levels were found to be increased slightly, indicating an incomplete manifesation of the heriditary disorder. A moderately elevated serum cholesterol has been reported in three cases of Werner's syndrome (Zucker-Franklin et al., 1968). A case of progeria was treated by controlling lipid uptake for a long period, in which hypertrigliceridemia with elevated B-lipoprotein and pre-B-lipoprotein was reported by Macnamara et al. (1970). An abnormally high level of serum lipoprotein was reported by Rosenthal et al. (1956) in a case of progeria. At necropsy at the age of 10, left ventricular dilatation and atherosclerosis of the coronary arteries and aorta were detected. Atherosclerosis was found in progeria and in Werner's syndrome (Keay et. al., 1955).

The present study clearly indicates that a possibility of the disorder of lipid metabolism and liver function cannot be ruled out in Werner's syndrome. The elevation of triglyceride and B-lipoprotein had been shown in a case of progeria. Such a lipid disorder would be an erroneous expression of Werner's syndrome. Even so, much attention should be paid to lipid metabolism and enzymatic activity in Werner's syndrome, since the disease shows a high prevalence of atherosclerosis, diabetes mellitus, and calcium deposition in the various connective tissues (Keay et al., 1955; Epstein et al., 1966; Murata and Nakashima, 1982).

SUMMARY

In a clinical study of patients with Werner's syndrome, it became apparent that careful observation of numbers of patients could result in the addition of new or modified signs and symptoms to those already known. In addition of flat feet and hyperreflexibility, it was observed that the irregular disarrangement of the teeth and thin, sparse and colour-faded hair were frequently occurences in patients with Werner's syndrome.

In the laboratory survey, disorders of lipid metabolism and liver function were detected in 3 out of 24 cases of Werner's syndrome. It was concluded that the disturbances of lipid metabolism result in part from moderate liver dysfunction.

Acknowledgements. The authors are grateful to Drs. T. Motokura, R. Abe, H. Matsuo, T. Ishi, K. Togawa and M. Sugioka for valuable suggestions. We express our thanks also to Misses K. Yamakita and Y. Kira for secretarial assistance.

REFERENCES

Epstein, C.J., Martin, G.M., Schultz, A.L., and Motulsky, A.G., 1966, Werner's syndrome: a review of its symptomatology, natural history, pathologic features, genetics and relationship to the natural aging process, Medicine, 45:177.

Irwin, G.W., and Ward, P.B., 1953, Werner's syndrome with a report of two cases, Am. J. Med., 15:266.

Goto, M., and Murata, K., 1977, Clinical and biochemical studies of Werner's syndrome, J. Jap. Geriatr. Soc., 14:450.

Keay, A.J., Oliver, M.F., and Boyd, G.S., 1955, Progeria and atherosclerosis, Arc. Dis. Child., 30:410.

Macnamara, B.G.P., Farm, K.T., Mitra, A.K., Lloyd, J.K., and Fosbrooke, A.S., 1970, Progeria case report with long-term studies of serum lipids, Arch. Dis. Childh., 45:553.

Murata, K., 1982, Urinary glycosaminoglycans in Werner's syndrome, Experientia, 38:313.

Murata, K., 1983, A disturbance of serum lipids in three cases of Werner's syndrome, Gerontology, 29:131.

Murata K., and Nakashima, H., 1982, 24 cases of Werner's syndrome: with a clinical review of the Japanese medical literature, Am. Geriatr. Soc., 30:303.

Nakazawa, K., and Murata, K., 1981, Epidemiological study of serum high density lipoprotein cholesterol with respect to risk factors against ischemic heart disease and atherosclerosis, Tohoku J. Exp. Med., 133:197.

Oppenheimer, B.S., and Kugel, V.H., 1934, Werner's syndrome: heredofamilial disorders with scleroderma, bilateral juvenile cataract, precocious greying of the hair and endocrine stigmatization, Trans. Assn. Am. Physns., 49:358.

Oppenheimer, B.S., and Kugel, V.H., 1941, Werner's syndrome: Report of the first necropsy and of findings in a new case, Am. J. Med. Sci., 202:629.

Reaven, G.M., and Vernstein, R.M., 1978, Effects of obesity on the relationship between very low density lipoprotein production rate and plasma triglyceride concentration in normal and hypertriglyceridemic subjects, Metab. Clin. Exp., 27:1047.

Rosenthal, L.M., Bernstein, I.P., Dallenbach, F.D., Pruzansky, S., and Rosenwald, 1956, Progeria: report of a case with cephalometric roentgenograms and abnormally high concentrations of lipoproteins in serum, Pediatrics, 18:565.

Thannhauser, S.J., 1945, Werner's syndrome (progeria of adults) and Rothmund's syndrome: 2 types of closely related herodofamilial atrophic dermatoses with juvenile cataracts and endocrine features: critical study iwth 5 new cases, Ann. Intern. Med., 23:559.

Valero, A., and Gellei, B., 1960, Retinitis pigmentosa, hypertension and uremia in Werner's syndrome: report of a case, with necropsy findings, Br. Med. J., 2:351.

Werner, C.W., 1904, Uber Katarakt in Verbindung mit Sklerodermie, Diss., Kiel.

Zackai, A.H., and Noth, R., 1974, cardiac findings in Werner's syndrome, Geriatrics, 29:141.

Zucker-Franklin, D., Rifkin, H., and Jacobson, H.G., 1968, Werner's syndrome. An analysis of ten cases, Geriatrics, 23:123

GROWTH CHARACTERISTICS OF WERNER SYNDROME CELLS IN VITRO

Darrell Salk*, Eileen Bryant*, Holger Hoehn+, Patricia
Johnston*, and George M. Martin*

* Department of Pathology, University of Washington
+ Department of Human Genetics, University of Wuerzburg

INTRODUCTION

Cultured skin fibroblast-like (FL) cells from patients with
Werner syndrome grow poorly: reduced growth potential has been
reported by more than 11 laboratories for cultures from more than
26 patients, using many different tissue culture media. This
characteristic is of importance to research in Werner syndrome for
several reasons. It remains to be determined whether poor growth
is a primary or a secondary manifestation of the basic molecular
defect, and the relationship is not yet clear between reduced
growth of cultured skin fibroblasts and the other manifestations of
Werner syndrome in vitro and in vivo. This characteristic also
makes it difficult to obtain sufficient growth for clonal studies
or for biochemical studies that require a large number of cells.

When evaluating the results of studies using Werner syndrome
FL cells, it is important to bear in mind several caveats about the
relationships among experimental models. Although Werner syndrome
patients appear superficially to be prematurely aged, it is evident
that Werner syndrome is not actually a condition of rapidly
progressive, but otherwise normal aging. Similarly, the in vitro
behavior of Werner syndrome FL cells appears superficially to be a
rapidly progressive form of the in vitro senescence of normal FL
cells, but it is not yet known whether Werner syndrome FL cell
"senescence" is really due to the same or a different process; it
is possible that Werner syndrome FL cells cease proliferation as a
result of some defect or injury that is different from the causes

305

of normal in vitro senescence. Finally, the relationship between
aging in vivo and cell senescence in vitro remains to be fully
understood. Thus, while it is likely that studies of Werner
syndrome in vivo and in vitro will yield information that is
relevant to an understanding of biological aging, specific
geriatric diseases, and the control of cellular growth, one should
be wary of considering it an exact model for either aging in vivo
or cellular senescence in vitro until these processes are more
fully understood.

In our laboratory we previously studied the growth of 20
independently derived skin FL cell strains from three patients with
Werner syndrome in comparison with the growth of ten FL cell
strains from non-Werner patients (Salk et al, 1981a). Population
growth rates and total replicative lifespans of Werner syndrome
strains averaged 55 percent and 27 percent, respectively, of the
growth rates and lifespans of non-Werner strains. In the first few
passages, four Werner syndrome cultures had population growth rates
in the low normal range, but the longest lived Werner syndrome
strain had only 75 percent of the total replicative lifespan of the
shortest lived normal strain.

Exponential growth rates, cloning efficiencies, and saturation
densities of Werner syndrome FL cell strains were also reduced,
whereas cell attachment was normal. Viable cells, identified by dye
exclusion, were maintained in postreplicative Werner syndrome and
control cultures for periods of at least ten months: there was no
evidence of accelerated postreplicative senescence or cell death of
Werner syndrome FL cells. Co-cultivation of Werner syndrome and
normal strains did not influence population growth rates of either
strain. Two proliferating hybrid clones were obtained from fusions
of normal and Werner syndrome FL cells and these hybrids displayed
the reduced growth potential typical of Werner syndrome FL cells.
These and other studies related to growth control of Werner
syndrome FL cells have been recently reviewed (Salk, 1982).

We describe here preliminary results that shed some light on
two questions regarding the growth of Werner syndrome cells: the
similarities and differences between the in vitro senescence of
Werner and non-Werner FL cells, and whether reduced growth
potential is manifested by any tissue other than FL cells.

IN VITRO SENESCENCE AND NUCLEAR MORPHOLOGY

As normal FL cells senesce in vitro, they gradually become
larger, less regular in shape, and accumulate cytoplasmic fibrils.
Werner syndrome FL cells assume this "senescent morphology" more
rapidly than normal cells. Normal proliferating FL cells can be
induced to assume a senescent morphology by depriving them of serum

and thus arresting their growth. Not only do serum starved cells
appear senescent, but they behave like senescent cells in fusions
with proliferating diploid FL cells and with heteroploid
(neoplastoid) HeLa cells (Rabinovitch and Norwood, 1980). It has
been suggested that the mechanisms of arrest in senescent and serum
starved cells may share a final common pathway.

   We had previously noted, but not quantitated, abnormal nuclear
morphology developing in aging cultures of both normal and Werner
syndrome cells as the thymidine labeling index declined. Matsumura
et al. (1979) reported an increase in abnormal nuclear morphology,
principally binucleation, in aging cultures of WI-38 and WI-26. To
explore the question of the relationship between the "senescence"

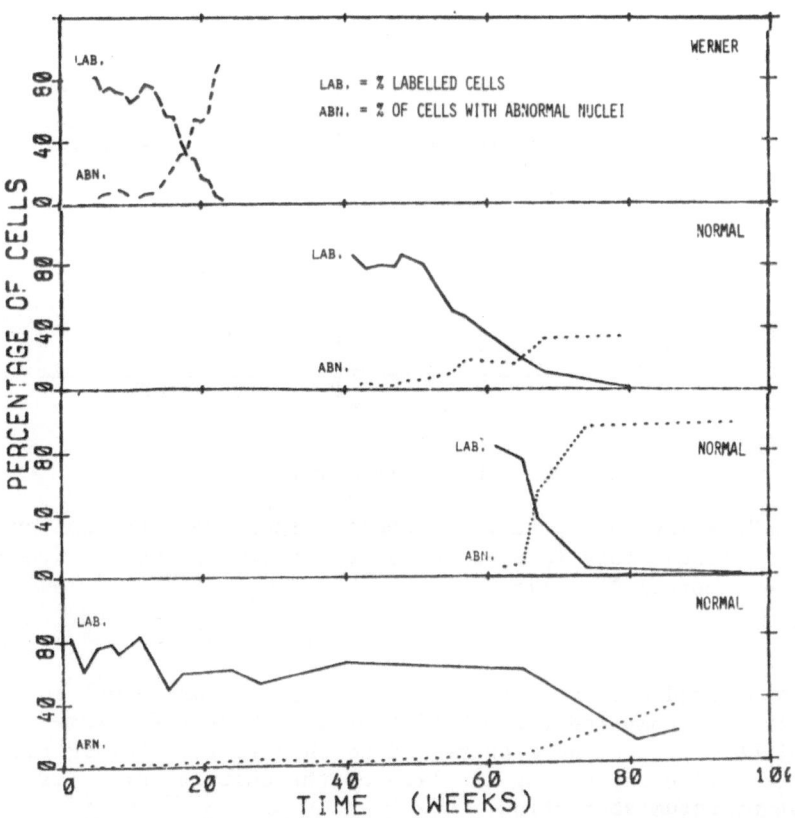

Figure 1. Tritiated thymidine labeling index and the percentage of
          abnormal nuclei in representative strains of Werner
          syndrome and normal FL cells during in vitro aging.

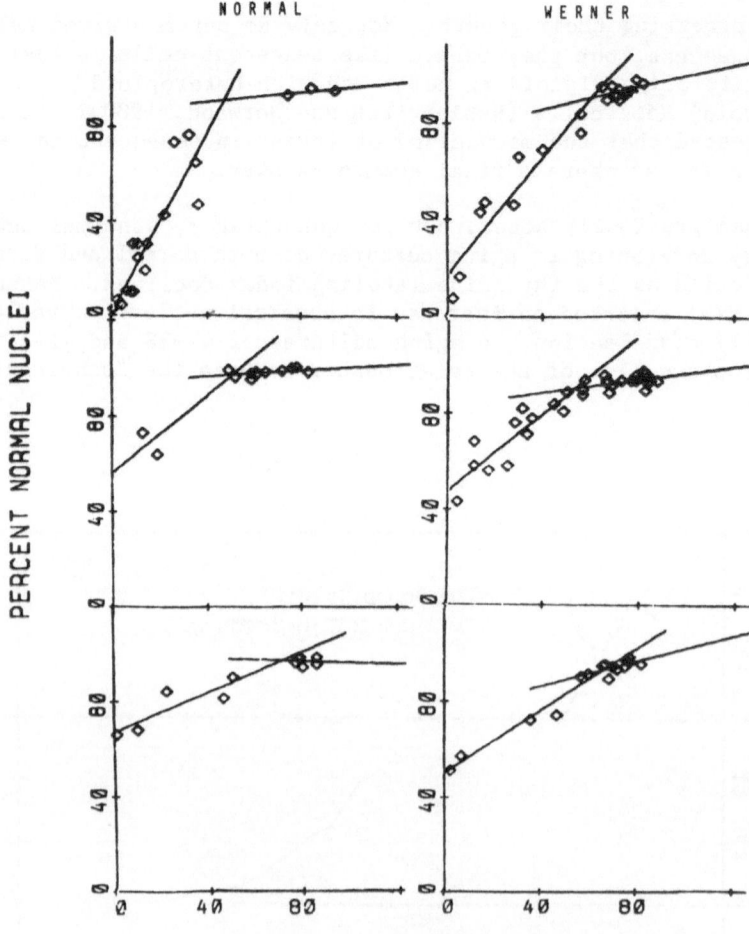

Figure 2. Relationship between labeling index and abnormal nuclear
          morphology in representative strains of Werner syndrome and
          normal FL cells.

of Werner syndrome FL cells and the senescence of normal FL cells
in vitro, we compared the behavior of five Werner syndrome and ten
normal FL cell strains with regard to changes in labeling index and
nuclear morphology during the life of the cultures or after growth
arrest by serum starvation.

     Cultures were maintained by regular weekly passage using
routine tissue culture techniques. In some normal strains,

passaging was routinely performed when confluence was achieved. At
the time of passaging, 35 mm plastic petri dishes containing
sterile coverslips were seeded with 5,000 to 10,000 cells. For
serum starvation studies, these cells were allowed to attach
overnight, then rinsed with serum-free medium and maintained in
medium containing 0.1 percent fetal calf serum until labeling.
Cells from routine aging cultures were allowed to attach overnight
and then were pulsed with tritiated-thymidine (1 microcurie/ml) for
48 hours. The coverslips were serially dehydrated in ethanol,
fixed with Bouin's fixative, and processed by routine
autoradiographic techniques. After developing, the slides were
stained with hemotoxylin-eosin and scored microscopically for
nuclear morphology and nuclear labeling. Cells were scored as
having normal nuclear morphology, binucleation, polynucleation,
micronucleation, or other aberrant nuclear shape.

    Both normal and Werner syndrome FL cells demonstrate an
increase in abnormal nuclear morphology with increasing in vitro
age (Figure 1). In early passages two to ten percent of cells have
aberrant nuclear morphology, compared with 50-90 percent in late
passage cells. There is a marked change in the accumulation of
cells with aberrant nuclear morphology after the labeling index of
a culture becomes less than 50 percent (Figure 2). Strains differ
with respect to the relationship between labeling index and nuclear
morphology, as indicated by the different slopes in the left-hand
portions of the scattergrams in figure 2.

    The development of abnormal nuclear morphology is not simply
related to a reduction in replication activity. Early passage
normal cells that are growing poorly due to serum starvation for
many weeks may show normal nuclear morphology despite their low
labeling indices and the otherwise "senescent" appearance of their
cytoplasm (Table 1). After two to four weeks in medium with 0.1%

Table 1.   Percentage of normal nuclei in cultures derived from a
           single tissue sample. Results are shown when cultures were
           growing normally during routine aging and when cultures
           were growing poorly after serum deprivation for one to six
           weeks.

Labeling index	Aging	Serum starved
	(N=21)	(N=7)
0-20%	15	94
20-40%	61	--
40-70%	--	--
>70%	94	--

serum, some FL cell strains do show a reduction in the number of cells with normal nuclear morphology, but others show only a gradual change even after six to nine weeks of serum deprivation; typical senescent morphology appears after one to two weeks (data not shown).

In summary, in aging cultures of skin FL cells, nuclear morphology becomes increasingly aberrant when fewer than 50 percent of cells enter S-phase during a 48 hour period. The cause-effect relationship between decreasing labeling index and aberrant nuclear morphology is unclear, but the relationship differs quantitatively from strain to strain. Werner syndrome FL cells behave similarly to normal FL cells, albeit more rapidly. These studies do not reveal any qualitative difference between the processes of senescence in Werner syndrome and normal FL cell cultures.

Changes in nuclear morphology in serum starved cells do not occur concomitantly with changes in cytoplasmic morphology; proliferation ceases long before nuclear morphology degenerates, unlike the situation in senescing cells. In spite of similar microscopic and ultrastructural appearances of the cytoplasm, and in spite of similar behavior in heterokaryon fusions, serum starved cells appear to undergo a process that is not identical to that of senescing cells, although some steps in the processes might be shared.

Table 2. Growth of EB virus transformed lymphoblastoid cell lines. All cultures except for the normal established line ceased replication after the number of doublings and number of days indicated.

	Population doublings per day	Cumulative population doublings	Cumulative days in culture
Normal	0.72	180+	256+
Werner syndrome brother	0.64	158	254
Werner syndrome patients			
(DC)	--	--	66
(KL)	0.44	54	106
(TB)	0.44	88	193

REDUCED GROWTH OF LYMPHOBLASTOID CELL LINES

EB virus transformed lymphoblastoid cells are generally considered to be continuously propagating cell lines with an indefinite in vitro lifespan. Nevertheless, two such lines derived from patients with Werner syndrome grew poorly and ceased replicating while we were maintaining them for cytogenetic studies.

We subsequently repeated the observation using cells that had been cryogenically preserved shortly after we obtained the original cultures and by using a third cell line derived from another Werner patient. Although an established line derived from a non-Werner patient grew continuously in the laboratory at the same time, all Werner lymphoblastoid cell lines died out (Table 2.) In addition, one cell line derived from the brother of a Werner patient ceased replicating; siblings of Werner patients have a 67% chance of being heterozygous for the Werner syndrome gene. The growth rates of the Werner cultures were less than those of the normal and the Werner syndrome sibling.

We are currently obtaining additional Werner and normal lymphoblastoid cell lines to determine if these preliminary observations can be confirmed. If so, this will be evidence that reduced growth potential is manifested by more than one tissue type in Werner syndrome. If the gene defect is expressed by lymphoblastoid cell lines, they may prove to be useful for studies aimed at elucidating the basic molecular defect in Werner syndrome.

REFERENCES

Matsumura, T., Zerrudo, Z., Hayflick, L. (1979). Senescent human diploid cells in culture: Survival, DNA synthesis and morphology. J. Gerontol. 34:328-334.
Rabinovitch, P. S., Norwood, T. H. (1980). Comparative heterokaryon study of cellular senescence and the serum-deprived state. Exp. Cell Res. 130:101-109.
Salk, D., Bryant, E., Hoehn, H., Martin, G. M. (1981), Systematic growth studies, cocultivation, and cell hybridization studies of Werner syndrome cultured skin fibroblasts. Hum. Genet. 58:310-316.
Salk, D. (1982). Werner's syndrome: A review of recent research with an analysis of connective tissue metabolism, growth control of cultured cells, and chromosomal aberrations. um. Genet. 62:1-15.

STUDIES OF SV40-INFECTED WERNER SYNDROME FIBROBLASTS

Toshiharu Matsumura, Masato Nagata, Ryuji Konishi*
and Makoto Goto**

Department of Cancer Cell Research*
Institute of Medical Science
University of Tokyo
Shirokanedai, Minato-ku, Tokyo 108

Department of Internal Medicine and Physical Therapy**
Faculty of Medicine
University of Tokyo
Bunkyo-ku, Tokyo 113, Japan

ABSTRACT

Skin fibroblasts from patients with the Werner syndrome (WS) and fibroblasts from normal donors were infected with SV40 of a wild type strain (777) or of a temperature-sensitive mutant strain (tsA900). The infected WS cells and the infected normal cells proliferated at permissive temperatures, and then entered into "crisis" in which state they ceased proliferation. In their proliferative phase, both WS and normal cells infected with tsA900 proliferated rapidly at 34°C, but their proliferation slowed down at 39°C. Some lines of infected WS cultures accrued more population doublings before they entered into "crisis" than uninfected WS cells. Among 13 series of infected cultures, one line, which had been infected with 777, passed through "crisis" and proliferated indefinitely. This line (PSV811) was from a 29-year-old female WS patient. We compared a cloned line of PSV811 with a permanent line of SV40-infected WI-38 normal human fibroblasts (VA13 2RA). Cells of both lines, PSV811 and VA13, were epithelioid, did not shed viruses into the culture medium, and their chromosome number distributed broadly across the diploid range. An autoradiographic study suggested that both lines are capable of unscheduled DNA synthesis. In both

313

cultures, the rate of proliferation depended on the concentration
of fetal bovine serum in culture medium. However, the PSV811
cells grew slower, and produced colonies with fewer cells than
did VA13 cells. The frequency of sister chromatid exchange was
about 70% higher in PSV811 than in VA13. In an adjunct paper,
Murata and others report that the percentage of hyaluronic acid
in total acidic glycosaminoglycans released into culture medium
was larger in PSV811 than in VA13. We concluded from these
results that PSV811 is not a contaminant of VA13, that an SV40
infection partly modify the proliferative characteristics of WS
cells, and that SV40-infected WS cells and permanent lines
obtained therefrom, are useful in furthering the study of WS.

INTRODUCTION

     For the study of the Werner syndrome, skin fibroblasts
grown in tissue culture are useful. WS fibroblasts differ from
normal fibroblasts in several respects: Their doubling potential
is less than that of normal fibroblasts (Martin et al., 1965,
1970). Some of their enzymes are more heat-sensitive that those
of normal cells (Holliday et al., 1974; Goldstein and Moerman
1975). They synthesize DNA slower than normal cells (Fujiwara et
al., 1977). They have a longer S phase than normal cells
(Shimada, 1977; Takeuchi et al., 1983). The distance between
initiation points of DNA synthesis is longer than that of normal
cells (Takeuchi et al., 1982). They show variegated
translocation mosaicism (Hoehn et al., 1975; Salk et al., 1981a).
Furthermore, the lineage of the stem cells changes during serial
passages of an WS cell population more frequently than during
those of a normal cell population (Salk et al., 1981a, 1981b).
Although the results of genetic analysis are compatible with WS
being inherited as autosomal recessive trait (Epstein et al.,
1966; Goto et al., 1981), the molecular mechanisms involved in
these diverse defects (all of which as a result from single-gene
mutation) have not been clarified.

     Our current approach to the problem of WS is to perturb the
genetic background of WS cells by infecting them with SV40. An
introduction of SV40 genes into non-permissive or semi-permissive
cells is known to enhance the activity of several cellular
enzymes, and to transform them either transiently or permanently
(Topp et al., 1981). In case of human fibroblasts, an SV40
infection enhances the rate of their proliferation, and sometimes
leads them into indefinitely proliferative (permanent) cell lines
(Shein et al., 1964; Moyer et al., 1964; Girardi et al., 1965,
1966). A permanent cell line may be useful in the study of WS,
because uninfected WS cells have only limited potential to
proliferate by themselves. Infecting several lines of WS cells,
we have obtained one permanent line so far. In this paper, we

partly characterize the infected WS cells and the permanent WS
cell line.

MATERIALS AND METHODS

Fibroblast Cultures

The clinical features of WS patients and materials for
fibroblast-like cell cultures from these patients were described
previously (Table 1. Refer also to Goto et al., 1978, 1981;
Matsumura et al., 1980). Skin cells were grown either in
plastic dishes or in T25 flasks containing Eagle's MEM
supplemented with 10 v/v per cent heat-inactivated fetal bovine
serum (FBS, Gibco, Grand Island, NY), nonessential amino acids
(Gibco), and 60 μg/ml kanamycin (growth medium). GRC202 and
GRC196 were from Dr. Youji Mitsui, TMIG.

Infection with SV40

Stocks of a wild type SV40 (strain 777) and its temperature-
sensitive mutant (tsA900) were from Dr. Nobuo Yamaguchi, IMS
(Yamaguchi and Kuchino, 1975). For infection, an T25-flask
culture was incubated for 2 h with viruses of approximately 10
multiplicity of infection, and then incubated in the growth
medium. A culture infected with tsA900 was incubated at 34°C
(permissive temperature). Other cultures were incubated at 37°C.

Infected or uninfected cultures were transferred by
trypsinization. Some infected cultures at their early stages
were exceptionally transferred by the use of dispase (Godo Shusei
Co., Tokyo) instead of trypsin. Dispase was used because it is
active in the growth medium and less toxic to cells than trypsin
during prolonged incubation with this protease (Matsumura et al.,
1975a, b). When a culture did not grow after a split during two
to four weeks of succeeding incubation, the culture was
considered to have attained its highest population doublings
(HPDs). 777-infected lines of S770811, S771216, S781005,
S790305M, S790305W, GRC196, and GRC202 (Refer to Table 1) will
respectively be designated as SV811, SV1216, SV1005, SV305M,
SV305W, SV196, and SV202. tsA900-infected lines of S781005,
S790305M, S790305W, GRC196, and GRC202 will respectively be
designated as TS1005, TS305M, TS305W, TS196, and TS202.

To examine culture fluid for the presence of infectious
viruses, we exposed CV1 African green monkey kidney cells,
supplied from Dr. Paul Berg, Stanford University School of
Medicine, to the spent medium of an infected culture. The CVI
culture was incubated and then examined for the presence of
cytopathy. We examined cells for the presence of T antigen by

the method of indirect immunofluorescence, using anti-SV40-T
hamster serum (from Dr. Sumio Sugano, IMS), and FITC conjugated
anti-hamster IGG (rabbit, Med. Biol. Lab., Ltd., Nagoya).

Infected Cell Lines

The permanently growing WS line, which was obtained after
777 infection in this study, will be referred to tentatively as
PSV811. A clone of PSV811 (PSV811 el) was obtained by the use of
a colony-isolation technique, and was used in most experiments in
this study. VA13 2RA, which was obtained from SV40-transformed
WI-38 human diploid lung fibroblasts (Girardi et al., 1966), was
from Dr. Leonard Hayflick, Center for Gerontological Studies,
University of Florida.

To determine the distribution of clonogenicity among cells,
we grew cells in colonies in 6-cm plastic dishes for two weeks,
fixed them, stained them with Giemsa solution, and counted the
cells in each and every colony in a dish.

To estimate the ability of unscheduled DNA synthesis, we
inoculated cells into chambered slides (no4804 Lab Tek Product,
Naperville), incubated them for one day in a subconfluent state
in the growth medium and again for an additional one day in the
growth medium supplemented with 10 mM hydroxyurea. On the third
day of incubation, the cultures were incubated in hydroxyurea-
containing medium, with or without 10^{-5}M 4-nitroquinoline-N-oxide
(4NQO), and with tritiated thymidine (0.5 μCi/ml or 2.0 μCi/ml
[^{3}H]-TdR, 47 μCi/mmole, Amersham Int. Ltd., Amersham, U.K.) for 3
h. The medium with 4NQO and the control medium without it
contained 0.1% ethanol as solvent for 4NQO. After the
incubation, the chambered slides were fixed in Carnoy's solution,
washed, dried, and covered with nuclear emulsion (NR-M2,
Konishiroku Photo Ind., Tokyo). After exposure for 8 days in the
dark, the slides were processed for autoradiography. The number
of grains in a nucleus and the area of the nucleus were
respectively determined on these slides by means of a microscopic
image analyser (VIP-21CH, Olympus, Tokyo).

The frequency of sister-chromatid exchange (SCE) was
determined by a modification of the previously described method
(Perry and Wolff, 1974; Schneider et al., 1978). Cells plated in
dishes were proliferated for two cell cycles in growth medium
supplemented with bromodeoxyuridine (BrdU) of varying
concentration. The cells were incubated for additional 3 h in
the presence of colcemide (0.1 μg/ml), and then subjected to a
routine procedure of chromosome preparation. A chromosome
preparation on a slide glass was stained with Hoechst 33258 (Wako
Pure Chem. Inc., Osaka), exposed to ultraviolet light, and then
stained with Giemsa solution for the determination of the number
of SCE in mitotic figures.

RESULTS

Evidence for Transformation

Table 1 shows the population doublings (PDs) accrued by the cell lines infected with either 777 or tsA900, or not infected. We studied SV811, SV305M, TS305M, and TS305W mostly, because their considerable lifespan was before they entered "crisis". In these infected cultures, foci of densely proliferative cells appeared after a few weeks of incubation. In an early transfer after infection, we incubated cells in a high density in order for transformed cells to proliferate on top of untransformed cells. In a couple of serial transfers, small and proliferative cells predominated in these infected cultures. They produced acids more rapidly than did cells in uninfected cultures. Thereafter, we transferred them at high split ratios. In as many infected cell cultures as were tested, i.e., SV811, TS305W, SV305M, and TS305M, T antigen-positive cells dominated the cell populations. The tsA900-infected lines, TS305M and TS305W, grew at 34°C. However, their proliferation slowed down at 39°C (non-permissive temperature) (Fig. 1). When a tsA900-infected culture ceased proliferation at 39°C, we noticed that the cells did not reach confluency, but became large. Results from the above two lines show that the lines infected with tsA900 were transformed by the viruses and that the proliferation of transformed cells depended on A-gene expression.

We did not examine SV1216, SV1005, and SV202 in detail. However, because of the similarity in morphology, acid production, and growth characteristics among these infected lines, we considered all these infected cell lines, except for infected GRC196 cells, as transformed at their permissive temperatures. SV40-infected GRC196 did not proliferate vigorously after infection. They might have contained some transformed cells, but were not studied in detail.

Proliferative Potential of Infected Cell Lines

We noticed that some infected WS cell lines proliferated for more than 30 PDs (Table 1). The highest population doubling (HPD) reached 56 in one cell line, a value never reported for an uninfected culture of WS fibroblasts. Sometimes we transferred two or more lines of cultures from one infected culture. The HPD values varied among them. Table 1 lists the highest values. As described above, an infected culture contained only a small number of infected foci in an early phase of infection. In addition, to make transformed cells, we transferred a culture at small split ratios in its early phase of infection. Therefore, an HPD value in Table 1 gives an estimation of the minimum potential of population doublings for an infected cell line.

Table 1. HIGHEST POPULATION DOUBLINGS (HPDs) ATTAINED BY CELLS WITH OR WITHOUT SV40 INFECTION

	Donor age	Sex	Patient code	Clinical data[a]	Pedigree chart[b]	Sample code	HPD (PD at the time of infection)		
							No infection	777 infection	tsA900 infection
WS	19	M	WS1TYO	1	1	S790305W	14[c]	30 (7)	38 (7)
	29	F	WS2TYO	4	4	S770811	9	56[d](3)	-
	42[e]	M	WS3TYO	9	9	S770715	22	-	-
	43	M	WS6TYO	-	16	S781005	-	19 (4)	25 (4)
	48	M	WS4TYO	11	11	S770926	9	-	-
	60	M	WS5TYO	15	15	S771216	-	24 (6)	-
	64	M	WS8TYO	-	18	S800703	15[c]	-	-
Normal	26	F				S790305M	47[c]	45 (4)	40 (13)
	40	M				GRC202	-	55 (29)	48[f](29)
	83	M				GRC196	-	35 (32)	37 (32)

a. Patient number in Goto et al., 1978.

b. Pedigree chart number in Goto et al., 1981.

c. Determined by Dr. Tadao Ohno.

d. This line, i.e., SV811 resumed proliferation after "crisis" as a permanent line, i.e., PSV811.

e. Estimated age.

f. This line was terminated close to, but before, "crisis."

Establishment of a Permanent WS Cell Line

Fig. 2 shows the passage profile of an SV811 line. This line entered into "crisis" and then proliferated again. After being released from "crisis", this line continued proliferation for more than 100 PDs. We refer to this line after it passed through "crisis" as PSV811. Because we kept the VA13 cell line in our laboratory, we needed to check whether PSV811 is a contaminant of VA13 or not.

Comparison of VA13 and PSV811

PSV811 grew slower than VA13 in the growth medium. The population doubling times, as averages determined from two independent replicate culture experiments, were 22.8 h for VA13 and 24 h for PSV811. VA13 cells formed larger colonies than did PSV811 cells; this was evident during the serial transfers of the two cell lines. Histograms of the number of cells in a colony were obtained after 2 weeks of colony formation, showing that the average number of cells in an PSV811 colony is smaller than that in a VA13 colony (Fig. 3). In addition, PSV811 contained a larger percentage of cells that did not form colonies and were lost from the culture during incubation than did VA13 (refer to the legends for Fig. 3). When the cells were incubated in medium containing FBS, the concentration of which ranged between 1 and 10 per cent, the proliferation of both PSV811 and VA13 increased with the concentration of serum (Fig. 4). The two profiles, one for PSV811 and the other for VA13, of the rate of the proliferation were parallel within this range of FBS concentration. This result did not support the possibility that VA13 and PSV811 have different sensitivities to the growth-enhancing effects of FBS.

In the distribution of chromosome number, the two lines were similar (Fig. 5). In both, the distribution was broadly across the diploid range. In morphology, both VA23 cells and PSV811 cells were epithelioid (Fig. 6). We noticed that PSV811 cells were subtly smaller than VA13 was, although their cell volume was not determined. Neither VA13 cells nor PSV811 cells shed infectious viruses into the culture medium, as could be detected by the method described earlier. We noticed, however, that during the proliferative phase of SV811 infectious viruses were shed into culture medium. In both cultures of PSV811 and VA13, T antigen-positive cells predominated (Fig. 6). These results show that PSV811, like VA13, is a non-producing cell line containing at least a part of the SV40 genes.

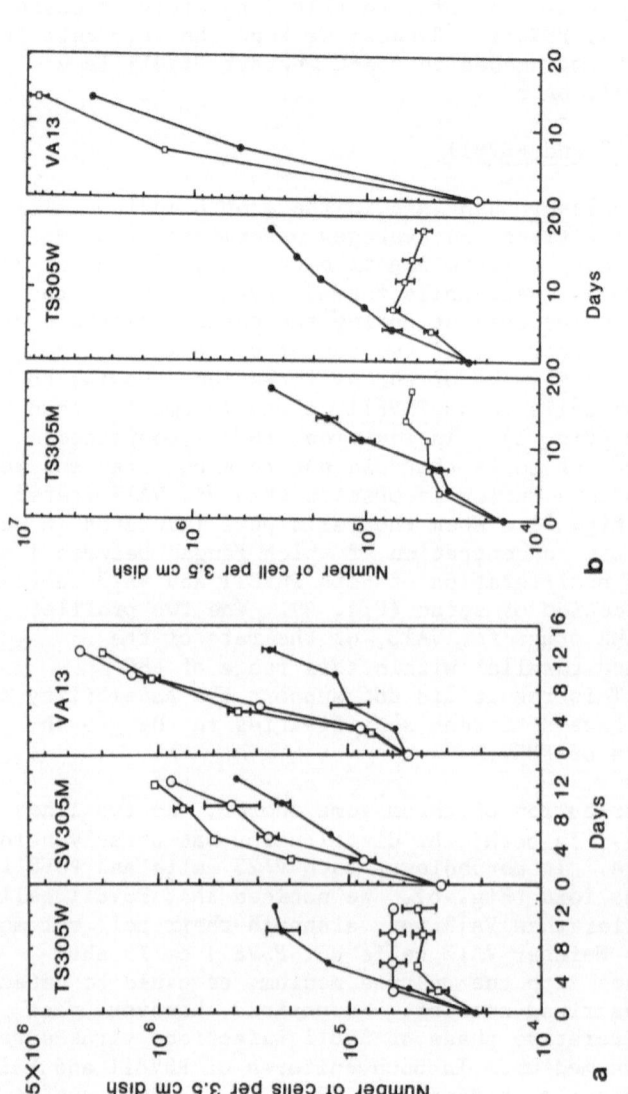

Fig. 1 Proliferation profiles of SV40-infected cells. The first three columns and the last three columns of this figure are from independent experiments. The columns represent, respectively: cultures of TS305M, SV305W and TS305M in their growing phase (left and center), and of permanently growing VA 13 (right). ● , at 34°C; ○ , at 37°C; □ , at 39°C.

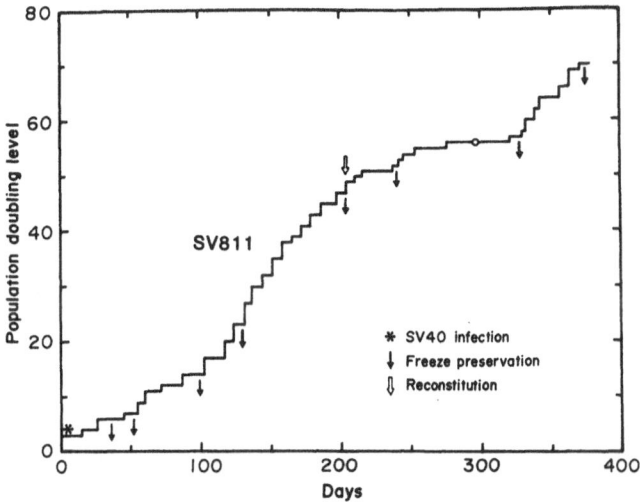

Fig. 2. Passage profile of SV811. *, the time when the cells
were infected with 777; ↓ , the time when a part of the
culture was kept frozen; ⇓ , the time when the culture
was reconstituted from a frozen ampule; -o-, 1:1 split.
After a period of crisis, cells of this line resumed
proliferation. These cells proliferated indefinitely as
described in text, and are referred to thereafter as
PSV811.

The grain numbers, which were counted from radioautograms
after exposure of the cells to [3H]-TdR in the presence of
hydroxyurea, are shown in Fig. 7. In both lines, PSV811 and
VA13, the grains per unit area of nucleus were distributed
broadly. Exposure of cells to 4NQO increased the number of grain
in both cell lines, but we did not notice any difference between
the two lines either in the distribution or in the mean number of
grains per unit area. These results did not suggest any
difference between the two lines in their ability to undergo
unscheduled DNA synthesis.

Because the number of chromosomes varied among the cells of
both lines, we show in Fig. 8 the frequency of SCE by the number
of SCE per chromosome. This value fluctuated also among the
cells in both lines. We observed, however, that the frequency of
SCE was about 70% higher in PSV811 cells than in VA13 cells
within the range of the BrdU concentration used, and that the
frequency distributed more widely in PSV811 than in VA13 (Table
2).

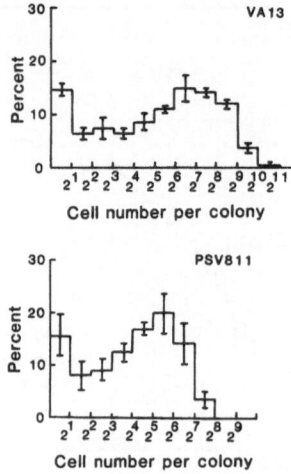

Fig. 3.   Histograms of the number of cells in a colony. The
         number of cells in a colony (± SE) is an average from
         those from three dishes. Four hundred cells were
         inoculated into each of the 6-cm dishes. The numbers of
         colony counted in a dish were 113, 126, and 151 for
         PSV811, and 151, 158, and 217 for VA13. These
         histograms are from one of two independent experiments.
         The results from the other experiment were very similar
         and are not shown.

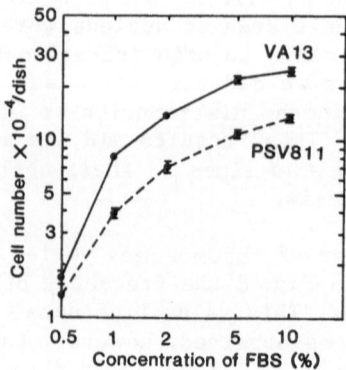

Fig. 4.   Dependency of the rate of cell proliferation on the
         concentration of FBS in the culture medium. Cells
         (2×10^4) were inoculated into each of the 3.5-cm dishes
         and incubated for 7 days for cell counting.

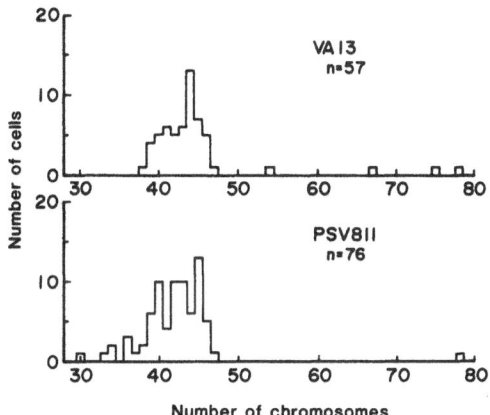

Fig. 5. Histograms of chromosome number.

Results of a routine bacteriological test for mycoplasma were negative for both PSV811 and VA13 cultures.

DISCUSSION

Establishment of a Permanent WS Line

As shown in RESULTS, PSV811 was similar in many respects to VA13. Both are epithelioid, do not produce SV40, and have chromosome numbers ranging broadly in the diploid range. Their proliferation depended similarly on the concentration of FBS in the culture medium. In addition, the present results suggest that the two lines have a similar ability to undergo unscheduled DNA synthesis after being exposed to 4NQO. The two lines, however, differed in their rates of proliferation, in clonogenicity, in the frequency of SCE and, although subtly, in morphology. The passage profile with which PSV811 was established was typical of that for an SV40-transformed human fibroblast line (Girardi et al., 1965). Because of this, we regard PSV811 in this paper not as a contaminant of VA13 but as a permanent line of WS origin. However, characterization of PSV811 is still only partial. This cell line awaits detailed analysis, particularly regarding its karyology and its virology.

As an established WS cell line, PSV811 showed several properties (see RESULTS) that are possibly related to the genetic defects in WS and could serve as a useful material for furthering

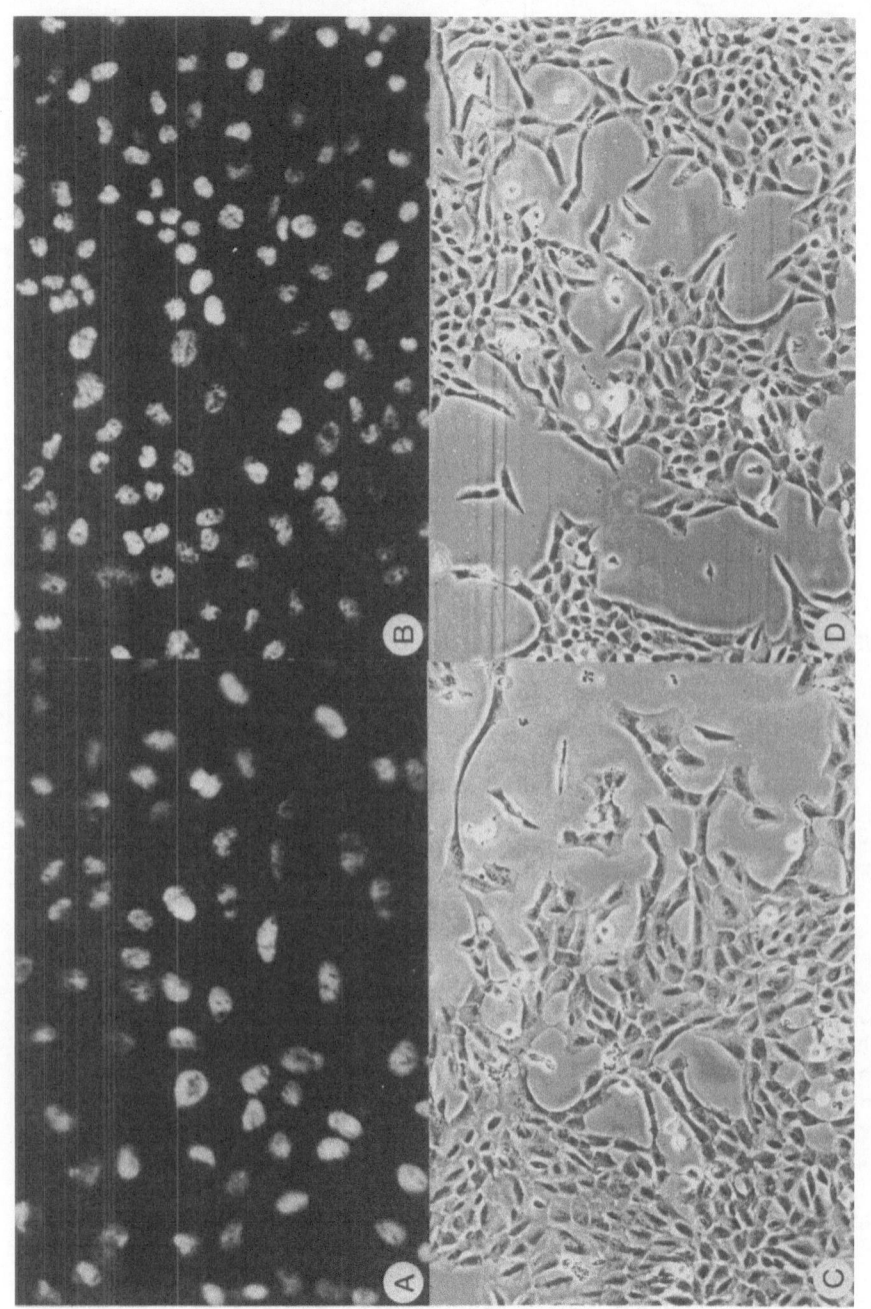

Fig. 6 Micrographs showing fluorescent T antigen-positive cells in (A), VA13; (B), PSV811; and phase-contrast micrographs of (C), VA13; and (D), PSV811.

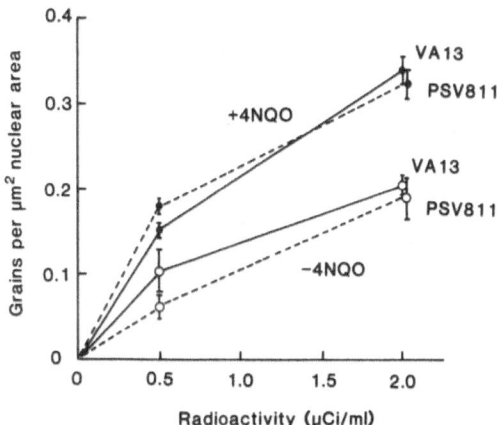

Fig. 7.   The number of grains per unit nuclear area in
          autoradiograms expressed as a function of radioactivity
          of [³]-TdR to which cells were exposed in the presence
          of hydroxyurea.

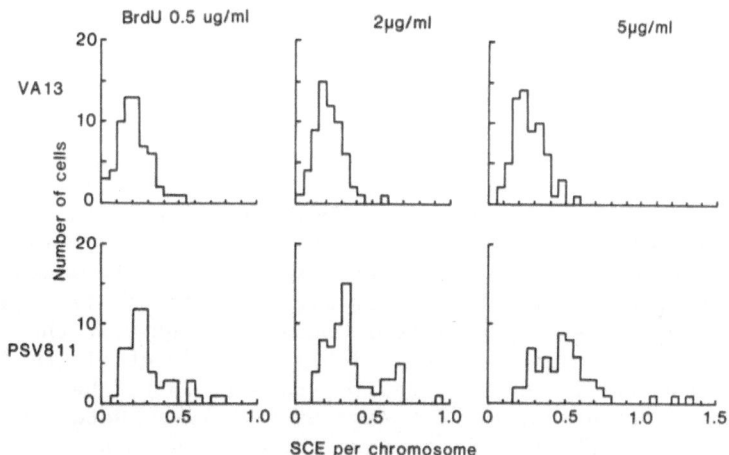

Fig. 8.   Histograms of the frequency of sister chromatid
          exchange. Data in this figure and those of Exp. 2 in
          Table 2 are from the same experiment.

the study of WS. It has been reported that untransformed WS
fibroblasts have a longer cell cycle time than that of normal
fibroblasts (Shimada, 1977; Takeuchi et al, 1983). The slow rate
of proliferation and the low clonogenicity of PSV811 in
comparison with those of VA13 may be related to this property of
untransformed cells. No significant difference in unscheduled

Table 2. FREQUENCY OF SISTER CHROMATID EXCHANGE

Exp.no.	BrdU concentration (μg/ml)	Incidence of SCE per chromosome ± SE[a]	
		VA13	PSV811
1	2	0.124 0.010(23)	0.211 0.025(20)
2	0.5	0.211 0.013(61)	0.292 0.020(57)
	2	0.220 0.012(61)	0.354 0.022(66)
	5	0.263 0.013(64)	0.493 0.029(60)

[a] Number in parenthesis is the number of cells examined.

DNA synthesis between PSV811 and VA13, as estimated from the autoradiographic experiment (see RESULTS), may coincide with the fact that untransformed WS and normal fibroblasts do not differ in their rates of unscheduled DNA synthesis (Fujiwara et al., 1977; Higashikawa and Fujiwara, 1978). As reported in an adjunct paper, acid glycosaminoglycans (AGAGs) were isolated from the culture fluids of the two lines of cells and were examined electrophoretically for their relative contents of AGAG species. The relative content of hyaluronic acid was higher in the culture fluid of PSV811 cells than that of VA13 (Murata et al. in this issue). The difference may possibly be related to the hyaluronuric nature of WS (Tokunaga et al., 1975; Goto and Murata, 1978). There are, however, at least two other possibilities to be considered: One is that immortalization by itself disturbs the gene expressions characteristic of WS; another is that the introduction of SV40 genes interferes, partly or wholely, with the defects of WS. As long as the genetic defects of WS are not known, neither possibility can be excluded. We do not mean, therefore, that any difference found between PSV811 and VA13 is related to the difference between WS and the normal. For example, the frequency of SCE in WS cells is reported to be normal (Bartram et al., 1976), but it differed (see RESULTS) between PSV811 and VA13. In fact, evidence suggesting the interference by SV40 gene expression of WS defects is shown in RESULTS, as will be discussed below.

Perturbation of Growth by SV40 Infection

As reported in RESULTS, the rate of proliferation of tsA900-
infected fibroblasts, either from WS or from normal origin, was permissive temperature. The decrease in the rate of proliferation by
this temperature up-shift for the infected WS cells was remarkable.
Previous studies using SV40-transformed permanent cell lines showed
that A-gene expression regulates cell phenotypes. Cells of some tsA-
mutant SV40-mutant SV40-transformed lines are freed from postconflu-
ence inhibition of proliferation at a nonpermissive temperature, but
are not freed from it at a permissive temperature (Topp et al., 1981).
However, our knowledge of the regulation by A-gene expression in a
finite cell population is limited (Butel et al., 1974). We regard
the present results as showing that A-gene expression markedly regulates the cell proliferation of a finitely proliferative human
fibroblast population. In addition, because SV40-infected WS cells
grew vigorously at a permissive temperature, we speculate that A-
gene expression may compensate for some of the WS defects. Among the
properties known about A-gene function are that its product, e.e.,
SV40-T antigen, is capable of initiating SV40 DNA synthesis and of
initiating DNA synthesis of G1-arrested cells to which it is introduced
(Tjian et al., 1978). It is known, on the other hand, that the distance between initiation points of DNA synthesis is longer in WS
fibroblasts than in normal fibroblasts (Takeuchi et al., 1982). Recently, we have obtained evidence that this distance is reduced toward that of normal cells in SV40-infected WS cells (Hanaoka et al.,
1983). Therefore we further speculate that the A-gene product could
compensate for some of the defects of WS through its participation
in DNA-synthesizing mechanisms.

Some lines of SV40-transformed WS cells had a longer
lifespan than untransformed WS cells (see RESULTS). This was not
at all unexpected: SV40-infected human cells sometimes have an
extended proliferative lifespan (Moyer et al., 1964). Human
cells transformed by BK virus also have a longer lifespan (Dr.
Seijiro Uchida, IMS, personal communication). Human cells
transformed by Rous sarcoma virus (RSV) have reduced doubling
potentials (Ponten, 1970). These previously obtained results,
together with the present results showing the extension of
proliferative lifespan in some SV40-infected WS cells, suggest
that mechanisms responsible for viral transformation modify the
proliferative lifespan of cells. It is totally unevaluated how
these mechanisms participate in the modification of proliferative
lifespan; however, we believe that this modification could
provide a clue to the study of WS as well as the evolution of
aging.

ACKNOWLEDGEMENT

The authors thank Professor Y. Nagai, IMS for his continuous interest and encouragement during this work, Professor H. Shimojo for permitting us to use his cancer virus laboratory for the SV40 infection study, Professors G.M. Martin, D.J. Salk, and Y. Fujiwara for inviting them to this seminar, Dr. T. Yamanaka, Serum Inst. of Chiba Pref. for mycoplasma testing, and Miss Noriko Munesawa and Mrs. Mieko Ninagawa for their help in preparing the manuscript and figures. This work was in part supported by a grant from the Institute of Physical and Chemical Research.

REFERENCES

Bartram, C.R., Koske-Westphal, T., and Passarge, E., Chromatid exchanges in ataxia telangiectasia, Bloom syndrome, Werner syndrome, and xeroderma pigmentosum, Ann. Hum. Genet., Lond., 40:79 (1976).

Butel, J.S., Brugge, J.S., and Noonan, C.A., Transformation of primate and rodent cells by temperature-sensitive mutants of SV40, Cold Spring Harbor Symposium on Quantitative Biology., 39, Part I:25 (1974).

Epstein, C.J., Martin, G.M., Schultz, A.L., and Motulsky, A.G., Werner's syndrome. A review of its symptomatology, natural history, pathologic features, genetics and relationship to the natural aging process, Medicine., 45:177 (1966).

Fujiwara, Y., Higashikawa, T., and Tatsumi, M., A retarded rate of DNA replication and normal level of DNA repair in Werner's syndrome fibroblasts in culture, J. Cell. Physiol., 92:365 (1977).

Girardi, A.J., Jensen, F.C., and Koprowski, H., SV40-induced transformation of human diploid cells: Crisis and recovery, J. Cell. Comp. Physiol., 65:69 (1965).

Girardi, A.J., Weinstein, D., and Moorhead, P.S., SV40 transformation of human diploid cells. A parallel study of viral and karyologic parameters, Ann. Med. Exp. Fenn., 44:242 (1966).

Goldstein, S., and Moerman, E.J., Heat-labile enzymes in Werner's syndrome fibroblasts, Nature., 255:159 (1975).

Goto, M., Horiuchi, Y., Tanimoto, K., Ishii, T., and Nakashima, H., Werner's syndrome: Analysis of 15 cases with a review of the Japanese literature, J. Am. Geriatr. Soc., 26:341 (1978).

Goto, M., and Murata, K., Urinary excretion of macromolecular acidic glycosaminoglycans in Werner's syndrome, Clin. Chim. Acta., 85:101 (1978).

Goto, M., Tanimoto, K., Horiuchi, Y., and Sasazuki, T., Family analysis of Werner's syndrome: A survey of 42 Japanese families with a review of the literature, Clin. Genetics., 19:8 (1981).

Hanaoka, F., Takeuchi, F., Matsumura, T., Goto, M., Miyamoto, T., and Yamada, M., Decrease in the average size of replicons in Werner's syndrome cells by simian virus 40-infection, Exp. Cell Res., 144:463 (1983).

Higashikawa, T., and Fujiwara, Y., Normal level of unscheduled DNA synthesis in Werner's syndrome fibroblasts in culture, Exp. Cell Res., 113:438 (1978).

Hoehn, H., Bryant, E.M., Au, K., Norwood, T.H., Boman, H., and Martin, G.M., Variegated translocation mosaicism in human skin fibroblast cultures, Cytogenet. Cell Genet., 15:282 (1975).

Holliday, R., Porterfield, J.S., and Gibbs, D.D., Premature aging and occurrence of altered enzyme in Werner's syndrome fibroblasts, Nature, 248:762 (1974).

Martin, G.M., Gartler, S.M., Epstein, C.J., and Motulsky, A.G., Diminished lifespan of cultured cells in Werner's syndrome, Fed. Proc., 24:678 (1965).

Martin, G.M., Sprague, C.A., and Epstein, C.J., Replicative life-span of cultivated human cells. Effects of donor's age, tissue, and genotype, Lab. Invest., 23:86 (1970).

Matsumura, T., Mitsui, Y., Fujiwara, Y., Ishii, T., and Shimada, H., Cell, tissue and organ banks in Japan with special reference to the study of premature aging, Japan. J. Exp. Med., 50:321 (1980).

Matsumura, T., Nitta, K., Yoshikawa, M., Takaoka, T., and Katsuta, H., Action of bacterial neutral protease on the dispersion of mammalian cells in tissue culture, Japan. J. Exp. Med., 45:383 (1975a).

Matsumura, T., Yamanaka, T., Hashizume, S., Irie, Y., and Nitta, K., Tissue dispersion, cell harvest and fluid suspension culture by the use of bacterial neutral protease, Japan. J. Exp. Med., 45:377 (1975b).

Moyer, A.W., Wallace, R., and Cox, H.R., Limited growth period of human lung cell lines transformed by simian virus 40, J. Natl. Cancer Inst., 33:227 (1964).

Murata, K., Kudo, M. and Matsumura, T., Acidic glycosaminoglycans in SV40-transformed Werner syndrome cells, in this issue.

Perry, P., and Wolff, S., New Giemsa method for the differential staining of sister chromatids, Nature, 251:156 (1974).

Ponten, J., The growth capacity of normal and Rous-virus-transformed chicken fibroblasts in vitro, Int. J. Cancer, 6:323 (1970).

Salk, D., Au, K., Hoehn, H. and Martin, G.M., Cytogenetics of Werner syndrome cultured skin fibroblasts: Variegated translocation mosaicism, Cytogenet. Cell Genet., 30:92 (1981a).

Salk, D., Au, K., Hoehn, H., Stenchever, M.R., and Martin, G.M.,
    Evidence of clonal attenuation, clonal succession, and
    clonal expansion in mass cultures of aging Werner syndrome
    skin fibroblasts, Cytogenet. Cell Genet., 30:108 (1981b).

Schneider, E.L., Tice, R.R., and Kram, D., Bromodeoxyuridine
    differential chromatid staining technique: A new approach to
    examining sister chromatid exchange and cell replication
    kinetics, Methods in Cell Biology, 20:379 (1978).

Shein, H.M., Enders, J.F., Palmer, L., and Grogan, E., Further
    studies on SV40-induced transformation in human renal cell
    cultures. I. Eventual failure of subcultivation despite a
    continuing high rate of cell division, Proc. Soc. Exp. Biol.
    Med., 115:618 (1964).

Shimada, H., The growth properties of Werner's syndrome cells and
    repair deficient cells, in: "Proceedings of the 5th
    Symposium of Basic Research on Aging, Aug. 1977, Tokyo", H.
    Tauchi, and S. Yamagata, eds., Ministry of Science,
    Education and Culture, Japan, pp. 43-51 (1977).

Takeuchi, F., Hanaoka, F., Goto, M., Akaoka, I., Hori, T.,
    Yamada, M., and Miyamoto, T., Altered frequency of
    initiation sites of DNA replication in Werner's syndrome
    cells, Hum. Genet., 60:365 (1982).

Takeuchi, F., Hanaoka, F., Goto, M., Yamada, M., and Miyamoto,
    T., Prolongation of S phase and whole cell cycle in Werner's
    syndrome fibroblasts, Exp. Gerontol., 17:473 (1983).

Tjian, R., Fey, G., and Graessmann, A., Biological activity of
    purified simian virus 40 T antigen proteins, Proc. Natl.
    Acad. Sci. USA., 75:1279 (1978).

Tokunaga, M., Futami, T., Wakamatsu, E., Endo, M., and Yosizawa,
    Z., Werner's syndrome as "Hyaluronuria", Clin. Chim. Acta.,
    62:89 (1975).

Topp, W.C., Lane, D., and Pollack, R., Transformation by simian
    virus 40 and polyoma virus, in: "DNA Tumor Viruses", 2nd
    Ed., J. Tooze, ed., Cold Spring Harbor Laboratory, Cold
    Spring Harbor, pp.205-296 (1981).

Yamaguchi, N., and Kuchino, T., Temperature-sensitive mutants of
    simian virus 40 selected by transforming ability, J. Virol.,
    15:1297 (1975).

EXPERIMENTAL STUDIES ON WERNER'S SYNDROME FIBROBLASTS

R. Holliday, K. V. A. Thompson, L. I. Huschtscha,
S. I. S. Rattan, S. G. Sedgwick, and A. Spanos

Genetics Division, National Institute for Medical
Research, The Ridgeway, Mill Hill, London, NW7 1AA
England

INTRODUCTION

The complex phenotype of Werner's syndrome is the result of a
single recessive mutation, which suggests that the product of the
normal gene plays an important role in the maintenance of several
types of body tissue. The mutation is pleiotropic in that it
appears to accelerate changes related to ageing in these tissues.
It would therefore be surprising if the identification of the
nature of the biochemical defect in Werner's syndrome did not yield
important information about the origins of similar age-related
changes in normal individuals. As full a characterization as
possible of the biological phenotype of Werner's syndrome fibroblasts may suggest specific biochemical investigations, but on the
other hand the slow and limited growth of these cells makes many
such studies almost impossible. For this reason, we have obtained
an SV40 transformed derivative of Werner's syndrome fibroblasts,
which must still inherit the genetic defect, even though it no
longer shows in vitro ageing. We have also carried out a series of
studies with diploid fibroblasts from four Werner's syndrome
patients.

Growth and Longevity of Werner's Syndrome Fibroblasts

Information about the donors of skin biopsies is given in
Table 1. The methods we have used have been published elsewhere
(Thompson and Holliday, 1983). Cultures were normally split 1:2,
so each passage is approximately equal to one population doubling.
In all cases, the fibroblast populations grew more slowly than
control cultures. After the establishment of primary cultures, the

Table 1. The Sources of Werner's Syndrome Fibroblasts and Their In Vitro Life Span

Donor, Age, Sex	Diagnosis	No. of Fibroblast Cultures Examined	Population Longevities: Range in Passages
D.D., 45, male	D. D. Gibbs, Sutton Coldfield Hospital, Warwick	5	9 – 10
C.A.W., 45, male	D. D. Cracknall, Addenbrooks Hospital, Cambridge	19	5 – 25
E.R., 42, male	H. Zade, Haddassah Hospital, Jerusalem	2	24 – 25[a]
H.B., 50, male	H. Cohen, Hope Hospital, Salford, Lancashire	8	10 – 29

[a]These cultures showed morphological features of senescence at passage 13 but subsequently recovered to reach the passage levels indicated.

doubling time during serial passaging averaged about 7 days compared with 3-4 days for normal skin fibroblasts. However, the
growth rate of Werner's cultures often did not remain constant.
The cultures frequently slowed down but later recovered to their
previous growth rate. This suggests that cultures are very heterogeneous in growth potential and that the cessation of growth of
most of the population is followed by the selection of the sub-
fraction of cells with greater growth potential. If this is the
case, one would expect considerable variability in life span of
parallel populations established from a single primary culture.
This was found to be the case for three out of four of the Werner's
syndrome strains (Table 1). In the one which was most thoroughly
studied (C.A.W.), 19 parallel cultures were established and these
achieved longevities of 5-25 population doublings. The growth of
14 of these cultures is represented in Figure 1. Each dot represents a 1:2 split, unless otherwise indicated. It can be seen that
fairly rapid subculture is often followed by a period of very slow
subculture, which may then be superseded by further fairly rapid
growth (Fig. 1, D and E). Sister cultures often vary enormously in
their growth potential (Fig. 1, A and B; C and D); in two cases
growth proceeded very slowly for a very long period of time (Fig.
1, B and F). This longevity experiment took over 16 months to
complete. If cellular selection is the explanation for the "stop-
start" growth of Werner's cultures, then it is quite possible that
the longest-lived cells have a growth potential comparable to
control cultures. Nevertheless, most of the cells must have a much
shorter life span. Results with cells from the first biopsy obtained (D.D.) showed that growth potential was increased at 33°.
At this temperature several cultures achieved 18-19 populations
compared with 9-10 at 37° (Thompson and Holliday, 1983). This
raised the very interesting possibility that the normal gene product might be indispensable for development and that only individuals with leaky or temperature-sensitive alleles with some activity
at 37° could survive to produce the clinical features of the disease. However, studies of cells from the other patients did not
bear this out since their growth potential was less at 33° than at
37°.

Chromosome Abnormalities

Metaphases were examined in three of the strains and the
results (Thompson and Holliday, 1983) were in agreement with the
much more extensive studies of Salk et al. (1981a, this volume).
The proportion of polyploid and subdiploid cells was higher than
controls, and there was a significantly increased frequency of
chromosome abnormalities, especially breaks. In one case (E.R.),
an abnormal marker chromosome (probably a translocation) was seen
in about 50% of metaphases, which provides evidence for a clonal
origin of this proportion of the population. In another case
(D.D.), 10/68 metaphases had endoreduplicated chromosomes. Since

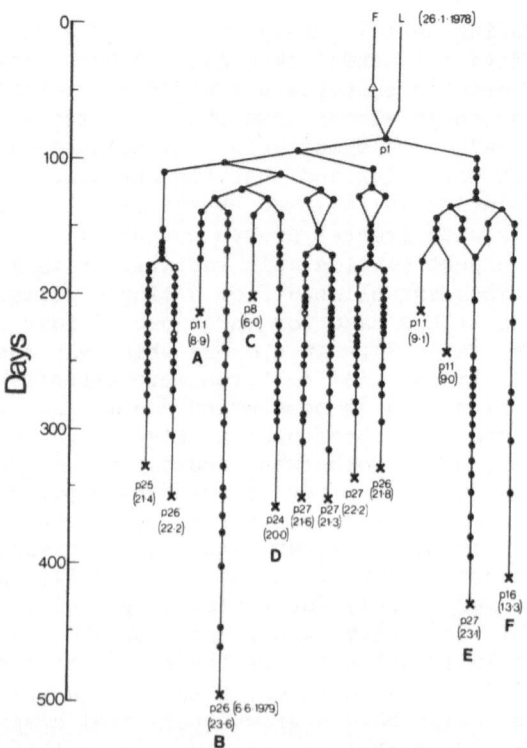

Fig. 1.   The growth and longevity of 14 subpopulations derived from
a passage 1 culture of Werner's syndrome fibroblasts
(patient C.A.W.).   Closed circles indicate the time when
cultures were split 1:2; open circles were 1:4 splits.
The primary culture was initiated from a skin biopsy
fragmented in a 25 cm^2 Falcon flask (F), which was subsequently trypsinised (Δ), and a Leighton tube (L).   Cultures were sometimes combined before they became fully
confluent.   They were terminated (X) when they failed to
become confluent after many changes of media.   Longevities
are indicated by passage level (P) and population
doublings (in brackets).   A-F, see text.

phase III fibroblasts have a reduced proportion of diploid metaphases and an increased level of chromosome abnormalities (Saksela
and Moorhead, 1963; Thompson and Holliday, 1975), the results are
consistent with the view that Werner's cells do, indeed, age prematurely in vitro.

Autofluorescence

The use of a fluorescent-activated cell sorter (FACS II) has demonstrated that fibroblasts contain a measurable quantity of autofluorescence (AF), which can be attributed to the "age-pigment," lipofuscin. The amount of AF increases exponentially with serial passage and therefore provides a useful index of physiological age. In the case of foetal lung strain, MRC-5, the AF increases 50-fold from passage 19 to passage 70 (Rattan et al., 1982). Werner's syndrome cells of early passage had a very high level of AF (Table 2), suggesting that they are indeed physiologically senescent.

Table 2. The Amount of Autofluorescence in Cultured Fibroblasts Measured by a Fluorescence-Activated Cell Sorter (FACS II)[a]

Cells	Passage Level[b]	Autofluorescence (arbitrary units)
MRC-5, foetal lung fibroblasts	19 - 70	15 - 800
MRC-5V1, SV40 transformed	>650	<10
Control, adult skin fibroblasts	20	40 - 50
Werner's syndrome (C.A.W.), skin fibroblasts	17	>400
Werner's syndrome, SV40 transformed	275	<35

[a]Information about the methods used and the quantitation is published elsewhere (Rattan et al., 1982).
[b]Passages are approximately equivalent to population doublings.

SV40-Induced Transformation

Using the methods described elsewhere (Huschtscha and Holliday, 1983), a permanent transformed line was obtained from strain C.A.W. After SV40-infection of human fibroblasts, many of the phenotypic features of the transformation are seen, including loss of contact inhibition, presence of T-antigen, growth in low serum and soft agar. However, we refer to these cells as pretransformed, because in most experiments the cells enter crisis and the

cultures subsequently die out. Occasionally a permanent line
emerges which retains most of the phenotypic features of the pretransformed population. The origin of the transformed Werner's
culture is shown in Figure 2. This culture has now achieved more
than 300 population doublings, so it is presumed to be a permanent
line. When we examined the amount of AF in these cells, we found
that a very low level was present (Table 2), suggesting that the
cells had become physiologically rejuvenated. Isoenzyme typing on
this transformed line has been carried out by Dr. S. M. Povey
(Galton Laboratory, University College, London), and this shows
that it cannot be contaminated with transformed MRC-5, Lesch-Nyhan
or HeLa cells, which are the only other permanent human lines we
have in the laboratory.

Evidence for Altered Glucose-6-Phosphate Dehydrogenase (G6PD)

We previously reported that senescent human fibroblasts have a
significantly increased level of heat-labile G6PD (Holliday and
Tarrant, 1972) and several lines of evidence suggest that these
altered molecules may arise from errors in protein synthesis (for a
review, see Holliday and Thompson, 1983). If Werner's syndrome
fibroblasts are prematurely senescent in vitro, then it would be
expected that they would contain heat-labile enzyme molecules.
This was confirmed for strain D.D. some years ago (Holliday et al.,
1974). Subsequently, G6PD was examined in cultures from the other
three Werner's strains and in each case there was a significant
fraction of heat-labile enzyme (19-22%). Early passage control
skin fibroblasts had only 3-9% heat-labile enzyme (Holliday et al.,
1974; Holliday and Thompson, 1983).

DNA Synthesis

Studies on replicon elongation using ^{3}H thymidine autoradiography had indicated that Werner's syndrome cells synthesize DNA in
vivo significantly more slowly than normal cells (unpublished
results of T. D. Petes). We have followed up this observation by
examining DNA polymerase α from Werner's syndrome cells. An SDS
polyacrylamide gel procedure has been developed which makes it
possible to examine the activity and molecular weight of the enzyme
in cell-free extracts. Proteins are first separated on SDS gels
and then the SDS is removed to allow the enzymes to renature
in situ. The activity of DNA polymerase is revealed by incubating
the gel in an assay mix containing nicked DNA substrate, deoxyribo-
nucleotides (one of which is ^{32}P labeled) and Mg^{++}. Using this
procedure, several active forms of DNA polymerase can be visualized
by autoradiography, the number of bands depending on the degree of
partial proteolysis of the enzyme. When freshly prepared extracts
from Werner's syndrome fibroblasts were used, the main active forms
of the enzyme had molecular weights of approximately 120K and 75K
(Spanos et al., 1981). The distribution of activities was not

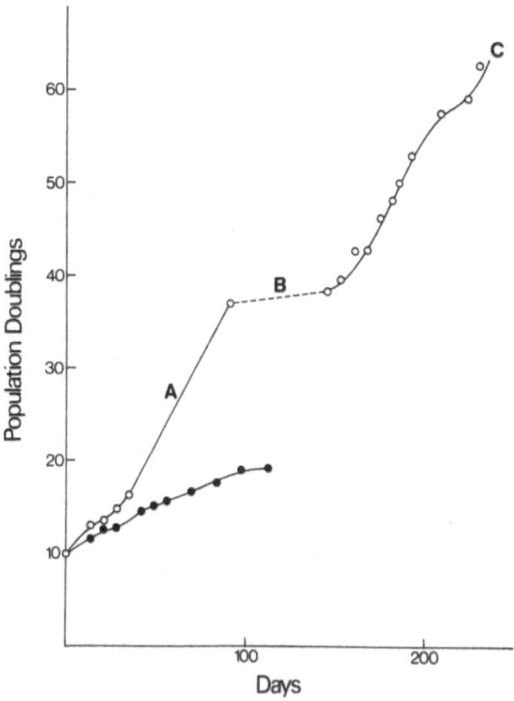

Fig. 2. The emergence of an SV40 transformed line from Werner's
        syndrome diploid fibroblasts, strain C.A.W. Cells were
        treated at passage 10 with SV40 virus. After several sub-
        cultures, a focus of vigorously growing cells was isolated
        and this eventually produced a confluent Falcon flask (25
        cm^2). A indicates the amount of growth, assuming the focus
        arose from a single cell. The cells ceased growth for 55
        days, during the period of crisis (B). Subsequently, a
        permanent line emerged which has achieved over 300 popula-
        tion doublings (C). The methods are based on those used to
        obtain transformed lines from MRC-5 (Huschtscha and
        Holliday, 1983). The close circles indicate the total
        cumulative growth of the untreated cells.

different from DNA polymerase α from normal cells examined under
these conditions or when limited proteolysis was allowed to occur
(Hübscher et al., 1981). There were also no obvious quantitative
differences between control and Werner's syndrome cell-free
extracts.

CONCLUSIONS

    We have carried out a number of experiments on fibroblasts

from skin biopsies from four Werner's syndrome patients aged 42-50.
In all cases, the in vitro longevity of the cells was significantly
shorter than controls, but there was considerable heterogeneity in
growth potential in parallel populations. The results support the
evidence from chromosome studies that clonal succession and expansion is a frequent occurrence in these populations (Salk et al.,
1981b). By the time Werner's cells are established in culture,
they resemble late passage normal cells by the following three
criteria: 1) They contain a high level of AF; 2) there is a substantial fraction of heat-labile G6PD, and 3) they have an increased frequency of chromosome abnormalities. Since Werner's
syndrome patients have many of the symptoms of premature aging, it
is obvious that these and other results obtained with cultured
fibroblasts provides support for the view that such cells provide
an appropriate model system for studies on the molecular basis of
cellular aging.   However, it is difficult to carry out biochemical
studies on diploid Werner's fibroblasts, since the number of cells
which can be obtained is very limited. We have used a sensitive
method for the study of DNA polymerase α, but have detected no
qualitative or quantitative differences between Werner's syndrome
and controls in the several molecular weight forms of the enzyme.
To facilitate further investigations of the possible biochemical
defect in the cells, we have obtained an SV40-induced permanent
transformed line. This has clearly escaped from senescence, but
since it presumably still retains the mutant gene, it opens up a
number of possibilities for further experimental investigations.

REFERENCES

Holliday, R., and Tarrant, G. M., 1972, Altered enzymes in ageing
    human fibroblasts, Nature, 238:26-30.
Holliday, R., and Thompson, K. V. A., 1983, Genetic effects on the
    longevity of cultured human fibroblasts. III. Correlations
    with altered glucose-6-phosphate dehydrogenase, Gerontology,
    29:89-96.
Holliday, R., Porterfield, J. S., and Gibbs, D. D., 1974, Premature
    ageing and occurrence of altered enzyme in Werner's syndrome
    fibroblasts, Nature, 248:762-763.
Hübscher, U., Spanos, A., Albert, W., Grummt, F., and Banks, G. R.,
    1981, Evidence that a high molecular weight replicative DNA
    polymerase is conserved during evolution, Proc. Natl. Acad.
    Sci. USA, 78:6771-6775.
Huschtscha, L. I., and Holliday, R., 1983, The limited and un-
    limited growth of SV40 transformed cells from human diploid
    MRC-5 fibroblasts, J. Cell Sci., 63:77-99.
Rattan, S. I. S., Keeler, K. D., Buchanan, J. H., and Holliday, R.,
    1982, Autofluorescence as an index of ageing in human fibro-
    blasts in culture, Bioscience Rep., 2:561-567.
Saksela, E., and Moorhead, P. S., 1963, Aneuploidy in the degenera-

tive phase of serial cultures of human cell strains, <u>Proc.</u>
<u>Natl. Acad. Sci. USA</u>, 50:390-395.

Salk, D., Au, K., Hoehn, H., and Martin, G. M., 1981a, Cytogenetics
of Werner's syndrome cultured skin fibroblasts: variegated
translocation mosaicism, <u>Cytogenet. Cell Genet.</u>, 30:92-107.

Salk, D., Au, K., Hoehn, H., Stenchever, M. R., and Martin, G. M.,
1981b, Evidence of clonal attenuation, clonal succession and
clonal expansion in mass cultures of ageing Werner's syndrome
skin fibroblasts, <u>Cytogenet. Cell Genet.</u>, 30:108-117.

Spanos, A., Sedgwick, S. G., Yarranton, G. T., Hübscher, U., and
Banks, G. R., 1981, Detection of the catalytic activities of
DNA polymerases and their associated exonucleases following
SDS-polyacrylamide gel electrophoresis, <u>Nucl. Acid Res.</u>, 9:
1825-1839.

Thompson, K. V. A., and Holliday, R., 1975, Chromosome changes
during the in vitro ageing of MRC-5 human fibroblasts, <u>Exp.</u>
<u>Cell Res.</u>, 96:1-6.

Thompson, K. V. A., and Holliday, R., 1983, Genetic effects on the
longevity of cultured human fibroblasts. I. Werner's syndrome, <u>Gerontology</u>, 29:73-82.

CELL FUSION STUDIES IN THE WERNER SYNDROME

Kiyoji Tanaka, Ken-ichi Yamamura, Kenichiro Fukuchi,
Kazuhiko Kawai and Yuichi Kumahara

Department of Medicine and Geriatrics
Osaka University School of Medicine
Fukushima-ku Osaka 553 Japan

INTRODUCTION

Werner syndrome (WS) is an autosomal recessive hereditary disease characterized by a reduced lifespan and with symptoms of premature senility (Epstein et al. 1966). Skin fibroblast cells from patients with Werner syndrome (WS cells) have a greatly reduced lifespan in vitro and showed marked retarded DNA synthesis even at early ages in culture (Goldstein, 1969; Martin et al., 1970; Danes, 1971; Fujiwara et al., 1977). One approach for the study of senescense of WS cells in vitro is to introduce gene product(s) or a gene itself and to observe changes in DNA synthesis. Norwood et al. (1974, 1975, 1979) demonstrated that DNA synthesis of senescent fibroblasts could be stimulated when these cells were fused with HeLa cells. On the other hand, when these cells were fused with young fibroblasts, no recovery of DNA synthesis was observed. They therefore suggested that the senescent cells have a 'senescent factor(s)' that inhibits their DNA synthesis. We also applied cell hybridization techniques in order to define the genetic defect of WS cells. In this article we will discuss the mechanism of aging in WS in comparison with senescent cells.

MATERIALS AND METHODS

Cell strains and cell culture

Strain NHKT is a human diploid fibroblast cell strain derived from the skin of a normal 29-year-old man. Strain WS10S

was derived from a skin biopsy of a 36-year-old man with WS.
Strain WS11KO derived from a skin biopsy of a 37-year-old man
with WS. Strain CRL1253 (WS-HMG, WS cells) was obtained from the
American Type Culture Collection, Rockville, Md. HeLa S3 9IV
cells were gifts from Dr. Y. Fujiwara, Kobe University School of
Medicine. Fibroblast cells were grown in Eagle's minimum
essential medium (MEM) supplemented with 10% fetal calf serum
(FCS) (Flow Lab.) in Falcon plastic Petri dishes under 5% CO_2 in
air in an incubator at 37°C. Cultures of normal and WS cells
were subcultured at split ratios of 1 : 4 and 1 : 2, respectively, and
the initial confluent monolayers were designated as the first cell
population doubling (CPD). The passage numbers of the cells used
were 6 or 9 CPD for NHKT cells and 4 or 7 CPD for WS10S cells,
which were in phase II.

Enucleation

     WS cells were inoculated into Falcon plastic Petri dishes (9
cm in diameter) containing 8 discs (2.5 cm o) at a density of 6-
8×10^5/dish and were labeled with [^{3}H] methionine (1 μCi/ml, spec.
act. 8.8 Ci/mmol) for about 36 h. WS cell discs were suspended in
5 ml 10 μg/ml cytochalasin B (CB) solution in 50 ml round-bottom
centrifuge tube and spun at 14000 rpm for 20 min at 37°C in a type
4 rotor on a Tominaga centrifuge. For preparation of cytoplasts,
the discs were recovered from the centrifuge tube and then cultured
in MEM supplemented with 10% FCS (10ECSMEM) for 3-4 h and
cytoplasts were collected from the discs by trypsinization. For
preparation of karyoplasts, the pellets formed at the bottom of
centrifuge tube were resuspended in 10FCSMEM.

Cell fusion

     Cells of two strains or suspension mixtures of whole cells and
karyoplasts (cytoplasts) in approx. 1 : 1 ratio were incubated with
UV-irradiated HVJ, first for 10 min in an ice bath and then for 20
min at 37°C with shaking. After fusion, the cell suspensions were
seeded sparsely in Petri dishes containing coverslips and cultured
in 10FCSMEM.

Prelabeling and autoradiography

     WS cells were labeled with [^{3}H] methionine (1 μCi/ml, spec.
act. 8.8 Ci/mmol) for about 36 h and normal young cells or HeLa
cells were labeled with [^{14}C] TdR (0.075 μCi/ml, spec. act. 60
mCi/mmol) for about 48 h. These prelabeled NH cells and HeLa cells
were then fused with whole WS cells, WS karyoplasts, or WS
cytoplasts, divided into three groups, and labeled with [^{3}H] TdR
(1 μCi/ml, spec. act. 5.0 μCi/mmol) for two or three sequential
24-h pulse periods. At the end of each pulse period, the
cultures were washed in PBS and fixed in methanol and acid-

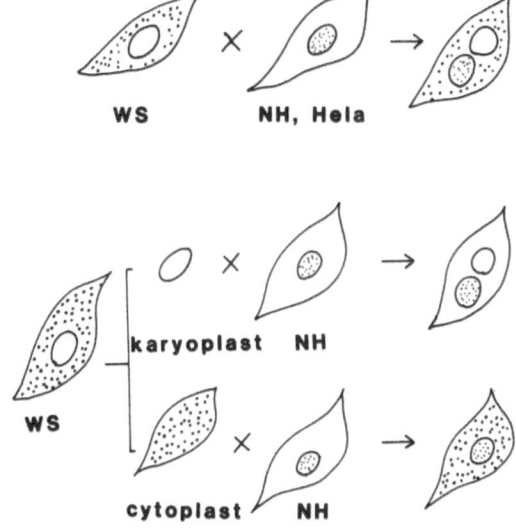

Fig. 1.   Identification of WS x NH (or HeLa) heterodikaryons, WS
karyoplast x NH heterodikaryons, and WS cytoplast x NH
cybrids according to the type of autoradiogram.

soluble materials were removed by washing the cells with 5% TCA
(trichloroacetic acid) at 4°C.   The double-layer autoradiographic
technique was then applied.   Details of this technique have been
described elsewhere (Norwood et al., 1974; Tanaka et al., 1979).
In each preparation WS X NH (or HeLa) heterodikaryons, WS
karyoplast X NH heterodikaryons, and WS cytoplast X NH cybrids
were identified according to the type of autoradiogram shown in
Fig. 1.   When both nuclei were heavily labeled with [3H] TdR, the
dikaryons were scored as DNA synthesizing cells.   When nuclei in
the cybrids were heavily labeled with [3H] thymidine, they were
scored as DNA-synthesizing nuclei.   The relative frequency of DNA
synthesizing cells was expressed as the [3H] TdR labeling index (%
of [3H] thymidine-labeled cells to total cells in the respective
classes, i.e. cells, cybrids, and dikaryons).

Difference in [3H] TdR labeling indices was tested by
parametrical statistics.

RESULTS

1.   Effect of prelabeling on DNA synthesis in NH cell

As shown in Fig. 2, the labeling incices of [14C] TdR
prelabeled NH X [3H] methionine prelabeled NH heterodikaryons,

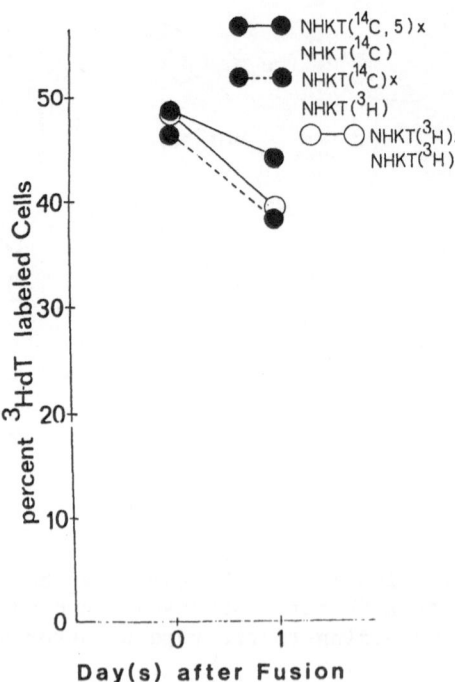

Fig. 2.   [3H] TdR labeling indices of NH x NH heterodikaryons.

[14C] TdR prelabeled NH homodikaryons, and [3H] methionine
prelabeled NH homodikaryons were 46.2, 48.5, and 48.4%,
respectively, in the first labeling period, 38.1, 44.2, and 39.4%
in the second period. Thus the prelabeling procedure has no
effect on the labeling indices of the heterodikaryons.

2.   DNA synthesis of WS X NH heterodikaryons

The labeling indices of WS homodikaryons were 5.4 and 13.3%
in the first and second [3H] TdR labeling periods, respectively,
while those of NH homodikaryons were 48.9 and 50.3%, respectively
(Fig. 3A). Thus, the labeling indices of NHKT homodikaryons were
higher than those of WS10S homodikaryons in all the [3H] TdR
labeling periods. The labeling indices of NHKT X WS10S
heterodikaryons were 17.1 and 19.5%, respectively. These results
indicate that although the labeling indices of the
heterodikaryons were considerably reduced as compared with normal
homodikaryons (p < 0.002), they were significantly higher than
those of WS10S homodikaryons (p < 0.01) in the first labeling
period. But in the second period the difference in labeling
indices between heterodikaryons and WS homodikaryons was not
statistically significant. When the WS11KO cells (passage number

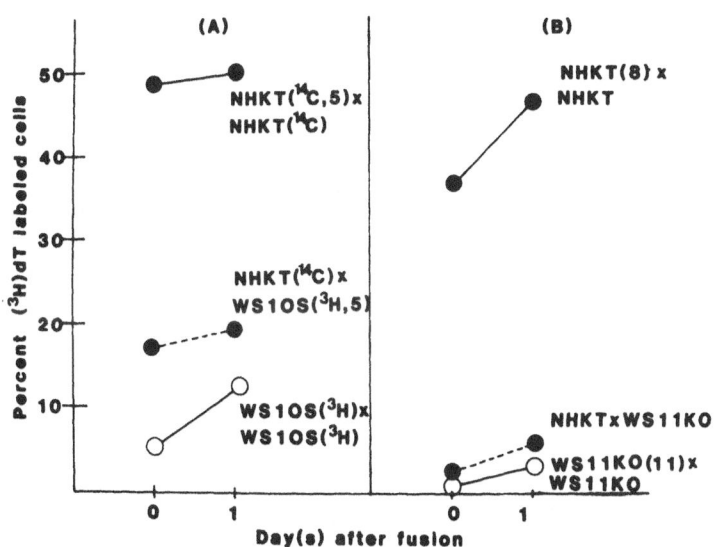

Fig. 3. [3H] TdR labeling indices of WS10S x NH heterodikaryons
(A) and WS11KO x NH heterodikaryons (B).

was 11) were used instead of WS10S cells, the labeling indices of
WS11KO homodikaryons were 1.0 and 3.3% in the first and second
[3H] TdR labeling periods, respectively, while those of WS11KO X
NHKT heterodikaryons were 2.4 and 6.2%, respectively (Fig. 3B).
These differences in labeling indices between WS homodikaryons
and heterodikaryons were not statistically significant.

3.   DNA synthesis of WS X HeLa heterodikaryons

The labeling indices of WS-HMG homodikaryons, HeLa
homodikaryons, and WS-HMG X HeLa heterodikaryons were 14.9, 96.6,
and 92.5% in the first [3H] TdR labeling period, respectively,
and were 10.4, 97.7, and 91.4% in the second labeling period,
respectively (Fig. 4). Thus, the labeling index of WS cell
nuclei increased markedly, indicating that the DNA synthesis was
initiated actively by the fusion with HeLa cells.

4.   DNA synthesis in WS karyoplast X NH heterodikaryons

The labeling indices of unfused parent normal cells were
28.0, 74.5 and 52.1% in the pulse periods 1, 2 and 3,
respectively, and those of NH karyoplast X NH homodilaryons were
19.1, 53.3 and 2.2%, respectively (Fig. 5A). Those of WS
karyoplast X NH heterodikaryons were 16.3, 12.5 and 0%,
respectively (Fig. 5B). These results showed that the labeling
indices of WS karyoplast X NH heterodikaryons were lower than

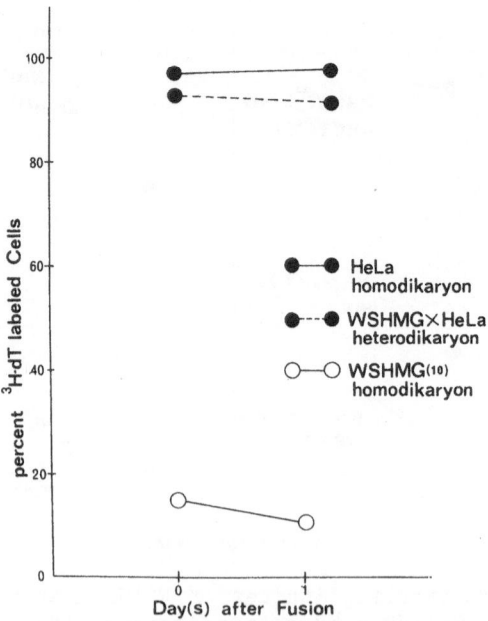

Fig. 4.   [³H] TdR labeling indices of WSHMG x NH heterodikaryons.

those of NH karyoplast x NH homodikaryons in the pulse period 2
(p < 0.01). The labeling indices of NH karyoplast X NH
homodikaryons were significantly lower than those of unfused NH
cells in the pulse period 2 and 3 (p < 0.001).

5.   DNA synthesis in WS cytoplast X NH cybrids

     The labeling indices of unfused parent normal cells were
24.6, 65.3 and 56.7% in the pulse periods 1, 2 and 3,
respectively, and those of NH cytoplast X NH cybrids were 15.6,
31.1 and 6.4%, respectively (Fig. 6A). Those of WS cytoplast X
NH cybrids were 2.3, 11.1 and 7.0%, respectively (Fig. 6B).
Thus, the labeling indices of WS cytoplast X NH cybrids are
significantly lower than those of NH cytoplast X NH cybrids in
the pulse periods 1 and 2 (p < 0.01). The labeling indices of NH
cytoplast X NH cybrids were also significantly lower than those
of unfused NH cells in the pulse period 1 (p < 0.01) and in the
pulse period 2 and 3 (p < 0.001).

DISCUSSION

     Our strategy for the study of senescence of WS cell in vitro
is to introduce gene product(s) or a gene itself by various
methods such as cell fusion and to see whether retarded DNA

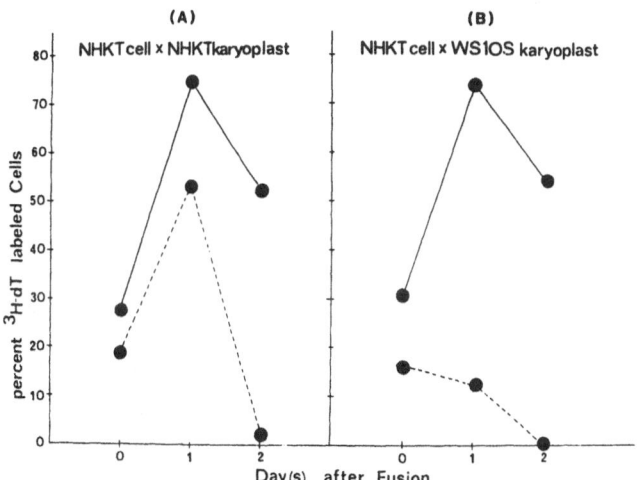

Fig. 5.   [³H] TdR labeling indices of NH karyoplast x NH
          heterodikaryons (A) and WS karyoplast x NH
          heterodikaryons (B).

synthesis in WS cells can be recovered or not. For the gene-
transfer experiment it is essential to establish the cell line.
The gene-transfer experiment could not be done by using the WS
cell line, because the retarded DNA synthesis is the only useful
marker of senescence in vitro and this is restored completely in
the established cell line. Thus the distinguishing markers,
which can still be detected in the established WS cell line,
should be found before the gene transfer experiment is designed.

    We first observed changes of labeling indices of WS cells
after fusing them with young NH cells or HeLa cells. As shown in
Fig. 3, DNA synthesis in younger WS cells was increased when they
were fused with young NH cells. On the other hand, those in
older WS cells did not increase at all. In both cases DNA
synthesis in NH cells decreased significantly. When WS cells
were fused with HeLa cells, DNA synthesis in WS cells increased
to approximately the same level as that of HeLa cells. These
phenomena can be explained in two ways. One explanation focuses
on the inhibition of DNA synthesis in NH cells. That is, WS
cells are producing 'senescent factor(s)' that inhibit DNA
synthesis in NH cells. Another explanation focuses on the
recovery of DNA synthesis in WS cells after they are fused with
NH or HeLa cells. In this case, WS cells are deficient of a
specific gene product that is necessary for DNA synthesis. If
the former is the case, the DNA synthesis in NH cells should be
inhibited when these cells are fused with WS cells or senescent
NH cells. Norwood et al. (1974, 1975) demonstrated that DNA

synthesis of old X young NH heterodikaryons did not increase at
all.   However those of old NH x HeLa heterodikaryons increased
considerably but not to the same level of HeLa homodikaryons.
They therefore suggested that the senescent cells have a
'senescent factor(s)' that inhibits DNA synthesis and that
certain cell lines of unlimited replicative potential may
inactivate this factor.   There is, however, no direct evidence to
support this assumption.   In 1979 Norwood et al. demonstrated the
marked depression of DNA synthesis in the HeLa nuclei after
fusion with WS cells and only minimal stimulation of the WS
nuclei.   They suggested that the mechanism of senescence in WS
cells was different from that in normal somatic cells.   However,
we observed the nearly complete recovery of DNA synthesis in WS x
HeLa heterodikaryons (Tanaka et al. 1979, 1980).   This
discrepancy may be caused by the difference between the HeLa
cells that we used and those that Norwood et al. used.   As the
recovery of DNA synthesis in old NH x HeLa heterodikaryons was
not complete in their experiments, their HeLa cells may have
produced less of the factor that is needed to rescue the DNA
synthesis of the senescent cell than our HeLa cells.   Our
results, shown in Fig. 3A, suggest that even young NH cells can
rescue DNA synthesis in WS cells if these WS cells are at low
PDL.   Thus, the younger WS cells were, the more obvious was the
increase in DNA synthesis.   If the retarded DNA synthesis were a

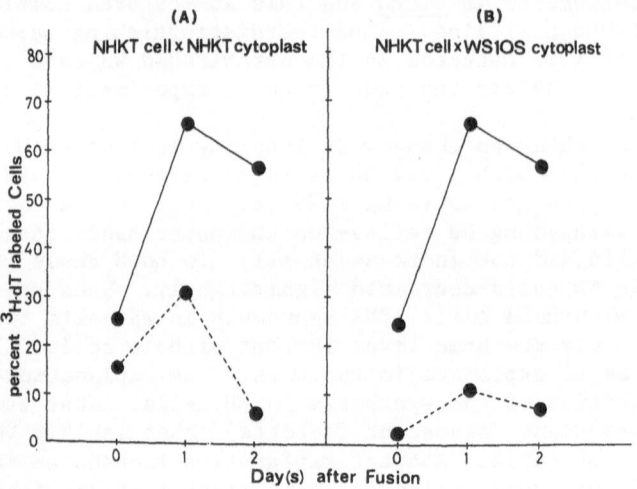

Fig. 6.   [3H] TdR labeling indices of NH cytoplast x NH cybrids
           (A) and WS cytoplast x NH cybrids.

primary consequence, this should be observed without any relation to the aging process. From this standpoint, it is not unlikely that WS cells are somewhat similar to senescent NH cells, and the main cause of senescence in NH cells is the same as that in WS cells.

Maggleton-Harris et al. (1976) examined the replicating ability in the reconstituted cells derived from fusions of the cytoplasts from young and senescent cells with reciprocal karyoplasts. They showed that karyoplasts were involved more than cytoplasts in cellular aging, although both carried the information for cellular aging.

To elucidate the roles of nuclear and cytoplasmic environments in senescence, the [3H] TdR labeling indices of NH cells fused with either WS karyoplasts or WS cytoplasts were investigated. For identification of the WS karyoplast x NH heterodikaryons or WS cytoplast x NH cybrids, we used prelabeling methods described in Materials and Methods. As shown in Fig. 5 and 6, the [3H] thymidine labeling indices of WS karyoplast x NH heterodikaryons and WS cytoplast x NH cybrids were significantly lower than those of NH karyoplast x NH homodikaryons and NH cytoplast x NH cybrids, respectively. Thus, both nuclear and cytoplasmic environments are responsible for the decreased DNA synthesis in NH nuclei in heterodikaryons and cybrids. As the [3H] TdR labeling indices of NH karoplast x NH homodikaryons and NH ctyoplast x NH cybrids were lower than those of parent cells, experimental procedures such as enucleation could affect the DNA synthesis. Consequently, it is hard to conclude which environment, nucleus or cytoplasm, plays the more important role in retarding DNA synthesis.

Another strategy to define the senescence factor(s) or deficient gene product is to introduce cell components to WS cells. These experiments are now in progress.

Certainly, senescence of normal cells in vitro is influenced by many factors. These factors can be classified into two groups, genetic factors and environmental factors. It is very hard to define each factor if the normal senescent cells are used as materials. It is one of the best strategies to choose WS cells, because only one gene is involved in the senescence of these cells. However, the restriction of distinguishing markers makes it difficult to study senescence in WS cells in vitro. Recent development in DNA technology made it possible to isolate human genes. This DNA technology will be applied to the study of senescence in vitro in the near future.

ABSTRACT

The mechanism of retarded DNA synthesis was investigated by the cell fusion method. The [^{3}H] TdR labeling index of young cells from patients with Werner syndrome (WS cells) X young normal human diploid fibroblast cells (NH cells) was considerably lower than that of NH homodikaryons, but was significantly higher than that of WS homodikaryons. The labeling index of old WS X young NH heterodikaryons was as low as that of WS homodikaryons. The labeling index of WS X HeLa heterodikaryons was the same as that of HeLa homodikaryons. These results indicate that WS cells are somewhat similar to senescent NH cells. The labeling indices in both WS karyoplast X NH heterodikaryons and WS cytoplast X NH cybrids were lower than those in normal karyoplast X NH heterodikaryons and normal cytoplast X NH cybrids, respectively. These results indicate that both nuclear and cytoplasmic environments are involved in the retarded DNA synthesis in WS cells. The most plausible interpretation of all our data is that the retarded DNA synthesis in WS cells could be caused by either the 'senescent factor(s)' or the deficiency of gene product(s) that is necessary for DNA synthesis and could be a secondary consequence of the genetic defect.

ACKNOWLEDGEMENTS

This work was supported by a research grant from the Ministry of Education, Japan, by a life science grant-in-aid from the Institute of Physical and Chemical Research, and by a research grant from the Japan Medical Research Foundation.

REFERENCES

Danes, B.S., 1971. Progeria: A cell culture study on aging, J. Clin. Invest., 50:2000.

Epstein, C.J., Martin, G.M., Schultz, A.S., and Motulsky, A.G., 1966. Werner's syndrome: A review of its symptomatology, natural history, pathology features, genetics, and relationships to the aging process. Medicine (Baltimore) 45:177.

Fujiwara, Y., Higashikawa, T., and Tatsumi, M., 1977. A retarded rate of DNA replication and normal level of DNA repair in Werner's syndrome fibroblasts in culture. J. Cell Physiol. 92:365.

Goldstein, S., 1969. Lifespan of cultured cells in progeria. Lancet 1:424.

Martin, G.M., Sprague, C.A., and Epstein, C.J., 1970. Replicative life-span of cultivated human cells: Effects of donor's age, tissue and genotype. Lab. Invest. 23:86.

Muggleton-Harris, A. and Hayflick, L., 1976. Cellular aging studied by the reconstruction of replicating cells from nuclei and cytoplasms isolated from normal human diploid cells. Exp. Cell Res. 103:321.

Norwood, T.H., Pendergrass, W.R., Sprague, C.A., and Martin, G.M., 1974. Dominance of the senescent phenotype in heterokaryons between replicative and post-replicative human fibroblast-like cells. Proc. Natl. Acad. Sci. (USA) 71:223.

Norwood, T.H., Pendergrass, W.R., and Martin, G.M., 1975. Reinitiation of DNA synthesis in senescent human fibroblasts upon fusion with cells of unlimited growth potential. J. Cell Biol. 64:551.

Norwood, T.H., Hoehn, H., Salk, D. and Martin, G.M., 1979. Cellular aging in Werner's syndrome: a unique phenotype? J. Invest. Derm. 73:92.

Tanaka, K., Nakazawa, T., Okada, Y., and Kumahara, Y., 1980. Increase in DNA synthesis in Werner's syndrome cells by hybridization with normal human diploid and HeLa cells. Exp. Cell Res. 123:261.

Tanaka, K., Nakazawa, T., Okada, Y., and Kumahara, Y., 1980. Roles of nuclear and cytoplasmic environments in the retarded DNA synthesis in Werner syndrome cells. Exp. Cell Res. 127:185

CELL FUSION STUDIES AND BIOCHEMICAL ANALYSIS OF DNA SYNTHESIS IN WERNER AND NON-WERNER CULTURED CELLS

William Pendergrass, Darrell Salk and Thomas Norwood

Department of Pathology
University of Washington
Seattle, WA 98195

INTRODUCTION

Cell fusion has been used extensively to determine whether DNA synthesis can be reinitiated ("rescued") in senescent human diploid fibroblast-like (HDFL) cells. These experiments have shown that temporary resumption of DNA synthesis can occur after fusion of senescent cells to some, but not all, continuously propagated cell lines. In contrast, fusion of senescent HDFL cells to early passage HDFL cells, never results in rescue. In this monograph, the literature describing these experiments is reviewed. In addition, we propose a model which predicts that DNA synthesis is initiated in heterokaryons between senescent HDFL cells and other cell types only when the proliferating parental cell types donate enough DNA replication factors to the common pool to exceed the threshold concentration required for initiation of DNA synthesis. Evidence is presented indicating that senescent HDFL cells cultured from patients with Werner syndrome (referred to here as Werner cells) possess an increased requirement for these replication factors. However, we will describe studies indicating that DNA polymerase alpha remains inducible following mitogen stimulation senescent cultures derived from both normal and Werner donors. Thus, senescent HDFL cells may be in a metabolic state distinct from other quiescent cell types.

BACKGROUND AND LITERATURE REVIEW

When HDFL cells are passaged in vitro until they cease dividing, they do not die immediately but rather fail to enter S phase and are arrested in the G1 phase of the cell cycle. This phenomenon is referred to as in vitro senescence (see reviews by Yanishevsky and Stein, 1981; Norwood and Smith, 1985). Werner cells undergo a similar but accelerated senescence (Salk et al., 1981; Salk, 1982; Goldstein, 1979; Aso et al., 1980; Schonberg, 1981; Scappaticci et al., 1982). The mechanism responsible for the in vitro senescence phenomena in either normal or Werner HDFL cells is unknown. Also, it is not known if the same mechanism(s) regulate the growth potential of cells derived from normal individuals and Werner patients. Theoretical proposals have generally centered around either a genetic regulatory mechanism (similar or identical to terminal differentiation), or, alternatively, that growth failure is the result of the random accumulation of damage (Orgel, 1963, 1970; Martin, 1977).

A variety of experimental approaches have been utilized to probe the mechanism(s) which limit the growth potential of cultured HDFL cells. Cell hybridization is one experimental technique which has been employed by a number of laboratories to probe the nature of the G1 block which occurs with senescence. Three types of cell fusion experiments have been used in the analysis of in vitro senescence: 1) heterokaryon studies in which DNA synthesis is identified by autoradiographic measurement of [^{3}H]-TdR uptake into bi- or poly-nucleated fusion products; 2) synkaryon studies in which the life span of proliferating hybrid clones is scored; and 3) cell reconstruction studies in which the growth potential of cells is determined after reconstitution of whole cells from nuclear and cytoplasmic components obtained by enucleation.

We and other investigators have suggested that specific regulatory factors may be involved in the G1 arrest in post-mitotic cultures derived from both Werner patients and normal individuals (Rabinovitch and Norwood, 1980; Burmer et al., 1982; Stein et al., 1982). In this chapter we shall discuss the observations derived from each of these types of cell fusion studies and how these observations can be interpreted in terms of the mechanism(s) of in vitro senescence. Although Werner HDFL cells have been less extensively studied by this approach, phenomenological differences between these cells and HDFL cells derived from normal individuals have been observed (Norwood et al., 1979a). We discuss possible interpretations of these differing observations.

Heterokaryon Fusions

The major thrust of heterokaryon studies has been to examine the interaction between the parental cells with different proliferative behaviors with respect to nuclear DNA synthesis that occurs immediately following cell fusion. In the earliest studies of this type Norwood et al. (1974) reported that nuclear DNA synthesis is inhibited in young HDFL cells following fusion to non-proliferating, senescent nuclei. Later studies in our laboratory (Rabinovitch and Norwood, 1980) and by Yanishevsky and Stein (1980) revealed that inhibition of cell cycle progression occurs on those HDFL cells in the early or mid G1 phase at the time of fusion, while cells that have already begun DNA synthesis or are in the last 2-3 hrs. of G1 continue to progress through the cell cycle apparently to the end of the S phase.

In contrast to the preceding observations, DNA synthesis is reinitiated in senescent nuclei following fusion to some permanently established cell lines such as HeLa and SV-40 transformed HDFL cells (Norwood et al., 1975). Norwood and Zeigler (1977) subsequently demonstrated that chromosomes from the senescent cells are completely replicated in these hybrids. In a more extended analysis of the capacity of established cell lines to stimulate synthetic activity in senescent nuclei, Stein and Yanishevsky (1979) demonstrated that, like low passage HDFL cells, a number of permanent cell lines do not stimulate DNA synthesis in senescent nuclei in the heterokaryons. The property or properties of transformed cell lines which confer dominance (i.e. stimulatory activity) or recessiveness (i.e. are inhibited) in this assay is unknown at the present time. Stein et al. (1982) have suggested that dominance may be associated with transformation by DNA oncogenic viruses that provide the necessary gene products capable of neutralizing putative inhibitory factors.

Other quiescent cell types such as serum starved and contact inhibited HDFL cells (Rabinovitch and Norwood, 1980; Stein and Yanishevsky, 1981) are able to inhibit DNA replication in early passage cells. Similarly, chemically damaged HDFL cells treated with mitomycin C or amino acid analogues inhibit young HDFL cells after fusion (Norwood et al., 1979b). Thus most quiescent cell types inhibited DNA replication in young HDFL cells. The only quiescent cell type that is known to be rescued by fusion with young HDFL is terminally differentiated chick erythrocytes (Rao, 1976). The very small size of these cells may account for this different response (see below).

The behavior of the Werner cells in the heterokaryon experimental system has not been entirely elucidated. Studies have been published showing that senescent Werner cells, like senescent normal cells, inhibit DNA synthetic activity in nuclei from actively proliferating HDFL cells following fusion (Tanaka et al., 1979). It is not yet clear, however, whether Werner cells also inhibit HeLa and other normally dominant transformed cell types. Norwood et al. (1979a) reported that senescent Werner cells were not rescued by fusion with HeLa cells and

actually inhibited initiation of DNA synthesis in the HeLa
nucleus. In contrast, Tanaka et al. (1979, 1980) reported that
senescent Werner cells are rescued by HeLa cells. The possible
basis for these differing observations will be discussed below.

Based on these heterokaryon studies a number of
investigators have proposed that senescence HDFL cells contain an
inhibitor that prevents young HDFL and recessive transformed
cells from entering S-phase (Rabinovitch and Norwood, 1980; Stein
et al., 1982; Burmer et al., 1982). Continuous cell lines such
as HeLa which exhibit dominance in heterokaryons are postulated
to possess an "anti-inhibitor" activity capable of neutralizing
the inhibitor (Stein et al., 1982). Recent studies in our
laboratory suggest that the dominance of certain cell types may
be due to the presence of higher concentrations of, rather than
unique inducers, of DNA synthesis (Pendergrass et al., 1982).

Synkaryon studies

The heterokaryon studies discussed above have examined only
one aspect of cell cycle activity (i.e., DNA synthesis)
immediately following fusion. In contrast sequential cell cycle
activity can be examined in hybrid cells which have progressed to
form synkaryons (hybrids with fused nuclei) and which are capable
of extended proliferation. By this methodology one can examine
the growth potential of hybrids derived from parental cell types
with different proliferative behaviors.

The first intraspecific (human-human) hybridization experiments with ambiguous identification of the hybrid clones were
reported by Hoehn et al. (1975, 1978). These investigators used
a non-selective technique to isolate the hybrids and
electrophoretic analysis of glucose-6-phosphate dehydrogenase
isozymes to confirm their parental origin. The growth potential
of clones isolated following hybridization of long and short-
lived strains was intermediate to those of the parental cultures.
It was concluded that the regulation of growth potential is co-
dominant. Pereiera-Smith and Smith (1982) also addressed this
question using hybridization studies of a somewhat different
design. They exploited a long-lived strain of fetal lung HDFL
cell which contained dominant and recessive selective markers,
thus permitting selective isolation of hybrid clones (Duthu et
al., 1982). The growth potential of hybrid clones isolated under
these conditions was similar to the shorter-lived parental
culture. The basis for different observations in these synkaryon
studies is not clear at the present time. Differences in methods
of selection (selective vs. non-selective) may be a factor.
However, both observations are inconsistent with the notion that
cellular senescence in vitro is the result of the accumulation of
recessive mutations.

In contrast to the euploid-euploid intraspecific fusions described above, intra- and interspecific hybridization studies using HDFL cultures and established or neoplastoid cell lines have yielded results which are seemingly different from the heterokaryon studies. The earliest reports describing the results of this type of hybridization studies were interpreted as showing dominance of the immortal phenotype (Goldstein and Lin, 1972; Croce and Kaprowski, 1974; Stanbridge, 1976). However, subsequent studies, in which cell hybrids were quantitatively recovered and their growth potential determined, have shown that the majority of such hybrids exhibits a finite growth potential (Pereira-Smith, 1981; Bunn and Tarrant, 1980). Pereira-Smith and Smith (1981) estimated that "transformation" to apparently unlimited proliferative capacity occurs at a frequency of about 10^{-5}. Such a low recovery of permanent lines may indicate that development of fused lines with an indefinite lifespan is possible only after loss of genetic information, possibly via chromosomal loss or rearrangement. This finding would also argue against the presence of any stable "anti-inhibitors" in dominant (HeLa or SV-40 transformed HDFL) cells that prevent or reverse the in vitro aging process. Interestingly, it was noted that clones of non-dividing synkaryons derived from senescent and SV-40 transformed HDFL remained positive for T-antigen indicating that this virally encoded factor by itself is not capable of permanently reversing in vitro senescence (Pereira-Smith and Smith, 1981).

There has been only one published synkaryon study with Werner cells. After multiple attempts, Salk et al. (1981) reported isolation of two proliferating hybrid clones following fusion of low passage Werner cultures and HDFL cells from a non-Werner donor. These clones exhibited low growth capacity, indicating that the Werner cell phenotype was not rescued by the normal cells. Studies attempting to isolate proliferating hybrids after fusion of Werner cells with established cell lines have not been reported.

Cell Reconstruction Experiments

The principle objective of cell reconstruction experiments has been to determine if the proliferative potential of cultured cells is regulated primarily by cytoplasmic or nuclear functions. These experiments became feasible with the development of techniques of enucleation of mass cultures. This enucleation is accomplished by exposure of the cultured cells to cytochalasin B and centrifugation which yields a nuclear pellet (karyoplasts) and enucleate cytoplasms (cytoplasts) adherent to the substrate (Wright, 1973a and b). These cell components can then be independently fused with whole cells or with each other to form reconstituted whole cells; such fusion products using karyroplasts and/or cytoplasts are referred to as "cybrids."

Two experimental designs have been used in these studies, similar to those used in heterokaryon and synkaryon studies. DNA synthetic activity has been examined in the cybrids immediately following fusion of a cell component (karyoplast or cytoplast) with a whole cell, and the growth potential of cybrids reconstructed from cell components derived from parental cells with different growth potential has been determined. Using the former approach, Burmer et al. (1983) and Dresher-Lincoln and Smith (1983) have recently demonstrated that nuclear DNA synthesis is depressed immediately following fusion to senescent, but not to young, cytoplasts. While these results are consistent with the presence of a diffusible inhibitory factor(s), the presence of toxic or inappropiate products of cell metabolism (e.g., free radicals or abnormal proteins) in the senescent cytoplasm could account for these observations.

A single study has been reported in which DNA synthesis was examined following fusion of cell components from a transformed cell type with whole senescent HDFL cells (Nette et al., 1982). In this study, both karyplasts and cytoplasts from L cells were capable of stimulating at least one round of DNA synthesis in the senescent nuclei immediately following fusion. This indicates that the stimulatory factor or factors are diffusible.

Cybridization studies in which the growth potential of proliferating cybrids was determined have produced somewhat variable results. Wright and Hayflick (1975a and b) isolated cybrid clones by complementation of chemically induced cytoplasmic and nuclear lesions and observed that clones resulting from the fusion of young cells and senescent cytoplast displayed a growth potential similar to that observed in cybrids constructed from young cells and cytoplasts. This indicates that the regulation of growth potential is primarily a nuclear function. However, in later studies in which cybrids were reconstructed from young and senescent cell components and isolated under direct visual observation, Muggleton-Harris and Hayflick (1976) reported data indicating that the growth potential is regulated by cytoplasmic, as well as by nuclear functions. The latter conclusion is also supported in subsequent studies of Muggleton-Harris (Muggleton-Harris and Desimone, 1980) in which cybrids constructed by the fusion of karyoplasts from SV-40 transformed HDFL cells and cytoplasts from a non-transformed HDFL cell exhibited a finite growth potential. The nature of this cytoplasmic control is unknown. However, the cytoplasm may be an important site for the storage of regulatory information in view of the recent reports documenting cytoplasmic modulation of specific genes (Gopalakrishnan and Anderson, 1979; Lipsich et al., 1979; Kahn et al., 1981).

Cybridization studies with Werner cells have been limited. Tanaka et al. (1980) have shown that fusion of either cytoplasts or karyoplasts from Werner cells suppress DNA synthesis in actively proliferating HDFL cells from normal donors. Again, the observations are consistent with the presence of an inhibitor, but do not rule out the presence of toxic products from aberrant cell metabolism.

Regulation of DNA Synthesis in Heterokaryons -- A Hypothesis

The observation described above provides some evidence for the presence of a factor or factors in senescent cells which prevents these cells from entering S phase and can inhibit nuclear DNA synthetic activity in certain cell types following fusion. The nature and target of this factor(s) are unknown. The mechanism by which certain cell types (e.g., HeLa and SV-40 transformed HDFL cells) are able to overcome the inhibitory activity of the senescent cell and reinitiate DNA synthetic activity in heterokaryons remains unclear. The observation that dominant cell types in the heterokaryon assay do not suppress senescence in proliferating hybrids suggests that these cells do not contain a stable "anti-inhibitor." Thus, some other explanation for the transient rescue of the senescence cells in heterokaryons must be sought.

A modified hypothesis has been proposed by Pendergrass et al. (1982) that initiation of DNA synthesis in heterokaryons is positively regulated by the concentration of factor(s) responsible for the initiation and maintenance of DNA synthesis. This model assumes that these initiation and replication factors, (or mRNA coding for them) are diffusible between nuclei in heterokaryons and that a threshold level of these factors is required for induction of DNA synthetic activity. Permanent cell lines which are able to initiate DNA synthesis in senescent cells (e.g., are dominant in fusions) are postulated to possess excess replication factors, which equilibrate at a concentration above the threshold level required for reinitation of DNA synthesis in both nuclei. In contrast, recessive cell types (unable to rescue senescent cells) have low endogenous levels of these factors such that, after equilibration between the heterologous nuclei and cytoplasms, subthreshold concentrations are present in both nuclei, and DNA synthesis does not occur. Recessive cells in late G1 or S phase are not inhibited by fusion to senescent cells. This may indicate that cells in these stages of the cell cycle are irreversibly committed to initiation and completion of chromosome replication.

The most direct test of this "dilution" hypothesis would be to measure the activities of initiation and replication factors in dominant and recessive cell types. At the present, the

mechanism of the initiation of DNA synthesis is unknown and the
factors involved in this aspect of cell metabolism are only
beginning to be identified. However, a number of enzymes
directly or indirectly involved in DNA synthesis is induced just
prior to the onset of DNA synthesis. There is some evidence to
suggest that these enzymes are organized into a supermolecular
complex, the concentration and organization of which may be
critical for entry into S-phase (Baril et al., 1974; Reddy and
Pardee, 1980; Noguchi et al., 1983). Thus the activity of these
enzymes may provide an indirect estimate of the levels of
putative regulatory factors. We have measured the specific
activity of DNA polymerase alpha in a series of cultivated cell
lines that display different behaviors in the heterokaryons assay
(Pendergrass et al., 1982) (Fig. 1) This enzyme is believed to
be the principal enzyme mediating chromosomal DNA synthesis
(Kornberg, 1980; Fry, 1983). These studies show that a
correlation exists between the specific activity of this enzyme
and dominance in the heterokaryon assay. All the dominant cell
types (6) tested exhibited higher specific activities (per mg.
protein) than the recessive cell types. Furthermore, one cell
line (RK13) derived from a rabbit kidney was found to alter
during serial passaging from a low polymerase recessive type to a
high polymerase dominant type (Pendergrass et al., 1982).

A recently published study by Rao and Satya-Prakash (1983)
provides further evidence that levels of inducers of DNA
synthesis vary with the cell type. These investigators assayed
"inducer" activity by measuring the rapidity of induction of DNA
synthesis in a synchronized G1 population following fusion with
unsynchronized populations of cell types with different
proliferative behaviors. Inducer concentrations ascertained by
this method are remarkably similar to the activities of
polymerase alpha described above (Fig. 1). HeLa cells induced
synthetic activity most rapidly and the HDFL cells induced
activity least rapidly. The rapidity of induction after fusion
with T98G cells was intermediate.

The induction of DNA synthesis in senescent nuclei by
dominant cell types is transient. As we indicated above, it now
appears that the majority of proliferating hybrids recovered from
continuous cell lines and HDFL cells exhibits a finite growth
potential (Bunn and Tarrant, 1980; Pereira-Smith and Smith,
1982). This suggests that the concentration of inducers in the
hybrids is gradually reduced by the euploid genome. To date the
levels of polymerase alpha or other enzymes involved in DNA
synthesis have not been examined in these proliferating hybrids.

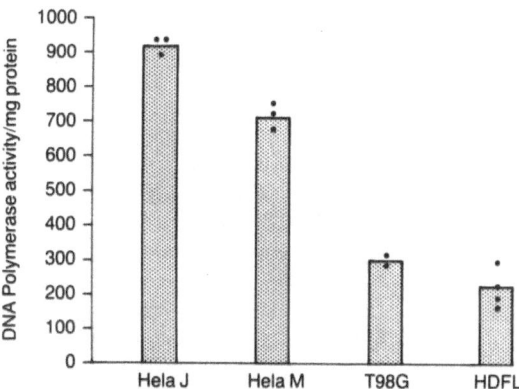

Fig. 1. The DNA polymerase alpha activity (pmoles TTP
incorporated/60 min/mg protein) in logarithmically
growing HeLa, T98G, and HDFL cells. Cell assays were
performed in triplicate. The cell culture conditions as
well as methods of polymerase and protein assay were
carried out as described previously (Pendergrass et al.,
1982) except that the cells were lysed by sonication
rather than homogenization (three two-second bursts on a
Branson Sonifier on a setting of "6", Branson Sonic
Power Company, Danbury, Connecticut). The origin of the
three transformed cell lines HeLa J, HeLa M, and T98G is
described in the text. The HDFL cell strain (82-6) was
examined at 31 population doublings, approximately 40%
of its maximum life span. Each data point represents a
triplicate determination in independent cultures.

EXPERIMENTAL OBSERVATIONS

Is the Extent of Reactivation of DNA Synthesis in Heterokaryons
Involving the Werner cell diminished?

There are conflicting reports regarding the capacity of HeLa
cells to reinitiate nuclear DNA synthesis in senescent Werner
cells following fusion. We observed a lower frequency of
reinitiation of synthetic activity of Werner cells compared with
cells derived from normal donors (Norwood et al., 1979a). In
contrast, Tanaka et al., (1979, 1980) observed that reactivation
of Werner nuclei under these conditions was comparable to that
observed in nuclei from "normal" cells. While a number of
reasons for these differing observations are conceivable, it
occurred to us that these results may be explained by the use of
different HeLa sublines in the two laboratories. We used a HeLa
subline designated "HeLa M" (Fialo and Kenny, 1966) which has
been continuously propagated in our laboratory since 1974; Tanaka
et al. (1979) used another subline designated as "HeLa J."

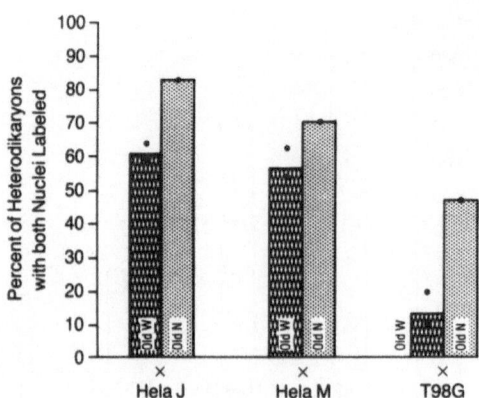

Fig. 2. The percent of heterokaryons labelled with ³H thymidine
after fusion of senescent Werner to normal HDFL cells,
T98G cells, or HeLa cells. Labeling index is defined as
the percent of heterokaryons with both nuclei labelled
following a 24-hour [3H]-thymidine pulse started
immediately after fusion. The methods of
autoradiography and cell fusion have been previously
described (Pendergrass et al., 1982). The hatched bars
represent the results of fusions to two different
strains of senescent Werner cells. The shaded bars
represent the results of fusions to normal senescent
cells. Approximately 100 heterokaryons were counted per
point. HeLa and T98G homodikaryons displayed [3H]-
thymidine labeling indices in excess of 95%; the
labeling indices of the senescent Werner and normal HDFL
homodikaryons were 5% and 7%, respectively. The two
Werner strains 78-80 KS and 78-78 were derived from
post-mortem from a 51-year-old female (patient 2 in Salk
et al., 1981). The normal (non-Werner) strain (76-109)
was derived from newborn foreskin. The Werner and
normal HDFL cells had expended nearly 100% of their
doubling potential when used in these studies.

    In an attempt to resolve this issue, we have systemically
measured the DNA polymerase alpha levels in these two HeLa
sublines, T-98G, and in a line of HDFL cells. In addition, we
examined the extent to which these cell lines stimulate nuclear
DNA synthesis following fusion with senescent cells derived from
Werner patients and from normal donors. T-98G was chosen because
it has an DNA polymerase specific activity only slightly higher
than HDFL cells (Fig. 1), and because it displays an intermediate
capacity to stimulate DNA synthesis in senescent nuclei in
heterokaryon fusions (Pendergrass et al., 1982). The methodology
for these experiments has been described in previous publications
(Pendergrass et al., 1982; Rabinovitch and Norwood, 1980). These

assays revealed that the HeLa J subline exhibits 30% more DNA polymerase alpha activity than the HeLa M subline (Fig. 1). On the other hand, the T98G cultures displayed less than 50% of the specific activity of either HeLa line. Although the activity of DNA polymerase alpha in this particular control HDFL cell line was the highest we have observed in HDFL cells, it was nonetheless lower than that observed in the T98G cultures.

Cell fusion studies revealed that the nuclear ^{3}[H]-thymidine labeling indices of the Werner nuclei in heterokaryons with Hela were modestly but consistently lower than those of nuclei from normal donors (Fig. 2). However, the T98G cells exhibited a significantly diminished capacity to reinitiate DNA synthesis in the Werner cells. In these recent studies the labeling indices of the Werner cells in heterokaryons with HeLa M were higher than those observed in the previous studies (Norwood et al., 1979a). The reason(s) for these differing observations is unclear. It is possible that variations in the biological properties between the specific strains of Werner cells used in the two studies are responsible for the differing extent of stimulation of DNA synthetic activity in the heterokaryons.

A variety of mechanisms can be invoked to explain the observation that Werner cells are relatively refractory to reinitiation of DNA synthesis under the conditions of heterokaryosis. Taking into consideration the constraints imposed by the hypothesis that we have proposed above, then two possible mechanisms merit discussion at this time: 1) Werner cells contain increased concentrations of inhibitors of initiation of DNA synthesis; and/or 2) the concentrations of initiators of DNA synthesis are diminished in senescent Werner cells.

Induction of DNA Polymerase Alpha in Senescent Normal and Werner Cells.

The first mechanism cannot be tested at the present time since the putative inhibitors have not been chemically defined. However, as discussed above, the second mechanism proposed above can be indirectly tested by examining the basal levels and inducibility of enzymes involved in DNA replication. We have examined the activities of DNA polymerase alpha at successive time points following serum stimulation of quiescent (serum deprived) cultures of normal and Werner cells. In these studies inducibility of this enzyme was demonstrable in the Werner strain and in both early and late passage non-Werner cultures (Fig. 3A and 3B). The peak levels of DNA polymerase alpha activity occurred 30-40 hours after serum stimulation. However, the relative levels of activity of this enzyme in early and late passage cultures were observed to be dependent upon the

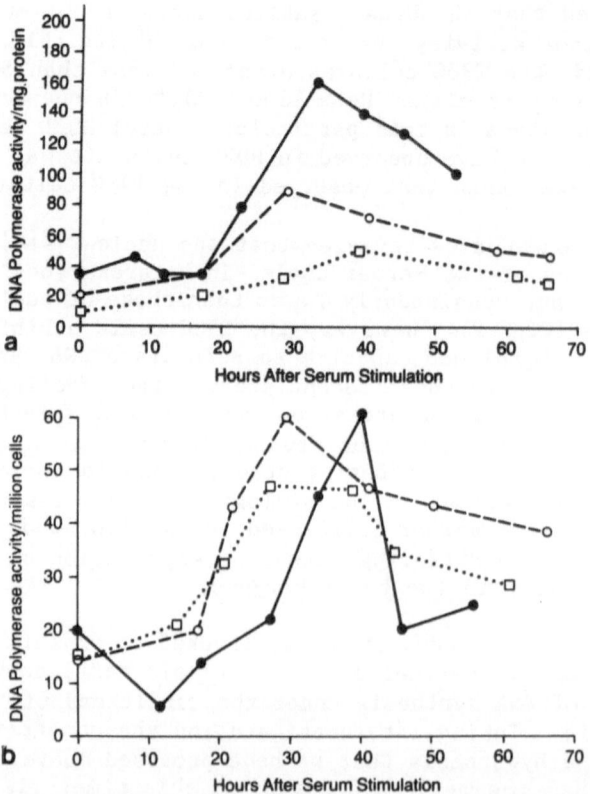

Fig. 3 (A and B). The specific activity of DNA polymerase alpha
          following serum stimulation normalized to millgrams
          of protein (A) and cell number (B). The cultures
          were plated at low density (4x10⁵ cells per 150 cm2
          flask). After approximately 48 hours the cultures
          were subjected to 10 days of serum deprivation as
          described in footnote "a" of Table 1. Fresh media
          containing 16% fetal calf serum was then added, at
          time "0", and DNA polymerase assays, cell counts,
          and protein determinations were performed at the
          time points indicated. Cell counts were performed
          with a hemocytometer. The methods for polymerase
          assays and protein determinations have been described
          previously (Pendergrass et al., 1982). (●--●) strain
          82 - 6 young normal (non-Werner) after 0.55 of its
          life span was completed; (□--□) strain 82-6, old
          normal (non-Werner), after 0.91 of its life span
          was completed; (O--O) strain 78-80, senescent Werner
          after 0.97 of its life span was completed. The tissue
          origins of these cell lines are described in footnote b
          of Table 1.

Table 1: Growth characteristics and maximum DNA polymerase-alpha activities following serum stimulation in early and late passage cultures from normal donors and late passage Werner cultures. (a)

Cell line (b)	% lifespan completed	Maximum population doubling achieved by cell line (c)	Max. Polymerase S.A. Pmols TTP incorp. per mg. protein	Pmols TTP incorp. per 10^6 cells	Maximum % cells in S phase(d)
71-95					
early passage	42	49	90	36	57
late passage	95	49	26	31	17
82-6					
early passage	41	71	202	54	55
late passage	88	71	90	60	33
78-80 KS	87	26	51	47	13

(a) Quiescence induced by incubating for one week in MEM medium supplemented with 0.5% fetal bovine serum, then for 3 days in MEM with 0.25% FBS. Stimulation was achieved by addition of MEM with 16% fetal bovine serum.

(b) The origins of the strains used are as follows: 78-80 KS, explanted post mortem from skin of right scapular region of 51-year-old patient with Werner syndrome; 82-6 explanted from foreskin of normal newborn; 71-95 explanted post mortem from mesial aspect of upper arm.

(c) "Senescence" is defined as a 24 hr (^{3}H)-thymidine labeling index <20%.

(d) The fraction of cells in S-phase was determined by autoradiography of replicate cultures pulsed for 15 minutes with [^{3}H]-thymidine and fixed at the same time as the polymerase assays were performed.

Table 2

Protein content of cultured HDFL cells

Cell strain	% lifespan completed	Maximum lifespan population doublings	Pg protein per million cells
71–95	17	49	330+28 (8)
71–95	98	49	804+75 (5)
71–95	100	49	960+59 (8)
82–6	41	71	488+42 (8)
82–6	88	71	711+48 (8)
82–6	91	71	781 – (2)
78–80 KS	87	26	1146+230 (7)
78–80 KS	97	26	1747+304 (4)

a) See footnote b,Table 1,for description of cell lines. Cells
were prepared as described in the legend to Fig. 3. After
serum stimulation, cells were counted and aliquots were
analyzed for protein (Pendergrass et al., 1982).
b) Mean values + standard error; number of experimental
observations in parenthesis

parameter utilized for normalization of the activity levels
polymerase alpha. When the activity of DNA polymerase is
normalized to protein content, the peak levels in senescent
cultures from both Werner and normal donors are 1/2 – 1/3 those
values observed in two strains of low passage active
proliferating HDFL cells (Fig. 3A, Table 1). In contrast, when
the specific activity of DNA polymerase alpha is normalized to
cell number, the peak levels of low passage and senescent
cultures are almost identical (Fig. 3B, Table 1). Similar
specific activities per 10^6 cells are maintained despite a
precipitous drop in the labelling indices of the senescent cells
(Fig. 4). This indicates induction of DNA polymerase alpha is
uncoupled from DNA synthesis in senescent cells.

    The reduced activity per unit amount of cellular protein is
almost certainly a reflection of increased cell size in the
senescent cultures. Measurements of the protein content per cell
support this interpretation (Table 2). The protein content is
increased over two-fold in the senescent cultures. Moreover, the
senescent Werner cultures have a protein content three to five
times that of the young actively proliferating cells from normal
donors. The observations indicate that DNA polymerase alpha
remains as inducible in post-mitotic, senescent cultures.

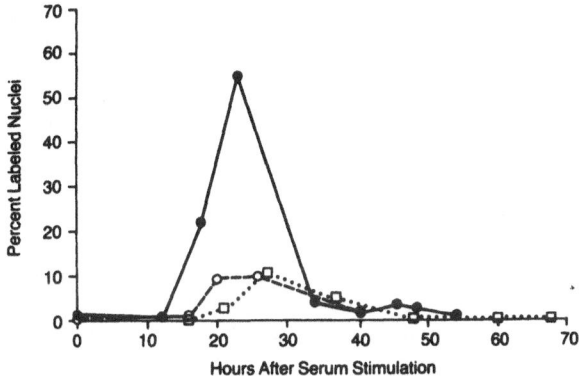

Fig. 4. Percent [3H]-thymidine labeled nuclei following serum
stimulation. The cells were plated in 25 cm2 flasks at
identical densities as the cultures used for the
polymerase assays in Fig. 3. The cultures were pulsed
with [3H]-thymidine for 15 minutes (2 μCi/ml, SA
6.76/mMole) at the times indicated following stimulation
with medium containing 16% fetal bovine serum. (●--●)
strain 82-6: young normal (non-Werner), (◻--◻) strain
82-6: senescent normal (non-Werner), FLC=0.91; (O--O)
strain 78-80: senescent Werner.

However, the reduced activity per unit protein raises the
possibility that the intra cellular concentration of factors
involved in the initiation and maintenance of DNA synthesis may
be reduced to subfunctional levels.

Discussion of Experimental Findings

We have proposed an hypothesis which could provide a partial
explanation for the loss of DNA synthetic activity in senescing
HDFL cells derived from normal and Werner donors. This
hypothesis predicts that endogenous levels of factors required
for initiation of DNA synthesis may be an important property
influencing the growth and possibly the life span potential of a
given cell type. The reduction of activity of DNA polymerase in
senescent cells may in part or entirely be due to dilution
resulting from increased cell size, or alternatively to the
presence of an "inhibitor" of DNA synthesis. These alternatives
are not mutually exclusive. For example, the observed dilution
of DNA polymerase may be due to cell enlargement secondary to
inhibition of cell cycle function by this putative inhibitor.

The phenomenon of cell enlargement following disruption of
coordination between cell growth and division cycles has been
termed unbalanced growth (Mitcheson, 1971). This has been well

documented in mammalian cells and appears to result from continued accumulation of RNA and protein in the absence of key regulatory molecules that trigger DNA synthesis and/or karyokinesis (Mitchison, 1971; Fournier and Pardee, 1975; Mitsui and Schneider, 1976). Unbalanced growth is also observed in lower organisms such as yeast and bacteria. This phenomenon is also observed in certain mutations which are associated with clonal senescence (i.e. loss of growth potential) - an example of which is the "nibbled" mutant in yeast. This strain displays a clonal decline of growth capacity which is associated with overproduction of the two micron plasmid DNA (Holm, 1982). It is postulated that initiation sites on these plasmids compete with chromosomal DNA initiation sites for replication factors finally diminishing the pool of available factors below the threshold level required for cell cycle function. Thus, this mutant strain is a potentially important model for the study of clonal senescence.

The senescent Werner cells were observed to have a significantly higher protein content than senescent cells derived from normal donors (Table 2). This correlated with increased sizes as assessed by visual inspection via phase contrast microscopy. Clearly, more extensive cell sizing studies will have to be completed in multiple strains derived from Werner patients from different pedigrees to determine if increased cell size is indeed a part of the phenotype of these cultures. However, in these studies we did observe that the level of DNA synthesis activity was lower in heterokaryons resulting from the fusion of the Werner cells and the transformed cell types used in these experiments (Fig. 2). This was most evident in the case of the heterokaryons studies in which the Werner and normal strains were fused to T98G cells. Thus, these observations suggest that the stimulation of DNA synthesis in senescent nuclei in these heterokaryons is conversely correlated with cell size, as assessed by protein content. This is consistent with the notion that critical replication factors are "diluted" in the larger cells which resulted in reduced DNA replicative capacity.

Finally, the demonstration of the inducibility of DNA polymerase alpha in these cultures provides further evidence that, in the presence of mitogens, senescent HDFL cells are lodged at G_1/S boundary. This was originally suggested by Olashaw et al (1983). These authors demonstrated that thymidine kinase activity and the thymidine triphosphate pool size in senescent HDFL cells, like DNA polymerase alpha, remain inducible following mitogen stimulation. This interpretation assumes that inducibility of the enzymes remains a valid marker of cell cycle position in these senescent cultures. Clearly further knowledge of the basic biology of the cell cycle is required before this interpretation can be accepted without question.

REFERENCES

Aso, K., Kondo, S., and Amano, M., 1980, A case of Werner's
    syndrome in which lowered activity of platelet-dependent serum
    factor for cell growth and reduced growth potential of
    fibroblasts and epidermal cells were demonstrated, Nippon
    Hifuka Gakka Zasshi, 90:929.
Baril, E., Baril, B., Elford, H., and Luftig, R.B., 1974, DNA
    polymerase and a possible multi-enzyme complex for DNA
    biosynthesis eukaryotes, in: "Mechanism and Regulation of DNA
    Replication," A. Kolber and K. Kohigam eds. Plenum
    Publishing Corp., New York, pp. 276-293.
Bunn, C.L. and Tarrant, G.M., 1980, Limited lifespan in somatic
    cell hybrids and cybrids, Exp. Cell Res., 127:385.
Burmer, G.C., Motulsky, H., Zeigler, C.J., and Norwood, T.H.,
    1983, Inhibition of DNA synthesis in young cycling human
    diploid fibroblast-like cells upon fusion to enucleate
    cytoplasms from senescent cells, Exp. Cell Res., 145:79.
Burmer, G.C., Zeigler, C.J., and Norwood, T.H., 1982, Evidence for
    endogenous polypeptide-mediate inhibition of cell-cycle
    transit in human diploid, J. Cell Biol., 94:187.
Croce, C.M. and Koprowski, H., 1974, Positive control of
    transformed phenotype in hybrid between SV-40 and normal
    human cells, Science, 184:1288.
Drescher-Lincoln, C.K. and Smith, J.L., 1983, Inhibition of DNA
    synthesis in proliferating human diploid fibroblasts by
    fusion with senescent cytoplasts, Exp. Cell. Res., 144:445.
DePamphilis, M.L. and Wassarman, M.L., 1980, Replication of
    eukaryotic chromosomes: A close-up of the replication fork,
    Annu. Rev. Biochem., 49:627.
Duthu, G.S., Braunschweiger, K.I., Pereira-Smith, O.M., Norwood,
    T.H., and Smith, J.R., 1982, A long-lived human diploid
    fibroblast line for cellular aging studies: applications in
    cell hybridization, Mech. Ageing Devel. 20:243.
Fialo, M. and Kenny, G.E., 1966, Enhancement of rhinovirus plaque
    formation in human heteroploid cell cultures by magnesuim
    and calcium, J. Bacteriol. 92:1710.
Fry, M., 1983, in: "Eukaryotic DNA Polymerases," L.S. Hnilica, ed.,
    CRC Press Series in Biochemistry and Molecular Biology of the
    Cell Nucleus, CRC press.
Gopalakrishman, T.V. and Anderson, W.F., 1979, Epigenetic
    activation of phenylalinine in mouse erythroleukemia cells
    by the cytoplast of rat hepatoma cells, Proc. Natl. Acad.
    Sci., 76:3922.
Goldstein, S., 1979, Studies on age-related diseases in cultured
    skin fibroblasts. J. Invest. Dermatol., 73:19.
Goldstein, S. and Lin, C.C., 1972, Rescue of senescent human
    fibroblasts by hybridization with hamster cells in vitro,
    Exp. Cell. Res., 70:436.

Hoehn, H., Bryant, E.M., Johnston, P., Norwood, T.H. and Martin, G.M., 1975, Non-selective isolation, stability and longevity of hybrids between normal human somatic cells, Nature 258:608.

Hoehn, H., Bryant, E.M. and Martin, G.M., 1978, The replicative life spans of euploid hybrids derived from short-lived and long-lived human skin fibroblast cultures, Cytogenet. Cell Genet., 21:282.

Holm, C., 1982, Clonal lethality caused by the yeast plasmid 2ᵐDNA, Cell, 29:585.

Johnston, L.H. and Nasmyth, K.A., 1978, Saccharomyces Cerevisiae cell cycle mutant cdc 9 is defective in DNA, Lyare. Nat., 274:891.

Kahn, C.R., Gopalakrishman, T.V., and Weiss, M.C., 1981, Transfer of heritable properties by cell cybridization: Specificity and the role of selective pressure, Somat. Cell. Genet., 7:547.

Kornberg, A., 1980, Eukaryotic DNA polymerases, in: "DNA Replication," A. Kornburg, ed., W.H. Freeman and Co., San Francisco, pp. 210-229.

Lipsich, L.A., Kates, J.R., and Lucas, J.J., 1979, Expression of a liver-specific function by mouse fibroblast nuclei transplanted into rat hepatoma cytoplasts, Nature, 281:74.

Martin, G.M., 1977, Cellular aging - clonal senescence, Amer. J. Path., 89:484.

Mitcheson, J.M., 1971, The Biology of the Cell Cycle, Cambridge University Press, London, pp. 29-33, 244-249.

Mitsui, Y. and Schneider, E.L., 1976, Increased nuclear sizes in senescent human diploid fibroblast cultures, Exp. Cell. Res., 100:147.

Muggleton-Harris, A.L. and Hayflick, L., 1976, Cellular aging studied by the reconstruction of replicating cells from nuclei and cytoplasms isolated from normal human diploid cells, Exp. Cell. Res., 103:321.

Muggleton-Harris, A.L. and DeSimone, D.W., 1980, Replicative potentials of various fusion products between WI-38 and SV-40 transformed WI-38 cells and their components, Somat. Cell Genet. 6:689.

Muggleton-Harris, A.L. and Aroian, M.A., 1982, Replicative potential of individual cell hybrids derived from young and old donor human skin fibroblasts, Somat. Cell Genet. 8:41.

Nette, E.G., Sit, H.L., King, D.W., 1982, Reactivation of DNA synthesis in aging diploid human skin fibroblasts by fusion with mouse L karyoplasts, cytoplasts and whole L cells, Mech. Age. Dev. 18:75.

Noguchi, H., Reddy, G.P., and Pardee, A.B., 1983, Rapid incorporation of label from ribonucleoside disphosphates into DNA by a cell-free high molecular weight fraction from animal cell nuclei, Cell 32:443.

Norwood, T.H., Hoehn, H., Salk, D., and Martin, G.M., 1979a, Cellular aging in Werner's syndrome: A unique phenotype, J. Invest. Dermatol. 72:92.

Norwood, T.H., Pendergrass, W.R., and Martin, G.M., 1975, Reinitiation of DNA synthesis in senescent human fibroblasts upon fusion with cells of unlimited growth potential, J. Cell Biol. 64:551.

Norwood, T.H., Pendergrass, W., Bornstein, P., and Martin, G.M., 1979b, DNA synthesis of sublethally injured cells in heterokaryons and its relevance to clonal senescence, Exp. Cell Res. 119:15.

Norwood, T.H., Pendergrass, W.R., Sprague, C.A., and Martin, G.M., 1974, Dominance of the senescent phenotype in heterokaryons between replicative and post-replicative human fibroblast-like cells, Proc. Natl. Acad. Sci., 73:223.

Norwood, T.H. and Smith, J.R., 1985, "The cultural fibroblast-like cell as a model for the study of aging." In Handbook of the Biology of Aging, Eds., C.E. Finch and E.L. Schneider, Van Nostrond Reinhold, New York, in press.

Norwood, T.H., Zeigler, C.J., 1979c, Complementation between senescent human diploid cells and a thymidine kinase deficient murine cell line, Cytogenet. Cell Genet. 19:355.

Orgel, L.E., 1963, The maintenance of the accuracy of protein synthesis and its relevance to aging, Proc. Natl. Acad. Sci., 49:517.

Orgel, L.E., 1970, The maintenance of the accuracy of protein synthesis and its relevance to aging: A correction, Proc. Natl. Acad. Sci., 67:1476.

Pendergrass, W.R., Saulewicz, A.C., Burmer, G.C., Rabinovitch, P.S., Norwood, T.H., and Martin, G.M., 1982, Evidence that a critical threshold of DNA synthesis in mammalian cells heterokaryons, J. Cell. Physiol. 133:141.

Pereira-Smith, O.M. and Smith, J.R., 1981, Expression of SV-40 T antigen in finite life-span hybrids of normal and SV-40-transformed fibroblasts. Somat. Cell. Genet. 7:411.

Pereira-Smith, O.M. and Smith, J.R., 1982, The phenotype of low proliferative potential is dominant in hybrids of normal human fibroblasts. Somat. Cell Genet..

Rabinovitch, P.S. and Norwood, T.H., 1980, Comparative heterokaryon study of cellular senescence and the serum-deprived state. Exp. Cell. Res. 130:101.

Rao, M.V.N., 1976, Reactivation of chick erythrocyte nuclei in young and senescent WI38 cells, Exp. Cell Res., 102:25.

Rao, P.N., Satya-Prakash,K.L. 1983, Inducers of DNA synthesis: Levels higher in transformed cells than in normal cells, J. Cell Biol. 96:571.

Reddy, P.V. and Pardee, A.G., 1980, Multienzyme complex for metabolic channeling in mammalian DNA replication, Proc. Natl. Acad. Sci., USA, 77:3312.

Salk, D., 1982, Werner's syndrome: A review of recent research
     with an analysis of connective tissue metabolism, growth
     control of cultured cells and chromosomal aberrations, Human
     Genetics, 62:1.
Salk, D., Bryant, E., Au, K., Hoehn, H., and Martin, G.M., 1981,
     Systematic growth studies, cocultivation, and cell
     hybridization studies of Werner syndrome cultured skin
     fibroblasts, Hum. Genet. 58:310.
Scappaticci, S., Cerimele, D., Fraccaro, M., 1982, Clonal
     structural chromosomal rearrangements in primary fibroblast
     cultures and in lymphocytes of patients with Werner's
     syndrome, Hum. Genet. 62:16.
Schonberg, S.A., Henderson, E., Niermeijer, M.F., and German, J.,
     1981, Werner's syndrome: preferential proliferation of clones
     with translocations, Am. J. Hum. Genet. 33:120A.
Stanbridge, E.J., 1976, Suppression of malignancy in human cells,
     Nature, 260:17.
Stein, G.H. and Yanishevsky, R.M., 1981, Quiescent human diploid
     cells can inhibit entry into S phase in replicative nuclei in
     heterodikaryons, Proc. Natl. Acad. Sci. 78:325.
Stein, G.H. and Yanishevsky, R.M., 1979, Entry into S phase is
     inhibited in two immortal cell lines fused to senescent human
     diploid cells, Exp. Cell. Res. 120:155.
Stein, G.H., Yanishevsky, R.M., Gordon, L., and Beeson, M., 1982,
     Carcinogen-transformed human cells are inhibited from entry
     into S phase by fusion to senescent cells but cells
     transformed by DNA tumor viruses overcome the inhibition,
     Proc. Natl. Acad. Sci. 79:5287.
Tanaka, K., Nakazawa, T., Okada, Y., and Kmahara, Y., 1979,
     Increase in DNA synthesis in Werner's syndrome cells by
     hybridization with normal human diploid and hela cells, Exp.
     Cell Res. 123:261.
Tanaka, K., Nakazawa, T., Okada, Y., and Kumahara, Y., 1980, Roles
     of nuclear and cytoplasmic environments in the retarded DNA
     synthesis in Werner's syndrome cells, Exp. Cell Res. 127:185.
Wright, W.E. and Hayflick, L., 1975a, Nuclear control of cellular
     aging demonstrated by hybridization of anucleate and whole
     cultured normal human fibroblasts, Exp. Cell Res. 96:113.
Wright, W.E. and Hayflick, L., 1975b, The regulation of cellular
     aging by nuclear events in cultured normal fibroblasts (WI-
     38), Adv. Exp. Mol. Biol, 61:39.
Yanishevsky, R.M. and Stein, G.H., 1981, Regulation of the cell
     cycle in eukaryotyic cells, Int. Rev. Cytol. 69:223.
Yanishevsky, R.M. and Stein, G.H., 1980, Ongoing DNA synthesis
     continues in young human diploid cells (HDC) fused to
     senescent HDC, but entry into S phase is inhibited, Exp. Cell
     Res. 126:469

HISTONE H1 IN G1 ARRESTED, SENESCENT, AND WERNER SYNDROME FIBROBLASTS

Youji Mitsui, Hiroshi Sakagami and Masa-atu Yamada

Fermentation Research Institute*
Chief, Division of Cell Science and Technology
Agency of Industrial Science and Technology
Higashi 1-1-3, Yatabe-machi, Ibaraki, 305
Japan

ABSTRACT

Histone H1 content and synthesis were examined in normal, Werner-syndrome, and transformed fibroblasts. Analysis of ^{3}H-lysine incorporation indicated that senescent cells, but not G1-arrested young cells, had a lower ratio of molar synthesis of H1 histone to nucleosome histones than did growing young cells or gamma-ray-transformed cells. Furthermore, a biochemical study of histone H1 content plotted as a function of DNA synthesis activity and an immunocytological study using antiserum against histone H1 revealed that senescent cells had a lower histone H1 content than did young cultures at all stages of cell proliferation. Werner syndrome skin fibroblasts at early passage, however, had amounts of histone H1 comparable to those of age-matched normal control fibroblasts. We conclude that a decline, with increasing passage number, in content and synthesis of H1 histone relative to nucleosomal histones (Mitsui et al., 1980) was not simply due to passage-related accumulation of G1-arrested cells, but actually reflected age specific changes of cultured human fibroblasts. The depletion of histone H1 in the chromatin of senescent cells is a possible cause of DNA strand breakage or relaxation of gene repression.

INTRODUCTION

A decrease in replication capacity and cell function is the most basic phenomenon of human cellular aging in vitro. Chromatin, composed of repeating structural units termed nucleosomes, has an important role in DNA replication and gene expression. Histones H2a, H2b, H3 and H4 form an octamer constituting the nucleosome core, whereas a single molecule of histone H1 is found in association with both the nucleosome core and with the spacer DNA between two adjacent nucleosomes. Thus, H1 is involved in DNA synthesis and in the higher order organization of chromatin structure. Several papers demonstrate a decrease in the amount of histone H1 in relation to altered genetic activity or proliferation capacity (Grimes et al., 1975; Shirley and Anderson, 1977; Pehrson and Cole, 1980; Seale and Alonson, 1975; Gorovsky and Keevert, 1975; D'Anna et al., 1982).

We have previously reported a decrease in histone H1 relative to nucleosomal histones with cellular aging of human diploid fibroblasts in vitro, and we concluded that the decrease was due to a decline in the synthesis rate and an increase in the degradation rate of histone H1 in senescent cultures (Mitsui et al., 1980a). Senescent cultures, however, contain rapidly dividing cells with an increased proportion of slowly dividing or non-dividing cells (Cristofaro and Sharf, 1973; Mitsui and Schneider, 1976c). Some aging indices are simply a reflection of the decreased potential for DNA synthesis rather than being specific characteristics of in vitro aging (Mitsui and Schneider, 1976c: Mitsui et al., 1979). Synthesis of the major histones in G1-arrested cells is uncoordinated with respect for each other (Taranowka et al., 1978; Herve et al., 1979). Thus the question arose whether the relative decrease in histone H1 synthesis in senescent cultures was due to the presence of an increasing number of resting cells with lower synthesis rate of histone H1.

The Werner syndrome is a rare genetic disease that shows many features similar to changes that occur during normal aging. It involves major segments of the senescent phenotype rather than being a true acceleration of the aging process, as pointed out by Martin (1978). Werner syndrome fibroblasts have a shortened life span in vitro than do donor-age matched control fibroblasts and they display chromosome instability (Salk et al., 1981) and defects in DNA replication (Fujiwara et al., 1977; Takeuchi et al., 1982). Thus, an interest has been aroused as to whether a decline of histone H1 content is seen at early passage of Werner fibroblasts. In the present studies, the effects of G1-arrest and of a genetic defect on histone H1 content and synthetic molar ratio were examined by study of normal and Werner-syndrome fibroblasts using biochemical and immunocytological procedures.

MATERIALS AND METHODS

Cell culture

The cell lines used in the present paper were TIG-1, a human fetal lung fibroblast strain established at the Tokyo Metropolitan Institute of Gerontology (Mitsui et al., 1980b; Ohashi et al., 1980), WI-38 fibroblasts transformed with Co-60 gamma rays (Co-transformed WI-38)(Namba et al., 1978), Werner-syndrome fibroblasts (57 year-old donor) and donor-age matched skin fibroblasts. Cells were cultured in Eagle's Minimum Essential Medium (MEM, Gibco) supplemented with glutamine, non-essential amino acids, 10% fetal bovine serum (Gibco), streptomycin sulfate (100 μ g/ml) and penicillin G potassium (100 U/ml). Routine subcultivations were performed at a 1:4 split ratio once a week, with one intervening change of medium, and population doubling levels (PDL) calculated.

Radioisotope incorporation

To examine serum concentration effects on DNA and histone synthesis, growing young cells cultivated in 15-cm diameter dishes were rinsed twice with culture medium containing 0.1, 1 or 10% serum and then cultured in medium containing the same concentration of serum for 48 hours. These cultures were incubated with 1 μCi/ml of ^{3}H-lysine (76.4 Ci/mmole) or 0.05 μCi/ml ^{3}H-thymidine (21 Ci/mmole) for the last 24 hours. To see the effect of contact inhibition of cell growth, young and senescent cells at various phases of cell growth were labeled with 2 μCi/ml ^{3}H-thymidine or 2 μCi/ml ^{3}H-lysine in lysine-free MEM containing 10% serum for one hour. For the measurement of DNA synthesis, parallel cultures containing coverglasses were used and the acid-insoluble radioactivity of tritium in cells on the coverglasses was counted with a gas-flow counter (Aloka FC-22B). The amount of DNA was determined by the diphenylamine reaction. Histones were isolated as described below.

Isolation of histones

Detailed procedures for histone isolation have been described in a previous paper (Mitsui et al., 1980a). Briefly, young and senescent cells were harvested after being scraped off with a rubber policeman and washed with buffer A [10 mM Tris-HCl, pH 7.4; 10 mM KCl; 5 mM CaCl; 1 mM phenylmethyl sulfonyl flouride (PMSF)] and then collected by spinning at 1500 rpm for 5 min. The cells were suspended in 2 ml of buffer B (0.5% Triton X-100 in buffer A), homogenized with 20 strokes in a teflon-glass homogenizer and centrifuged. The recovered crude nuclei were washed twice with 1 ml of buffer C (0.25 M sucrose; 10 mM Tris-HCl, pH 7.4; 5mM CaCl; 0.25 % Triton X-100; 1 mM PMSF) and twice with 1 ml of buffer D (0.15 M NaCl; 10mM Tris-HCl, pH 8.0; 1 mM PMSF) to remove 0.15 M

NaCl soluble proteins. Histones were extracted twice with 10
volumes of 0.4 N H_3SO_4 with 1 mM PMSF. The extracted histones
were precipitated with trichloroacetic acid (final concentration
25%) and washed with acidified acetone, then three times with
acetone.

Polyacrylamide gel electrophoreses of histones

The histones were solubilized in solution F (7 M urea, 5% 2-
mercaptoethanol, 0.9 N acetic acid) and subjected to
electrophoresis on 0.5 x 15 cm, acid-urea (15%) according to the
method of Panyin and Chalkley (1969). To measure histone content,
the gels were stained with 0.05% amido black 10 B solution for 3
hours. The stained gels were scanned at 560 nm with a Cosmo D-101
densitometer (Cosmo Co., Tokyo) with gel scanning attachment. For
the measurement of histone synthesis, the one-dimensional acid-urea
gels were equilibrated for 2 hours in SDS sample buffer and
subjected to electrophoresis in the second dimension on 10%
acrylamide SDS gels as described by O'Farrell (1975). The areas
corresponding to each histone were cut into slices of 1 mm
thickness and kept at 50°C overnight in vials with 1 ml of Soluene-
350 (Packard).

Radioactivity was measured in 10 ml of scintillation liquid
containing 10 ml toluene, 50 mg PPO and 3 mg dimethyl POPOP using a
scintillation spectrophotometer. To determine the molar ratio of
histone H1 synthesis, the sum of the radioactivity in the areas of
histone H1, H2a + H2b + H3, and H4 were divided by the respective
lysine content in the histone fractions [62 for H1, 15.7 for H2a +
H2b + H3, and 11 for H4 as described by Tarnowka et al. (1978)] and
then the relative rates of synthesis were calculated, normalizing
the rate of H2a + H2b + H3 to 3.

Immunocytological staining of histone H1

Rabbit antiserum against calf thymus histone H1 and FITC-
conjugated antiserum against rabbit immunoglobulin were obtained
from Dr. Tutsui, Hamamatsu Medical School. The indirect method to
show the binding of fluorescent antibody to histone H1 was used.
Co-cultivation of early and late passage cells was performed by
inoculating a drop of each cell suspension onto a coverglass in a
culture dish.

RESULTS

Effects of serum depletion

Early passage cells were cultured in medium with 10, 1, or
0.1% serum and labeled with ^{3}H-lysine for 24 hours. As seen in
Fig. 1, ^{3}H-lysine incorporation into histone fractions markedly

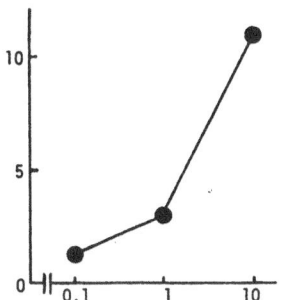

Fig. 1:   Histone synthesis under serum depletion. [Abscissa: serum
           concentration (%); ordinate: radioactivity in histones
           (dpm x 10^{-4}/dish).]   Young cells (18 PDL) were cultured
           in different concentrations of serum (0.1, 1 and 10%
           fetal bovine serum in MEM) for 48 hours and labeled with
           1 μCi/ml (^{3}H)-lysine for the last 24 hours.

declined in cultures grown at reduced serum concentration. When
corrected for differences in cell number, histone synthesis per
cell in 0.1% serum cultures decreased to 20% of that in 10% serum
cultures and was accompanied by a decline in the cycling cell
population.

      DNA synthesis was monitored by labeling parallel cultures with
^{3}H-thymidine for the same periods, and newly synthesized histone
versus newly synthesized DNA was examined at various degrees of
cell proliferation.   Fig. 2 indicates that an excess amount of
histones was synthesized relative to DNA with the accumulation of
resting cells in 0.1% serum cultures, suggesting the presence of
histone turnover in the resting cells.

      The extracted histones were separated by acid-urea polyacryl-
amide gel electrophoresis, and the sum of the radioactivities of
each histone fraction was divided by the respective lysine content
to determine the relative molar ratio of histone synthesis. As
shown in Fig. 3, the molar synthesis ratio of histone H1 relative
to the other nucleosomal histones did not decrease with the
accumulation of resting cells.

Effects of contact inhibition of cell growth

      To confirm the above findings, histone and DNA synthesis were
examined in contact-inhibited cultures in which G1-arrested cells
were also expected to accumulate. Young and senescent cultures
were incubated with radioactive thymidine or lysine for one hour in
lysine-depleted MEM containing 10% fetal bovine serum. Histones
were then extracted and subjected to two-dimensional

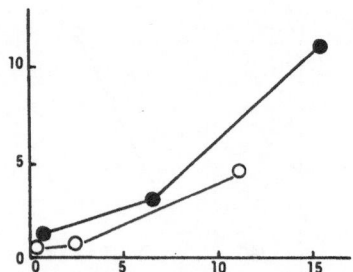

Fig. 2:   Histone synthesis as a function of DNA synthesis
           activity. [Abscissa: radioactivity in DNA
           (cpm x 10^{-3}/coverglass); ordinate: radioactivity in
           histones (dpm x 10^{-4}/dish).] Young cells (18 PDL, solid
           circles) and senescent cells (52 PDL, empty circles) were
           cultured and labeled as described in Fig 1; parallel
           cultures containing coverglasses were labeled with 0.05 μ
           Ci/ml (^{3}H-)thymidine for 24 hours. Acid-insoluble
           radioactivity was measured with a gas flow counter to
           determine DNA synthesis.

electrophoresis to exclude any possible contamination of other
proteins in the histone fractions. Fig. 4 shows histone H1
synthesis as a function of DNA synthesis in young and senescent
cultures. The extrapolated values of lysine incorporation at zero

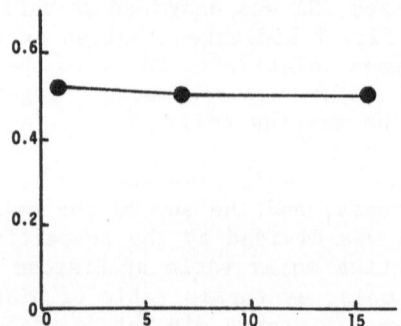

Fig. 3:   Relative histone H1 synthesis in serum depleted cultures.
           [Abscissa: radioactivity in DNA (cpm x 10^{-3}/cover-
           glass); ordinate: molar synthetic ratio of histone H1.]
           Labeled histones were extracted from young cells in Fig.
           2 and subjected to acid-urea polyacrilamide gel electro-
           phoresis. Distribution of the total radioactivities into
           the peaks corresponding to H1, (H3 + H2b + H2a), and H4
           (see Fig. 7 for a sample) were counted, and molar synthe-
           sis ratio of histone H1 relative to other nucleosomal
           histones was determined.

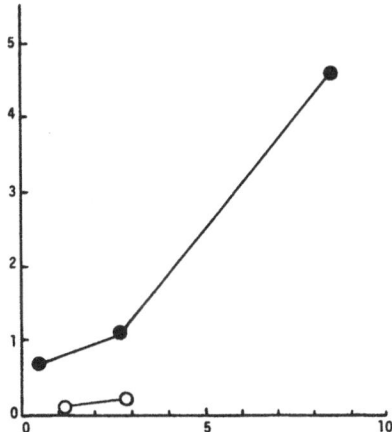

Fig. 4:   Histone Hl synthesis in contact-inhibited young and
           senescent cells. [Abscissa: radioactivity in DNA
           (cpm x 10^{-4}/ µg DNA); ordinate: radioactivity in histone
           Hl (dpm x 10^{-2}/ µ g DNA).] At different stages of growth,
           young cells (solid circles) and senescent cells (empty
           circles) were labeled with 2 µ Ci/ml (^{3}H)-lysine in
           lysine-depleted medium for one hour. Parallel cultures
           with a coverglass in each dish were labeled with 2 µCi/ml
           (^{3}H)-thymidine for one hour. Separation of histone Hl
           fraction was performed by two-dimensional gel
           electrophoresis (acid-urea/SDS) to minimize any possible
           contamination by other proteins. For the determination
           of DNA synthesis, total radioactivity of the TCA
           insoluble fraction from each coverglass was divided by
           the amount of DNA in the dish.

DNA synthesis indicate that there is some turnover synthesis of
histone Hl in Gl-arrested cells. The data also demonstrate that
histone Hl synthesis in senescent cultures was lower than that in
young cultures (similar data were obtained in the serum-depleted
cultures). The molar ratio of histone Hl synthesis was again found
not to decline with the accumulation of non-cycling cells (Fig. 5).

    It is noticeable that the molar ratio of histone Hl synthesis
in senescent cultures was lower than that in growth-retarded or
rapidly-growing young cultures. Relative amounts of histone Hl at
various stages of cell growth were determined by ^{3}H-thymidine
incorporation into DNA and densitometric analysis of histones
subjected to electrophoresis. Fig. 6 reveals that the histone Hl
content in senescent cultures was lower than that in young
cultures, irrespective of their growth activity, although some
decline in histone Hl content was observed in the highly contact-
inhibited young cultures.

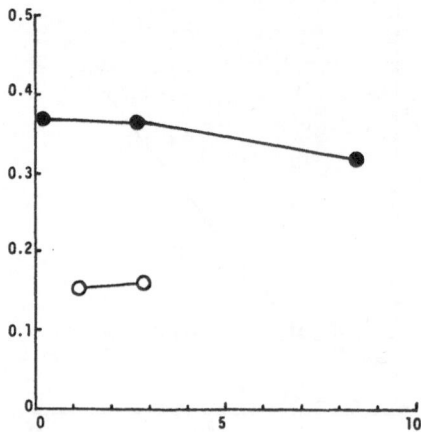

Fig. 5:   Relative histone H1 synthesis in contact-inhibited
           cultures. [Abscissa: radioactivity in DNA (cpm x 10⁻⁴/
           μg DNA); ordinate: molar synthesis ratio of histone
           H1.]   Young (solid circles) and senescent cells (empty
           circles) were cultured and labeled as in Fig. 4.   The
           molar synthesis ratio of histone H1 was determined from
           the distribution of radioactivity in each histone
           separated by two dimensional electrophoresis.

Table 1

Molar ratio of histone H1 in normal
and transformed human fibroblasts

Cell strain	(Population doubling level)	Maximum life span	Molar ratio H1: (H3 + H2b + H2a): H4				
TIG-1	(18 PDL)	65 PDL	0.46	:	3	:	1.15
TIG-1	(56 PDL)	65 PDL	0.26	:	3	:	1.27
^{60}Co- transformed WI-38	(>200 PDL)	Infinite	0.47	:	3	:	1.18

Growing cells were labeled with 1 μ Ci/ml (³H)-lysine or
0.1 μCi/ml (¹⁴C)-lysine for 24 hours.   Histones were
extracted, analyzed by acid-urea gel electrophoresis, and
molar ratio of histone H1 synthesis was determined as
shown in Fig. 7.

Histone H1 synthesis in transformed human cells

The above results indicate that a decrease in histone H1 synthesis with increasing passage number is an age-specific phenomenon rather than a growth-related one. Thus, transformed human fibroblasts at high population doubling levels were expected to have as high a molar ratio of histone H1 synthesis as that in young diploid fibroblasts. Therefore, ^{3}H-lysine incorporation into histone fractions of growing young, senescent, or gamma-ray transformed human cells was examined (Fig. 7). As seen in Table 1, the molar ratio of histone H1 synthesis in transformed cells even at their high population doubling levels was identical to that in normal early passage cells and much higher than that in normal late passage cells.

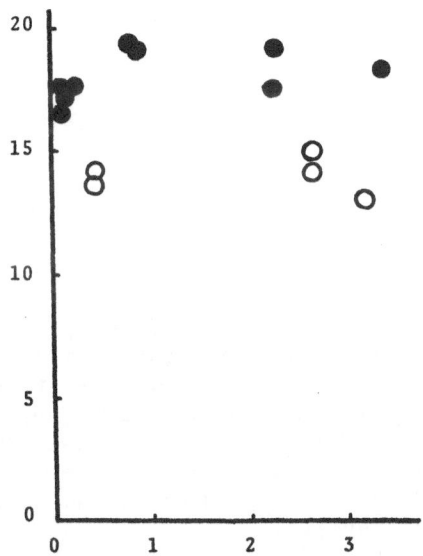

Fig. 6:   Histone H1 content in growth-inhibited young and
            senescent cultures. [Abscissa: radioactivity in DNA
            (cpm x 10^{-4}/ μg DNA); ordinate: relative amount of
            histone H1 (% of total histones).] At different stages
            of cell growth, young (solid circles) and senescent
            (empty circles) cells were harvested for histone
            isolation. Relative amount of histone H1 was determined
            by densitometric analysis of histones separated by acid-
            urea gel electrophoresis. For the determination of DNA
            synthesis, parallel cultures containing coverglasses were
            labeled with 2 μCi/ml (^{3}H)-thymidine.

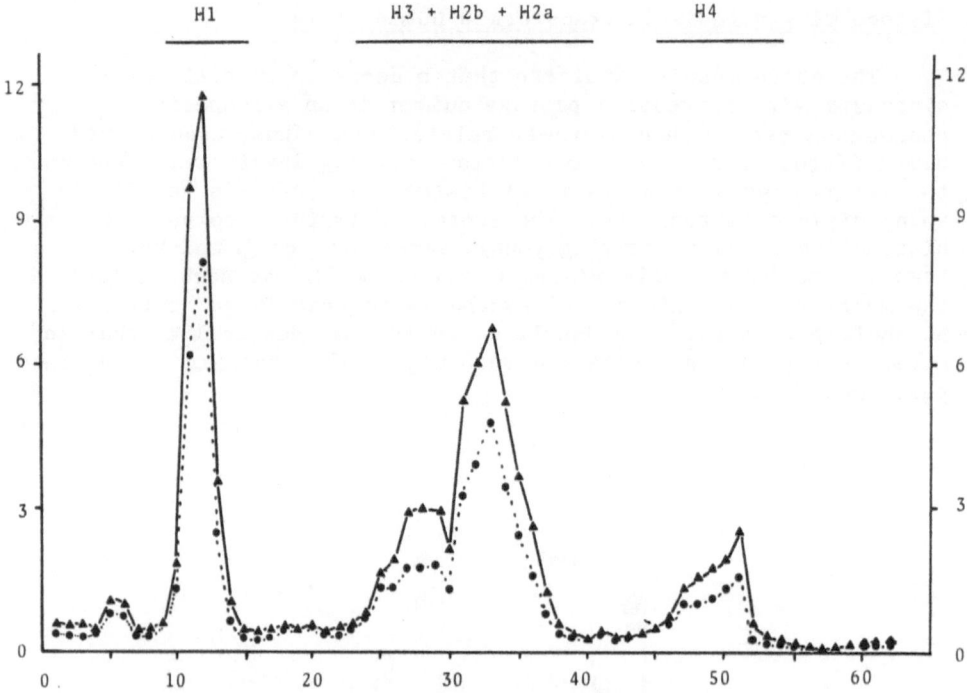

Fig. 7:   Distribution of radioactivity of lysine in histone
           fractions from young diploid fibroblasts and transformed
           fibroblasts. [Abscissa: slice number of electrophoretic
           gel; ordinate: (left, circles) radioactivity of (^{3}H)-
           lysine (dpm x 10^{-3}/slice); (right, triangles)
           radioactivity of (^{14}C)-lysine (dpm x 10^{-2}/slice).]
           Growing young diploid fibroblasts (18 PDL) and
           transformed WI-38 cells (200 PDL) were labeled for 24
           hours with ^{14}C-lysine and ^{3}H-lysine, respectively, and
           mixed immediately after cell collection. Histones were
           extracted from the mixed cells and collectively subjected
           to electrophoresis.

Immunofluorescence cytological study of histone H1

        To avoid the possibility that an artificial degradation or
loss of histone H1 might occur during histone preparation, we also
used immunocytological procedures to confirm the differences in the
amount of histone H1 between early- and late-passage cells.

        Figures 8 and 9 are photomicrographs of fluorescent-stained
histone H1. Early-passage cells (Fig. 8, left) had a higher
intensity of flourescence in their nuclei than did late-passage

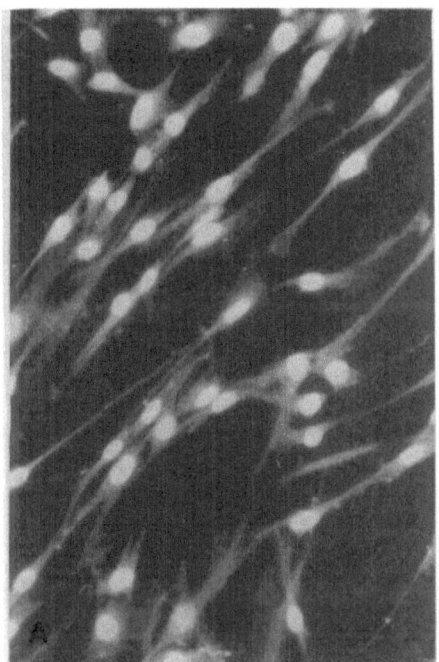 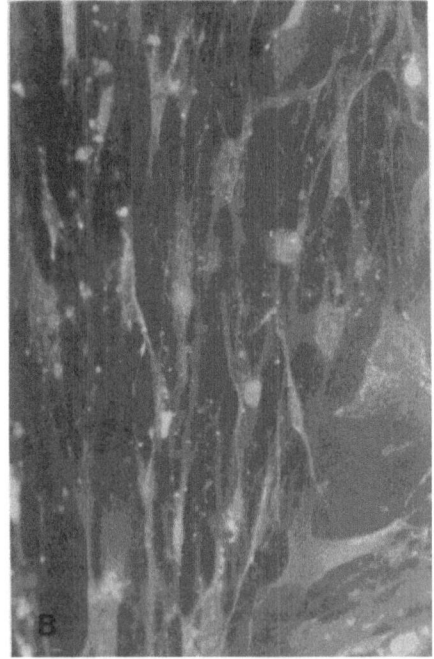

Fig. 8:   Photomicrographs of immunocytologically stained TIG-1
            cells. Left: 15 PDL, right: 62 PDL. Early- and
            terminal-passage cells were cultivated side by side on a
            same coverglass. Anti-histone H1 antiserum and FITC-
            conjugated anti-immunoglobulin were used to show the
            amount of histone H1 in cell nuclei.

cells (Fig. 8, right). G1 arrest by either contact inhibition or
inhibition of DNA-synthesis by short-term hydroxyurea treatment did
not apparently reduce the fluorescence intensity of early-passage
cells (data not shown). Werner-syndrome fibroblasts at early
passage (Fig. 9, left) had an intensity of fluorescence in their
nuclei equivalent to that in donor-age matched normal fibroblasts
(Fig. 9, right).

DISCUSSION

     Some of the aging indices of cultured human diploid
fibroblasts are closely related to retardation of cell
proliferation and simply reflect the accumulation of non-dividing
cell populations in aging cultures. Rapidly dividing cells in
senescent cultures, however, resemble young cells in terms of cell

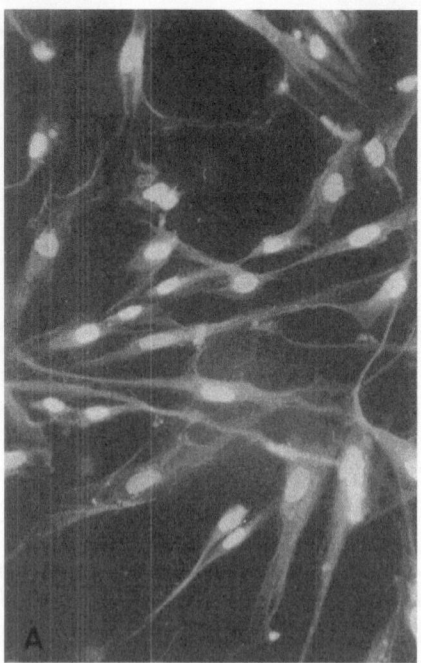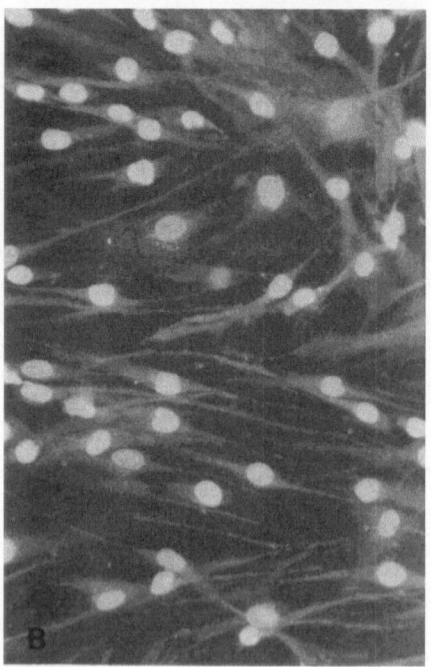

Fig. 9:   Photomicrographs of immunocytologically stained skin
          fibroblasts. Left: fibroblasts from Werner-syndrome
          patient (56 years old), 10 PDL. Right: Donor-age
          matched normal control fibroblasts, 12 PDL.

volume (Mitsui and Schneider, 1976a), nuclear size (Mitsui and
Schneider, 1976), cell-cycle traverse time (Bowman et al., 1975)
and DNA repair (Hart and Setlow, 1976); however, they acquire
senescent cell characteristics and lose proliferative capacity very
soon after isolation and reintroduction into culture (Mitsui et
al., 1980b). Age-specific characteristics of cycling cells or of
whole populations in senescent cultures, therefore, rather than
growth-related cell changes, are very important in elucidating the
mechanisms of cellular aging. Since a tight coupling between
histone and DNA synthesis has been generally accepted (Elgins and
Weintraub, 1975), our previous finding of a decline in histone H1
synthesis in senescent cultures seems to reflect age-specific
differences in cycling cell populations. However, turnover
synthesis of histones, especially of histone H1, was recently
suggested in BHK cells (Tarnowka et al., 1978) and lens cells
(Herve et al., 1979). Thus, examination of histone H1 synthesis in
resting cells is also required in human diploid fibroblast system.

As shown in the present paper, there was some turnover synthesis of histone H1 in growth-retarded human diploid fibroblasts (Fig. 2 & 4) and the molar ratio of histone H1 synthesis was not lower in resting cell cultures than in cycling cell cultures (Fig. 3 & 5). Therefore, a decrease in histone H1 synthesis in senescent cultures (Fig. 5 and Mitsui et al., 1980a) was not due to an increase of the number of resting cells in senescent cultures, but reflects an age-specific difference in cycling cell populations. In addition, the lower content of histone H1 in older cultures was found at all stages of cell growth, suggesting a lack of histone H1 in non-cycling cell populations (Fig. 6). The lower intensity of immunofluoresence in senescent cell nuclei (Fig. 8) confirmed these findings. However, a recent study (D'Anna et al., 1982) suggests that the histone H1 content of CHO cells arrested at early S phase markedly declined. Confirmation by long-term arrest of human diploid cells at Gl or early S phase might be needed to draw a definite conclusion.

The significance of decreased histone H1 in senescent human fibroblasts remains to be determined. A complete loss of histone H1 is seen in post-mitotic chick erythrocytes, and a transfer of histone H1 from the transformed cell nucleus to the chick erythrocyte nucleus in heterokaryon hybrid cells occurred in company with reinitiation of DNA synthesis in the erythrocyte nucleus (Appels et al., 1974). Thus, histone H1 depletion might cause cessation of DNA synthesis in senescent human cells.

One of the results of lack of histone H1 in chromatin might be an increase in the susceptibility of linker DNA to nuclease or other enzymes leading to DNA strand breakage. In fact, Beaupain et al. have recently reported that the number of alkali-sensitive sites of single-strand DNA from human diploid fibroblasts in creased with aging in vitro (1980). The accumulation of more DNA strand breaks than the cells could repair would result in cell death (Berger et al., 1979). This idea is consistent with the findings of increased number of DNA strand breaks in vivo (Price et al., 1971; Ono et al., 1976) and loss of brain cells (Peng and Lee, 1979) in aged rats and mice.

The other possible result of the lack of histone H1 in chromatin is the relaxation of gene repression, leading to disordered cell function. Evidence for the role of histone H1 in the regulation of gene expression is increasing (Lohr et al., 1977; Wircek and Benyajuti, 1977). Histone H1 is absent in transcriptionally active chromatin from cultured cells (Chiu et al., 1977) as well as from animal tissues (Berlowitz and Doty, 1975). In senescent human diploid fibroblasts, an increase in RNA synthesis (Schneider et al., 1975) and a higher basal level of transcription (Pochran et al., 1978), but decline in collagen synthesis activity (Houck et al., 1972) have been reported.

Examinations in vivo also suggested an increase in gene expression in aged mouse brain (Ono and Cutler, 1978). Thus, we consider the possibility that depletion of histone H1 might cause relaxation of gene repression and DNA strand breakage, resulting in dysfunction and death of senescent human diploid fibroblasts. The hypothetical role of histone H1 as a target of cellular aging certainly needs to be tested by further investigation.

Acknowledgement

We wish to thank Dr. Namba (Kawasaki Medical University) for providing us with ^{60}Co-transformed WI-38 cells and Dr. Fujiwara (Kobe University, School of Medicine) for providing Werner-syndrome fibroblasts. This work was supported by a project grant from the Institute of Physical and Chemical Research, and by a grant-in-aid from the Ministry of Education, Science and Culture, Japan.

REFERENCES

Aizawa, S. and Mitsui, Y. (1979), A new cell surface marker of aging in human diploid fibroblasts, J. Cell. Physiol., 100:383.

Aizawa, S., Mitsui, Y., Kurimoto, F. and Matuoka, K. (1980), Cell surface changes accompanying aging in human diploid fibroblasts. III. Division age and senescence revealed by concanavaline A-mediated red blood cell adsorption, Expl. Cell Res., 125:297.

Appels, R., Bolund, L. and Ringertz, N.R. (1974), Biochemical analysis of reactiviated chick erythrocyte nuclei isolated from chick/HeLa heterokaryons, J. Mol. Biol., 87:339.

Beaupain, R., Icard, C., and Maciera-Coelho, A. (1980), Changes in DNA alkalin-sensitive sites during senescence and establishment of fibroblasts in vitro, Biochim Biophys Acta, 606:251.

Berlowitz, E.M. and Doty, P. (1975), Chemical and physical properties of fractionated chromatin, Proc. Natl. Acad. Sci. USA, 72:328.

Berger, N.A., Petzold, S.J. and Berger, S.J. (1979), Association of poly (ADP-rib) synthesis with cessation of DNA synthesis and DNA fragmentation. Biochim Biophys Acta, 564:90.

Bowman, P.D., Meek, R.L. and Daniel, C.W. (1975), Aging of human fibroblasts in vitro., Exp. Cell Res. 93:184.

Chiu, N., Baserga, R. and Furth, J.J., (1977), Composition and template activity of chromatin fractionated by isoelectric focusing, Biochemistry, 16:4796.

Christofalo, V.J. and Sharf, B.B. (1973), Cellular senescence and DNA synthesis, Exp. Cell Res. 76:419.

D'Anna, J., Gurley, L. and Tobey, R., (1982), Synthesis and modulations in the chromatin contents of histones H1 during G1 and S phases in Chinese hamster cells, Biochem., 21:3991.

Elgins, S.C.R. and Hood, L.E. (1973), Chromosomal Proteins of Drosophila, Biochem., 12, 4984.

Elgins, S.C.R. and Weintraub, H. (1975), Chromosomal proteins and chromatin structure, Annu. Rev. Biochem. 44:725.

Greenaway, P.J. and Murray, K. (1971), Heterogeneity and polymorphism in chicken erythrocyte histone fraction V. Nature, 229:233.

Grimes, S.R. Jr., Chae, C-B and Irvin, J.L. (1975), Effects of age and hypophysectomy upon relative proportions of various histones in rat testis, Biochem. Biophys. Res. Commun., 64:911.

Gorovsky, M.A. and Keevert, J.B. (1975), Absence of histone F1 in a mitotically dividing, genetically inactive nucleus, Proc. Natl. Acad. Sci. USA, 72:2672.

Hart, R.W. and Setlow, R.B. (1976), DNA repair in late-passage human cells, Mech. Ageing Dev., 5:67.

Herve, B., Jacquemin, E. and Courtois, Y. (1979), Histones biosynthesis and turnover in epithelial lens cells cultured in vitro, Cell. Biol. Intern. Rep., 3:271.

Houck, J.C., Sharma, U.K. and Hayflick, L. (1972), Functional failures of cultured human diploid fibroblasts after continued population doublings, Proc. Soc. Exp. Biol. Med., 137:331.

Kraus, M.O. and Stein, G.S. (1974), Modifications in the chromosomal proteins of SV-40 transformed WI-38 human diploid fibroblasts, Biochem. Biophys. Res. Commun., 59:796.

Linder, S., Zuckerman, S. and Ringertz, N. (1982), Distribution of histone H5 in chicken erythrocyte-mammalian cell heterokaryons, Exp. Cell Res., 140:464.

Lohr, D., Tatchell, K. and Van Holde, K.E. (1977), On the occurrence of nucleosome phasing in chromatin, Cell, 12:829.

Macieira-Coelho, A. (1974), Are non-diving cells present in ageing cell cultures? Nature, 248:421.

Martin, G.M. (1978), Genetic syndromes in man with potential relevance to the pathology of aging, Birth Defects, Orig. Article Series, 14:5.

Mitsui, Y. and Schneider, E.L. (1976), Increased nuclear sizes in senescent diploid fibroblast cultures, Exp. Cell Res., 100:147.

Mitsui, Y. and Schneider, E.L. (1976), Characterization of fractionated human diploid fibroblast cell populations, Exp. Cell Res., 103:23.

Mitsui, Y. and Schneider, E.L. (1976), Relationship between replication and volume in senescent human diploid fibroblasts, Mech. Ageing Dev., 5:45.

Mitsui, Y., Aizawa, S. and Matuoka, K. (1979), The relation of cell nuclei and surface membranes to the capacity of cell proliferation in human diploid fibroblasts. In Recent Advances in Gerontology, Orimo, H., Shimada, K., Iriki, M. and Maeda, D., editors, Excerpta Medica, Amsterdam, 108-110.

Mitsui, Y., Sakagami, H, Murata, S. and Yamamada, M. (1980), Age related decline in H1 histone fraction in human diploid fibroblast cultures, Exp. Cell Res., 126:289.

Mitsui, Y. Matuoka, K., Aizawa, S. and Noda, K. (1980), New approaches to the characterization of aging human diploid fibroblasts at individual cell level, Adv. Exp. Med. Biol., 129:5.

Namba, M., Nishitani, K. and Kimoto, T., (1978), Carcinogenesis in tissue culture 29: Neoplastic transformation of a normal human diploid cell strain, WI-38, with Co-60 gamma rays, Japan J. Exp. Med., 48:303.

O'Farrell, P.H. (1975), High resolution two-dimensional electrophoresis of proteins, J. Biol. Chem, 250:4007.

Ohashi, M., Aizawa, S., Ooka, H., Ohsawa, T., Kaji, K., Kondo, H, Kobayashi, T., Noumura, T., Matsuo, M., Mitsui, Y., Murata, S., Yamamoto, K., Ito, H., Shimada, H. and Utakoji, T. (1980), A new human diploid cell strain, TIG-1, for the research on cellular aging, Exp. Gerontol., 15:121.

Ono, T., Okada, S. and Sugahara, T. (1976), Comparative studies of DNA size in various tissues of mice during the aging process, Exp. Gerontol., 11:127.

Ono, T. and Cutler, R.G. (1978), Age-dependent relaxation of repression: Increase endogenous murine leukemia virus-related and globin-related RNA in brain and liver of mice, Proc. Natl. Acad. Sci. USA, 75:4431.

Panyim, S. and Chalkley, R. (1969), High resolution acrylamide gel electrophoresis of histones, Arch. Biochem. Biophys. 130:337.

Pehrson, J. and Cole, D.R. (1980), Histone H1 accumulates in growth-inhibited cultured cells, Nature, 285:43.

Peng, M.T. and Lee, L.R. (1979), Regional differences of neuron loss of rat brain in old age, Gerontology, 25:205.

Pochran, S.F., Omeara, A.R. and Kurtz, M.J. (1978), Control of transcription in ageing Wl-38 cells stimulated to divide, Exp. Cell Res., 116:63.

Price, G.B., Modak, S.D. and Makinodan, T. (1971), Age-associated changes in the DNA of mouse tissue, Science, 171:917.

Sakagami, H., Mitsui, Y., Murata, S. and Yamada, M. (1982), Effect of growth stage on histone H1 metabolism in human diploid fibroblasts, J. Cell Physiol. 110:213.

Salk, D., Au, K., Hoehn, H. and Martin, G.M. (1981), Cytogenetics of Werner syndrome cultured skin fibroblasts: Variegated translocation mosaicism, Cytogenet. Cell Genet., 30:92

Schneider, E.L., Mitsui, Y., Tice, R., Shorr, S.S. and Braunschweiger, K. (1975), Alteration in cellular RNAs during the in vitro lifespan of cultured human diploid fibroblasts, Mech. Ageing Dev., 4:449.

Seale, R.L. and Alonson, A.I. (1973), Chromatin-associated proteins of the developing sea-urchin embryo. 11 Acid-soluble proteins, J. Mol. Biol., 75:647.

Shirley, M.A. and Anderson, K.M. (1977), Electron-microscopic visualization of transcriptionally active and less active chromatin fractions from the rat ventral prostate and their content of histones, Can. J. Biochem., 55:9.

Takeuchi, F., Hanaoka, F., Goto, M., Yamada, M. and Miyamoto, T. (1982), Prolongation of S phase and whole cell cycle in Werner syndrome fibroblasts, Exp. Geront., 17:473.

Tarnowka, M.A., Baglioni, C. and Basilico, C. (1978), Synthesis of H1 histones by BHK cells in G1, Cell., 15:163.

Worcel, Z. and Benyajuti, C. (1977), Higher order coiling of DNA chromatin, Cell., 12:83.

GENOME REORGANIZATION DURING AGING OF DIVIDING CELLS

A. Macieira-Coelho[1] and F. Puvion-Dutilleul[2]

[1] Institut de Cancerologie et d'Immunogenetique
(INSERM)
[2] Institut de Recherches Scientifiques sur le
Cancer (CNRS), 94804 Villejuif (Cedex), France

SUMMARY

The study of the effect of low dose rate ionizing radiation on the long-term proliferation of fibroblasts led to the observation that radiation accentuated the growth potential of the cells, favoring events which normally take place during division. These events could be related to the genome reorganization taking place during division. Hence, it was hypothesized (Macieira-Coelho, 1979; Macieira-Coelho, 1980; Macieira-Coelho, 1981) that the long-term proliferation of fibroblasts depends upon the potential for reorganization of the genome, the latter being a self-limiting process. At each division residual quantitative and qualitative changes would accumulate in chromatin, limiting the long-term potential for further rearrangements.

The hypothesis was checked looking for quantitative and qualitative changes in DNA through the in vitro lifespan of human fibroblast populations.

It was found that at each population doubling in 20% of the cells there is unequal distribution of DNA between sister cells. Results show that this could be due to errors in chromosome assembly and segregation, to loss of DNA, to errors during semi-conservative DNA synthesis and to multiple rounds of DNA replication at a single origin.

An increased alkali- and thermo-lability of chromatin was found during in vitro aging. At the ultrastructural level after mild decondensation, chromatin fibers were spaced and shorter. After Miller's spreading, most of the chromatin of old cells had lost the nucleosome organization and was fragmented. These chromatin changes became apparent only towards the end of the life span of human embryonic fibroblasts but were already present in a significant fraction of low population doubling level (PDL) fibroblasts from human adults.

Almost all cells of low-PDL fibroblasts from the Werner syndrome presented these chromatin changes. In addition, short, unbeaded DNA fragments could be seen in these fibroblasts, occasionally forming circles; they could correspond to transposable elements which detach during the division cycle and fail to reintegrate into chromosomes because of the age-related chromatin structural changes.

PREMISE

In order to test the somatic mutation theory of aging, we studied the effect of low dose rate ionizing radiation on the lifespan of human fibroblasts in vitro. With embryonic cells it was found that if the irradiation was started early during the life span, it would either prolong or have no effect on the doubling potential depending on the dose applied; if radiation was started later, the division potential was reduced (Macieira-Coelho et al., 1977). With postnatal fibroblasts irradiation could either prolong or shorten the life span depending on the donor (Azzarone et al., 1980; Diatloff and Macieira-Coelho, 1979; Macieira-Coelho et al., 1978). Hence the data could not be interpreted in terms of the somatic mutation hypothesis. Later it was found that the different effects of radiation were related to the potential of chromosome rearrangements of the respective fibroblast populations and to their long-term division potential (Macieira-Coelho et al., to be published). When chromosome changes were analyzed in the irradiated cells, it was found that most sites involved in breaks were also involved in chromosome exchanges and were mainly localized in the centromeric and acrocentric regions (Bourgeois et al., 1981). These regions are known to be the site of highly repetitive DNA which has been implicated in recombinational events. Furthermore, the irradiation of cells with different growth potentials, originated from different species, suggested that low dose rate ionizing radiation accentuates the intrinsic growth potential of fibroblasts, accelerating changes in the cell genome which anyway take place during cell replication (Macieira-Coelho et al., 1976). Hence on one hand, the long-term effect of radiation was related to the potential for chromosome rearrangements and on the other it seemed to accentuate cellular changes that occur normally during division and are determinant for cell aging.

Irradiation is known to accelerate genome reorganization through sister chromatid exchanges (SCE), DNA strand switching and dislocation of transposable elements (Macieira-Coelho, 1980). SCE and DNA strand switching occur during division of mammalian cells; the dislocation of transposable elements has been described in different types of cells and it would be surprising if they were not a general phenomenon. Hence, we hypothesized that aging of dividing cells is the result of the reorganization of the genome which leaves behind changes leading to a progressive decrease of the plasticity of the genome and a disorganization of chromatin template activity and gene interaction (Macieira-Coelho, 1980); furthermore, the long-term growth of the cell population would overcome these changes occurring during genome reorganization.

Pertinent to the hypothesis is the finding that the capacity to exchange chromatids in the presence of drugs declines during cellular aging (Schneider and Monticone, 1978).

The changes caused by the genome reorganization on DNA and chromatin could be of a quantitative and qualitative nature (Fig. 1). The former could be due to loss or unequal distribution of DNA during cell division or from the integration of new DNA. Qualitative changes could be caused by changes in chromatin structure and conformation, by the mutual relationship between chromatin regions coming together, by the transposition of controlling elements, by breaks, and also by the loss or integration of new DNA.

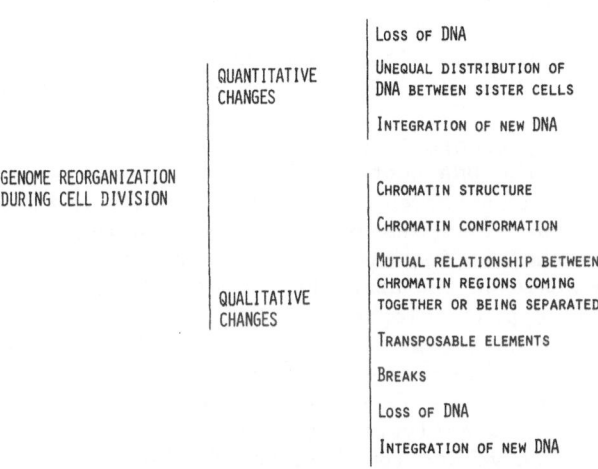

Fig. 1.   Schematic representation of eventual changes taking place during reorganization of the genome.

Thus we attempted to determine if indeed quantitative and
qualitative changes take place in DNA and chromatin during
cellular senescence.

PARTITION OF DNA BETWEEN SISTER CELLS

It is well known that measurements of DNA with
cytophotometry above interphases show two peaks corresponding to
cells in the G_1 and G_2 periods and intermediate values
corresponding to the cells in the S period. The spread of the G_1
and G_2 DNA contents could be due to quantitative differences
between cells in the amount of DNA, to cells that are engaged in
DNA synthesis, to different afffinities of the stain to DNA of
cells at different stages of the cycle, or to methodological
errors.

To see if DNA values are the same regardless of the stage of
the cell cycle, the cytophotometric measurements found on
interphases were compared with those found for cells in mitosis.
Figure 2 illustrates the distribution of the amount of DNA
measured cytophotometricaly after ethidium bromide staining
(Macieira-Coelho et al., 1982), for interphases, metaphases and
anaphases plus telophases of a human embryonic lung fibroblast-
like population. The distribution of the DNA content of
anaphases plus telephases and of metaphases accords with the G_1
and G_2 peaks found for interphases. The distribution of DNA of
tetraploid anaphases and telophases corresponds to the DNA
content of diploid metaphases. The amount of DNA of tetraploid
metaphases corresponds to that of octaploid interphases. Thus
the same amount of DNA is found by this method regardless of the
period within the cell cycle. The same results were obtained
measuring the DNA content with a computer-assisted program for
scanning cytophotometry after staining with Feulgen-
pararosaniline (SO_2) (Macieira-Coelho et al., 1982).

Since DNA synthesis is semi-conservative, the scatter of the
distribution of the DNA content of each half anaphases and
telophases should be the same as that of metaphases when the
latter is halved. This was evaluated by plotting on probit paper
the DNA distributions for these two classes of cells in such a
way that the scale of the abscissa for metaphases is twice that
of the anaphases plus telophases (Fig. 3). The values
corresponding to each half of anaphases and telophases and to
metaphases overlap; this suggests that the spread in DNA values
is due to quantitative differences in the DNA content of the
cells. This type of analysis was performed at different PDL
(Fig. 4). The DNA values found in the different classes of cells
were tested by an analysis of variance which showed that they
never were significantly different; for the sample with the
largest difference, F=33 at the 0.05 level.

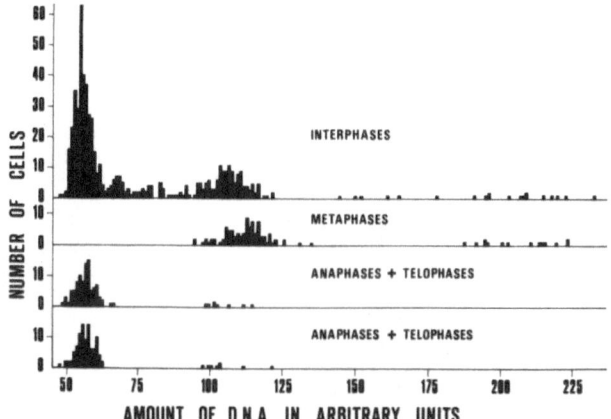

Fig. 2. Distribution of the relative amount of DNA in a human
embryonic lung fibroblast population, after ethidium
bromide staining, measured for 500 interphases, 100
metaphases, and 100 anaphases plus telophases. The
upper and lower values of the latter correspond to the
respective daughter cells (A. Macieira-Coelho et al.,
1982).

The DNA content of each half of anaphases and telophases
(Fig. 5) was also compared to determine the frequency of sister
cells with significant differences. The differences were
expressed as the percentage of the mean value of each pair. With
both ethidium bromide (Fig. 6) and Feulgen-pararosaniline (Fig.
7), large differences in the DNA content between sister cells
were found for some pairs. A total of 4000 anaphases plus
telophases were analyzed after ethidium bromide staining and 350
after Feulgen pararosaniline staining at different PDL; the
distribution of the differences were identical throughout the
life span and only at the terminal 2-3 doublings an increase was
noted in the number of pairs with large differences (Fig. 8).
This is not surprising since the life span of embryonic
fibroblast populations are characterized by a terminal stage with
abrupt events (Macieira-Coelho and Taboury, 1982).

Repeated measurements were made on the samples stained with
Feulgen-pararosaniline to evaluate the differences attributable
to methodology. The white area in Figure 7 represents these
differences with three standard deviations. According to these
data, in approximately 20% of the cells, differences between
sister cells are not due to methodological errors.

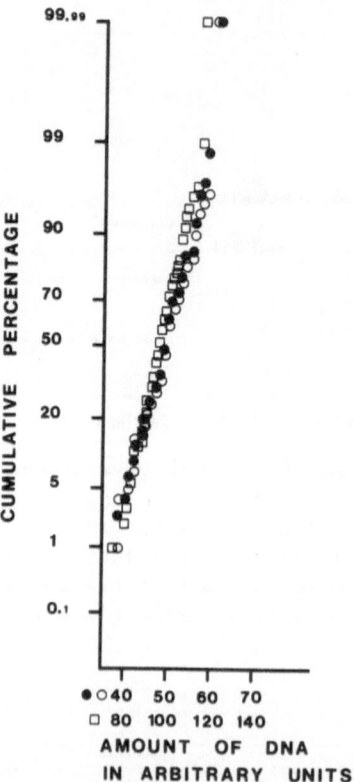

Fig. 3. Plot on probit paper of the distribution of the amount
         of DNA of a human embryonic lung fibroblast population,
         measured for metaphases (□) and for each half of
         anaphases and telophases (O•) (Macieira-Coelho et al.,
         1982).

Microscopical observations showed that the cells were not
contaminated by mycoplasma. In addition control DNA measurements
were made repeatedly in areas above the cytoplasm to ensure
absence of aberrant DNA. With ethidium bromide, the total
background was below 5% of the mean DNA diploid value and after
Feulgen-pararosaniline below 0.1%. Thus the data show that
continuous rearrangements in DNA content originate during serial
divisions without changing the spread and the mode of the
distribution.

Results of an unequal distribution of DNA during division
identical to those described above were found through the
life span of three different human embryonic lung fibroblast

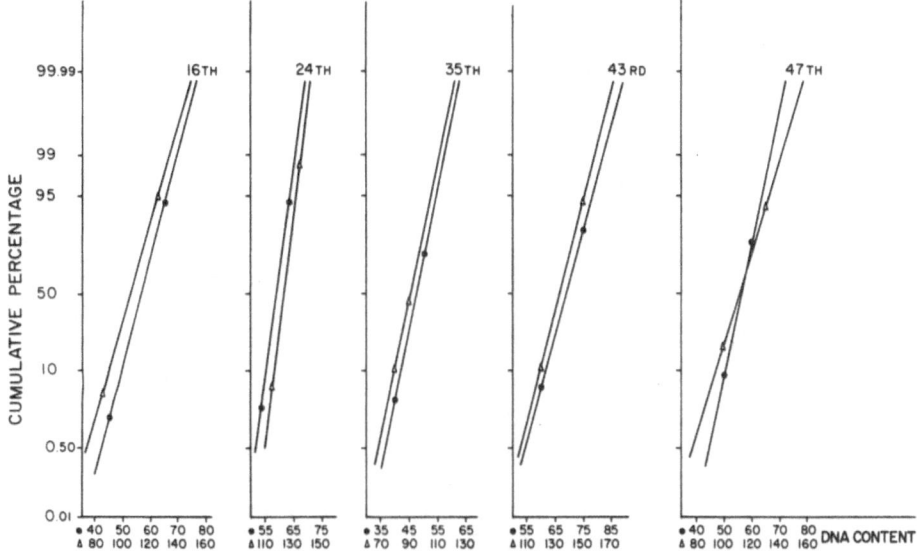

Fig. 4.   Regression lines, computed by the least square method,
          of the distribution of DNA contents of a human embryonic
          lung fibroblast population at different PDLs, measured
          for metaphases (△) and for anaphases plus telophases
          (●) (Macieira-Coelho et al., 1982).

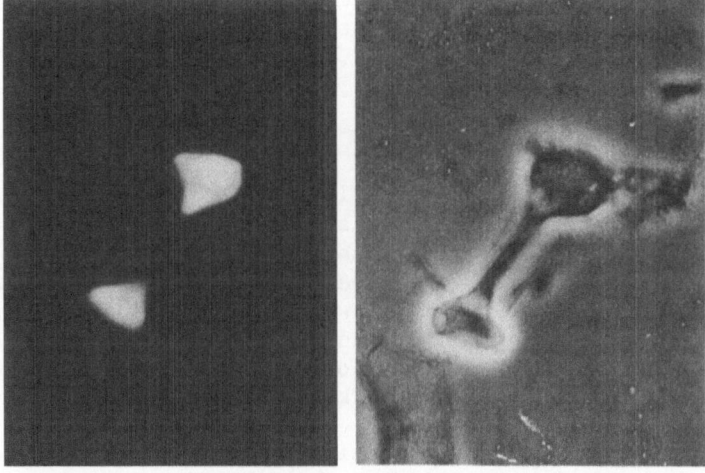

Fig. 5.   Anaphase photographed after ethidium bromide staining
          under visible and UV lights (Macieira-Coelho et al.,
          1982).

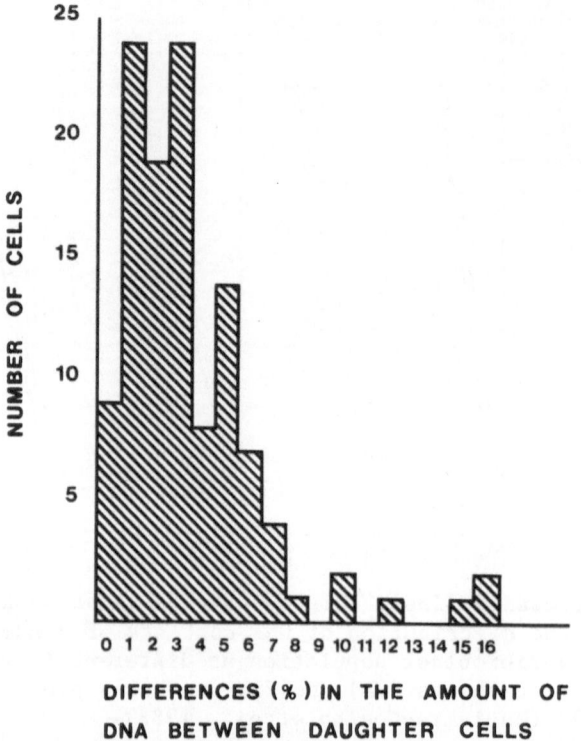

Fig. 6.   Distribution of the differences in the amount of DNA
          after ethidium bromide staining found between daughter
          cells and expressed as percentage of the mean of the
          pair in a sample of a human embryonic lung fibroblast
          population (Macierira-Coelho et al., 1982).

populations (Macieira-Coelho et al., 1982). The three lines used
differed in the chromosome changes taking place through their
life span; in all three there were oscillations in the number of
aneuploid cells, but towards the end, there was a considerable
number of aneuploid cells in two while the other line remained
predominantly diploid until the end (Macieira-Coelho et al.,
1982). Thus uneven DNA segregation at cell division can take
place simultaneously with a remarkable stability of diploidy.

     Differences in DNA distribution between sister cells could
be due to errors during semi-conservative DNA synthesis. To
determine whether DNA synthesized during the preceding S period
is unequally distributed, the number of grains on each half of
anaphases and telophases was measured after labeling the DNA with

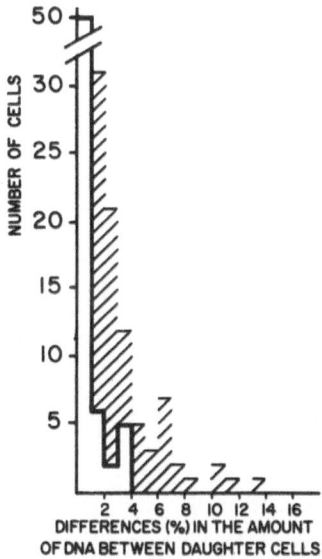

Fig. 7. Distribution of the differences in the amounts of DNA
         after Feulgen-pararosaniline staining, found between
         daughter cells in a sample of human embryonic lung
         fibroblasts. The area limited by the continuous line
         corresponds to the differences with three standard
         deviations, found between repeated measurements of the
         same samples. Each sample was measured twice (Macieira-
         Coelho et al., 1982).

tritiated thymidine (^{3}H-TdR). To check if ^{3}H-TdR would disturb
the distribution of DNA between daughter cells, cultures were
labeled with different concentrations of the radioactive
precursor and the DNA in each half of anaphases and telphases was
measured (Fig. 9). Concentrations between 0.01 and 0.2 Ci/ml
did not change the distributions of the differences in DNA
content between sister cells, beyond that there was a decline in
the number of pairs with less than 5% difference from the mean
and an increase in the number of pairs with larger differences.
Thus radioactivity increased the differences between daughter
cells in the upper 20% of the distribution, i.e., the same
percentage that normally shows a significant unequal distribution
of DNA.

Since 0.01μ Ci/ml ^{3}H-TdR gives a grain spread over the
nucleus with a good resolution, this concentration was considered
safe for the experiment. The number of grains on sister cells
was measured after labeling the DNA with ^{3}H-TdR during a whole S

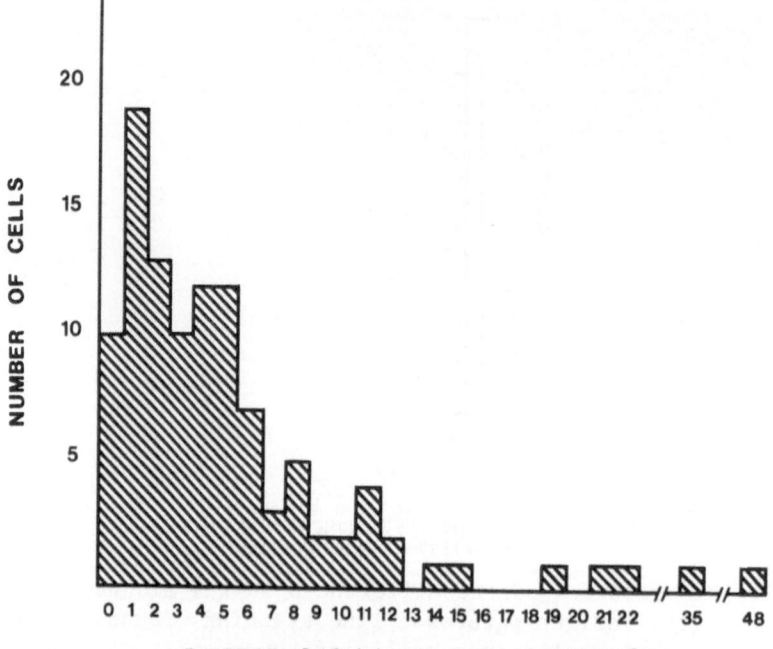

Fig. 8.   Distribution of the differences in the amount of DNA
          after ethidium bromide staining found between daughter
          cells and expressed as percentage of the mean of the
          pair in a sample of a human embronic lung fibroblast
          population in phase IV.

period. The time after labeling when most cells had gone through
a whole S period in the presence of the labeled precursor was
measured as previously described (Macieira-Coelho et al., 1982).
The number of grains found on each daughter cell was plotted
(Fig. 10) so that all halves with less grains were represented on
the ordinate and all halves with a higher number of grains were
represented on the abscissa. If each daughter cell had the same
number of grains, the plot should fall on the diagonal of the
chart (solid line). A Monte Carlo simulation was performed on
the data to determine whether the differences between daughter
cells which deviate from the ideal line were significant (Fig.
11). The experimental and theoretical data were compared
plotting the distribution of the differences in the number of
grains between daughter cells found with both methods (Fig. 12).
The plot shows a significant fraction of cells in which the DNA
synthesized during the preceding S period was not distributed

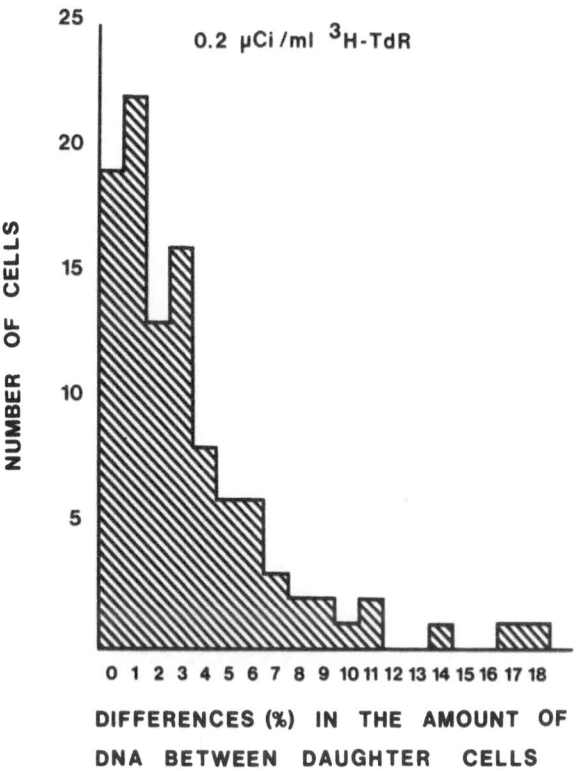

Fig. 9A.

Figs. 9A and 9B.   Distribution of the differences in the amount of DNA after ethidium bromide staining found between daughter cells in cultures of human embryonic lung fibroblasts labeled during a full S period with different concentrations of ^{3}H–TdR (Macieira-Coelho et al., 1982).

evenly between daughter cells. The fraction of significant differences is smaller when one measures the distribution of ^{3}H–TdR incorporated on each half than when one measures the DNA content, which is to be expected since the precursor is incorporated in a limited number of sites (Fig. 13). Cytophotometry, on the contrary, evaluates the whole DNA content. The differences in grain counts between daughter cells cannot be due to geometrical errors in the two halves during anaphase or telophase since the grain count distribution and the peak grain count for these cells are the same as for metaphases (Macieira-Coelho et al., 1982).

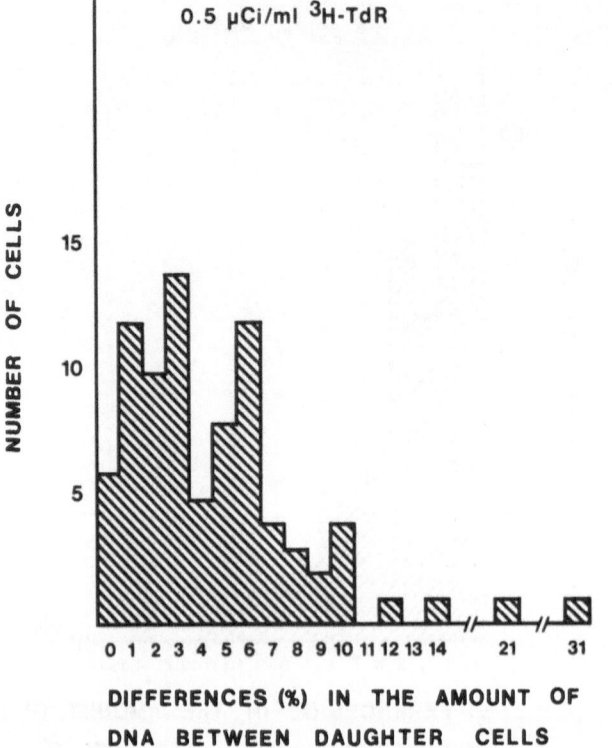

Fig. 9B. (See figure caption on preceding page.)

An event that can contribute to unequal distribution of
newly synthesized DNA is asymmetric DNA synthesis. Human
fibroblasts were stained with Hoescht 33258 and Giemsa as
previously described (Perry and Wolff, 1974); after two rounds of
replication in the presence of bromodeoxyuridine (BrdU) small
regions with BrdU incorporated in the two DNA strands facing a
bifilarly substituted chromatid were seen (Fig. 14a) with a
frequency which oscillates through the population life span
(Table I). It could be due to multiple rounds of replication at
a single origin. Chromosome deletions and gaps (Fig. 14b) is
another possible explanation for unequal distribution of DNA at
the time of division. In addition, errors in chromosome assembly
or segregation and loss of DNA (Fig. 15) can also be the cause of
unequal DNA distribution.

Pertinent to our results is the finding (Shmookler-Reis and
Goldstein, 1980) that cultured human fibroblasts lose 0.6-1.2%
per population doublings of highly repetitive DNA; it was
proposed that this loss occurs by unequal recombination.

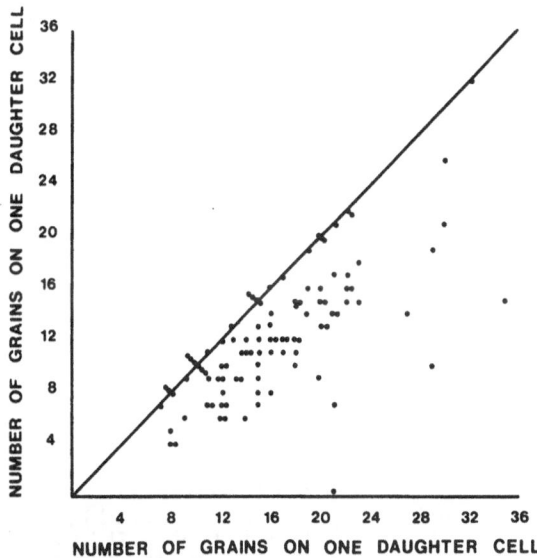

Fig. 10. Number of grains for daughter cells of human embryonic
lung fibroblasts when the grain count saturated after
growing in the presence of ^{3}H-TdR. The diagonal
corresponds to the ideal line where the number of
grains should fall if each half would have the same
grain count (Macieira-Coelho et al., 1982).

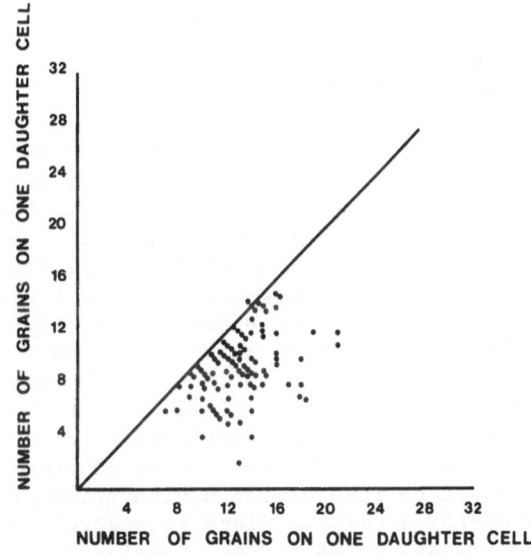

Fig. 11. Number of grains for daughter cells computed with a
Monte Carlo stimulation (Macieira-Coelho et al., 1982).

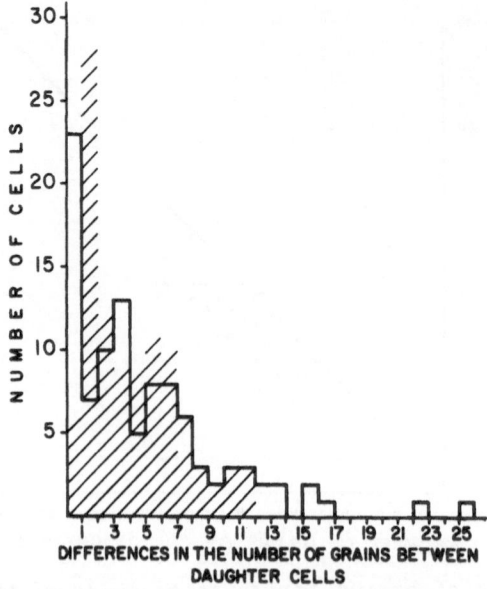

Fig. 12.   Computed (dashed area) and experimental (continuous
           line) distributions of the differences in the number of
           grains found for daughter cells (Macieira-Coelho et
           al., 1982).

CHANGES IN CHROMATIN ORGANIZATION

     DNA single strand breaks which have been claimed to
accumulate in the cells of certain tissues during aging
(Chetsanga et al., 1977; Karran and Ormerod, 1973; Ono and Okada,
1978; Price et al., 1971; Wheeler and Lett, 1972) could also
accumulate in dividing cells during genome reorganization. This
was checked by centrifuging chromosomal DNA from human embryonic
lung fibroblasts at different PDL in alkaline sucrose gradients
(Icard et al., 1979). The results showed that DNA from old cells
sedimented in a dispersed fashion as compared to that of young
cells, suggesting the presence of small molecular weight DNA.
The data however did not allow the distinction between single
strand breaks, apurinic sites or replication intermediates,
either due to a decreased rate of chain elongation or to the
presence of slow dividing cells. Since in neutral sucrose
gradients DNA was monodispersed, it was concluded that double
strand breaks were not present (Icard et al., 1979). We have now
found that most of the small molecular weight DNA found during

Table 1. Number of isolated asymmetries per 100 mitoses at
          different PDL of MRC-5 Cells.

PDL	ASYMMETRIES
33	51
41	9
46	99

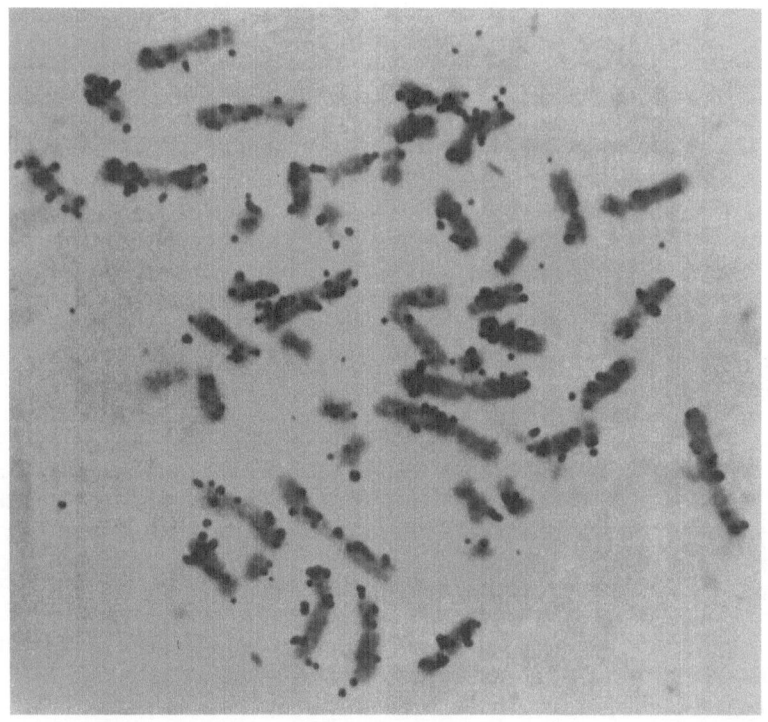

Fig. 13. Chromosome spread after autoradiography of the same cells
          used in the experiment illustrated in Fig. 10, with the
          grains corresponding to the sites where ^{3}H-TdR was
          incorporated.

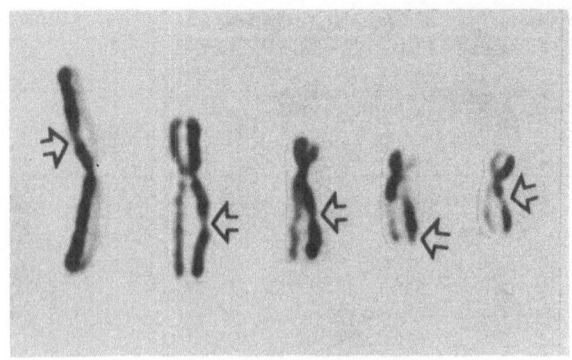

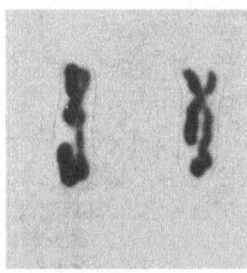

Fig. 14.   Chromosomes of human embryonic lung fibroblasts after
            bromodeoxyuridine incorporation and stained with
            Hoechst 33258 and Giemsa. (a) The arrows indicate the
            sites of asymmetric DNA synthesis, (b) gaps.

aging originates during cell lysis through breakage of alkali-
and temperature-labile sites.

    Resting stage human embryonic fibroblasts in phase II, III
and IV (Fig. 16) on plastic 15 mm discs were stimulated with a
medium change and labeled during 15 hr with 0.5 μCi/ml ^{14}C-TdR
(s.a. 50 Ci.mM). Then after a 30 min chase in cold TdR, the
discs were laid during 5 hr on an alkaline lysing solution
containing 0.1% lauryl sulfate, the lysing solution itself being
on top of an alkaline 5-20% sucrose gradient (Icard et al.,
1979). Half of the cultures were lysed at room temperature and
the other half at 37ºC. After lysis the gradients were
centrifuged during 2 hr in an SW41 rotor at 40,000 rpm. Fig. 17
illustrates the radioactivity found in the different fractions
collected after centrifugation; it shows that most of the DNA of
the cells lysed at room temperature sediments as a single peak.
A small amount of radioactivity from cells in phases II and III
remains on the top of the gradient; this small molecular weight

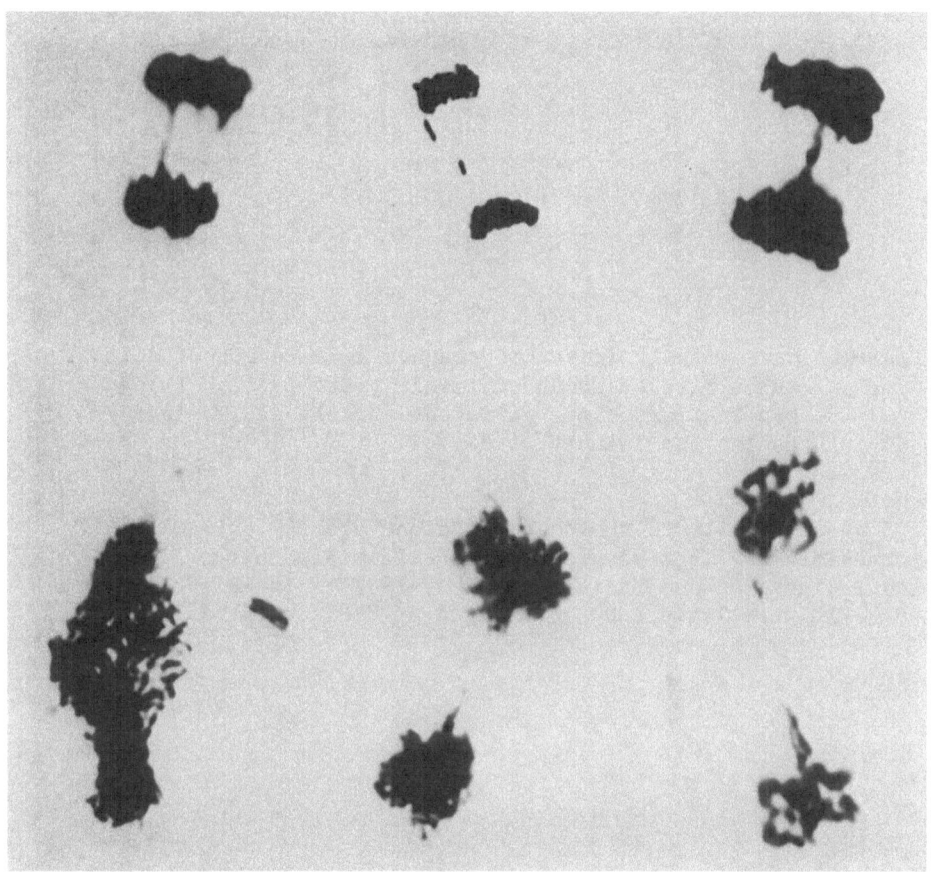

Fig. 15. Mitoses found in cultures of human embryonic lung
          fibroblasts, showing losses of chromosome and errors in
          chromosome segregation.

material increases in phase IV. When cells in phases II and III
were lysed at 37oC most of the DNA still sedimented as a single
peak but had a smaller molecular weight. The decrease in
molecular weight after lysis at 37oC was more pronounced in phase
III. In phase IV, the DNA was even more thermolabile since it
sedimented in several peaks. Hence the results show that at all
PDL most of the DNA has no breaks but that with serial division
it becomes more labile. It seems though that some small
molecular weight material is always present and increases in the
final stages.

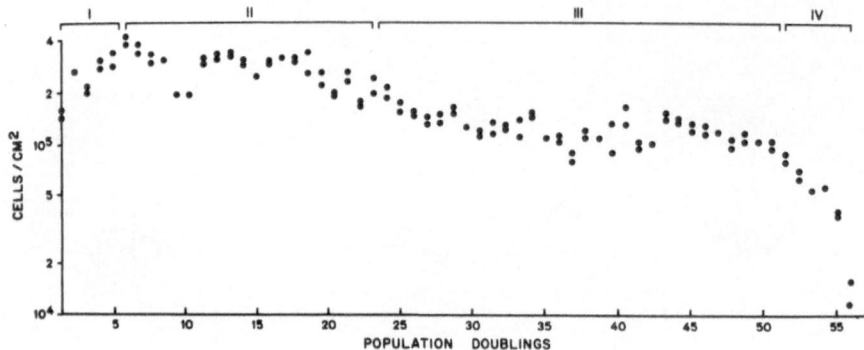

Fig. 16.   Maximum cell densities reached at each PDL of serially
           subcultivated human embryonic fibroblasts. For an
           explanation of the different phases, see Macieira-
           Coelho and Taboury, 1982.

     We also followed the sedimentation velocity of newly
synthesized DNA from young and old cells heated before lysis
(Icard-Liepkalns and Macieira-Coelho, 1982). In this experiment
the cells were lysed and centrifuged at different times after

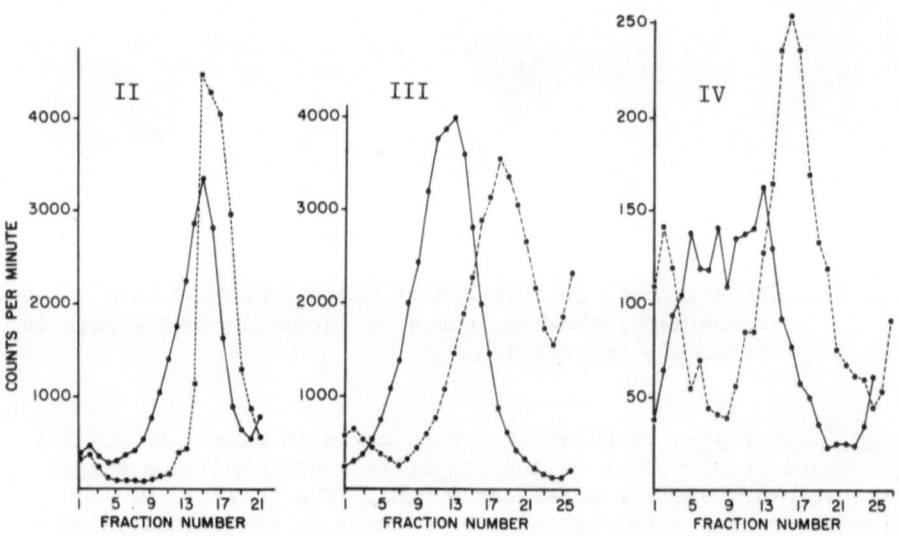

Fig. 17.   Radioactivity (14C-TdR) found in the different
           fractions collected from alkaline sucrose gradients.
           Cells in phases II, III, and IV were lysed on top of
           the gradients at 20oC (●---●) and 37oC (●____●).
           The sedimentation direction is from left to right.

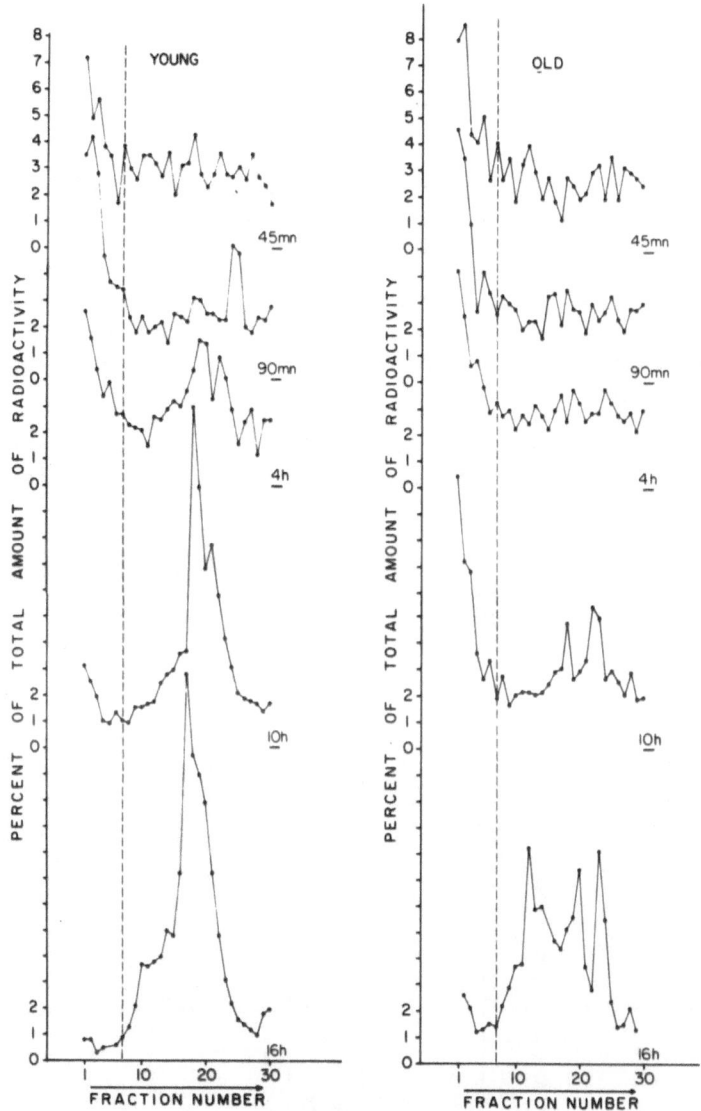

Fig. 18. Radioactivity found in the different fractions
collected from alkaline sucrose gradients. Cells in
phase II (young) and phase IV (old) were lysed on top
of the gradients. The sedimentation direction is from
left to right. The dashed line indicates the fraction
where denatured lambda phage DNA (40.5 S) sedimented
(C. Icard-Liepkalns and A. Macieira-Coelho, 1982).

addition of ^{14}C–TdR (Fig. 18). In both young and old cultures 45 min after labeling, the radioactivity is distributed in small peaks throughout the gradient. Then DNA from young cells progressively sediments as a single peak which is completed 10 hr after labeling, while in old cells even at the 16th hr after adding ^{14}C–TdR, DNA sedimented in several peaks with different sedimentation velocities.

The length of the S period was also measured in young and old cultures determining the time when the peak metaphase grain count saturates (Icard-Liepkalns and Macieira-Coelho, 1982). Results illustrated in Figure 19 show that the peak metaphase grain count saturated 7 and 10 hrs after labeling in young and old cells respectively. Hence in old cells although most of the cells have completed DNA synthesis, labile sites remain which break with heating in an alkaline medium. These results would be compatible with a deficient maturation of the gap-filling step between DNA replication intermediates with the persistence of labile sites, may be due to alterations in histone binding to DNA.

In order to analyze further these age-related changes, chromatin studies were done at the ultrastructural level (Puvion-Dutilleul and Macieira-Coelho, 1982) with a mild loosening procedure which preserves the nucleoproteins and allows the in situ observation of the transcriptional complexes (Puvion-Dutilleul and Puvion, 1980), and with the standard Miller spreading technique (Miller and Bakken, 1972). The experiments were first performed on a cell line of human embryonic lung

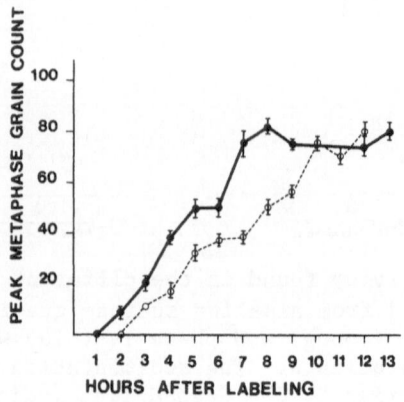

Fig. 19. Peak metaphase grain count determed in young (●) and old (O) cultures (C. Icard-Liepkalns and A. Macieira-Coelho, 1982).

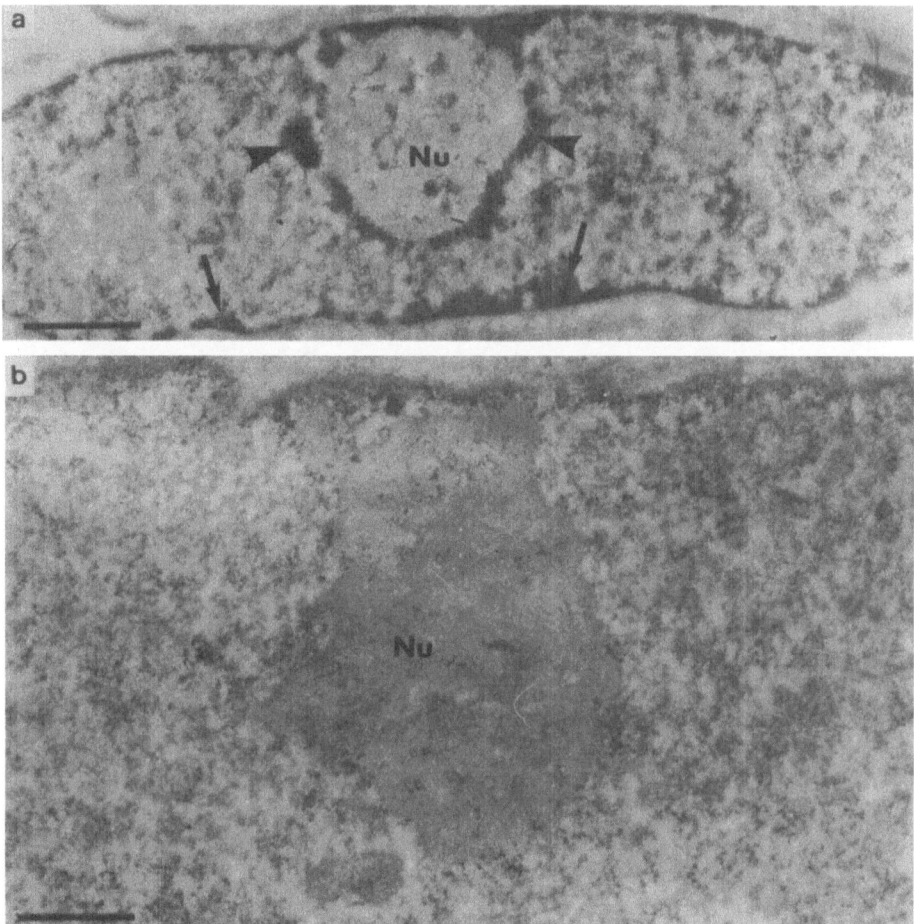

Fig. 20. Nuclei of human embryonic lung fibroblasts after
specific DNA staining. (a) Early PDL; dense chromatin
is observed along the nuclear membrane (arrows) and
around the nucleolus (arrowheads). The nucleoplasm
contains dispersed chromatin as well as the nucleolar
body (Nu). (b) Late PDL; dense chromatin is absent
from both nuclear and nucleolar peripheries. In
addition, the reaction fails to reveal chromatin inside
the large nucleolus (Nu). Bar, 1 µm x 18 000 (F.
Puvion-Dutilleul and A. Macieira-Coelho, 1982).

fibroblasts (Fig. 16). Up to the 41st PDL, cells fixed with
glutaraldehyde alone (Fig. 20a) had the chromatin condensed at
the nuclear periphery and around the nucleolus and largely
dispersed in the nucleoplasm. Beyond the 41st PDL an increasing
number of nuclei was enlarged and abnormally clear (Fig. 20b).

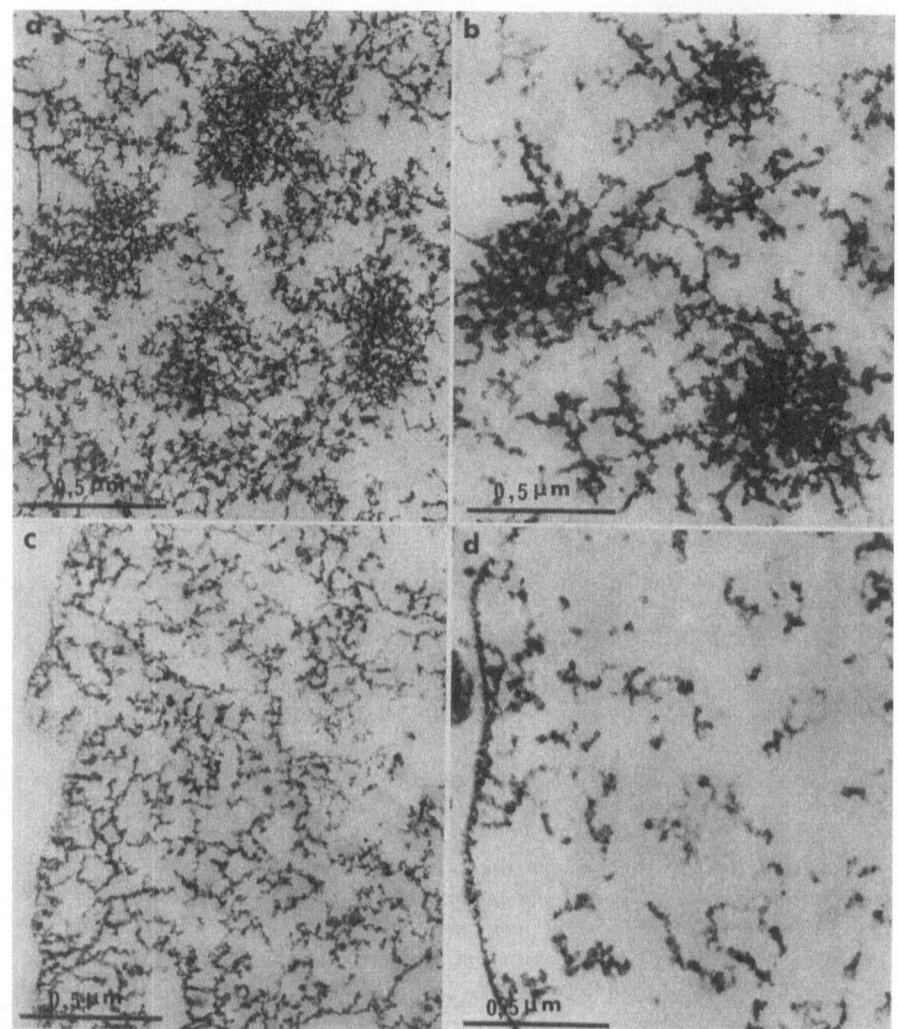

Fig. 21. Nuclear ultrastructure following mild loosening of
          early (a and c) and late (b and d) PDL human embryonic
          lung fibroblasts. Nucleolar (a and b) and peripheral
          (c and d) regions (F. Puvion-Dutilleul and A. Macieira-
          Coelho, 1982).

Chromatin was neither accumulated along the nuclear envelope nor
around the nucleolus and displayed a highly dispersed pattern.
The loosening procedure induced a swelling of each nucleus and
the disappearance of most of the cytoplasmic components. In
young cells the nucleolar regions contained highly contrasted
filamentous masses and clusters of packed granules which were

related to the RNP components (Fig. 21a). Chromatin appeared as
individual threads homogeneously distributed within the nuclei
(Fig. 21c), with a single or small clusters of perichromatin
granules attached to the chromatin threads. Beyond the 41st PDL
in an increasing number of nuclei (Table 2), the nucleolar
filamentous masses displayed a granular appearance due to the
knoby configuration of their entangled filaments (Fig. 21b). The
chromatin threads were rarer especially at the nuclear periphery
where the threads were shorter and unusually spaced along the
lamina densa which sometimes were entirely devoid of chromatin
threads (Fig. 21d).

The increase in the fraction of old cells with altered
nuclei and nucleoli was found to be related with some of the
changes in the kinetics of cell proliferation occurring during
the life span of human fetal lung fibroblasts in vitro (Puvion-
Dutilleul et al., 1982).

The same techniques were used to compare embryonic with
postnatal fibroblasts from normal donors and from a donor with
Werner syndrome (Puvion-Dutilleul and Macieira-Coelho, 1983).
The results are summarized in Table 3. They show that cells with
altered chromatin which are only seen in embryonic fibroblasts at
the end of their life span are already present in early PDL
postnatal cultures. In addition, most of the cells from the
Werner syndrome have altered nucleoli and chromatin.

Chromatin fibers were further analyzed in detail with
Miller's spreading technique. As can be seen in Figure 22, DNA
fibers from young type chromatin displayed a typical nucleosomal
organization whereas in old type chromatin most of the DNA fibers
were punctuated by highly spaced nucleosomes or were entirely
extended. In addition to spreads of the Werner syndrome nuclei,

Table 2. Percentage of nuclei with altered nucleoli and
          chromatin at different PDL of the human embryonic lung
          fibroblast line ICIG-7, revealed by the loosening
          procedure (F. Puvion-Dutilleul and A. Macieira-Coelho,
          1983).

PDL	%
10th to 40th	0
41st to 49th	5
50th to 56th	98

Table 3. Percentage of altered nuclei found after the loosening
          procedure in human skin fibroblasts of embryonic and
          postnatal origin (F. Puvion-Dutilleul and A. Macieira-
          Coelho, 1983).

CELLS	ORIGIN	PDL	% ALTERED NUCLEOLI	% ALTERED CHROMATIN	MAXIMAL NUMBER OF DOUBLINGS
ICIG-9	Fetal	4th	0	0	
AG-4525[+]	Fetal	6th	0	0	
MVL	Adult (30 yrs)	12th	0	17	30
AG-4353[+]	Adult (59 yrs)	6th	0	7	40
AG-780[+] (Werner's syndrome)	Adult (60 yrs)	6th	89	89	19

[+]NIA Aging Cell Repository (USA).

short pieces of unbeaded DNA fibers with length distributed
between 0.1 and 0.2 μm were frequently seen, occasionally forming
a circle.

    Since after the mild loosening procedure chromatin fibers
maintain the nucleosomal organization, the disappearance of the
latter must take place during the spreading technique; this
suggests an increased fragility of the DNA with aging and fits
the results described above after alkaline sucrose gradient
centrifugation. Thus it seems that the fragile sites are located
at the level of the nucleosomes. Previous results on the action
of nucleases on chromatin (Dell'Orco and Whittle, 1982)
suggesting a change in histone binding in the nucleosome core
could be germane to our data.

    As revealed by Miller's spreads, transcription complexes did
not become rarer on "old" type chromatin (Fig. 23). Ribosomal
matrix units always exhibited widely spaced RNP transcripts whose
density was only 6-10 fibrils per m of DNP axis (Fig. 23). The
few spacer intercepts that we could detect measured about 5 m.

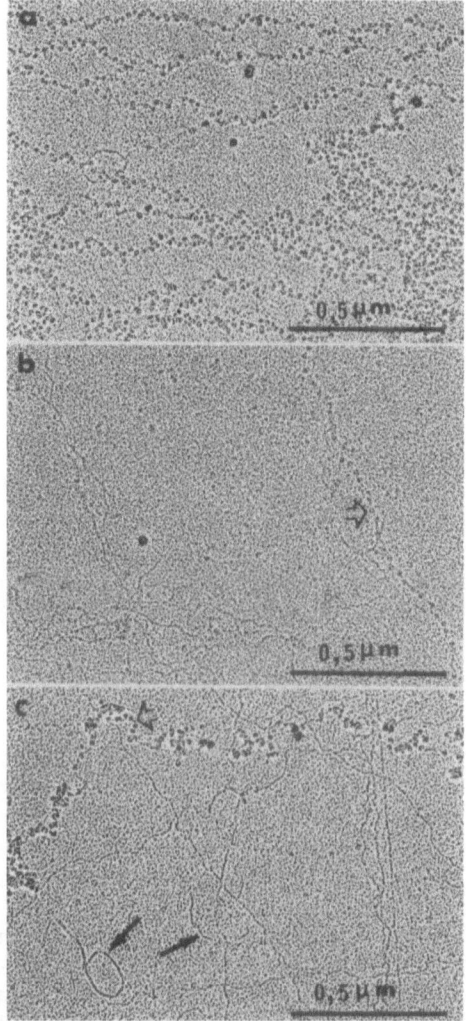

Fig. 22. Miller spreads of embryonic (a) and adult (b and c)
          human skin fibroblasts. Normal 59-year-old (b) and 60-
          year-old (c) donor with the Werner syndrome. (a)
          Beaded chromatin fibers are abundant in young-type
          nuclei; (b) most of the DNA of old-type nuclei is
          extended, however, chromatin fibers with a "bead-on-a-
          string" configuration (empty arrow) could be found; (c)
          most of DNA fibers are fully extended without any
          nucleosomes in Werner syndrome cells although typical
          beaded chromatin fibers can be found (empty arrow). In
          addition, short pieces of unbeaded DNA fibers are
          dispersed, sometimes forming a circle (arrow). Bars =
          0.5 μm (F. Puvion-Dutilleul and A. Macieira-Coelho, 1983).

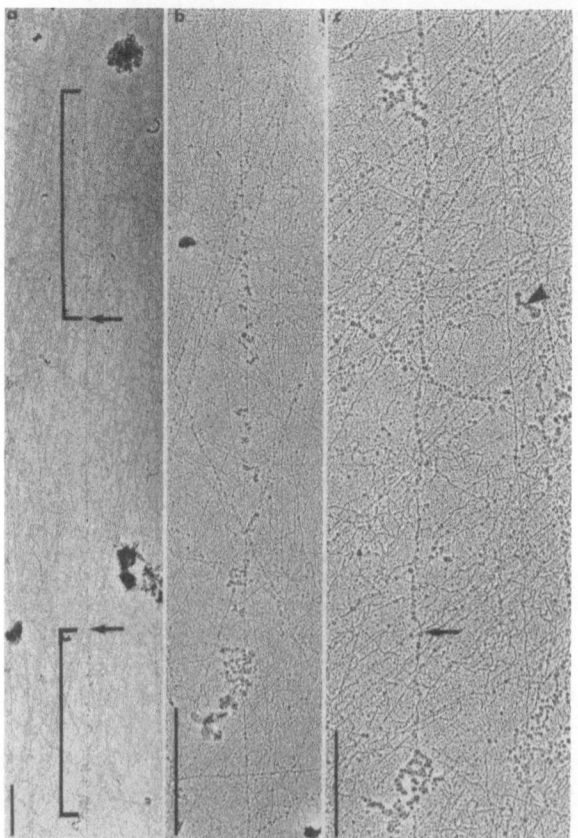

Fig. 23. Miller spreads of human embryonic lung fibroblasts in
Phase IV. Platinum shadow casting. (a) Ribosomal
repeating units. The spacer intercept (between the two
arrows) is longer than the corresponding matrix units
(brackets) x 12 000. Bar is 1 μm. (b) Higher
magnification of the ribosomal matrix unit located at
the bottom of (a). RNP fibrils are widely spaced x 30
000. Bar is 1 μm. (c) Non nucleolar RNP fibrils are
either solitary (arrowhead) on the DNA axis or
clustered in arrays with a low density of RNP
transcripts. Note the beaded aspect of the DNP fiber
carrying the array (arrow) x 50 000. Bar is 0.5 μm (F.
Puvion-Dutilleul et al., 1982).

A finding of circular DNA in a high fraction of Werner
syndrome cells is interesting. Shmookler-Reis et al. (1982) have
also found with other methodologies an increased amount of extrachromosomal circular copies of an Inter-Alu sequence. It is
possible that transposable elements detach from and reintegrate

into chromosomes at each cell division. The short linear and circular DNA that is found in old cells could correspond to elements which do not reintegrate because of the chromatin changes that accumulate with aging. This interpretation would fit the hypothesis described above which was previously proposed to explain senescence of dividing cells (Macieira-Coelho, 1979; Macieira-Coelho, 1980; Macieira-Coelho, 1981).

REFERENCES

Azzarone, B., Diatloff-Zito, C., Billard, C., and Macieira-Coelho, A., 1980, Effect of low dose rate irradiation on the division potential of cells in vitro. VII. Human fibroblasts from young and adult donors, In Vitro, 16:634.

Bourgeois, C.A., Raynaud, N., Diatloff-Zito, C., and Macieira-Coelho, A., 1981, Effect·of low dose rate ionizing radiation on the division potential of cells in vitro. VIII. Cytogenetic analysis of human fibroblasts, Mech. Age. Dev., 17:225.

Chetsanga, C.J., Tuttle, M., Jacoboni, A., and Johnson, C., 1977, Age-associated structural alterations in senescent mouse brain DNA, Biochem. Biophys. Acta., 474:180.

Dell'Orco, R.T. and Whittle, W.L., 1982, Micrococal nuclease and DNase I digestion of DNA from aging human diploid cells, Biochem. Biophys. Res. Commun., 107:117.

Diatloff, C., and Macieira-Coelho, A., 1979, Effect of low dose rate irradiation on the division potential of cells in vitro. V. Human skin fibroblasts from donors with a high risk of cancer, J. Nat. Cancer Inst., 63:55.

Icard, C., Beaupain, R., Diatloff, C. and Macieira-Coelho, A., 1979, Effect of low dose rate irradiation on the division potential of cells in vitro. VI. Changes in DNA and in radiosensitivity during aging of human fibroblasts, Mech. Age. Dev., 11:269.

Icard-Liepkalns and Macieira-Coelho, A., 1982, Aging and hydrocortisone effects on transient structures of replicative DNA of human fibroblasts, Proc. Soc. Exp. Biol. Med., 170:373.

Karran, P. and Ormerod, M.G., 1973, Is the ability to repair damage to DNA related to the proliferative capacity of a cell? The rejoining of X-ray-produced strand breaks, Biochem. Biophys. Acta., 299:54.

Macieira-Coelho, A., 1979, Reorganization of the cell genome as the basis of aging in dividing cells, in: "Recent Advances in Gerontology," Proceedings of the XIth International Congress of Gerontology, Excerpta Medica, Amsterdam.

Macieira-Coelho, A., 1980, Implications of the reorganizaion of the cell genome for aging or immortalization of dividing cells in vitro. Gerontology, 26:276.

Macieira-Coelho, A., 1981, Possible implications of the
    reorganizaion of the cell genome for the transfer of
    information in dividing cells, in: "Aging: a Challenge to
    Science and Society, Vol. I., Biology," D. Danon, N.W. Shock
    and M. Marois, eds., Oxford University Press, Oxford.
Macieira-Coelho, A., Bengtsson, A. and Van Der Ploeg, M., 1982,
    Distribution of DNA between sister cells during serial
    subcultivation of human fibroblasts. Histochemistry, 75:11.
Macieira-Coelho, A., Diatloff, C., Billardon, C., Brougeois, C.A.
    and Malaise, 1977, Effect of low dose rate ionizing
    radiation on the division potential of cells in vitro.   III.
    Human lung fibroblsts, Exp. Cell Res., 104:215.
Macieira-Coelho, A., Diatloff, C., Billard, M., Fertil, B.,
    Malaise, E., and Fries, D., 1978, Effect of low dose rate
    irradiation on the division potential of cells in vitro.
    IV. Embryonic and adult human lung fibroblast-like cells, J.
    Cell. Physiol., 95:235.
Macieira-Coelho, A., Diatloff, C. and Malaise, 1976, Doubling
    potential of fibroblasts from different species after
    ionizing radiation, Nature, 261:586.
Macieira-Coelho, A., and Taboury, F., 1982, A re-evaluation of
    the changes in proliferation in human fibroblasts during
    ageing in vitro, Cell Tissue Kinet., 15:213.
Miller, O.L., Jr., and Bakken, B.R., 1972, Morphological studies
    of transcription, in: "Gene Transcription in Reproductive
    Tissue," E. Diczfaluzy, ed., Karolinska Institutet,
    Stockholm.
Ono, T., and Okada, S., 1978, Does the capacity to rejoin
    radiation induced DNA breaks decline in senescent mice? Int.
    J. Radiat. Biol., 33:403.
Perry, P. and Wolff, S., 1974, New giemsa method for the
    differential staining of sister chromatids, Nature, 251:156.
Price, G.B., Modak, S.P. and Makinodan, T., 1971, Age-associated
    changes in the DNA of mouse tissue, Science, 171:917.
Puvion-Dutilleul, F., Azzarone, B. and Macieira-Coelho, A., 1982,
    Comparison between proliferative changes and nuclear events
    during ageing in human fibroblasts in vitro, Mech. Age.
    Dev., 20:75.
Puvion-Dutilleul, F., and Macieira-Coelho, A., 1982,
    Ultrastructural organization of nucleoproteins during aging
    of cultured human embryonic fibroblasts, Exp. Cell Res.,
    138:423.
Puvion-Dutilleul, F. and Macieira-Coelho, A., 1983, Aging
    dependent nucleolar and chromatin changes in cultivated
    fibroblasts. Cell Biol. Int. Rep., 7:61.
Puvion-Dutilleul, F. and Puvion, E., 1980, New aspects of
    intranuclear structures following partial decondensation of
    chromatin: A cytochemical and high-resolution
    autoradiographical study, J. Cell Sci., 42:305.

Schneider, E.L. and Monticone, R.E., 1978, Aging and sister
    chromatid exchange. II. The effect of the in vitro passage
    level of human fetal lung fibroblasts on baseline and
    mutagen-induced sister chromatid exchange frequencies, Exp.
    Cell Res., 115:269.
Shmookler-Reis, R.J. and Goldstein, 1980, Loss of reiterated DNA
    sequences during serial passage of human diploid
    fibroblasts, Cell, 21:739.
Shmookler-Reis, R.J., Lumpkin, C.K., McGill, J.R., Riabowol, K.T.
    and Goldstein, S., 1983, Extrachromosomal circular copies of
    an inter-Alu unstable sequence in human DNA are amplified
    during in vitro and in vivo aging, Nature, 301:394.
Wheeler, K.T. and Lett, J.T., 1972, Formation and rejoining of
    DNA strand breaks in irradiated neurones in vivo, Radiat.
    Res., 52:59

CELLULAR MECHANISMS OF AGING IN THE WERNER SYNDROME

Osamu Nikaido, Taka Nishida and Akihiro Shima[1]

Division of Radiation Biology
Faculty of Pharmaceutical Sciences
Kanazawa University, Kanazawa 920

[1]Department of Experimental Radiology
Shiga University of Medical Science
Ohtsu 520-21 Japan

INTRODUCTION

The Werner syndrome (WS) is a rare autosomal recessive disease with characteristic features of accelerated ageing such as gray hair, dwarfism, juvenile cataract[1]), urinary excretion of high levels of acidic glycosaminoglycans[2]) and a short life span. Many attempts to elucidate the relatively short life spans of patients with various progeroid syndromes by using cultured cells have been made in the past two decades[3,4]). Among them, the reduction in population doubling numbers (PDs) in cells derived from the patients with genetic disorders such as WS[3]) and Hutchinson-Gilford progeria[4]) gave us a clue to the finding of a causal relationship between the clinical symptoms and biological defects found in these cells.

Many investigations using WS cells in culture have focused on whether ageing processes in WS cells in vitro are different from those in normal cells or merely mimic those in normal cells in accelerated forms; in other words, whether or not WS cells could be a model cell system for elucidating ageing processes in vitro in normal cells.

The search for biological abnormalities in WS cells in culture revealed their chromosomal instability during culture[5]), high levels of the heat-labile fraction of glucose 6-dehydrogenase[6]), presence of "senescent factor(s)" that inhibit

DNA synthesis in the fused normal cell nucleus[7]) and slowed rates of DNA chain elongation, while DNA repair in WS cells following irradiation with ultraviolet light (UV) appeared at the same rate as that in normal cells[8]).

The cells derived from patients with Hutchinson-Gilford progeria were reported to have low PDs in culture[3]) and to be deficient in the repair of DNA-single strand breaks induced by gamma-rays[9,10]). The reduced reparability in progeroid cells is controversial[11]). However, these results have made many researchers investigate the relationship between the mechanisms of cellular ageing and DNA repair[12,13]).

We previously reported that the cells derived from patients with xeroderma pigmentosum and ataxia telangiectasia, which are known to be defective in DNA repair, attained the same PDs as age-matched normal cells[14]). In this study, we extended the experiment further to study the cellular reparability to DNA damage induced not only by UV- but also by gamma-irradiation. The results obtained revealed that cellular reparability of gamma-irradiation damage in viral DNA did not relate to the PDs attained by cells. Furthermore, WS cells attaining low levels of PDs in culture did not show any deficiency in repair of either UV- or gamma-irradiation damage when assayed by host-cell reactivation of herpes simplex virus.

On the other hand, cytokinetic analysis of ageing cells revealed the gradual accumulation of noncycling cells in cell populations with increasing passage numbers[15]). Noncycling cells, defined as the cells unlabeled after treatment with [3H]-TdR for a certain time, were reported to result from the heterogeneity in generation times[16]) and from non-proliferating cells that accumulated in G_1 phase[17]). The prolongation of the S phase and generation times were reported in WS cells[18]); however; the changes in distribution of cells in various cell-cycle phases with ageing in vitro has not been fully investigated.

In this study, we analysed WS cells at various passages by using Feulgen-DNA cytofluorometry simultaneously with autoradiography. The results revealed the accumulation of noncycling cells at the G_1 phase in WS cell population with increasing passage numbers and retarded DNA synthesis in both normal and WS cells at very late passages.

MATERIALS AND METHODS

Cells, Culture Method and Medium

Biopsy specimens were obtained from the femoral skin of patients with WS. Biopsy specimens of skin fragments from the patients with Cockayne syndrome (CS), xeroderma pigmentosum (XP) and ataxia telangiectasia (AT) were taken mainly from their upper arms. In the case of healthy donors, skin biopsy specimens were obtained from either their upper arms or femurs. In addition, skin fragments left over from the skin sheets transplanted to the burned wounds of healthy people were used as sources of normal cells with the donors' consent. These skin specimens were aseptically minced with blades to small fragments (0.5 X 0.5 mm) after removing the fat. Three pieces of these fragments were put onto a plastic dish (6 cm-diameter) which had been soaked with 0.5 ml of culture medium. The dishes were incubated in a CO_2-incubator at 37°C for 4 days, then another 4.5 ml of fresh medium containing alpha-MEM (Flow Laboratories, McLean, Virginia) supplemented with 10% fetal bovine serum (M.A. Bioproducts, Walkersville, Maryland) and 50 µg/ml Kanamycin sulfate (Yamanouchi Pharmaceutical Co. Ltd., Tokyo) was added to each dish. The medium was changed every 4 days. When the fibroblasts propagated from the skin fragments occupied two-thirds of the culture surface of a dish, they were treated with 0.1% trypsin (Difico Laboratories, Detroit, Michigan) and 0.01% EDTA (Wako Pharmacy Co. Ltd., Osaka) in phosphate buffer saline (PBS). At this time, the cell PD was designated as 0. An aliquot of 10^6 cells suspended in 12.5 ml culture medium was inoculated into a culture flask (75 cm^2/Tissue culture flask, Corning Glass Works, Corning, N.Y.). Three flasks of cells were successively cultured. Cells were fed every 2 days with fresh medium and subcultured from the 4th to the 7th day, before reaching confluency. The cessation of growth of a cell population was recognized when lower cell yields than the inoculum cell number (10^6 cells/flask) were obtained twice in successive subcultures. The number of population doublings (PDs) attained by the cells was calculated by the method published previously[14,19].

Measurement of Labeling Indices in Cells at Various Passages

    Aliquots of 10^5 cells at various passages were inoculated into a plastic dish (3.5 cm-diameter) and incubated in a CO_2-incubator at 37°C for 24 hours. The cells were treated with 1µ Ci/ml of [^{3}H]-thymidine ([^{3}H]-TdR, 5 Ci/mmol; Amersham, England) for 24 hours. Cells in the dishes were washed twice with PBS and fixed with absolute methanol for 30 min. After the dishes were dried at room temperature, the bottom of each dish was cut off and mounted on a glass slide with Eukitt (Kindler Co. Ltd., Freiburg, West Germany). The glass slides were dipped into predissolved Sakura NR-M2 nuclear emulsion (Konishiroku Photo Ind. Co. Ltd., Tokyo) and kept in a refrigerator at -20°C for a week. Then the slides were developed, fixed and washed with tap water. Finally, the slides were stained with Giemsa.

Preparation of Slides for Cytofluorometry

Aliquots of 2×10^4 cells at various passages were inoculated onto a cover slip (23 x 24 mm) housed in a plastic dish (3.5 cm-diameter) and incubated in a CO_2-incubator for 24 hours. The cells were treated with 0.01 μ Ci/ml of $[^3H]$-TdR (specific activity 2Ci/mmol) for up to 120 hours. Cells were refed with freshly prepared medium containing $[^3H]$-TdR on the 3rd day of labeling. After various hours of incubation, cells were washed twice with PBS and fixed with absolute methanol for 30 min. The experimental procedures for preparing the slides for assaying both cellular DNA content and labeling intensity were the same with those described by Fujita et al.[20] and Shima et al. [21]. Briefly, the cells on the cover slips were treated with 1N HCl at 60°C for 5 min, followed by the Feulgen nuclear reaction. Pararosanilline Schiff's reagent was diluted to 0.5% with glycine buffer (pH 2.3) and the cells were stained at 7°C for 10 min. The cover slips were then rinsed with three changes of pre-cooled (7°C) bisulfite solution and then washed in tap water for 1 hour and air dried. The cover slips were next dipped into Sakura NR-M2 nuclear emulsion prewarmed to 46°C. After 4 weeks of exposure at 4°C, the autoradiographs were developed, fixed, and mounted on clean glass slides with the cell side downwards, as described by Fujita et al.[20].

Feulgen-DNA Cytofluorometry and Measurement of Labeling Intensity

All the procedures were carried out in accordance with the methods described by Fujita et al.[20]. In brief, after at least 10 hours' irradiation of the slides with green light to diminish the non-specific fluorescence of the background, both the fluorescence from the Feulgen dye-complex, which is proportional to the nuclear DNA content, and the reflected red light, which is proportional to the number of grains, were measured by Automatic Digital-Microfluorometers (Olympus MMSP-RF-S). About 200 cell nuclei per slide were measured for their DNA content and labeling intensity. The data were further computed by an YHP-85 computer.

Host-Cell Reactivation of UV- or Gamma-Irradiated Virus

The experimental procedures used in this study were essentially identical to those published previously[14]. In brief, a stock suspension of herpes simplex virus (HSV), having a titer of 1.5 to 1.7×10^7 pfu/ml against a human amnion F1 cell line was used for all virus experiments. After diluting the virus suspension with PBS to the appropriate concentration, various doses of UV were given with germicidal lamps (10 watt x 2, Toshiba GL-10) at a dose rate of 1.65 J/m^2/sec., and monitored by a Topcon radiometer (Tokyo Kagaku Co. Ltd., Tokyo). For gamma-irradiation of the virus, a stock virus suspension was irradiated with ^{60}Co gamma-ray at a dose rate of 7.1×10^3 rad/min at $-75°C$. 0.5 ml of either UV- or gamma-irradiated virus suspension was delivered to freshly confluent cells in plastic dishes (6 cm-diameter), that had been previously washed once with PBS and incubated for 90 min at 37°C. Virus adsorption was stopped by adding 4.5 ml of complete medium containing 0.25% human gammaglobulin (human immunoglobulin; Midori-Juji Co. Ltd., Osaka). Plaques were scored on the 3rd day of incubation, and survival curves for HSV irradiated and infected to various cell strains were depicted as a function of either UV- or gamma-irradiation doses. The survival curves usually had two components[33]. In this study, D_0 values were obtained from the first component of the curves.

RESULTS

Relationship Between PDs and Donor Ages

        Cells derived from both healthy normal donors and patients of various ages with hereditary disorders were serially cultured to obtain their maximal PDs. The ages at biopsy of 32 normal healthy donors ranged from 3 months to 70 years. On the other hand, the WS patients at biopsy were mainly in their thirties. In Figure 1, the PDs attained by the various cell strains were plotted against donor ages. The inverted relationship between age of normal donor and the maximal PD attained by normal cells can be seen. It is noteworthy that PDs attained by WS cells were lower than those attained by the cells from age-matched normal healthy donors. On the other hand, the cells derived from both XP and AT patients, which are known to be defective in DNA

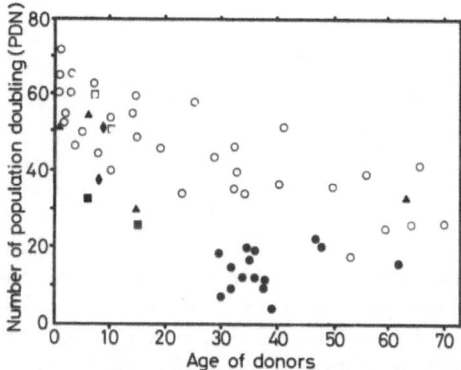

Fig. 1. The relationship between PDs attained by cells and age of donors, ■ BS cells, ◆ AT cells, ▲ XP cells, ● WS cells, □ CS cells and ○ cells derived from normal healthy donors.

repair, could attain PDs comparable to those of normal donors.
The PDs of cells derived from the patients with Cockayne syndrome
showing segmental progeroid characteristics[22] and repair
deficiency[23] were at the same levels as those of normal cells.

Changes in 24 Hours' Labeling Indices in Cells at Various Passages

Both normal and WS cells at various passages were labeled
with [3H]-TdR for 24 hours. Labeling indices obtained from
autoradiographs of cell strains were plotted against their
normalized PDs (NPDs), i.e. the maximum PDs attained by each cell
strain was designated to 1. In normal cells, labeling indices
decreased gradually to 0.8 NPD, followed by a drastic decrease
beyond this PD, as shown in Figure 2. These biphasic changes in
the labeling index were also observed in WS cells, although the
lower labeling indices in WS cells in vitro than in normal cells
were observed throughout their life spans. It is remarkable that
more than 10% of both WS and normal cells did synthesize DNA
during the 24 hours at the extreme end of their life spans.

DNA Content in Normal and WS Cells at Various Passages

Both WS and age-matched normal cells were labeled with low
concentrations of [3H]-TdR for up to 120 hours. DNA content and
labeling intensity of cells at various passages were assayed by
Feulgen DNA-cytofluorometry simultaneously with autoradiography.
Frequencies of both labeled and unlabeled cells, shown as percent
of total cells, were plotted as a function of cellular DNA con-

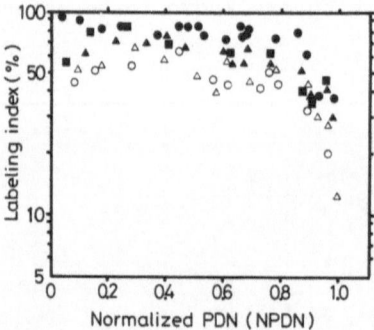

Fig. 2.   Changes in labeling indices in both WS and normal cells at
          various passages in vitro. △ Cells derived from 48-yr-old
          WS patient (max. PD; 20.7), ○ cells derived from a 47-yr-
          old WS patient (max. PD; 22.6), ● cells from a 1.8-yr-old
          normal donor (max. PD; 56.5), ▲ cells from a 32-yr-old
          normal donor (max. PD; 34.1) and ■ cells from a 60-yr-old
          normal donor (max. PD; 25.5).

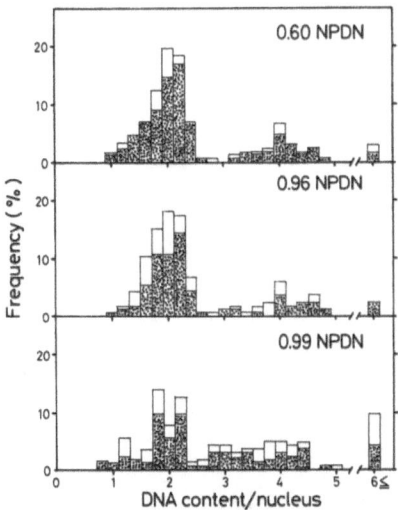

Fig. 3. Distribution of labeled and unlabeled DNA contents in
         normal cells at various passages. Cells were labeled with
         [3H]-TdR for 120 hours. Dotted area shows the fraction of
         labeled cells in each histogram. The number of the cells
         at each passage was labeled and is shown in each figure.

tents, which were assayed as intensity of fluorescence (Fig. 3).
Almost 80% of the actively growing normal cells at 0.6 NPD were
labeled with [3H]-TdR during 120 hours. The unlabeled cells
accumulated mainly at the G_1 phase, having 2C DNA content. The
fraction of unlabeled cells became more abundant with increasing
passage numbers. At the very end of their life spans, the
accumulation of unlabeled cells at various cell phases such as
G_1, S, and G_2 became evident; furthermore, distribution of
cellular DNA content in the cells deviated slightly from the
bimodal patterns which were seen in cells at young passages and
the cells showing DNA content more than 6C accumulated.

WS cells at 0.93 NPD were 43% labeled after treatment with
[3H]-TdR for 120 hours. Unlabeled G_1, S, and G_2 cells
accumulated as shown in Figure 4. At 0.96 NPD, unlabeled cells
at the G_1 phase increased. WS cell population at 0.99 NPD
contained a large fraction of unlabeled cells distributed across
all phases in the cell cycle. The fraction of unlabeled cells in
WS cells was larger than that in age-matched normal cells at the
same NPD.

Labeling Intensity in Cells at Various Passages

The distribution of labeling intensity in both WS and normal
cell nuclei is shown in Figures 5 and 6. The labeling intensity

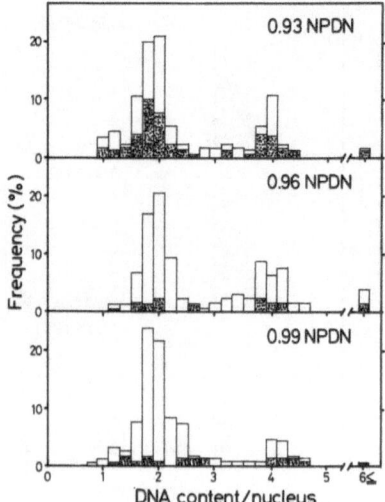

Fig. 4. Distribution of labeled and unlabeled DNA contents in WS
         cells at various passages. For details in this figure,
         see the legend for Figure 3.

in each nucleus was determined by assaying the intensity of red
reflected light from the grains on the nucleus, which is known to
be proportional to the number of the grains[20]). The distribution
patterns of the labeling intensities in normal cells at various
passages are somewhat different from each other. The mean
labeling intensity in the main peak of actively growing normal
cells at 0.6 NPD is 3.54 ±1.37. With increasing passages, the
labeling intensities of the main peaks decreased to 1.9 ±0.76
and 2.30 ±1.08, at 0.96 and 0.99 NPD respectively (Fig. 5).

On the other hand, the mean labeling intensity in the main
peaks of WS cells at various passages are comparable to those in
normal cells at very late passages such as 0.96 and 0.99 NPDs,
although the height of the main peaks is lower than that of those
in normal cells at the same NPD level, which seems to reflect the
lower labeling indices in WS cells compared with those in normal
cells. Furthermore, the lower labeling intensities observed in
WS and normal cells at late passages may reflect the decreased
amount of DNA synthesis during 120 hours (Fig. 6).

Repair of UV-damage in HSV by Various Cells

Various cells at 0.20 - 0.22 NPDs were assayed for the UV-
survival of HSV. Cells derived from normal healthy donors of
various ages, patients with ataxia telangiectasia, and patients

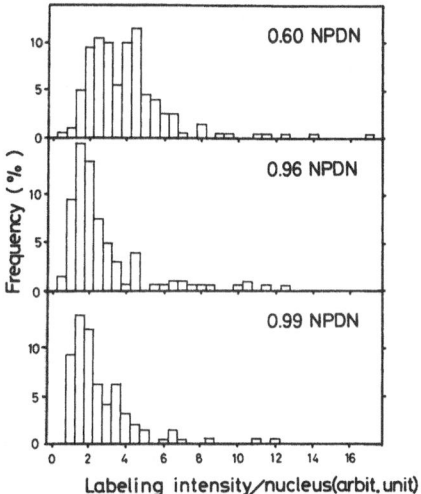

Fig. 5.   Distribution of labeling intensity in normal cell nuclei
labeled with [^{3}H]-TdR for 120 hours.

with the Werner syndrome were most efficient in host-cell
reactivation of UV-irradiated HSV as shown in Figure 7. On the
other hand, the cells from patients with xeroderma pigmentosum
(complementation group A) were slow in host-cell reactivation.
It is noteworthy that the cells derived from normal healthy
donors of various ages and WS cells attaining reduced PDs in
culture also showed the same activity in host-cell reactivation.
The mean D_0 values in J/m^2 for the first component of the
survival curves were 25 for normal, WS, and AT cells and 8 for XP
cells. Cells at various passages were assayed for host-cell
reactivation of the UV-irradiated HSV. The D_0 values of the
first component of the survival curves plotted against NPD are
shown in Figure 8. No remarkable changes in D_0 values were
observed in any cell population up to 80% of NPD, while low D_0
values were obtained in XP cells throughout their life span in
vitro.

Repair of Gamma-Damage in HSV by Various Cells

      Various cells at 0.32 - 0.43 NPDs were assayed for gamma-
irradiation survival of HSV. Normal and WS cells were not
different in reactivation of gamma-irradiated HSV (Fig. 9).
Furthermore, AT cells known to be gamma-ray sensitive revealed
the same host-cell reactivation as normal cells. AT3BI reported
to be repair-deficient when assayed by gamma-specific
endonuclease from Micrococcus luteus[24] were not different in

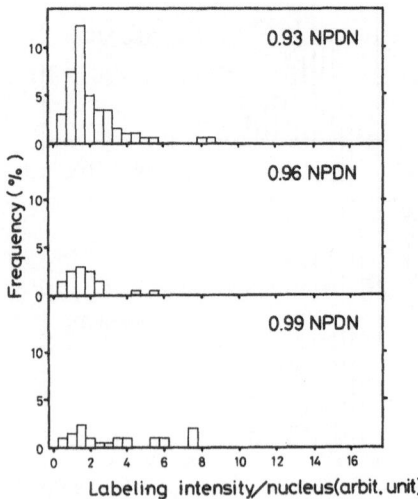

Fig. 6. Distribution of labeling intensity in WS cell nuclei
         labeled with [3H]-TdR for 120 hours.

reactivation from normal cells (data not shown). Cells at
various passages were assayed for reactivation of HSV gamma-
irradiated with 300 krad. The surviving fraction gamma-irradiated
HSV in various cells was plotted against their NPDs. No
remarkable changes in the surviving fractions were observed
throughout their lifespans in vitro up to 0.8 NPD (Fig. 10). It
can be therefore concluded that WS cells are proficient in the
repair of viral DNA irradiated with gamma-rays. Furthermore, we
failed to show any repair deficiency of AT cells by host cell
reactivation of HSV irradiated with gamma rays.

DISCUSSION

      Cellular kinetics in ageing cells in vitro have been well
discussed in the literature. Labeling indices[15,25] and
distributions of DNA content[17,26] in cells at various passages
have been frequently employed as markers to show the changes in
cell population with ageing in vitro. In this study, cytokinetic
comparison using autoradiography and Feulgen-DNA cytofluorometry
was carried out in both normal and WS cells. Fraction of cells
labeled with [3H]-TdR for 24 hours gradually decreased by 0.8 NPD
in both normal and WS cells. Beyond 0.8 NPD, labeling indices in
both cells drastically decreased (Fig. 2). These biphasic
changes in labeling indices in cellular aging were consistent
with the results reported by Vincent et al.[25].

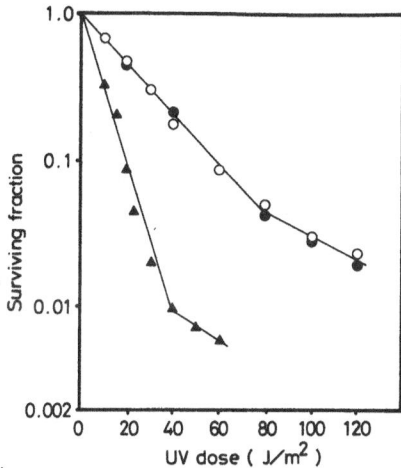

Fig. 7. Host cell reactivation of UV–irradiated herpes simplex
virus in ◯ normal, ● WS and ▲ XP cells at 0.20 - 0.22 NPD.

In preliminary results obtained from the measurement of
interdivision times (IDTs) by time-lapse microcinematography,
more or less constant IDTs up to 0.8 NPD followed by widely
divergent IDTs were observed in normal cells (data not shown).
From these results, we assumed that the first step in ageing in
vitro represented by a gradual decrease in the labeling indices
up to 0.8 NPD might reflect the accumulation of cells at certain
phases in the cell cycle, and that the second step in cellular
ageing, characterized by a sudden decline in labeling indices,
might result from both the heterogenous distribution of cell
generation times and the accumulation of cells at various phases.

In normal cells at 0.6 NPD, those not labeled with [^{3}H]–TdR
after 120 hours were distributed mainly in the G_1 and G_2 phases
(Fig. 3). At 0.96 and 0.99 NPDs, unlabeled cells distributed in
the G_1, S and G_2 phases. If noncycling cells can be defined as
cells unlabeled by [^{3}H]–TdR treatment after 120 hours, these
cells primarily accumulated in the G_1 phase, showing 2C DNA
content with increasing passage numbers and became distributed in
all phases of the cell cycle at the very end of their life spans.
On the other hand, a wider variation of DNA contents in both
normal and WS cells was observed at 0.99 NPD (Figs. 3 and 4).
It is noteworthy that the DNA contents of G_1 cells at very late
passages decreased slightly. Our results are quite consistent
with those reported by Schneider et al.[17] and Yanishevski et
al.[26]. The decrease of cellular DNA contents has been discussed
in terms of either the increase of aneuploid cells in the

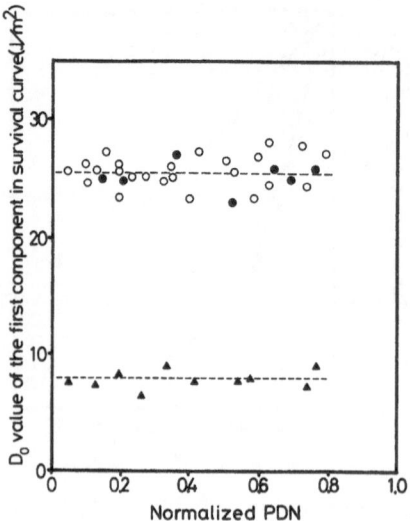

Fig. 8.   Changes in D_0 values of the first component in UV-
           irradiation survival curves of herpes simplex virus in
           various cells at various NPD. Symbols are the same as for
           Figure 8.

population, or the increased frequency of chromosomal deletion,
or the altered binding of Feulgen dye to cellular DNA at very
late passages. We can not define the cause of the apparent loss
of cellular DNA at this moment because the number of metaphase
cells from both normal and WS cell populations at late passages
is insufficient to analyse their karotypes.

     Essentially similar results were obtained in WS cells at
various passages although the accumulation of noncycling cells in
the G_1 phase was marked. Furthermore, labeling indices in WS
cells decreased with increasing passage numbers and noncycling
cells accumulated in all cell phases of the cell cycle (Fig. 4).
It is common to both normal and WS cells at the very end of their
life spans in vitro that noncycling cells were distributed into
all phases of the cell cycle; however, preferential accumulation
of noncycling cells at the G_1 phase was characteristic of WS
cells. The depressed levels of PDs attained by WS cells· may be
the result of the accumulation of noncycling cells at the G_1
phase that do not enter into the S phase within 120 hours. The
results, that labeling indices derived from 24 hours' labeling
with [3H]-TdR were lower in WS than normal cells from the
beginning of the culture to the end of their life spans, seem to
indicate that the fraction of noncycling cells in the WS cell
population is considerably larger than in normal cell population.
Furthermore, the fraction of cells departing the cell cycle and
becoming noncycling cells in each cell generation may be larger
in WS cells than in normal cells.

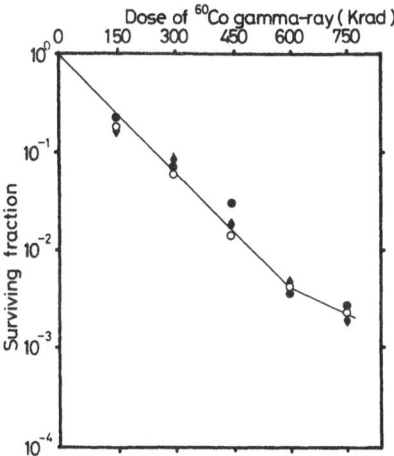

Fig. 9. Host-cell reactivation of gamma-irradiated herpes simplex virus in ◆ AT cells, ● WS cells and ◯ normal cells at 0.32 − 0.43 NPD.

The labeling intensity in cells is known to be proportional to the number of grains on the nucleus[20]. The labeling intensity in normal cells at various PDs is somewhat higher than that in WS cells and the frequency of cells expressed as the percent of total cells is lower in WS cells than those in normal cells. The latter result seems to reflect low labeling indices in WS cells. Since the difference in the distribution pattern of DNA contents between both cells was not so great (Figs. 3 and 4), the shift of peaks in the distribution of labeling intensities to lower values with increasing passage numbers seems to reflect the reduction of DNA synthesis in cells at late passages (Figs. 5 and 6).

An inverted relationship between the PDs attained by cells and ages of donors was established (Fig. 1). This relationship was first reported by Martin et al. in 1970[3] and later by Schneider et al. [27]. The decreases in PDs attained by cells with increasing age of donor may be the result of a gradual increase in the fraction of noncycling cells in the cell population. These results should be examined further from the point of view of how the steps of ageing in vivo apply to those of ageing in vitro. The experiment to approach the problems mentioned above is now under way.

Comparative studies on the relationship between the extent of unscheduled DNA synthesis (UDS) induced in cells by UV-irradiation and maximum life spans in a number of placental animals from which the cells were derived[28], and on the

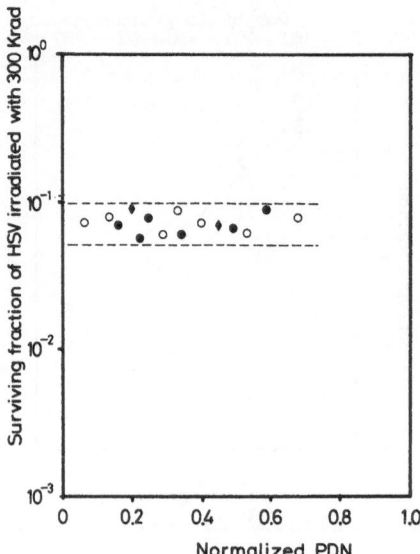

Fig. 10.   Changes of the surviving fractions of herpes simplex
           virus gamma-irradiated with 300 krads in various cells in
           culture.   Symbols are the same as for Figure 9.

relationship between the PDs attained by cells in culture and the
maximum life spans of the various animals from which cells were
derived[29), gave us the hypothesis that the ability of cells to
repair the DNA damage induced by environmental agents such as UV-
and X-radiation and chemicals determines not only the life spans
of the animals but also the PDs attained by cells derived from
those animals.   On the other hand, the cells derived from
patients with Hutchinson-Gilford progeria were reported to attain
low PDs in culture[3) and reduced ability to repair DNA single-
strand breaks[9) compared with normal cells.   Evidence supporting
the relationship between the extent of UDS and maximum life spans
was reported by Hall et al. in various primates[30) and by
Paffenholtz in mice with different lifespans[31).   However,
conflicting results were reported by Kato et al.[32).   In their
experiment no obvious relationship between the extent of UDS and
the maximum life spans was established.   Furthermore, the evidence
on repair proficiency in progeria cells was reported by Regan et
al.[11).   Thus, the contradictory evidence on the relationship has
accumulated.   In the present study, we examined the PDs attained
by the cells assumed to be repair-deficient.   XP cells that were
incapable of repairing UV-damaged HSV by host-cell reactivation

were able to attain the normal PDs levels. On the other hand, AT cells that were able to repair gamma-irradiation damage also attained the PDs comparable to those of normal cells. CS cells derived from patients with segmental progeroid syndromes also attained the same levels of PDs with those attained by age-matched normal cells. From these results, it may be concluded that cells defective in reparability of DNA damage can attain the same levels of PDs as age-matched normal cells and that damage assumed to accumulate in cellular DNA with aging in vitro are not the same types of DNA damage induced by UV- or gamma-irradiation.

Cellular repair of DNA damage, which was assayed by host-cell reactivation of HSV irradiated with either UV- or gamma-irradiation did not appreciably change, up to 0.8 NPD (Figs. 8 and 10). Host-cell reactivation of HSV in cells at more than 0.8 NPD was not carried out because of a lack of a sufficient number of cells. As shown in Figure 2, the number of cells synthesizing DNA during 24 hours were gradually decreasing to 0.8 NPD. These results clearly indicate that cellular reparability to DNA damage induced by either UV- or gamma-irradiation has nothing to do with the first step of cellular ageing in either normal or WS cells. Furthermore, we can exclude the possibility of the accumulation of such damage in cellular DNA with ageing in vitro. This study demonstrated that WS cells are proficient in repair of both UV- and gamma-irradiation damage when assayed by host-cell reactivation of HSV. These results are in good agreement with the data reported by Fujiwara et al.[8], who compared the extent of UDS induced by UV-irradiation in both WS and normal cells.

In conclusion, we found that WS cells were characteristic in preferentially accumulating noncycling cells at the G_1 phase and that the extent of DNA synthesis in cells decreased with increasing passage numbers. The cells at various passages up to 0.8 NPD maintained constant reparability of DNA damage induced by either UV- or gamma-irradiation. Neither UV- nor gamma-irradiation damage was a cause of cellular aging. WS cells were proved to be capable of repair of UV- and gamma-irradiation damage.

Acknowledgement.

The authors thank Miss Yoko Nanashima for her technical assistance. This work was supported partly by a Grant in Aid from the Ministry of Education, Sciences and Culture, Japan, and partly by a Life Science Grant from the Institute of Physical and Chemical Research, Tokyo, Japan.

REFERENCES

1. C.J. Epstein, G.M. Martin, A.S. Schultz, and A.G. Motulsky,
    Werner's syndrome. A review of its symptomatology, natural
    history, pathologic features, genetics and relationship to
    the aging process, Medicine. 45:177 (1966).
2. K. Murata, Urinary acidic glycosaminoglycans in Werner's syn-
    drome, Experientia. 38:313 (1982).
3. G.M. Martin, C.A. Sprague, and C.J. Epstein, Replicative life-
    span of cultured human cells. Effects of donor's age,
    tissue, and genotype, Lab. Invest. 23:86 (1970).
4. B.S. Danes, Progeria: a cell culture study on aging, J. Clin.
    Invest. 50:2000 (1971).
5. D. Salk, K. Au, H. Hoehn, and G.M. Martin, Cytogenetics of
    Werner's syndrome cultured skin fibroblasts: varigated
    translocation mosaicism, Cytogenet. Cell Genet. 30:92
    (1981).
6. R. Holliday, J.S. Porterfield, and D.D. Gibbs, Premature ageing
    and occurrence of altered enzyme in Werner's syndrome
    fibroblasts, Nature. 248:762 (1974).
7. K. Tanaka, T. Nakazawa, Y. Okada, and Y. Kumahara, Roles of
    nuclear and cytoplasmic environments in the retarded DNA
    synthesis in Werner syndrome cells, Exp. Cell Res. 127:185
    (1980).
8. Y. Fujiwara, T. Higashikawa, and M. Tatsumi, A retarded rate of
    DNA replication and normal level of DNA repair in Werner's
    syndrome fibroblasts in culture, J. Cell. Physiol. 92:365
    (1977).
9. J. Epstein, J.R. Williams, and J.B. Little, Deficient DNA re-
    pair in human progeroid cells, Proc. Natl. Acad. Sci. USA,
    70:977 (1973).
10. J. Epstein, J.R. Williams, and J.B. Little, Rate of DNA repair
    in progeric and normal human fibroblasts, Biochem.
    Biophys. Res. Comm. 59:850 (1974).
11. J.D. Regan and R.B. Setlow, DNA repair in human progeroid
    cells, Biochem. Biophys. Res. Comm. 59:858 (1974).
12. A.A. Francis, W.H. Lee, and J.D. Regan, The relationship of DNA
    excision repair of ultraviolet-induced lesions to the
    maximum life span of mammals, Mech. Ageing Dev. 16:181
    (1981).
13. R.T. Dell'Orco and W.L. Whittle, Evidence for an increased
    level of DNA damage in high doubling level human diploid
    cells in culture, Mech. Ageing Dev. 15:141 (1981).
14. O. Nikaido, S. Ban, and T. Sugahara, Population doubling number
    in cells with genetic disorders, Adv. Exp. Med. Biol.
    129:303 (1980).
15. V.J. Cristofalo and B.B. Sharf, Cellular senescence and DNA
    synthesis; Thymidine incorporation as a measure of
    population age in human diploid cells, Exp Cell. Res.
    76:419 (1973).

16. A. Maieira-Coelho, Kinetics of the proliferation of human fibroblasts during their life span in vitro, Mech. Ageing Dev. 6:341 (1977).

17. E.L. Schneider and B.J. Fowlkes, Measurement of DNA content and cell volume in senescent human fibroblasts utilizing flow multiparameter single cells analysis, Exp. Cell Res. 98:298 (1976).

18. F. Hanaoka and M. Yamada, Autoradiographic studies of DNA replication in Werner's syndrome, in: "Pathogenetic Mechanisms in Werner's Syndrome and Their Role in Human Aging," US-Japan cooperative seminar, Kobe, Japan (1982).

19. S. Ban, O. Nikaido, and T. Sugahara, Acute and late effects of a single exposure of ionizing radiation on cultured human diploid cell population, Radiat. Res., 81:120 (1980).

20. S. Fujita, T. Ashihara, and M. Fukuda, Simultaneous measurement of DNA content and grain count on an autoradiograph of Feulgen stained cells, Histochem. 40:155 (1974).

21. A. Shima and T. Sugahara, Age-dependent ploidy class changes in mouse hepatocyte nuclei as revealed by Feulgen-DNA cytofluorometry, Exp. Gerontol. 11:193 (1976).

22. C.A. Neill and M.M. Dingwall, A syndrome resembling progeria: a review of 2 cases, Arch. Dis. Child. 25:213 (1950).

23. M. Ikenaga, M. Inoue, T. Kozuka, and T. Sugita, The recovery of colony-forming ability and the rate of semi-conservative DNA synthesis in ultraviolet-irradiated Cockayne and normal cells, Mutation Res. 91:87 (1981).

24. M.C. Paterson, B.P. Smith, P.H.M. Lohman, A.K. Anderson, and L. Fishman, Defective excision repair of gamma-ray-damaged DNA in human (ataxia telangiectasia) fibroblasts, Nature. 260:444 (1976).

25. R.A. Vincent, and P.C. Huang, The proportion of cells labeled with tritiated thymidine as a function of population doubling level in cultures of fetal, adult, mutant, and tumor origin, Exp. Cell Res. 102:31 (1976).

26. R. Yanishevski, M.L. Mendelsohn, B.H. Mayall, and V.J. Cristofalo, Proliferative capacity and DNA content of aging human diploid cells in culture: cytophotometric and autoradiographic analysis, J. Cell. Physiol. 84:165 (1974).

27. E.L. Schneider and Y. Mitsui, The relationship between in vitro aging and in vivo human age, Proc. Natl. Acad. Sci. USA. 73:3584 (1976).

28. R.W. Hart and R.B. Setlow, Correlation between deoxyribonucleic acid excision-repair and life span in a number of mammalian species, Proc. Natl. Acad. Sci. USA. 71:2169 (1974).

29. L. Hayflick, The longevity of cultured human cells, J. Am. Geriatr. Soc. 22:1 (1974).

30. K. Hall, C. Albrightson, and R.W. Hart, A direct relationship
        among primates between maximum lifespan and DNA repair.
        Abstract of 11th Int. Congr. Gerontology, Tokyo, 1978.
31. V. Paffenholtz, Correlation between DNA repair of embryonic
        fibroblasts and different life span of 3 inbred mouse
        strains, Mech. Ageing Dev. 7:131 (1978).
32. H. Kato, M. Harada, K. Tsuchiya, and K. Moriwaki, Absence of
        correlation between DNA repair in ultraviolet irradiated
        mammalian cells and life span of the donor species,
        Japan J. Genetics. 55:99 (1980).
33. C.D. Lytle, O. Nikaido, V.M. Hitchins, and E.D. Jacobson, Host
        cell reactivation by excision repair is error-free in
        human cells, Mutation Res. 94:405 (1982).

AUTORADIOGRAPHIC STUDIES OF DNA

REPLICATION IN WERNER'S SYNDROME CELLS

Fumio Hanaoka, Masa-atsu Yamada[1], Fujio Takeuchi, Makoto
Goto, Terumasa Miyamoto[2], Tada-aki Hori[3]

[1] Department of Physiological Chemistry
Faculty of Pharmaceutical Sciences
University of Tokyo, Japan

[2] Department of Internal Medicine and Physical Therapy
Faculty of Medicine
University of Tokyo, Japan

[3] Division of Genetics
National Institute of Radiological Sciences
Chiba, Japan

ABSTRACT

We have compared cultured fibroblasts of early passage derived
from patients with the Werner syndrome and from normal subjects in
several aspects of cell cycle time and DNA replication. The
average cycle time was prolonged in Werner's syndrome cells
compared with normal cells because of changes in the duration of S
phase. The durations of G1 and G2 were unchanged. In addition,
the labeling index was lower in Werner's syndrome cells, suggesting
that there are two cell-cycle abnormalities in Werner's syndrome
cells. The cause of the prolongation of S phase was investigated
by DNA fiber autoradiography and alkaline sucrose density gradient
sedimentation. The rate of DNA chain elongation was not different
in Werner's syndrome cells from that in normal cells, but the
frequency of replication initiation was decreased in Werner's
syndrome cells.

INTRODUCTION

The Werner syndrome (WS) is a rare autosomal recessive
disorder clinically characterized by a distinctive habitus (short
stature and slender extremities), a variety of feature of premature
senescence (alopecia, arterioscrelosis, cataracts, etc.),
scleroderma-like skin changes and endocrinological abnormalities
(Epstein et al., 1966; Rabbiosi and Borroni, 1975; Björneerg, 1976;
Beadle et al., 1978; Martin, 1978; Nakao et al., 1978; Goto et al.,
1978; Goto et al., 1981). The syndrome has been described either
as a caricature of aging (Epstein et al., 1966) or as segmental
progeroid syndrome (Martin, 1978; Norwood et al., 1979).
Comparative studies of the growth properties of skin fibroblasts
from WS patients with those from normal subjects may provide
information about this genetic disease.

Normal human fibroblasts in culture have a limited lifespan
(Hayflick, 1965; Martin et al., 1970) and the changes in the cell-
cycle duration in the late passages in culture are primarily due to
changes in the G1 phase (Yanishevsky et al., 1974; Grove and
Cristofalo, 1977). The decreases in the labeling index (Cristofalo
and Sharf, 1973; Schneider and Mitsui, 1976; Nichols et al., 1977)
and in the rate of DNA elongation (Petes et al., 1974) have also
been reported. A striking diminution in lifespan (Martin et al.,
1970; Goldstein, 1979; Norwood et al., 1979; Salk et al., 1981a), a
decrease in the number of cells in S phase (Tanaka et al., 1979)
and a decrease in population growth rate (Salk et al., 1981a)
compared with normal fibroblasts are features of cultured
fibroblasts from WS patients. In addition, a slowed rate of DNA
replication has been reported in some WS fibroblasts (Fujiwara et
al., 1977). The duration of the interphase periods of the cell
cycle of WS cells, however, has yet to be determined.

We have compared WS skin fibroblasts with normal skin
fibroblasts in several aspects, including the duration of the
interphase periods, the rate of DNA chain elongation, and the
frequency for replication initiation.

MATERIALS AND METHODS

Cell strains

We used cultured skin fibroblasts from five WS patients (Goto
et al., 1978; Matsumura et al., 1980) and three normal subjects
(Table 1). Fibroblast lines were derived from biopsy samples from a
standard skin biopsy site (mesial aspect of the mid upper arm). All
cells were used for every experiment in early passages. Donor ages
were widely spread. Population doubling level (PDL) was calculated
from haemocytometer counts at the time of weekly passage as

described by Martin et al. (1970). Cells were maintained in
Eagle's MEM containing 10% fetal bovine serum (FBS) and antibiotics
in a water-saturated atmosphere of 5% CO_2 in air. Usually cultures
were split 1:4.

Cell cycle analysis

The duration of the interphase periods of the cell cycle was
determined by the percent labeled mitosis method of Quastler and
Sherman (1959), with minor modifications. Cells were inoculated
with 2 ml of the growth medium at a concentration of 1×10^4 cells
/ml into two-chambered tissue-culture chamber slides (Lab-Tek
Products). The cells were incubated at 37°C for 2 days, and were
exposed to [3H] thymidine at 0.5 µCi/ml (specific activity: 25
Ci/mmol, Amersham) for 30 min. Cells were then washed twice with
the growth medium, and were incubated continuously. Duplicate
cultures were stopped at one-hour intervals over the next 11 hours
and then at two-hour intervals for further 33 hours. Sampled slides
were washed with calcium, magnesium-free phosphate-buffered saline
(CMF-PBS), and were fixed with mixture of acetate and ethanol (1:3)
for 1 min. Air-dried slides were washed 4 times with 2% cold
perchloric acid and once with water, and then covered with Sakura
NR-M2 autoradiograpic emulsion. After exposure for 1-2 weeks,
autoradiographs were developed with Rendol and Renfix (Fuji Photo
Film Co.). A minimum of 100 mitoses throughout the slides were
scored for each sample. The duration of the interphase periods of
the cell cycle was determined by the method of Macieira-Coelho
(1973).

Labeling index

The percentage of nuclei synthesizing DNA (labeling index) for
a 30 min pulse period was determined by autoradiography. Samples
were prepared as described in "Cell cycle analysis" and about 1,000
cells were scored.

DNA fiber autoradiography

DNA elongation rate was measured by DNA fiber autoradiography
according to Huberman and Riggs (1968), Lark et al. (1971) and Hori
and Lark (1973) with minor modifications. 1×10^5 cells were
inoculated into ϕ35 mm plastic Petri dishes with 2 ml of the growth
medium and incubated at 37°C for 2 days. Before labeling, the cell
layers were washed once with MEM containing 10% dialysed FBS (dFBS),
2×10^{-6} M fluorodeoxyuridine and Eagle's non-essential amino acids,
and the cells were incubated at 37°C for 30 min in the same medium
in order to exhaust the endogenous thymidine nucleotide pools. The
cells were then labeled at 37°C in the above medium containing 250
µCi/ml [3H] thymidine (50-70 Ci/mmole, Amersham) for varying times.
After each labeling time, cells were washed with cold CMF-PBS

containing 1×10^{-4} M thymidine, and were collected with 0.05%
trypsin containing 0.02% EDTA and 1×10^{-4} M thymidine.
Approximately 5,000 cells resuspended in 4-fold diluted CMF-PBS
containing 1×10^{-4} M thymidine were mixed with lysis solution (2%
sodium dodecyl sulfate, 0.05 M EDTA, pH 8.0) on slides (BSA-coated),
and the DNA fibers released from the cells were spread with a glass
rod over the glass surface. Air-dried slides were washed with 10%
cold trichloroacetic acid (TCA), 5% TCA and ethanol successively,
and were covered with Sakura NR-M2 emulsion. Exposure time was 4-6
months. Lengths of about 300 tracks for each sample were measured
using a micrometric eyepiece and disregarding both end segments of
tandem arrays. Slides were coded before measurements ("blind"
procedure) to exclude the danger of personal bias.

The distance between initiation sites along DNA (center-to-
center distance, CCD) was also measured by DNA fiber autoradiography
(Huberman and Riggs, 1968; Hand and Tamm, 1974a). The methods were
the same as those for the measurement of DNA chain elongation rate,
except that the cells were labeled with 250 μCi/ml [^{3}H] thymidine
(50-70 Ci/mmol) for 10 min ("hot" pulse) and then nonradioactive
thymidine was added to reduce the specific activity of the isotope
to 1/5. The incubation was continued for 20 or 60 min ("warm"
chase). The CCDs between adjacent tracks in a tandem array were
measured using a blind procedure.

Alkaline sucrose gradient sedmentation

Alkaline sucrose gradient sedimentation of DNA was according to
the methods of Abelson and Thomas (1966) and Fujiwara et al. (1977),
with some modifications. Cells prepared as in the case of DNA fiber
autoradiography were incubated at 37°C for 3 min with MEM containing
10% dFBS, 2×10^{-6} M fluorodeoxyuridine, Eagle's non-essential amino
acids and 250 μCi/ml [^{3}H] thymidine (50-70 Ci/mmol, Amersham). The
labeling medium was then removed and was replaced by MEM containing
10% FBS and 5×10^{-5} M thymidine, and the incubation at 37°C was
continued for 10, 30, or 120 min. The cells were lysed with 0.25%
sodium dodecyl sulfate, 0.01 M EDTA and 0.15 M sodium bicarbonate,
pH 8.0, and digested with 1 mg/ml proteinase K (Boehringer-Mannheim)
for 16 hours at 37°C. After addition of 5N NaOH to make 0.3 N, the
lysate (0.2 ml of about 1.25×10^5 lysed cells/ml) was layered on
top of a 4.8 ml linear gradient from 5 to 20% (w/v) sucrose
containing 0.8 M NaCl, 0.2 N NaOH and 0.01 M EDTA, pH 12.5. The
gradients were centrifuged at 30,000 rpm for 2 hours at 20°C in
Hitachi RPS40-T2 rotor (90,100 x g) with [^{14}C] thymidine-labeled T4D
bacteriophage DNA (66×10^6 in the denatured form) as an internal
reference. After the centrifugation, 5-drop fractions were
collected onto Whatman-type 3MM filter-paper disks. Disks were
washed with 5% TCA and ethanol, dried, and assayed for
radioactivity. The average molecular weights (Mr) between fractions
1 and 32 or 33 in the sedimentation profiles were calculated from

the formula of Abelson and Thomas (1966). For the control study,
normal cells were labeled with 0.5 μCi/ml (25 Ci/mmol, Amersham)
[3H] thymidine for 24 hours and subjected to alkaline sucrose
gradient sedimentation.

RESULTS

Cell-cycle analysis

     Figure 1 shows the percent labeled mitosis curves for two
typical samples: one for normal and the other for WS fibroblasts.
The first peak almost reached 100% but the second peak was less
high, indicating in individual cells the variability of the cell
cycle time. The curve was the same regardless of the age of donors
of the cells, but the appearance of the second peak was delayed in
WS cells. Table 2 shows the duration of the interphase periods in
the cell cycle, calculated from these curves. T_C was 18.8 to 19.0
hours (mean = 18.9 hours) and T_S was 7.4 to 8.9 hours (mean = 8.2 hours
hours) in normal cells. In early population doublings, cells from

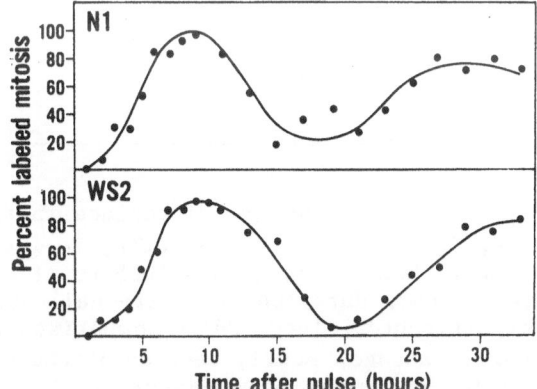

Fig. 1   Percent labeled mitosis of normal and Werner's syndrome
           cells (Takeuchi et al., 1982a). Only typical cases are
           shown (N1 and WS 2). From these kinds of figures, the
           duration of the interphase periods was calculated by
           the method of Macieira-Coelho (1973). Percent labeled
           mitosis curves were generated by plotting the
           percentage of labeled mitosis in log phase culture
           after a 30 min pulse exposure to [3H] thymidine. In
           details, methods are described in the text.

Table 1   Cells used in this study

Cell I.D. number	Donor age	Sex	Final PDL	PDL	Previously reported identification no. Goto et al. (1978)	Matsumura et al. (1980)
N*1	26	F	ND	4.0		
N 2	40	M	ND	13.4		
N 3	86	M	ND	6.2		
WS 1	19	M	6.7	2.5	1	1
WS 2	29	F	ND	3.0	4	2
WS 3	43	M	6.5	4.3	10	6
WS 4	60	M	9.8	2.7	15	5
WS 5	61	M	7.0	2.9		

```
*  N   = normal subject
   WS  = Werner syndrome
   PDL = population doubling level
   ND  = not determined
```

variously aged donors did not show any difference in the durations of T_C, T_S, T_{G1}, or T_{G2}. In WS cells, T_C was 20.4 to 22.4 hours (mean = 21.2 hours) and T_S was 10.5 to 11.4 hours (mean = 10.9 hours). Thus, duration of entire cell cycle of WS fibroblasts was significantly elongated in comparison with the normal cells of early passage, mostly because of the prolongation of S phase ($p < 0.05$). No appreciable change in the G1 and G2 phases was observed.

Labeling index

The percentages of cells incorporated [3H] thymidine during a 30-min labeling period are also shown in Table 2. In normal cells, the labeling index was 32.0 to 37.8 (mean = 35.3). The older the donor was, the lower was the labeling index in equally early passages. The data agree with the report by Schneider and

Table 2   The duration of the internal periods of the cell cycle
           and labeling index (Takeuchi et al., 1982a)

Cells	TG1* (h)	TG2[†] (h)	TS[‡] (h)	TC[§] (h)	L.I.[Π] (%)
N 1	5.8	4.8	8.4	19.0	37.8
N 2	4.8	5.1	8.9	18.8	36.2
N 3	6.7	4.8	7.4	18.9	32.0
mean	5.8+0.95	4.9+0.17	8.2+0.76	18.9+0.10	35.3+3.0
WS 1	6.3	4.7	11.4	22.4	26.7
WS 2	5.2	5.3	10.5	21.0	17.6
WS 3	5.5	5.1	10.5	21.1	21.5
WS 4	5.0	5.1	10.9	21.0	29.8
WS 5	4.7	4.6	11.1	20.4	29.5
mean	5.3+0.61	5.0+0.30	10.9+0.39	21.2+0.74	25.0+5.3

```
*  TG1 :  duration of G1 phase + 0.5 mitosis
†  TG2 :  duration of G2 phase + 0.5 mitosis
‡  TS  :  duration of S phase
§  TC  :  duration of entire cell cycle
Π L.I.:  labeling index
```

Mitsui (1976). On the other hand, the labeling index of WS cells
was 17.6 to 29.8 (mean = 25.0). No simple correlation between
labeling index and donor age was found in this case.

DNA chain elongation rate

Because prolongation of the S phase was observed in WS
cells, we tried to clarify the cause of the phenomenon. The
overall rate of DNA replication in nuclei is generally influenced
by two factors: the frequency of initiation of replication and

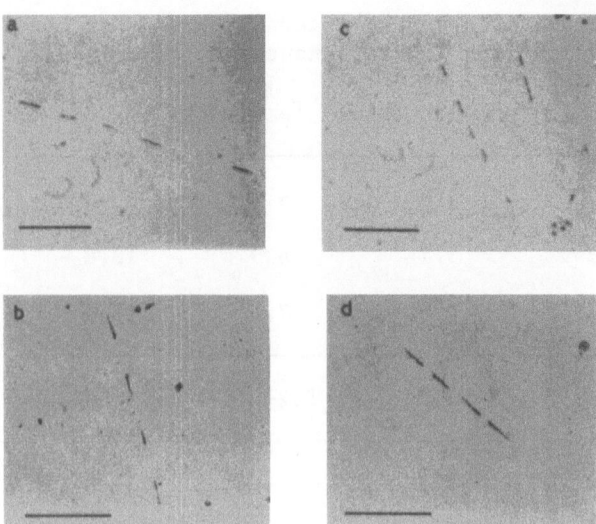

Fig. 2   Fiber autoradiographs of DNA from WS fibroblasts and
           normal fibroblasts (Takeuchi et al., 1982b). The samples
           were prepared as described in Materials and Methods.
           Bars represent 50 μm. a, WS2 cells, 30 min pulse; b, WS2
           cells, 20 min chase; c, N1 cells, 30 min pulse; d, N1
           cells, 20 min chase.

the rate of chain elongation (Hand and Tamm, 1974b; Sheinin et
al., 1978). We have therefore examined the rate of DNA chain
growth by means of DNA fiber autoradiography. Exponentially
growing cells were pulse-labeled with [3H] thymidine for varying
periods and DNAs from these labeled cells were subjected to DNA
fiber autoradiography. DNAs spread straight with no aggregation
were observed as tandem arrays of grain tracks in
autoradiographs. The lengths of individual tracks in tandem
arrays were measured on each sample. Figure 2a and c show the
DNA fiber autoradiographs of typical samples. The distribution
histograms of the track length of five WS cells and three normal
cells are shown in Figs. 3 and 4, respectively. As the pulse
time increased, the track length became longer. Short-sized DNA
was also observed in longer pulse samples because of the random
cultures. The histograms of track lengths of cells labeled for
60 min had the widest distribution in both WS and normal cells
(note the difference of the abscissa between various labeling
periods). There were no significant differences between the
track-lengths distribution of WS and normal cells. Figure 5
shows the mean grain-track length of each sample for different
labeling periods. The average track lengths (+ mean and standard

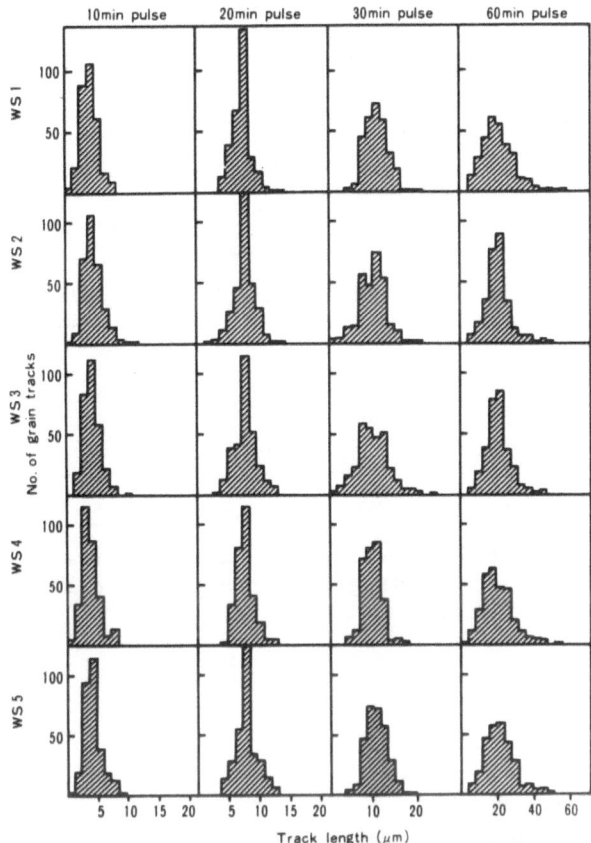

Fig. 3   The distribution histograms of the track length for
different labeling times in WS cells (Takeuchi et al.,
1982b).

deviations) of 10, 20, 30 and 60 min pulse labeling were
respectively 4.31 ± 1.35, 7.66 ± 1.70, 10.06 ± 2.97 and 20.74 ±
7.40 μm in the five WS cells, and 4.16 ± 1.45, 7.70 ± 1.65, 10.61
± 2.79 and 20.97 ± 8.12 μm in the three normal cells. Thus, the
track length increased almost linearly up to 60 min, and WS cells
showed similar means and distributions of track lengths to those
of normal cells for each labeling period.

The average DNA elongation rates estimated from Fig. 5 were
0.39 ± 0.007 μm/min (mean ± standard error) for WS cells, and
similarly, 0.38 + 0.008 μm/min for the normal cells. These
averages indicate that there is no difference in DNA chain
elongation rate within replicons between these two groups.

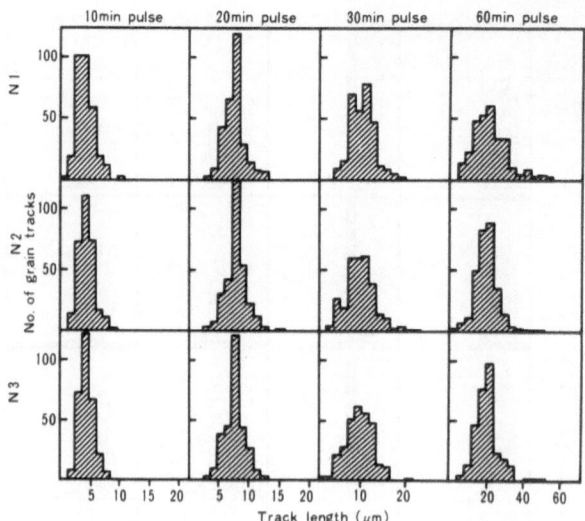

Fig. 4   The distribution histograms of the track length for
         different labeling times in normal cells (Takeuchi et
         al., 1982b).

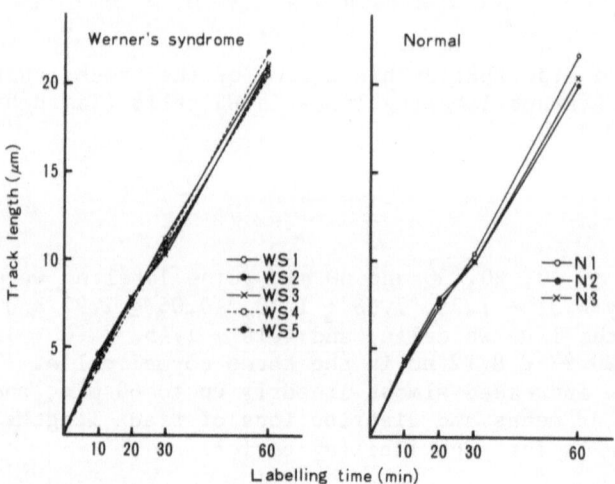

Fig. 5   Mean lengths of the grain track for different labeling
         times in WS and normal cells (Takeuchi et al., 1982b).
         Mean lengths were calculated from the histograms in Figs.
         3 and 4.

    To clarify this point further, we next examined the changes
in the sedimentation profiles of pulse-labeled DNA with chasing
time. In Fig. 6, sedimentation profiles of labeled DNA from two
typical cells, one normal and the other WS, are shown. The
sedimentation velocity of newly synthesized DNA in an alkaline
sucrose gradient increased rapidly with chasing time from 0 to
120 min. No difference was observed between these cells and
other normal and WS cells (data not shown). Calculated mean
molecular weights are plotted against the chasing time in Fig. 7.
After chasing for 120 min, newly synthesized DNA in normal and WS
cells was almost of the same size as the continuously labeled DNA
(Mr = 178 x 10^6). The Mr of single-stranded DNA labeled for 3
min with no chase was not zero but 68 to 80 x 10^6 both in normal
and WS cells because of the random culture. The Mr of 3-min
pulse-labeled DNA was slightly higher in WS cells than in normal
cells. This could be explained by the larger replicon size in WS
cells, which will be described in the next section. Thus, there
was no significant difference between WS and normal cells in the
rate of DNA elongation, studied both by DNA fiber autoradiography
and alkaline sucrose density gradient.

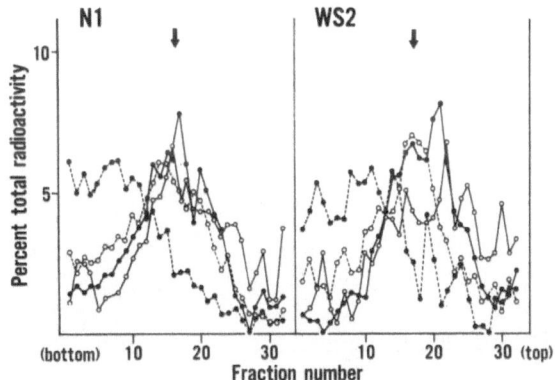

Fig. 6   Alkaline sucrose sedimentation profiles of pulse-labeled
          and chased DNA from normal and WS cells (Takeuchi et al.,
          1983). Only typical cases are shown (N1 and WS2).
          Methods were described in the text in detail. Arrows
          indicate the peak position of T4D DNA.

　　──○──   3 min pulse

　　──●──   3 min pulse and 10 min chase

　　----○----   3 min pulse and 30 min chase

　　----●----   3 min pulse and 120 min chase

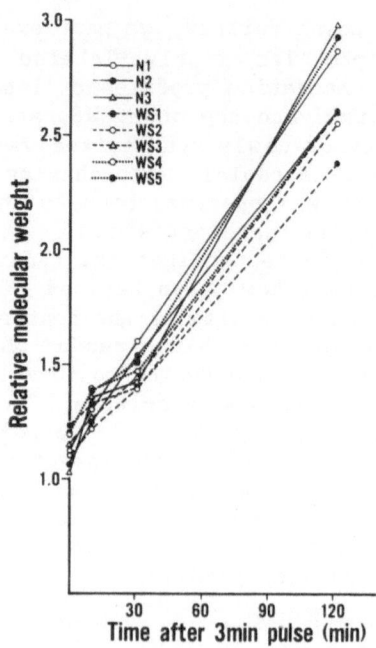

Fig. 7   The mean molecular weights of labeled DNA from three
           normal cells and five WS cells for different chasing time
           (Takeuchi et al., 1982a). The mean values were
           calculated from the formula of Abelson and Thomas (1966).

Replicon center-to-center distance

        We then examined the distance between initiation sites along
the DNA. DNA fiber autoradiographs made from the samples with
hot (high specific activity) pulses and warm (lower specific
activity) chases revealed the direction of DNA chain elongation
by the different density of grains (Fig. 2b and d). CCDs were
measured between adjacent tracks with a tandem array of at least
two sets of tracks. Figure 8 shows histograms of CCDs in five WS
cells and three normal cells. It is obvious that the
distribution of CCDs in WS cells resembled each other. The
arithmetic means and standard errors of CCDs was 55.6 ± 2.20 μm.
Histograms of the CCDs of normal cells were also similar to each
other, and the average of CCDs was 33.8 ± 1,40 μm. This
increase of CCD in WS cells was significant (Welch, 1949)
(p < 0.01) and could cause the delay of overall DNA synthesis.

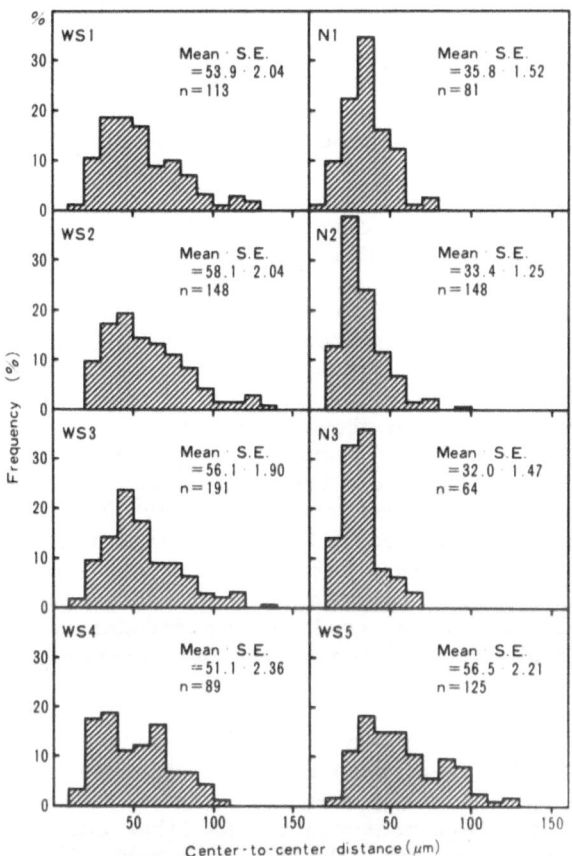

Fig. 8   Histograms of center-to-center distance in WS and normal
cells (Takeuchi et al., 1982b). CCDs were determined
with autoradiograms of 10 min pulse and 20 or 60 min
chase samples. Since no difference was observed in the
distribution of CCDs between samples of 20 min and 60 min
chases, the results were pooled.

DISCUSSION

    In this study, we analysed the cell cycle of WS cells,
comparing it with that of normal cells. The results indicated
that the S phase was specifically prolonged in WS cells and, as a
result, the whole cell-cycle time was prolonged. In the case of
normal human fibroblasts in culture, the prolongation of cell-

cycle duration in late passages has been reported as primarily due to changes in the G1 phase (Yanishevsky et al., 1974; Grove and Cristofalo, 1977) and partly due to changes in the G2 phase (Macieira-Coelho et al., 1966; Grove and Cristofalo, 1977). In this context, WS cells are somewhat different from normal cells in late passages.

As for the cause of the prolongation of the S phase, there are two conceivable explanations. First, the slower rate of DNA chain elongation could decrease the overall rate of DNA replication. Slowing of the rate of DNA chain elongation has been reported in Bloom's syndrome fibroblasts (Hand and German, 1975; Ockey, 1979) and in human basal cell carcinomas (Heenen and Galand, 1980). Among cultured fibroblasts from human fetal lung, a slower rate of DNA chain growth has also been described in senescent cultures than in younger cultures (Petes et al., 1974). However, we recently disputed the correctness of the conclusion drawn by these authors (Hasegawa et al., 1982). Fujiwara et al. (1977) reported that cultured WS cells derived from some WS patients showed slower than normal rate of DNA elongation, but other cultured WS cells had an almost normal rate of DNA chain growth by alkaline sucrose gradient centrifugation. They suggested this as a reflection of the heterogeneity of the syndrome.

In our present study, no clear difference between WS and normal cells in DNA elongation rate was observed either by DNA fiber autoradiography or by alkaline sucrose sedimentation study. The DNA elongation rate measured by DNA fiber autoradiography was the rate within a replicon. On the other hand, DNA chased for 120 min in an alkaline sucrose sedimentation experiment was close in size to our bulk DNA (about 2-3 replicon size) as calculated from the size of T4D marker DNA and the average replicon size (Huberman and Riggs, 1968). It is, therefore, possible that there is a change in the maturation step of these 2-3 replicon-sized DNAs or larger DNAs. So, we conclude that no difference between WS and normal cells was observed in the rate of DNA elongation at least up to 2-3 replicons.

Second, the decrease in the frequency of replicon initiation could be the cause of the prolongation of S phase. Our data show that this is indeed the case. The observed increase in average CCD in WS cells means that the frequency of initiation events per unit length at given time was reduced. We are unable to determine whether the replicon size itself has changed in WS cells or whether the frequency of initiation of adjacent replicons has decreased. Judging by the distribution profiles of CCDs in Fig. 8, however, the latter possibility seems the more plausible, because the distribution of CCDs was broader in the WS cells than in the normal cells with the same short extremities. Moreover, the data suggest a bimodality and occasionally a trimodality, of CCDs in the WS cells. This also supports the latter possibility.

Martin and Oppenheim (1977) reported that CCD distributions were usually log normal. When the frequency was plotted against CCD in log scale in our experiments, the skewness seemed to decrease and the CCD distribution looked log normal. After log transformation, the average CCDs (+ standard deviation) were 3.93 ± 0.44 for the WS cells and 3.43 ± 0.41 for the normal cells (log scale), and the difference between these two groups in CCDs was significant ($p < 0.01$). The arithmetic means and standard errors described under the "RESULTS" section, however, might be appropriate for empirically evaluating the significance of the difference, because of the large sample number. The distribution pattern is obviously different in the two groups.

It has been demonstrated that replicon size in eukaryotic cells is not uniform (Hand, 1978). For example, Hand and Tamm (1974a) reported that the distance between initiation sites labeled during a 10-min pulse increased in mouse fibroblasts infected with reovirus. Conversely, a decrease in replicon size was reported in SV40-transfromed Chinese hamster lung cells (Martin and Oppenheim, 1977). The new finding here is that CCD increases significantly in cells derived from patients with a genetic disease, the Werner syndrome. Since all five WS cell lines tested showed the increase in CCD, the measurement of CCD in WS cells in early passage might be useful in the diagnosis of this genetic disease.

About the cause of the increase of CCD in WS cells, there are two possibilities: one is a change in DNA sequence or in chromatin structure around the origin of the replicon; the other is a decrease in the proteins(s) essential for the initiation of replicons. Differing from prokaryotes and extrachromosomal elements in eukaryotic cells, initiation of DNA synthesis from fixed origins of DNA replication has not been demonstrated in eukaryotic chromosomal DNA. Recently, Heintz and Hamlin (1982) studied a mode of initiation of DNA replication in a methotrex-ate-resistant Chinese hamster ovary cell line, and demonstrated that replication of the amplified sequence initiates at specific sites within each repeated unit. Their data indicate that eukaryotic cells use genetically fixed nucleotide sequences as origins of replication; however, it is also possible that chromatin structure dictated by DNA sequences limits initiation of DNA synthesis to specific chromatin domains. In our DNA fiber autoradiographic experiments we used random culture, therefore we did not look at DNA fiber from any specific region. For these reasons, it is difficult to think that change in the CCDs in WS cells is due to the change in nucleotide sequence.

Little is known about the protein(s) needed for the replicon initiation in mammalian cells. Cell-to-cell hybridization experiments by Rao and Johnson (1970) suggested the presence of inducible factor(s) for DNA synthesis in S-phase HeLa cells. Using the same technique, Tanaka et al. (1979) demonstrated that DNA synthesis in WS cells was partly restored by fusing the cells with normal diploid cells, and was completely restored by HeLa cells. Although the nature of presumptive initiator protein(s) is not clear, it might be true that WS cells are deficient in the initiator protein(s) and, as a result, the frequency of initiation events per unit length at given time is reduced. On the other hand, the presence of a senescence factor(s) in WS cells that may suppress DNA synthesis of WS cells is also presumed by cell hybridization studies (Tanaka et al., 1979, 1980; Salk et al., 1981a).

In this study, skin fibroblasts in early passage were used to compare WS cells with variously aged normal cells in vivo. Whether like WS cells normal skin fibroblasts in late passage have increased CCDs is an interesting question with respect to aging in vitro. In our preliminary experiments using DNA fiber autoradiography, we observed no change in CCD during aging in vitro of human diploid fibroblasts derived from fetal lung (unpublished data). Similar observations had been made by Petes et al. (1974).

Considering the prolongation of S phase only, the increase of labeling index in such cells could be expected, but in WS cells, however, the labeling index decreased (Tanaka et al., 1979; and this study). This indicates that there are at least two kinds of abnormalities in the cell cycle of WS cells: the prolongation of the S phase and the increase of the proportion of non-cycling cells. We do not have any data about the cause of the decreasing proportion of cycling cells in WS cells. Recently, a chromosome instability in WS cells has been reported (Salk et al., 1981b), and this could be one explanation for the reduced growth. In any event, these two abnormalities would cause the decrease of population growth rate (Salk et al., 1981a), and the decrease of the overall rate of DNA replication (Fujiwara et al., 1977) in WS cells.

It remains unclear whether the prime cause of the disease in WS is the increase of CCD. At present, various unique clinical features of this syndrome could not be explained by an increase in CCD. Thus the increase in CCDs in WS cells might be a secondary phenomenon caused by another metabolic abnormality. We would like to emphasize, however, that the abnormality in DNA replication was observed among all cultures derived from five non-consanGuineous patients. WS should be considered as one of the metabolic disorders transmitted as an autosomal recessive trait. Therefore genetic and biochemical investigation of the replication initiation in WS cells might help us better understand the cause of the disease and the control mechanism of DNA replication.

ACKNOWLEDGEMENTS

This work was supported in part by a Grant-in-Aid for Cancer Research from the Ministry of Education, Science and Culture, Japan, and by a Life Science Grant from the Institute of Physical and Chemical Research, Tokyo, Japan. We thank Drs. T. Matsumura, K. Murata, A. Hashimota, Y. Nishida, T. Chihara, K. Ishihara, T. Horiuchi and N. Hasegawa for their advice.

REFERENCES

Abelson, J., and Thomas, C.A., Jr., 1966, The anatomy of the T5 bacteriophage DNA molecule, J. Mol. Biol., 18:262.

Beadle, G.F., Mackay, I.R., Whittingham, S., Taggart G., Harris, A.W. and Harrison, L.C., 1978, Werner's syndrome: A model of premature aging?, J. Med., 9:377.

Björneerg, A., 1976, Werner's syndrome and malignancy, Acta Dermatovener, 56:149.

Cristofalo, V.J. and Sharf, B.B., 1973, Cellular senescence and DNA synthesis. Thymidine incorporation as a measure of population age in human diploid cells, Exp. Cell Res., 76:419.

Epstein, C.J., Martin, G.M., Schultz, A.L. and Motulsky, A.G., 1966, Werner's syndrome: A review of its symptomatology, natural history, pathologic feature, genetics and relationship to the natural aging process, Medicine, 45:177.

Fujiwara, Y., Higashikawa, T. and Tatsumi, M., 1977, A retarded rate of DNA replication and normal level of DNA repair in Werner's syndrome fibroblasts in culture, J. Cell. Physiol., 92:365.

Goldstein, S., 1979, Studies on age-related disease in cultured skin fibroblasts, J. Invest. Dermatol., 73:19.

Goto, M., Horiuchi, Y., Tanimoto, K., Ishii, T., and Nakashima, H., 1978, Werner's syndrome: Analysis of 15 cases with a review of the Japanese literature, J. Am. Geriat. Soc., 16:341.

Goto, M., Tanimoto, K., Horiuchi, Y., and Sasazuki, T., 1981, Family analysis of Werner's syndrome: A survey of 42 Japanese families with a review of the literature, Clin. Genet., 19:8.

Grove, G.L., and Cristofalo, V.J., 1977, Characterization of the cell cycle of cultured human diploid cells: Effects of aging and hydrocortisone, J. Cell. Physiol., 90:415.

Hand, R., 1978, Eucaryotic DNA: Organization of the genome for replication, Cell, 15:317.

Hand, R., and German, J., 1975, A retarded rate of DNA chain growth in Bloom's syndrome, Proc. Natl. Acad. Sci., USA, 72:758.

Hand, R. and Tamm, I., 1974a, Initiation of DNA replication in mammalian cells and its inhibition by reovirus infection, J. Mol. Biol., 82:175.

Hand, R. and Tamm, I., 1974b, DNA replication: Initiation and rate of chain growth in mammalian cells, in: Cell Cycle Controls, G.M. Padilla, I.L. Cameron, and A. Zimmerman, eds., Academic Press, New York.

Hasegawa, N., Hanaoka, F., Hori, T., and Yamada, M., 1982, Reevaluation of DNA chain elongation rate in human diploid fibroblasts, Exp. Cell Res., 140:443.

Hayflick, L., 1965, The limited in vitro lifetime of human diploid cell strains, Exp. Cell Res., 37:614.

Heenan, M., and Galand, P., 1980, Decreased rate of DNA chain growth in human basal cell carcinoma, Nature, 285:265.

Heintz, N.H., and Hamlin, J.L., 1982, An amplified chromosomal sequence that includes the gene for dihydrofolate reductase initiates replication within specific restriciton fragments, Proc. Natl. Acad. Sci., USA, 79:4083.

Hori, T., and Lark, K.G., 1973, Effect of puromycin on DNA replicatioin in Chinese hamster cells, J. Mol. Biol., 77:391.

Huberman, J.A., and Riggs, A.D., 1968, On the mechanism of DNA replication in mammalian chromsomes, J. Mol. Biol., 32:327.

Lark, K.G., Consigli, R. and Toliver, A., 1971, DNA replication in Chinese hamster cells: Evidence for a single replication fork per replicon, J. Mol. Biol., 58:873.

Macieira-Coelho, A., 1973, Cell cycle analysis: a mammalian cells, in: Tissue Culture: Methods and Applications, P.F. Kruse Jr. and M.K. Patterson Jr. eds., Academic Press, New York.

Macieira-Coelho, A., Ponten, J., and Philipson, L., 1966, The division cycle and RNA synthesis in diploid human cells at different passage levels in vitro, Exp. Cell Res., 42:673.

Martin, G.M., 1978, Genetic syndromes in man with potential relevance to the pathobiology of aging, Birth Defects, 14:5.

Martin, G.M., Sprague, C.A., and Epstein, C.J., 1970, Replicative life span of cultivated human cells: Effects of donor's age, tissue and genotype, Lab. Invest., 23:86.

Martin, R.G., annd Oppenheim, A., 1977, Initiation points for DNA replication in nontransformed and simian virus 40-transformed Chinese hamster lung cells, Cell, 11:859.

Matsumura, T., Mitsui, Y., Fujiwara, Y., Ishii, T., and Shimada, H., 1980, Cell, tissue and organ banks in Japan with special reference to the study of premature aging, Japan J. Exp. Med., 50:321.

Nakao, Y., Kishihara, M., Yoshimi, H., Inoue, Y., Tanaka, K., Sakamoto, N., Matsukura, S., Imura, H., Ichihashi, M., and Fujiwara, Y., 1978, Werner's syndrome. In vivo and in vitro characteristics as a model of aging, Amer. J. Med., 65:919.

Nichols, W.W., Murphy, D.G., Cristofalo, V.J., Toji, L.H., Greene, A.E., and Dwight, S.A., 1977, Characterization of a new human diploid cell strain, IMR-90, Science, 196:60.

Norwood, T.H., Hoehn, H., Salk, D., and Martin, G.M., 1979, Cellular
    aging in Werner's syndrome: A unique phenotype?, J. Invest.
    Dermatol., 73:92.
Ockey, C.H., 1979, Quantitative replicon analysis of DNA synthesis
    in cancer-prone conditions and the defects in Bloom's syndrome,
    J. Cell Sci., 40:125.
Petes, T.D., Farber, R.A., Tarrant, G.M., and Holliday, R., 1974,
    Altered rate of DNA replication in aging human fibroblast
    cultures, Nature, 251:434.
Quastler, H., and Sherman, F.G., 1959, Cell population kinetics in
    the intestinal epithelium of the mouse, Exp. Cell Res., 17:420.
Rabbiosi, G., and Borroni, G., 1975, Werner's syndrome; Seven cases
    in one family, Dermatologica, 158:355.
Rao, P.N., and Johnson, R.T., 1970, Mammalian cell fusion: I.
    Studies on the regulation of DNA synthesis and mitosis, Nature,
    225:159.
Salk, D., Bryant, E., Au, K., Hoehn, H., and Martin, G.M., 1981a,
    Systemic growth studies, cocultivation, and hybridization
    studies of Werner syndrome cultured skin fibroblasts, Hum.
    Genet., 58:310.
Salk, D., Au, K., Hoehn, H., and Martin, G.M., 1981b, Cytogenetics
    of Werner's syndrome cultured skin fibroblasts: variegated
    translocation mosaicism, Cytogenet. Cell Genet., 30:92.
Schneider, E.L., and Mitsui, Y., 1976, The relationship between in
    vitro cellular aging and in vivo human age, Proc. Natl. Acad.
    Sci. USA, 73:3584.
Sheinin, R., Hubert, J., and Pearlman, R.E., 1978, Some aspects of
    eukaryotic DNA replication, Ann. Rev. Biochem., 47:277.
Takeuchi, F., Hanaoka, F., Goto, M., Yamada, M., and Miyamoto, T.,
    1982a, Prolongation of S phase and whole cell cycle in Werner's
    syndrome fibroblasts, Exp. Gerontol., 17:473.
Takeuchi, F., Hanaoka, F., Goto, M., Akaoka, I., Hori, T., Yamada,
    M., and Miyamoti, T., 1982b, Altered frequency of initiation
    sites of DNA replication in Werner's syndrome cells, Hum.
    Genet., 60:365.
Tanaka, K., Nakazawa, T., Okada, Y., and Kumahara, Y., 1979,
    Increase in DNA synthesis in Werner's syndrome cells by
    hybridization with normal human diploid and HeLa cells, Exp.
    Cell Res., 123:261.
Tanaka, K., Nakazawa, T., Okada, Y., and Kumahara, Y., 1980, Roles
    of nuclear and cytoplasmic environments in the retarded DNA
    synthesis in Werner syndrome cells, Exp. Cell Res., 127:185.
Welch, B.L., 1949, Further note on Mrs Aspin's Tables and on certain
    approximations to the tabled function, Biometrika, 36:293.
Yanishevsky, R., Mendelsohn, M.L., Mayall, B.H., and Cristofalo,
    V.J., 1974, Proliferative capacity and DNA content of aging
    human diploid cells in culture: A cytophotometric and
    autoradiographic analysis, J. Cell. Physiol., 84:165

ABNORMAL FIBROBLAST AGING AND DNA REPLICATION IN THE WERNER

SYNDROME

Yoshisada Fujiwara[1], Yoshio Kano[1], Masamitsu Ichihashi[2], Yoshinobu Nakao[3], and Toshiharu Matsumura[4]

Department of Radiation Biophysics[1], Department of Dermatology[2], and Department of Medicine III[3], Kobe University School of Medicine, Kusunokicho 7-5-1, Chuo-ku, Kobe 650, and Department of Pathobiochemical Cell Research[4], Institute of Medical Science, University of Tokyo, Shirokanedai, Minato-ku, Tokyo 108, Japan

ABSTRACT

Cell and DNA replicative potentials were studied in 10 strains of skin fibroblasts from unrelated patients with the Werner syndrome (WS) and in a progeric CRL 1277 strain. The lifespans of all WS strains and of CRL 1277 cells are greatly abbreviated in vitro, due to large fractions of non-cycling cells and the basic process of progressive clonal attenuation during Phase II. In some WS strains, the population-doubling rate per day and the cloning efficiency fluctuated concurrently in random fashion during the cellular aging process, indicating alternating successions of adaptively well and poorly growing clones, probably resulting from various chromosome translocations. No detectable defect in excision repair was found in WS or CRL 1277 cells. However, the rate of increase in the molecular weight of pulse-chased DNA involving overall rates of chain elongation and replicon fusion was retarded in WS and CRL 1277 cells. Also, pulse-labelled DNA in WS fibroblasts was less enriched in the nuclear matrix and was more slowly chased out than in normal cells. These results led us to postulate a misfiring or delayed initiation due to the sticky attachment of replicating DNA to the nuclear matrix in the replisomes of WS fibroblasts. A suggested model for abnormal DNA replication is presented and discussed to explain the loss of DNA and the chromosome abnormalities in WS cells. The abnormal DNA-synthetic profiles so derived appeared

to be normalized in SV40-transformed PSV811 (WS) cells as were in
gamma ray-transformed wild-type WI38CT-1 cells.

INTRODUCTION

The Werner syndrome (WS) is an autosomal recessive, typical
segmental progeroid syndrome (Martin, 1978) that manifests the
accelerated development of many age-associated disorders
expressed mainly in mesenchymal and connective tissues after
puberty in affected individuals (Epstein et al., 1966; Nakao et
al., 1978, Salk, 1982). Studies of cultured skin fibroblasts
derived from patients with WS have revealed many aspects of
cellular aging (Martin et al., 1970; Goldstein and Moreman, 1975;
Salk, 1982). The diminished lifespan and abnormal population
doubling potential are characteristic of WS cells in vitro
(Martin et al., 1970; Hoehn et al., 1975; Higashikawa and
Fujiwara, 1978; Norwood et al., 1979; Salk et al., 1981b).
Cytogenetically, WS fibroblasts exhibit the characteristic
chromosome instability of variegated translocation mosaicism
despite a low level of chromosome breakage (Hoehn et al., 1975;
Salk et al., 1981a). Also, their DNA synthesis is abnormal in
culture (Fujiwara et al., 1977a; Takeuchi et al., 1982) and they
suppress DNA synthesis in normal young cells when fused to them
as heterokaryons (Norwood et al., 1974; 1979; Tanaka et al.,
1979). However, neither the basic genetic defect nor the
mechanism of its interaction with the observed variety of
manifestations in vivo and in vitro in WS has been identified.

The study reported here is of abnormal fibroblast aging and
DNA replication in WS cells, which are then compared with those
of an SV40-transformed WS line, and then of DNA repair in WS
cells. A hypothetical model of abnormal replication is presented
in relation to the nuclear matrix and replicon initiation in WS
cells.

MATERIALS AND METHODS

Strains and Culture

The fibroblast strains used are listed in Table 1. Normal
human skin fibroblasts (NHSF), Werner syndrome (WS) and acrogeria
(ACG) cell series were obtained from skin biopsies taken from
similar sites of the upper arms of normal subjects, unrelated WS
patients, and ACG patients, respectively. TIG-1 cells (Ohashi et
al., 1980) of female fetal lung origin were kindly supplied by
Dr. M. Ohashi, Tokyo Metropolitan Institute of Gerontology. The
PSV811 line was an SV40-transformed permanent line (Matsumura et
al., this volume), and the WI38CT-1 line was a gamma ray-

Table 1. Characteristics of normal human, Werner syndrome, and
other strains.

Strains	Sex	Age[a] (yr)	Maximum Pop. Doub. (PD)	%[b]	%CE per PD[c]	UDS[d]	DNA repair Rejoining[e]
Normal							
NHSF6	F	6	56	120	-0.43	100	N[f]
NHSF5	F	5	53	110	-0.43	100	N
NHSF41	M	41	50	104	-0.50	100	nt[g]
NHSF46	M	46	48	100	-0.45	100	N
NHSF63	M	63	42	88	-0.41	nt	N
NHSF64	F	64	37	80	-0.42	nt	nt
TIG-1	F	Fetus	82	170	-0.41	100	N
Werner syndrome							
WS1KO	F	32	10	20	-0.43	100	N
WS2KO	M	34	not available				
WS3KO	F	40	11	23	-0.43	100	N
WS4KO	M	39	13	26	-0.68	100	N
WS5KO	M	45	28	59	-0.44	100	N
WS6KO	M	30	19	40	fluc.[h]	100	N
WS7KO	M	47	not available				
WS8KO	F	49	19	40	fluc.	100	nt
WS9KO	F	53	12	25	nt	100	nt
WS10KO	M	44	17	35	nt	nt	nt
WS11KO	M	37	26	54	-0.43	100	N
WS12KO	M	46	28	59	fluc.	100	nt
Progeric ATCC							
CRL1277	M	16	27	56	-0.50	100	N
Acrogeria							
AcG1KA			43	90	-0.41	100	N
AcG3KA			62	130	-0.45	100	N
AcGH1KA-F[i]			33	69	-0.43	100	nt

a Age at which skin biopsy was taken
b % of NHSF46
c Calculated from the cloning efficiency decline curves in Fig. 2
d Autoradiographically determined after incubation in 5 uCi/ml
  of [^{3}H] tymidine (5 Ci/mmole) for 4 hr following irradiation of 10 J/m^2 254 nm UV. Relative to NHSF6 and NHSF46.
e Detected by alkaline sucrose gradient centrifugation as shown in Fig. 5
f N, normal rejoining
g nt, not tested
h fluc, % CE/PD fluctuated during serial subcultivations (see Fig. 2)
i Heterozygous: Father of AcG1KA patient.

transformed WI38 cell line (Namba et al., 1980) supplied by
courtesy of Dr. M. Namba, Kawasaki Medical School. ACG strains
were a gift of Dr. M. Inoue, Kanazawa Medical School. A progeric
(ATCC) CRL1277 strain and a Cockayne syndrome GM739 strain were
purchased from ATCC and the Institute of Medical Research (NJ),
respectively. The cells were cultured in Eagle's MEM
supplemented with 1 x non-essential amino acids and 15% fetal
calf serum (Flow Lab.) under a water-saturated atmosphere of 5%
CO_2 in air, as described previously (Fujiwara and Tatsumi, 1976;
Fujiwara et al., 1982; Fujiwara and Satoh, 1981).

Population Doubling (PD), Cloning Efficiency (CE) and Average PD/Day

The fibroblast outgrowths from several small pieces (1 mm^3)
of skin explants were used as passage "zero" for further PD
experiments. After the initial inoculation of 2-5 x 10^4 cells
per 35 mm Corning dish (=No), the cells were cultured by renewing
the medium every 2 to 3 days and then the number of cells
remaining (=N) after trypsinization at pre-confluent growth were
counted. Using this regimen, the cells were repeatedly
subcultured until terminal cell senescence was attained. PD at
each subculturing was calculated by the empirical equation:
PD =log(N/No)/log 2, and cumulative PD by the sum of PD$_i$, thus the
maximum PD (MPD) was the cumulative PD at the final cell
senescence. The average number of PD per day was calculated
simply by dividing the PD increase at a given interval (4-10
days) during successive subcultures by the day required. In
parallel with the PD experiment, cloning efficiencies (CEs) were
assayed at desired PDs in cultures of 500-2000 cells per 60 mm
dish in triplicate Corning dishes incubated for 12-14 days to
develop clones with 50 cells or more (Fujiwara and Tatsumi,
1976). Such clone-forming experiments were also used to
establish X-ray and 254 nm-UV survival curves (Fujiwara and
Tatsumi, 1976; Fujiwara et al., 1977a; 1981; 1982).

Detection of non-cycling cells

Exponentially growing cells at various PDs were continuously
labelled with 0.05 uCi/ml [^{3}H-methyl] thymidine (5 Ci/mmole, The
Radiochemical Centre, UK) for 72 hr and processed for
autoradiography (Fujiwara et al., 1977b). After random counting
of a total of 300 cells, unlabelled cells, that did not enter S-
phase were taken as being non-cycling cells a priori.

Measurement of DNA repair

UV-induced unscheduled DNA synthesis was determined
autoradiographically described previously (Fujiwara and Tatsumi,
1976; see also Table 1 footnote). Rejoining of single-strand DNA

breaks induced by an X-ray dose of 15 krad was measured in [3H] thymidine-prelabelled cells, as described previously (Fujiwara et al., 1977a).

Molecular weight increase and replicating matrix-DNA

For weight-average molecular weight (Mw), exponentially growing cells were pulse-labelled with 5 uCi/ml [3H]-thymidine (5 Ci/mmole) and immediately lysed or otherwise incubated in 5 x 10$^-$5M non-radioactive thymidine for the lengths of time indicated in Fig. 7. After cell lysis, digestion with pronase, and alkalinization to pH 12.5 the Mw of the DNA in these lysates was analyzed by alkaline sucrose gradient centrifugation (Fujiwara and Tatsumi, 1976; Fujiwara et al., 1977a; see also legends to Figs. 5 and 7).

Replicating DNA attached to the nuclear matrix was detected by a minor modification of the method of Pardoll et al. (1980) and McCready et al. (1982). Exponentially growing cells were prelabelled uniformly with 0.01 uCi/ml [2-14C] thymidine (460 Ci/mole) for 4-5 days, washed, and incubated in non-radioactive medium for several hours. The cells were then pulse-labelled for 3 to 5 min with 20-50 uCi/ml [3H] thymidine with a high specific activity (46 Ci/mmole), washed, and chased in 5 x 10^{-5} M unlabelled thymidine for up to 30 min. All manipulations of cells were carried out at 37°C. Immediately after treatment, the cells were rapidly cooled and scraped, and the nuclei were isolated by addition of 0.2% NP40 (Fujiwara, 1972). Then, the nuclear matrix fraction was isolated by the sequential low and high salt (2 M NaCl) treatments in the presence of Mg^{++} and a protease inhibitor, then treated with 400 ug/ml pancreatic DNase 1 (Worthington) and centrifuged at 2000 X g for 20 min. Under such conditions, DNA attached to the matrix was constantly approximately 3% of the total radioactivity of [14C] DNA, which permitted the analysis of varying radioactivity of replicating matrix-[3H] DNA.

RESULTS AND DISCUSSION

1.   PD, MPD, and Replicative Potential of WS Fibroblasts

Fig. 1 illustrates the cumulative PDs against culture days in typical WS (3KO, 4KO, 5KO, 6KO, 11KO) strains in comparison with a roughly age and site matched normal strain (NHSF46) (Fig 1a) and in an unmatched CRL 1277 (KeHe) progeric strain (Fig. 1b). Control NHSF46 cells replicated rapidly until reaching the terminal phase III. However, the overall doubling rate of these WS strains was 1/2 to 1/3 retarded, except for that of a WS5KO strain from the patient with relatively mild clinical

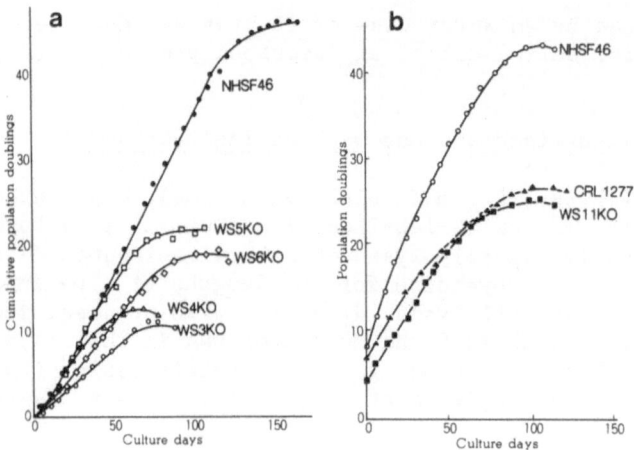

Figure 1. Population doubling (PD) kinetics of normal, WS, and
    progeric fibroblasts.

manifestations. All these WS strains entered so-called terminal
senescence earlier than did NHSF46 cells. The PD profile of the
progeric CRL 1277 strain was similar to that of the WS11KO cells
(Fig. 1b). Compared with the 48-50 MPDs of the NHSF46 cells, the
MPDs of the WS strains (=10-28) were significantly lower, being
as low as 20 to 60% of the matched normal MPDs (Table 1; Fig. 1).
Such a shortened lifespan or greatly diminished cell-replicative
potential in WS is consistent with the previous results (Martin
et al., 1970; Higashikawa and Fujiwara, 1978; Salk, 1981b). In
addition, the inverse relation of MPD and donor's age, including
a high MPD (=82) of TIG-1 lung cells, can be seen in Table 1, as
described previously (Hayflick, 1965; Martin et al., 1970;
Schneider and Mitsui, 1976). Therefore, the lifespan of the mass
culture populations of WS fibroblasts of connective tissue (skin)
origin is as greatly abbreviated in vitro as is the patients'
abnormally accelerated age change, which correlates with the
predominant connective tissue abnormalities and probably with the
shortened lifespan of the patients. ACG1KA and ACG3KA from
acrogeria patients showed near-normal level of MPD (Table 1).

2.   Change in CE as a Function of PD

In parallel to the PD experiments (Fig. 1), we also measured CE at
various PD levels in normal, WS, and CRL 1277 cells. The cloning
conditions are known to drop a large number of cells out of cycle (Absch
and Absher, 1976; Bell et al., 1978). However, we still expect a greate
CE reduction as a function of PD in WS cells, which may be a good indica

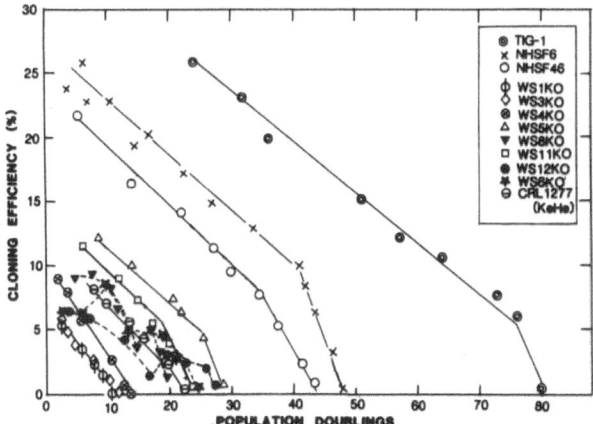

Figure 2. Changes in cloning efficiency as a function of population doubling.

of the sequential clonal attenuation. Fig. 2 shows the actual results based on our criterion of cycling cells (greater than or equal to 50 cells/colony). In fact, NHSF6, NHSF46 and TIG-1 cells demonstrated the linear reduction of CE as a function of PD during Phase II and the abrupt decline in the terminal Phase III, which agreed generally with the findings of Smith et al. (1978). The extent of parallel downward shift in such normal cells may be a function of donor's age (Fig. 2). The WS (1KO, 3KO, 4KO, 5KO and 11KO) cells revealed the remarkable similarity in such a PD-dependent CE reduction (Fig. 2). Moreover, the various parallel downward shifts of CE curves of WS cells from the normal cell curves are indicative of larger fractions of non-cycling cells at any PD level in WS populations, even though the cloning conditions may accentuate this effect to some extent. In these normal and WS strains, as well as in the ACG strains, the reduction rate estimated from regression lines (Fig. 2) was very similar, -0.43% CE per PD (range: -0.41 to -0.68) (Table 1). This indicates the constant loss of proliferative capacity during Phase II. Therefore, a large fraction of non-cycling cells in addition to the basic progressive clonal attenuation determines the retarded replicative potential of WS cells. Clone inactivation may arise by the stochastic mechanism of presumably terminal differentiation (Martin, et al., 1974; Bell et al., 1978; Smith and Whitney, 1980).

However, the three WS strains (6KO, 8KO and 12KO) exhibited the remarkable upward and downward fluctuations of the CE curves

(Fig. 2). This phenomenon may be an indication that in mass
cultures of some WS strains there are alternating successions of
adaptively well and poorly growing clones during cellular aging
in vitro. Table 2 shows several G-band analyses that indicate
that in WS12KO cells the stable type of variegated translocation
mosaicism without unstable aberrations predominates at 10 PDs
where a clonal expansion occurs (Fig. 2) and in lymphocytes from
a WS1NA patient (not shown). Hoehn et al. (1975) and Salk et al.
(1981a) analyzed extensively such translocations in WS cells.
However, the specific relationship between alternate successions
of selective clones with particular translocations and abnormal
growth property in WS cells has not be substantiated.

3. Proliferative Property of WS Fibroblasts during Cellular Aging

The abnormal growth pattern in some WS strains prompted us
to evaluate the sequential change in the PD per day. Figure 3
displays the profiles in the two normal and four WS strains. The
decline of the PD/day curve found in NHSF41 and NHSF46 cells was
smooth and linear. However, those for WS6KO, WS8KO and WS12KO
cells fluctuated markedly (Figs. 3c, d, and f), and as a whole,
the lower values of 0.41-0.04 PD/day were found than those of
normal cells (PD/day = 0.8-0.3 and 0.43-0.23 for NHSF41 and
NHSF46, respectively) during Phase II. In these WS6KO, WS8KO,
and WS12KO cells, the fluctuation time sequence of the PD/day
curves (Fig. 3) correlate well to the oscillating CE-decline
curves (Fig. 2). On the other hand, the smooth decline in the
PD/day curves in WS11KO cells is similar to that in normal cells
(Fig. 3) as is the linear CE-decline (Fig. 2). Although such a
clonal instablity occurs in some WS mass cultures, PD/day curve
of WS cells is still characteristically lower than normal.

Fig. 4a plots the percentage of labelled cells as a function
of PD, and Fig. 4b replots the percentage against normalized PD.
The NHSF46 population manifested only a minor constant fraction
of less than or equal to 5% non-cycling (non-S-entering) cells up
to 70% of its MPD, and thereafter they increased abruptly.
However, a considerably larger fraction of 20-40% non-cycling
cells persisted even before reaching 70% MPD in the WS5KO, WS8KO
and WS11KO cells tested. Therefore, all the above data indicate
that a large fraction of non-cycling cells is the firm basis of
the shortened lifespan of WS cells in vitro. CRL 1277 cells also
had a larger fraction of linearly increasing non-cycling cell
frequency (Fig. 4).

4. DNA Repair in WS and CRL 1277 Cells

Decreased or defective DNA repair may be related to
accelerated aging (Hart and Setlow, 1974; Epstein et al., 1974).

Table 2. Chromosomal translocations in WS12KO fibroblasts (10 PDs)

G-band No.	Karyotype	Translocations	Visible Deletions	Unstable Aberration[a]
1	46,XY		del 8(q12-qter)	-
2	46,XY	t(11;4)(q21;p16)		-
		t(11;12)(p14;q24)		-
3	46,XY	t(3;8)(q21;p23)	del 9	-
		t(12;4)(q15;p16)		-
		t(13;15)(q11;q16)		-
4	46,XY	t(8;4)(q22;p16)		-
5	46,XY	t(9;5)(p21;p25)		-
6	45,XY	t(9;5)(q13;p15(inv))	del 12	-
7	46,XY	t(2;4)(p21;p16)		-
		t(8;1)(p21;p36)		-
		t(18;17)(q21;q25)		-
8	46,XY	t(2;3)(p21;p27)		-
		t(9;22)(q21;q13)		-
		t(10;16)(q23;q24)		-

[a] less than 1.3% in 100 metaphases and comparable to normal cells.

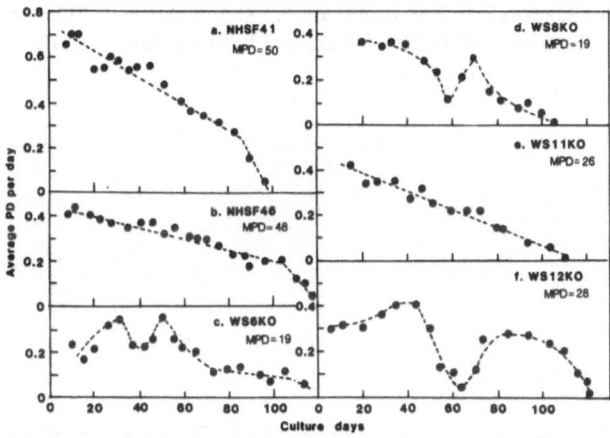

Figure 3. Sequential changes in mean population doubling per day as a function of culture day in normal (NHSF41, NHSF46) and WS (WS6KO), WS8KO, WS11KO, WS12KO) cells.

In this regard, Hutchinson–Gilford progeria and progeric CRL 1277
cells were found to be defective in rejoining of single strand
breaks induced by X-rays (Epstein et al., 1974). However, an
attempt to reproduce these results in CRL 1277 cells met with
only partial success (Regan and Setlow, 1974). Our results in
Fig. 5 demonstrate the normal rejoining of X-ray-induced single-
strand breaks in CRL 1277 and WS11KO cells. The same results
were obtained in the other WS and ACG strains (Table 1). UV-
induced unscheduled DNA synthesis in all the WS strains tested
and CRL 1277 cells was absolutely normal (Table 1). Further,
survival curves in NHSF46, WS11KO and CRL 1277 cells exhibited
the normal resistance to X-ray and UV killings (Fig. 6), as in
the other WS strains (Fujiwara et al., 1977a). Thus, we are
unable to find any detectable defect in excision repair
(incision, excision, repair synthesis, and ligation) or in its
correlation with shortened lifespan of these mutant strains (Fig.
1; Table 1).

Cockayne syndrome (CS) cells manifest a higher than normal
sensitivity to only UV and UV-mimetic agents, due primarily to
the defective recovery of DNA synthesis after UV irradiation
(Fig. 6) (Fujiwara et al., 1981; 1982). CS cells have a lower
than normal level of cellular NAD, which is required for poly
ADP-ribosylation of chromatin proteins in response to excision
breaks (Fujiwara et al., 1983) and for recovery of post-UV DNA
synthesis (Fujiwara et al., 1982).

5.   Abnormal DNA Replication in WS Cells – Increase in molecular weight and replication of matrix DNA

We have reported that an increase in M_w is retarded in
several WS strains (Fujiwara et al., 1977a). In the present
experiments, NHSF46, WS11KO, WS12KO, PSV811 and CRL1277

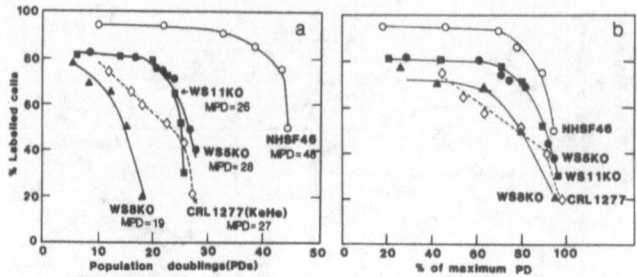

Figure 4. Non-cycling (unlabelled after a 72 hr labelling
     period) and labelled cell fractions as a function of
     population doubling (PD) (a) and as a function of normalized
     PD (b).

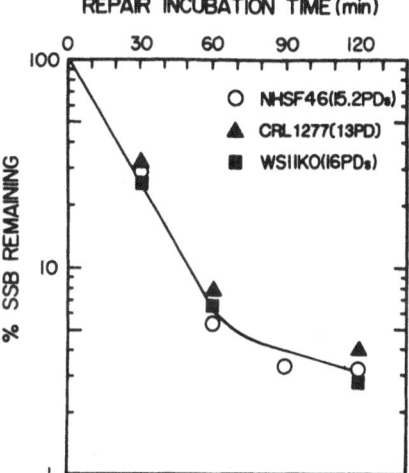

Figure 5. Rejoining kinetics of DNA single-strand breaks (SSB) induced by X-rays. Exponentially growing cells at the indicated PDs were labelled with [³H] thymidine for 2 days, exposed to an X ray dose of 15 krad at 0ºC, and immediately lysed or further incubated at 37ºC for the periods indicated. After cell lysis and pronase digestion, the alkalinized cell lysate was loaded on top of a 5-20% linear alkaline sucrose gradient and centrifuged in an SW50.1 head of a Beckman L5-50 centrifuge at 35,000 rpm for 1 hr at 20ºC, as described previously (Fujiwara et al., 1877a; 1977b). Then, the number of breaks per dalton was calculated by [1/average Mw at time t) - 1/average Mw at 5 = 0)].

cells were pulsed-labeled for 10 min and chased to measure the Mw increase rate of newly synthesized DNA (Fig. 7) from alkaline sucrose sedimentation profiles. In NHSF46 cells (PDs 15 and 30; 31 and 63 MPD, respectively) and GM739 cells (10 passages), Mw increased rapidly during the first hour and reached maximum at 2.8×10^8 within 2 hr. Characteristically, rates of Mw increase in WS12KO (8 PD; 29% MPD) and presenescent WS11KO (13 PD; 68% MPD) were retarded to various degrees. Rates of Mw increases in CRL1277 were also retarded during both middle and presenescent phases.

Mw ranged from 4×10^7 to 9×10^7 immediately after pulsing (Fig. 7), indicating that the majority of incorporations are end-added to already initiated elongating DNA. The maximum Mw of 2.8×10^8 is equivalent to the length of at least several replicons averaging 20 um long. Thus, it appears that a slowing of the Mw

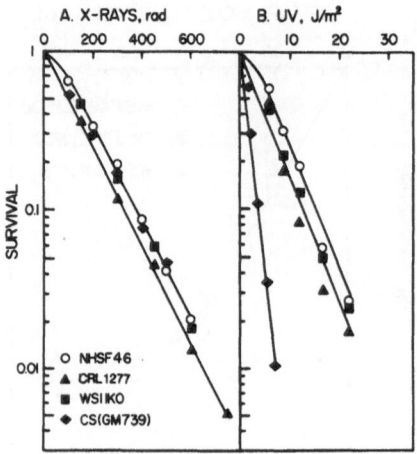

Figure 6.   X-ray and UV survival curves.

increase may arise either through a slowing of chain elongation
itself or through a delay in replicon fusion, presumably due to a
misfiring or delayed firing of one or more orgins in such
clusters.

       To elucidate either possibility, we devised a method to
detect the movement of replicating DNA at the nuclear matrix.
Briefly, cells previously labelled with the uniform ^{14}C-label
were pulse-labelled and chased; the DNA matrix was then analyzed.
In untransformed NHSF46 cells (Fig. 8a), % ^{3}H-cpm remaining in
the matrix after DNase I digestion immediately after a 3-min
pulse was enriched 7-fold, compared with approximately 3% ^{14}C-cpm
of the total radioactivity remaining. This is compatible with
the view that growing points of replicating DNA attach to the
nuclear matrix (Pardoll et al., 1980; McCready et al., 1982).
Then, ^{3}H-label disappeared very rapidly (half life of
approximately 5 min) from the nuclear matrix, and saturated at a
low level over roughly 10 min of chase, which is a time
appropriate to cover a replicon 20 um long by bidirectional
replication. In WS11KO and WS12KO cells at middle PD (Fig. 8a),
the initial enrichment at the anchorage sites appeared to be less
than in NHSF46 and the subsequent chase-out was slower. The
sticky movement of less replicating DNA in the matrix of WS cells
(Fig. 8a) may result from fewer than normal or delayed
initiations of some replicons.

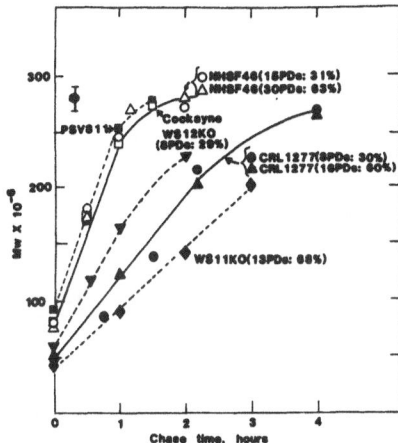

Figure 7. Molecular-weight increase of pulse-labelled DNA as a
     function of chase time. Exponentially growing cells at the
     indicated PD levels and % MPDs were pulse-labelled for 10
     min. with 5 uCi/ml of [3H] thymidine, washed, and incubated
     with 5 x 10^{-5} M non-radioactive thymidine for desired
     lengths of time. DNA in the cell lysate was sedimented as
     described in the legend to Fig. 6 and weight average
     molecular weight (Mw) was calculated as described previously
     (Fujiwara and Tatsumi, 1976). The symbol (⍟) indicates
     the present maximum Mw with standard error of NHSF46 cell
     DNA labelled for 2 days (Mw = 2.8 $\pm$ 0.15 x 10^8). The cell
     strains and PDs (%MPD) are indicated.

Such an event could cause the phenomenon of the delayed fusion of
replicon clusters apparent in the alkaline sucrose Mw-increase
prolifes (Fig. 7). We therefore suggest that misfiring takes
place in some initiations of tandemly arrayed replicon clusters
in WS fibroblasts; however, we cannot absolutely eliminate a
possibility of slow chain elongation occuring at sites of delayed
fusion.

    We made the further comparative study in transformed PSV811
and WI38CT-1 cells. Fig. 7 shows the normalized Mw-increase rate
in PSV811 cells. Figure 8b shows that in both types of
transformed cells, the initial enrichment of matrix [3] DNA is
high and the chase-out is comparably rapid. Thus, we assume that
acquisition of unlimited proliferative ability by transformation
normalizes the defect observed in untransformed WS cells (Fig.
7). Furthermore, a slightly larger amount of matrix [3H] DNA in
transformed cells (Fig. 8b) at 15 min. of chase than that in
NHSF46 cells (Fig. 8a) seems likely to arise from the greater
replicon length in transformed cells (Cleaver, 1978).

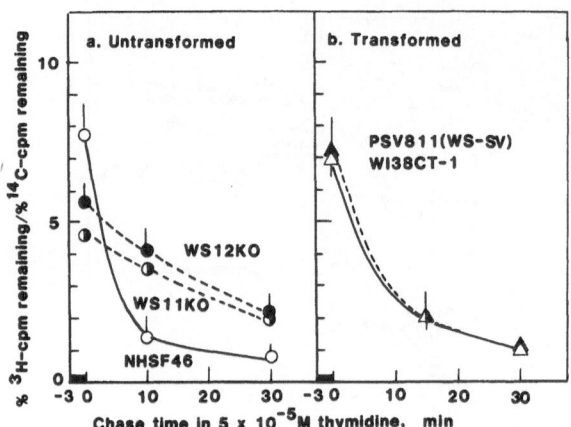

Figure 8. Replicating DNA at fixed anchorage sites of the
     nuclear matrix and chase-time effect. The methods are
     described in Materials and Methods. The matrix DNA was
     isolated after digestion with DNase I. Replicating matrix
     [^{3}H] DNA remaining was expressed relative to [^{14}C] DNA
     remaining. a) Untransformed fibroblasts: NHSF46 (12-15
     PDs): O --O; WS11KO (10 PDs, single determination): ◐ --
     ◐ ; WS12KO (9-13 PDs): ●--●. b) Transformed cells:
     WI38CT-1, △ --△ ; PSV8111, ▲--▲ .

A model for abnormal replication in WS cells

     Figure 9 illustrates our hypothetical model, which is based
on the above findings in WS cells and takes into account the new
model of bidirectional replication in the nucleoid matrix of
eukaryotic cells (Pardoll et al., 1980; McCready et al., 1982).
According to McCready et al. (1982), each replisome or a
replication domain consisting of several supercoiled replicons in
tandem is approximately 70 um long (220 kilobase pairs) (Fig.
9a). Upon replication, the initiation complex and origins attach
to the nuclear matrix under common regulation (McCready et al.,
1982) (Fig. 9b), and coordinated replication proceeds
bidirectionally in a replisome at each fixed anchorage site of
the nuclear matrix (Pardoll et al., 1980) (Fig 9c). Thus, the
replication bubbles, or eyes, are homogeneous in size in
undisturbed normal cells (Fig. 9c'). Finally, replicons are
fused to make replicated long segments (Fig. 9d).

     In WS cells, on the other hand, misfiring or delayed
initiation of at least one origin in such a replisome may cause
the imbalance of initiations (Fig 9q), which will result in the
creation of various eye forms (Fig. 9r'). The resultant replicon
fusions in a replisome are eventually delayed or arrested until

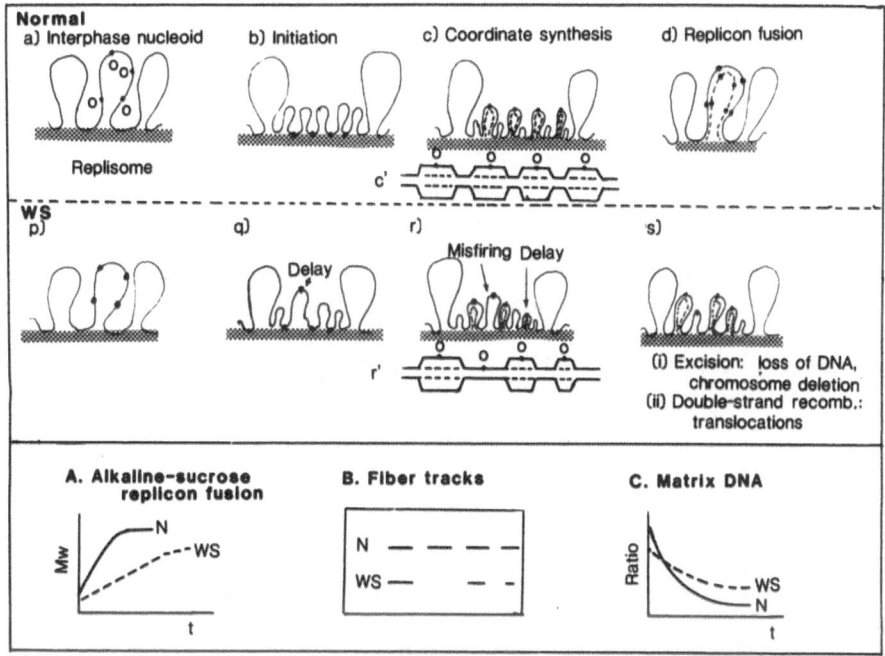

Figure 9. A hypothetical model for abnormal DNA replication in WS
    fibroblasts. See the detailed explanation in text.

synthesis proceeds beyond the termini or the backup synthesis
approaches (Fig. 9s).

The schematic profiles compatible with this mode (see Fig. 9
bottom) can now be predicted. Scheme A illustrates a slower Mw-
increase in WS cells than in normal cells as a result of delayed
replicon fusion with or without DNA chain elongation if large
segments of DNA are detected in alkaline sucrose (see Fig. 7).
Scheme B illustrates the heterogeneous track lengths in
autoradiographic fibers in WS cells, which contrasts with the
homogeneity seen in normal cells. This scheme correlates well
with the experimental data of Takeuchi et al. (1982) which have
indicated that the center-to-center distance in some DNA fiber
tracks is extended in WS cells. Scheme C illustrates the rapid
disappearance of pulse labelled DNA from the nuclear matrix in
normal cells, but the long persistence in WS cells of adherence
of growing points to the matrix identified as matrix DNA as shown
in Fig. 8a.

Furthermore, our model as applied to WS cells can also explain (1) the loss of DNA from chromosomes and the production of extra-chromosomal DNA with replicating origin that will allow autonomous amplification (Goldstein et al., this volume), and (2) chromosomal deletions and various random translocations (Hoehn et al., 1975; Salk et al., 1981a; Fraccarro, this volume). Explanation of our speculative mechanism would be that the stress points made by uncoordinated replicon synthesis and arrested replicon fusion may be subjected to the endonucleolytic attack and promote the excision of double strand DNA from the replisomal loops and to enhance the double strand recombinations of the ends with the ends of duplexes excised from other simultaneously replicating domains in different chromosomes. The latter random recombinations will produce the variegated translocation mosaicism in WS cells.

ACKNOWLEDGEMENTS

This work was supported in part by Grants-in-Aid for life science project from the Institute of Physical and Chemical Research and for scientific research from the Ministry of Education, Science and Culture, Japan. We thank Drs. M. Ohashi (Tokyo Metropolitan Institute of Gerontology) and M. Namba (Kawasaki Medical School) for supplies of TIG-1 and WI38CT-1 cells, respectively, and Miss A. Katanoda (Department of Radiation Biophysics, Kobe University) for her skillful technical assistance.

REFERENCES

Absher, P.M., and Absher, R.G. (1976) Clonal variation and aging of diploid fibroblasts. Exp. Cell Res., 103:247-255.

Bell, E., Marek, L.F., Levinstone, D.S., Merril, C., Sher, S., Young, I.T., and Eden, M. (1978) Loss of division potential in vitro: aging or differentiation. Science, 202:1158-1163.

Cleaver, J.E. (1978) DNA repair and its coupling to DNA replication in eukaryotic cells. Biochim. Biophys. Acta, 516:489-516.

Epstein, C.J., Martin, G.M., Schultz, A.L., and Motulsky, A.G. (1966) Werner's syndrome: A review of its symptomatology, natural history, pathological features, genetics and relationship to the natural aging process. Medicine, 45:177-221.

Epstein, J., Williams, J.R., and Little, J.B. (1974) Rate of DNA repair in progeric and normal human cells. Biochem. Biophys. Res. Commun., 59:850-857.

Fujiwara, Y. (1972) Effect of cycloheximide on regulatory protein for initiating mammalian DNA replication at the nuclear membrane. Cancer Res., 32:2089-2095.

Fujiwara, Y., Goto, K., and Kano, Y. (1982) Ultraviolet hypersensitivity of Cockayne's syndrome fibroblasts, effects of nictoniamide adenine dinucleotide and poly (ADP-ribose) synthesis. Exp. Cell Res., 138:207-215.

Fujiwara, Y. (1983) Roles of poly (ADP-ribose) synthesis in repair and replication in normal human, Cockayne syndrome and xeroderma pigmentosum cells after UV irradiation. In: ADP-Ribosylation, DNA Repair and Cancer, M. Miwa et al., (Eds.), Japan Sci. Soc. Press, Tokyo, pp. 209-218.

Fujiwara, Y., Higashikawa, T., and Tatsumi, M. (1977a) A retarded rate of DNA replication and normal level of DNA repair in Werner's syndrome fibroblasts in culture. J. Cell Physiol. 92:365-374.

Fujiwara, Y., Ichihashi, M., Kano, Y., Goto, K., and Shimize, K. (1981) A new human photosensitive subject with a defect in the recovery of DNA synthesis after UV irradiation. J. Invest. Dermatol., 77:256-263.

Fujiwara, Y., and Tatsumi, M. (1976) Replication bypass repair of ultraviolet damage to DNA of mammalian cells: caffeine resistant and sensitive mechanisms. Mutation Res., 37:91-110.

Fujiwara, Y., Tatsumi, M., and Sasaki, M.S. (1977b) Crosslink repair in human cells and its possible defect in Fanconi's anemia cells. J. Mol. Biol., 113:635-649.

Fujiwara, Y., and Satoh, Y. (1981) Age-dependent change in fibroblast cultures from xeroderma pigmentosum variant. J. Invest. Dermatol. 76:215-220.

Goldstein, S., and Moreman, E.J. (1975) Heat-labile enzymes in Werner's syndrome fibroblasts. Nature, 255:159.

Hart, R.W., and Setlow, R.B. (1974) Correlation between DNA excision-repair and life-span in a number of mammalian species. Proc. Natl. Acad. Sci. USA, 71:2169-2173.

Hayflick, L. (1965) The limited in vitro lifetime of human diploid cell strains. Exp. Cell Res., 37:614-636.

Higashikawa, T., and Fujiwara, Y. (1978) Normal level of unscheduled DNA synthesis in Werner's syndrome fibroblasts in culture. Exp. Cell Res., 113:438-442.

Hoehn, H., Bryant, E.M., Au, K., Norwood, T.H., Boman, H., and Martin, G.M. (1975) Variegated translocation mosaicism in human skin fibroblast cultures. Cytogenet. Cell Genet., 15:282-298.

Martin, G.M. (1978) Genetic syndromes in man with potential relevance to pathobiology of aging. Birth Defects Orig. Art. Ser., 14:5-39.

Martin, G.M., Sprague, C.A., and Epstein, C.J. (1970) Replicative lifespan of cultivated human cells: effects of donor's age, tissue and genotype. Lab. Invest., 23:86-91.

Martin, G.M., Sprague, C.A., Norwood, T.H., and Pendergrass, W.R.
    (1974) Clonal selection, attenuation and differentiation in
    in vitro model of hyperplasia. Am. J. Pathol. 94:137-150.
McCready, S.J., Kackson, D.A. and Cook, P.R. (1982) Attachment
    of intact superhelical DNA to the nuclear cage during
    replication and transcription. Prog. Mutat. Res. 4:113-130.
Nakao, Y., Kishihara, M., Yoshimi, M., Inoue, Y., Tanaka, K.,
    Sakamoto, N., Imura, H., Ichihashi, M., and Fujiwara, Y.
    (1978) Werner's syndrome: in vivo and in vitro
    characteristics as a model of aging. Am. J. Med., 65:919-
    932.
Namba, M., Nishitani, K., and Kimoto, T. (1980) Characteristics
    of WI-38 cells (WI38CT-1) transformed by treatment with Co-
    60 gamma rays. Gann, 71:300-307.
Norwood, T.H., Hoehn, H., Salk, D., Martin, G.M. (1979) Cellular
    aging in Werner's syndrome: a unique phenotype? J. Invest.
    Dermatol., 73:92-96.
Norwood, T.H., Pendergrass, W.R., Sprague, C.A., and Martin, G.M.
    (1974) Dominance of the senescent phenotype in the
    heterokaryon between replicative and post-replicative human
    fibroblast-like cells. Proc. Natl. Acad. Sci. USA, 71:2231-
    2235.
Ohashi, M., Aizawa, Ooka, H., Ohsawa, T., Kaji, K., Kondo, H. and
    T. Utakoji (1980) A new human diploid cell strain, TIG-1,
    for the research on cellular aging. Exp. Gerontol., 15:121-
    133.
Pardoll, D.W., Vogelstein, B., and Coffey, D.S. (1980) A fixed
    site of DNA replication in eukaryotic cells., Cell 19:527-
    536.
Regan, J.D., and Setlow, R.B. (1974) DNA repair in human
    progeroid cells. Biochem. Biophys. Res. Commun., 59:858-
    864.
Salk, D. (1982) Werner's syndrome: a review of recent research
    with analysis of connective tissue metabolism, growth
    control of cultured cells and chromosomal aberrations.
    Human Genet., 62:1-15.
Salk, D., Au, K., Hoehn, H., and Martin, G.M. (1981a)
    Cytogenetics of Werner's syndrome cultured skin fibroblasts:
    Variegated translocation mosaicism. Cytogenet. Cell Genet.,
    30:92-107.
Salk, D., Au, K., Hoehn, H., Stenchever, M.R., and Martin, G.M.
    (1981b) Evidence of clonal attenuation, clonal succession
    and clonal expansion in mass cultures of aging Werner's
    syndrome skin fibroblasts. Cytogenet. Cell Genet., 30:108-
    117.
Schneider, E.L., and Mitsui, Y. (1976) The relationship between
    in vitro cellular aging and in vivo human aging. Proc.
    Natl. Acad. Sci. USA, 73:3584-3588.

Smith, J.R., Pereira-Smith, O.M., and Schneider, E.L. (1978) Colony size distributions as a measure of in vivo and in vitro aging. Proc. Natl. Acad. Sci. USA, 75:1353-1356.

Smith, J.R., and Whitney, R.G. (1980) Interclonal variation in proliferative potential of human diploid fibroblasts: stochastic mechanism for cellular aging. Nature, 207:82-84.

Takeuchi, F., Hanaoka, F., Goto, M., Akaoka, I., Hori, T., Yamada, M., and Miyamoto, T. (1982) Altered frequency of initiation sites of DNA replication in Werner's syndrome cells. Human Genet., 60:365-368.

Tanaka, K., Nakazawa, T., Okada, Y., and Kumahara, Y. (1979) Increase in Werner's syndrome cells by hybridization with normal human diploid and HeLa cells. Exp. Cell Res., 123:261-267.

EXTRACHROMOSOMAL CIRCULAR DNA AND AGING CELLS

Charles K. Lumpkin, Jr., John R. McGill, Karl T. Riabowol, E. J. Moerman, Robert J. Shmookler Reis and Samuel Goldstein

Departments of Medicine and Biochemistry, University of Arkansas for Medical Sciences, and Geriatric Research Education and Clinical Center, Veterans Administration Medical Center, Little Rock, Arkansas 72206

ABSTRACT

A DNA sequence situated in the human genome between Alu-repeat clusters ("Inter-Alu" DNA) is progressively amplified in extrachromosomal DNA, including covalently closed DNA circles, during serial passage of diploid fibroblasts. A single size-class of Inter-Alu circles is also amplified in lymphocytes from 16 of 24 old donors and yet is not detected in cells from 18 young donors.

INTRODUCTION

Human diploid fibroblast-like cells exhibit a finite replicative lifespan in culture (Hayflick and Moorhead, 1961). This phenomenon, in vitro aging, is termed cellular senescence and may contribute in large or small part to organismic (in vivo) senescence (Walton, 1982). Fibroblasts from patients with Werner's syndrome consistently display reduced growth potential in culture (Norwood et al., 1979) which is consistent with the hypothesis that Werner's syndrome features many but not all of the manifestations of aging (Martin, 1982). It has recently been shown that the somatic genome of human fibroblasts displays marked instability during their replicative lifespan (Shmookler Reis and Goldstein, 1980, 1982). Specifically, highly reiterated DNA sequences, including the Eco RI family of centromeric tandem repeats and three smaller repetitive classes, become progressively depleted as the cells replicate toward senescence. More recently correlations have

been noted between a class of extrachromosomal circular DNA and
both "in vitro" and "in vivo" aging. Given the likely relevance to
organismic aging of genomic instability, we will review the most
recent findings concerning extrachromosomal circular DNA and aging.

In 1982 Calabretta et al. reported the construction and
hybridization of a 0.8 Kilo base (Kb) Eco RI fragment situated
between clusters of four and three units of Alu repeated sequences
(the largest class of repetitive sequences in the human genome).
This Inter-Alu probe was used to reveal extensive inter-tissue and
inter-individual heterogeneity of banding patterns due primarily to
bands of extrachromosomal circular DNA. We have used this probe in
a similar manner to examine genomic instability in human diploid
fibroblast-like cells during "in vitro" aging and in normal human
lymphocytes from young and old donors ("in vivo" aging).

Extrachromosomal Circles and In Vitro Aging of Fibroblasts

DNA from human diploid fibroblasts at several doubling levels
was digested to completion with Eco RI restriction endonuclease,
electrophoresed in agarose and transferred to nitrocellulose membrane filters for hybridization to Inter-Alu ^{32}P-DNA probe (plasmid
pλH15A of Calabretta et al., 1982) at 2-6 x 10^8 cpm/μg. The autoradiographs developed from these hybridizations revealed a slight
decline in chromosomal copies of the Inter-Alu sequence (0.8 Kb
Figure 1, a-c) and a progressive increase with culture age in
hybridization corresponding to extrachromosomal circular forms (4.8
Kb in Figure 1, a-c). DNA autoradiographs from three additional
fibroblast strains are shown in Figure 2. In each case after Bam
HI digestion the chromosomal Inter-Alu band appeared at 3.4 Kb
(Figure 2, a-f) as expected from the restriction map of the original 15 Kb genomic DNA clone (Calabretta et al., 1982). Also in
each case at late passage additional discrete DNA bands appeared or
increased (Figure 2, a-f) which are believed to represent DNA
species which are extrachromosomal and circular (see below). The
bands varied in size following Bam HI digestion: 4.2 Kb, 4.8 Kb,
6.6 Kb, and 8.0 Kb.

Generally the extent of "amplification" also varied between
cell strains increasing from 0 to 4 copies/cell in strain A2
(Figure 2, a and b), from 6 to 20 copies/cell in strains DS (Figure
2, c and d), and from 1 to 4 copies/cell in strain TM (Figure 2, e
and f). Restriction cleavage was complete in each case, since
further increase in enzyme/DNA ratio or incubation time had no
effect on the band patterns. Generally the sizes of extrachromosomal bands and their degree of "amplification" at late passage
varied from strain to strain of fibroblasts, and sometimes varied
between expansions of the same strain from different frozen
ampules.

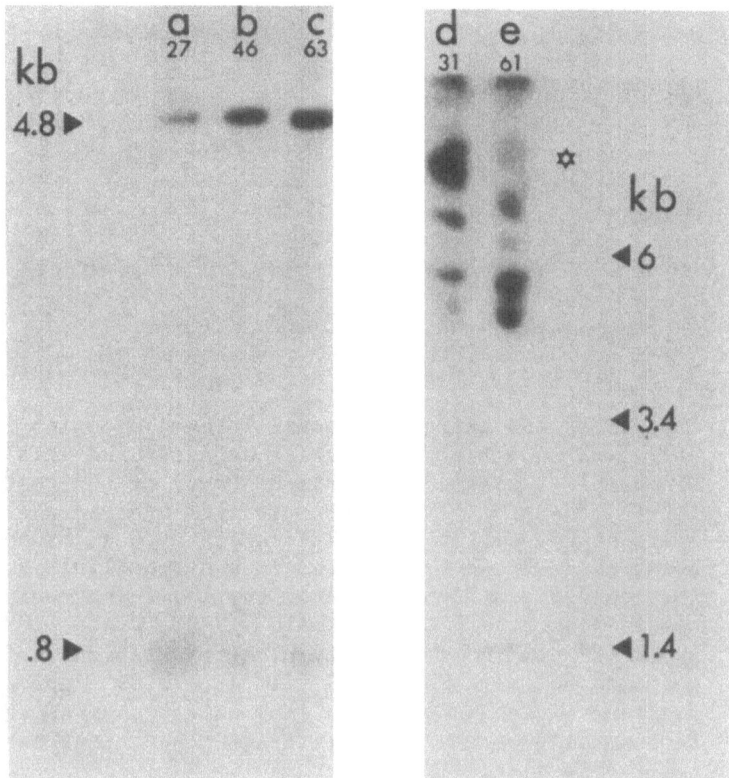

Fig. 1. Inter-Alu copies in the DNA of diploid human fibroblasts
at early, middle, and late passage. Inter-Alu ^{32}P-DNA
probe was hybridized to Southern-transferred DNA samples
following complete cleavage with Eco RI (a-c) or undigested (d, e). Approximate fragment sizes in Kilo base
(Kb) pairs, as indicated, were determined from PM2/Hind
III digested fragments. Loads were 3 μg per 0.5 cm slot.
DNA was prepared from DS-A cells at (a) 27 mean population
doublings (MPD); (b) 46 MPD, and (c) 63 MPD; or from DS-B
cells at (d) 31 MPD and (e) 61 MPD. (Reproduced from
Shmookler Reis et al., 1983a.)

It should be emphasized that all fibroblast strains reported
here were derived from forearm biopsies of healthy donors (Harley
and Goldstein, 1978), and retain the diploid karyotype even at late
passage (Shmookler Reis and Goldstein, 1980). They have been
maintained continuously in our laboratory, free of mycoplasma by
both fluorescent-staining and uridine/uracil incorporation assays
and without any use of antibiotics (which may lead to amplification
of circular extrachromosomal DNA (Smith and Vinograd, 1972;

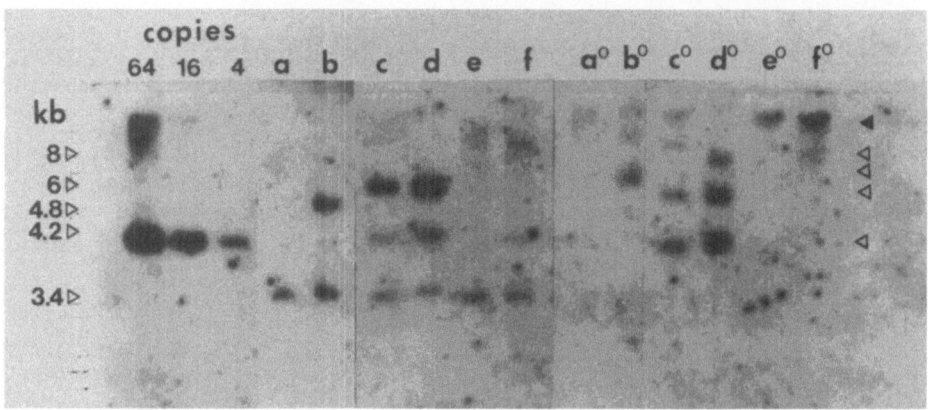

Fig. 2.   Integrated and extrachromosomal Inter-Alu copies in the
          DNA of three fibroblast strains at early and late passage.
          DNA samples, cleaved with Bam HI (a-f) or undigested
          (a°-f°), were electrophoresed in 1.5% agarose gel (16
          hours at 2 v/cm, in 40 mM Tris-acetate, 4 mM NaOAc, 1 mM
          EDTA, pH 7.9) and transferred to a nitrocellulose filter
          (Schleicher and Schuell, BA85) (6, 13). They were then
          hybridized (2, 13) to Inter-Alu ^{32}P-DNA probe (10^6 cpm/ml,
          2-6 x 10^8 cpm/μg, labeled by nick-translation) and auto-
          radiographed with Kodak XAR film at -70°C. Approximate
          fragment sizes in Kilo base (Kb) pairs, as indicated, were
          determined from PM2/Hind III fragments. Loads were 2 μg
          per 0.5 cm slot.

          DNA samples were from: strain A2, max. lifespan 62 MPD,
          at (a) 17 MPD and (b) 51 MPD; strain DS, max. lifespan 60
          MPD, at (c) 21 MPD and (d) 51 MPD; and strain Tm, max.
          lifespan 52 MPD, at (e) 15 MPD and (f) 49 MPD. Lanes
          a°-f° contain undigested DNA samples corresponding to a-f
          as above, i.e. lane a° = lane a without enzyme digestion,
          etc. Hybridization standards, corresponding to 4, 16, and
          64 copies of Inter-Alu per cell, were prepared by serial
          dilution of Eco RI-digested plasmid pλH15A.

Stanfield and Helinski, 1976). Control hybridizations against pure
mitochondrial DNA showed no homology to Inter-Alu probe (data not
shown), indicating that the circular DNA molecules in question were
not derived from the mitochondrial genome. The chromosomal/genomic
bands served as internal controls for hybridization efficiency,
since they either remained at constant intensity or altered slightly while the extrachromosomal bands increased at late passage
(Figure 2, a-f).

    The extrachromosomal nature of these variable, passage-

dependent bands was confirmed by hybridization of Inter-Alu probe
to undigested total cell DNA (Figure 2, a°-f°). While the bulk of
the DNA ran as a diffuse region near the top of the gel (Figure 1,
d and e, Figure 2, a°-f°), there were several discrete hybridizing
bands migrating faster than this (open triangles in Figure 2,
a°-f°). In addition, hybridization to DNA in the high molecular
weight region (◄) indicated integrated chromosomal copies of
Inter-Alu. Reconstruction experiments have shown that added circular DNA of probe size (plasmid pBR 322, 4.3 Kb) does not become
trapped by high molecular-weight DNA, while ^{32}P-DNA probes from
endogenous genes such as β- and γ-globin (Shmookler Reis and
Goldstein, 1982) hybridized exclusively to this chromosomal DNA
region in undigested samples (data not shown). Thus the observed
difference in mobility between "chromosomal" and "extrachromosomal"
sequences would not have arisen artefactually.

For each new Inter-Alu band in Bam HI digested DNA, there were
generally two bands in undigested DNA, presumably corresponding to
nicked and closed circular forms (Calabretta et al., 1982). Both
the number and intensity of discrete bands in undigested DNA were
well correlated with nongenomic bands in restriction-digested DNA.
Thus, the increase in Bam HI bands (other than 3.4 Kb) at late
passage was reflected in an increased number and intensity of
discrete hybridizing bands in undigested DNA, running ahead of the
high-molecular-weight linear DNA region (Figure 1, d and e; Figure
2, a°-f°). The close agreement between these two assays, using
cleaved and uncleaved DNA, indicates that most if not all of the
amplified Inter-Alu copies are extrachromosomal.

In order to demonstrate the presence of amplified Inter-Alu
sequences in covalently closed circular DNA (cccDNA), chromosomal
nucleoprotein was precipitated (Birnboim and Doly, 1979) from
nuclei of A2 fibroblasts at early and late passage, and the supernatants were centrifuged to equilibrium in CsCl gradients containing 200 μg/ml ethidium bromide (Smith et al., 1971). Hybridization
to fractions from these gradients (Figure 3, a and b) indicated
Inter-Alu hybridization to cccDNA molecules (density = 1.59 g/ml)
as well as to nicked circles and linear molecules (density = 1.55
g/ml). Moreover, extrachromosomal Inter-Alu sequences were greatly
enriched (>50-fold, per μg of DNA) in the cccDNA peaks from both
early- and late-passage cells, but were 8- to 10-fold more abundant
in cccDNA of cells at late passage (Figure 4, b, d, f, h), than at
early passage (Figure 4, a, c, e, g). These cccDNA molecules ran
predominantly at 4.8 Kb after cleavage with Hind III (a, b), Eco RI
(c, d), or Bam HI (g, h), consistent with a single cleavage site or
cluster for each enzyme on a circular molecule.

Extrachromosomal Circles and In Vivo Aging of Lymphocytes

If in vitro aging of cells is accompanied by a variable

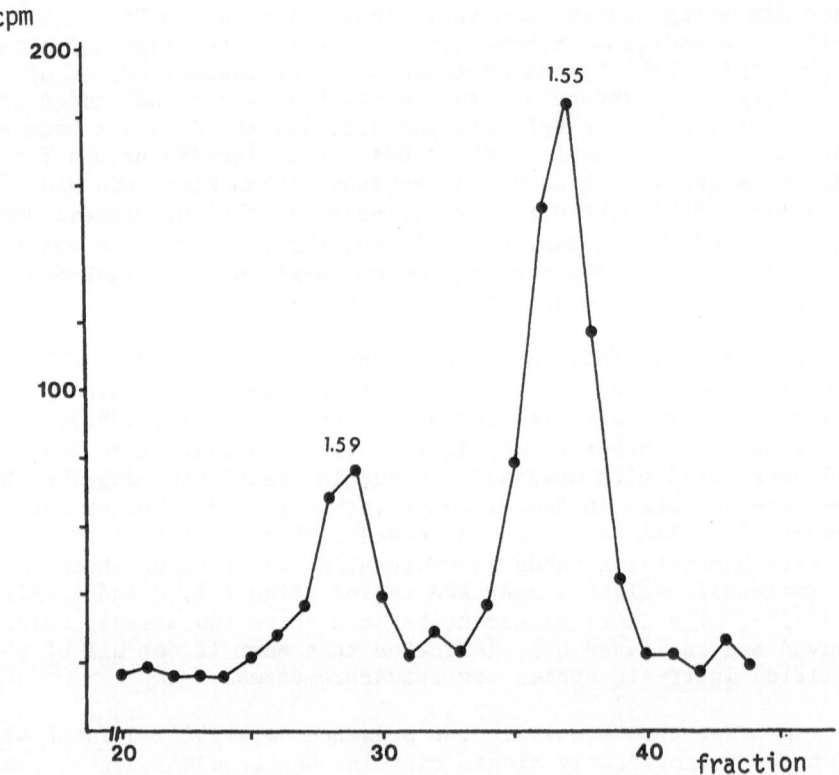

Fig. 3a. Identification of <u>Inter-Alu</u> sequences in cccDNA. ^{3}H-DNA
          banded in CsCl/ethidium bromide, isopycnic gradient.
          Very late-passage A2 fibroblasts (60 MPD) were labeled
          for 6 days (∿1 MPD) with 1 μCi/ml ^{3}H-TdR. Cells were
          harvested, rinsed twice, and lysed in hypotonic medium
          using a Dounce homogenizer. Nuclei were rapidly pelleted
          through 0.5 M sucrose and lysed in alkaline SDS; chromo-
          somal nucleoprotein was precipitated after neutralization
          and the supernatant was concentrated by ethanol-precipi-
          tation, for isopycnic centrifugation in CsCl (density
          1.57 g/ml) containing 200 μg/ml ethidium bromide. Frac-
          tions at densities 1.59 g/ml and 1.55 g/ml, as indicated,
          correspond to cccDNA and linear/nicked-circular DNA
          respectively. ^{3}H-DNA cpm per 10 μl aliquot are shown.

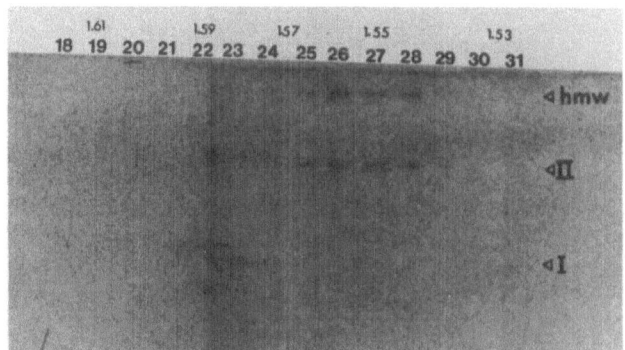

Fig. 3b. Hybridization of Inter-Alu ^{32}P-DNA probe to fractions
from a gradient (similar to that in a) containing A2 DNA
at 60 MPD. Following removal of ethidium bromide by
isopropanol extraction, 2-μl aliquots from 0.1 ml fractions were diluted to 10 μl in gel buffer and electrophoresed on a 1.5% agarose gel. DNA was blotted onto a
nitrocellulose filter, which was hybridized to Inter-Alu
probe as described in Figure 1. Densities of fractions,
determined from refractive indices, are indicated above
the fraction numbers. Positions are marked for Inter-Alu
form I (cccDNA) and form II (nicked-circular DNA) bands;
hmw indicates hybridization which may represent Inter-Alu
sequences in large linear molecules or in large nicked
circles (concatenates or oligomers).

increase in extrachromosomal copy number for the Inter-Alu
sequence, might aging of the organism have a similar effect? In
order to study the effects of in vivo aging, we prepared DNA from
peripheral lymphocytes of eighteen "young" normal donors aged 21-31
years, and of twenty-four "old" normal donors aged 61-91 years.
All donors were in apparent good health and were living at home at
the time of blood collection; their nutritional status is being
investigated currently. Lymphocytes were prepared from fresh blood
samples by standard procedures (Boyum, 1976), and their DNA was
purified. Samples of total lymphocyte DNA, either undigested or
digested with Bam HI endonuclease, were electrophoresed, Southern
blotted, and probed for Inter-Alu sequences. Results for four
young and four old donors are shown in Figure 5. All samples
contained the genomic (3.4 Kb) Inter-Alu band, for which the copy
numbers (estimated by comparison to hybridization standards, serial
dilutions of Eco RI cleaved Inter-Alu plasmid DNA) in both young
and old individuals ranged from 2 up to 30-40 copies per cell.
Several-fold variation in the chromosomal Inter-Alu copies had been
observed by Calabretta et al. (1982) within a smaller sample of
normal lymphocyte donors, but the extent of population heterogeneity we observed was unexpected.

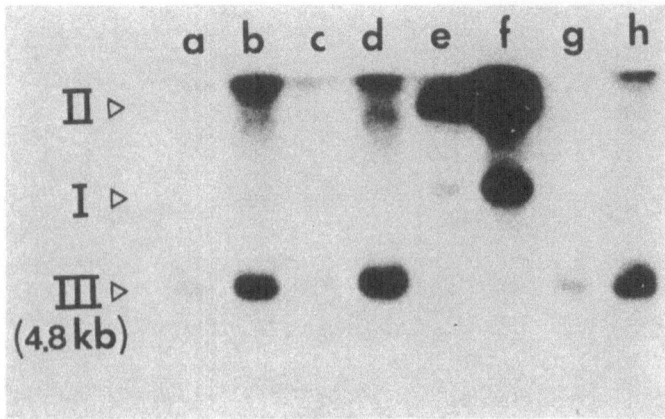

Fig. 4.   Analysis of cccDNA from human fibroblasts. Extrachromo-
          somal DNA from A2 fibroblasts at 28 and 53 MPD ($\sim$10^8 cells
          each) was prepared by alkaline-SDS lysis of nuclei and
          centrifuged in CsCl/ethidium bromide as described in
          Figure 2. The gradient fractions corresponding to cccDNA
          were pooled, ethidium bromide removed by isopropanol
          extraction, and DNA recovered by ethanol precipitation.
          These cccDNA preparations were electrophoresed in adjacent
          lanes of an agarose gel, Southern-transferred and probed
          with Inter-Alu. DNA samples (0.1 µg) each represent 5 x
          10^6 cells: (a and b) digested with Hind III; (c and d)
          digested with Eco RI; (e and f) undigested; and (g and h)
          digested with Bam HI. Restriction bands of genomic length
          were not seen in these fractions. Forms I (cccDNA), II
          (nicked circles), and III (linears) are indicated for the
          Inter-Alu 4.8 Kb extrachromosomal molecules.

          A2 cccDNA at 28 MPD: lanes a, c, e, and g.
          A2 cccDNA at 53 MPD: lanes b, d, f, and h.

     No Inter-Alu bands other than the genomic (3.4 Kb after Bam
HI) were seen in DNA samples derived from any of the eighteen young
donors' lymphocytes (Figure 5, a-d). In striking contrast, 16 of
24 old donors' samples had a single additional band at 4.8 Kb
(Figure 5, e-h), at levels ranging from 4-40 copies per cell. This
age-dependent Inter-Alu band was evidently extrachromosomal, since
undigested DNA samples from old donors' (but not young donors')
lymphocytes also showed two discrete bands of hybridization, in
advance of the unresolved chromosomal linear DNA (Figure 5, e°-h°).
These two bands, presumably corresponding to covalently closed
circular DNA (faster band) and nicked circular DNA (slower band),

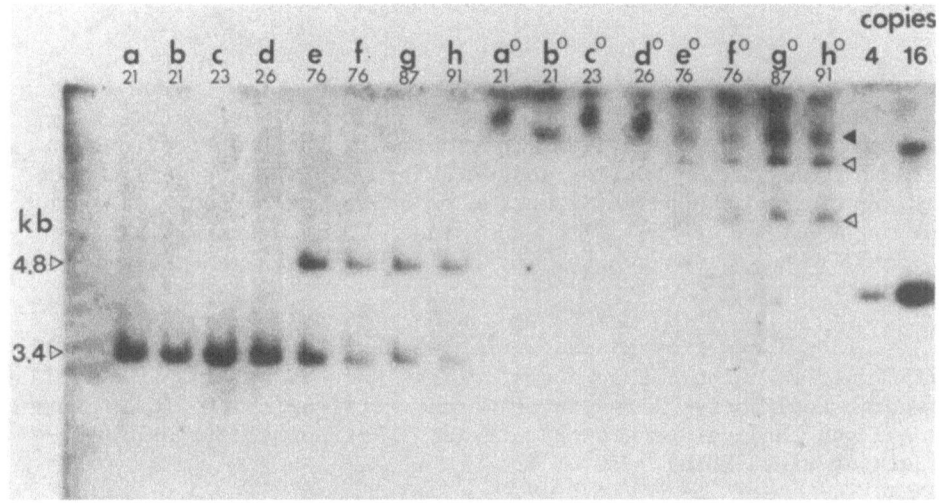

Fig. 5. Integrated and extrachromosomal Inter-Alu copies in human
lymphocyte DNA from young and old donors. Lymphocyte DNA
samples, digested to completion with Bam HI (a-h) or
undigested (a°-h°), were electrophoresed, transferred to
nitrocellulose, and hybridized to Inter-Alu ^{32}P-DNA probe
(see Figure 1).

DNA samples (2 µg each) were from donors of the indicated
ages (years): (a) 21, (b) 21, (c) 23, (d) 26, (e) 76, (f)
76, (g) 87, and (h) 91. Hybridization standards, on the
right, correspond to 4 and 16 Inter-Alu copies per cell.
Lanes a°-h° correspond to lanes a-h; that is, lane a° =
lane a without digestion, etc. (Figures 2-5 reproduced
from Shmookler Reis et al., 1983b.)

were consistently found at the same mobilities in lymphocyte DNA
samples from old donors. The close association between donor age
and extrachromosomal Inter-Alu copies, seen in Bam HI-digested DNA,
was thus confirmed by this assay on undigested DNA.

Lymphocytes from two of the older donors were fractionated
into T and B cells, and their DNAs were then isolated and probed
for Inter-Alu sequences. In both fractionations, the amplified
Inter-Alu circles were found predominantly in B lymphocyte DNA;
indeed, the residual level of circles apparent in our T-cell
preparations may be accounted for by B-cell contamination of this
fraction (manuscript in preparation).

DISCUSSION

Aging

The diploid human fibroblast has a limited replicative lifespan in vitro (Hayflick, 1977), measured by the number of cell
divisions undergone (Harley and Goldstein, 1978). The end of the
exponential growth phase is marked by a decline, gradual or abrupt,
in the capacity of the cells to divide. This phenomenon has been
termed "in vitro senescence," by analogy with the senescence of
organisms.

Fibroblasts from patients with Werner's syndrome are more
difficult to culture than normal cells (Norwood et al., 1979). The
average replicative lifespan of Werner strains is 27% of the normal
value and the average growth rate is 55% of normal fibroblasts
(Salk et al., 1981a).

We have examined normal fibroblasts at several points in their
replicative lifespans. An increase in extrachromosomal Inter-Alu
molecules per cell was observed at late passage, and in one
instance was shown to occur progressively (Figure 1). The increase
in extrachromosomal bands during in vitro aging ranged from two-
fold to more than ten-fold in different cell strains. Because the
size and number of extrachromosomal species varied between fibroblast strains and expansions, autonomous replication of specific
circular molecules would appear to be involved.

A striking correlation was also observed between the in vivo
age of donors and the appearance of 4.8 Kb Inter-Alu circles in
their lymphocyte total DNAs. This indicates that the age-depen-
dence of circular DNA amplification may be a quite general phenomenon, common to both in vitro and in vivo senescence. In peripheral
lymphocytes, however, the situation was less complex than in cultured fibroblasts, in that only one discrete size-class of
Inter-Alu hybridization (4.8 Kb) was found in 16 of 24 of the older
individuals tested (Figures 3 and 4). None of the younger donors
showed any hybridization apart from the genomic band, and the copy
number for that band was extremely heterogeneous between individuals, young or old. This population heterogeneity has been confirmed by Calabretta et al. (1982; personal communication), and
indirectly serves to corroborate the instability of the Inter-Alu/
Alu cluster in the human genome.

Therefore, in addition to extensive population heterogeneity
of genomic Inter-Alu copy numbers, we have found a remarkable
association between Inter-Alu circular forms and senescence, both
in terms of cellular replicative lifespan ("in vitro aging") and
organism lifespan ("in vivo aging"). These two model systems for
the study of senescence have both differences and similarities

which deserve emphasis. Neurohumoral changes in vivo may be involved in the age-correlation for lymphocytes, whereas in vitro cell cultures have the distinct advantage of isolation from such variables. In each case the amplification of extrachromosomal Inter-Alu copies accompanies senescence, suggesting a common molecular concomitant of aging in both systems. Despite the attractiveness of this parallel, we would caution that the two systems might "senesce" for different reasons, and could conceivably amplify Inter-Alu circles by different mechanisms. Thus far the principal difference we have noted is that amplified Inter-Alu molecules are polymorphic with respect to size in fibroblasts but not in lymphocytes.

Since both lymphocytes and the fibroblast cultures are heterogeneous mixtures of cells, it is possible that each contains minor subpopulations of circle-bearing cells which come to dominate the population during senescence. In the case of lymphocytes, our evidence indicates that Inter-Alu circles arise primarily in B rather than T cells. Since the proportion of B lymphocytes in human peripheral blood does not alter with age (Gupta and Good, 1979; Gillis et al., 1981), the age-dependent appearance of Inter-Alu 4.8 Kb circles cannot be attributed to B-lymphocyte hyperplasia. Fibroblasts, however, can undergo "clonal succession" during in vitro culture (Harley and Goldstein, 1978). We have found initial evidence of inter-clonal heterogeneity for Inter-Alu circle number, but none of the five clones assayed at early passage had as many Inter-Alu circles as the mass cultures at the same doubling level. If the increase in Inter-Alu circles were due to shifts in the clonal composition of the fibroblast mass culture, then some clones at early passage must contain at least as many circles per cell as the late-passage mass culture contains. Failure to find such clones would argue against clonal succession as a sole explanation for Inter-Alu amplification. Further investigations are in progress to pursue this question and to ascertain (a) whether circle numbers increase within each clone, (b) whether specific clones rich in circles plate more efficiently or proliferate more rapidly than others, and (c) whether an increasing proportion of clones acquire high numbers of circles at late passage.

Chromosomal Instability

In addition to the reduced growth potential characteristic of Werner's cells, a variety of non-constitutional, stable chromosomal rearrangements are also observed in their cultured skin fibroblasts (Salk et al., 1981b). This pattern has been termed variegated translocation mosaicism (VTM) (Hoehn et al., 1975). There are four genetic diseases that have classically been referred to as chromosome instability syndromes: ataxia telangiectasia, Fanconi anemia, Bloom syndrome, and xeroderma pigmentosum (German, 1972).

Skin fibroblasts from each of these categories have been recently obtained and grown in our laboratory. The preliminary results are that, as expected, all of the five classes of chromosomal instability syndromes display hybridization to the genomic band of Inter-Alu. A consistent pattern has not yet emerged concerning the extrachromosomal bands; however, so far four of the five syndromes do display these bands; the exception being a single patient with xeroderma pigmentosum. Further work is in progress to determine possible amplification during either in vitro or in vivo aging.

Mechanisms for Generating Inter-Alu Circles

Circular molecules could in principle arise by excision (via recombination) from linear chromosomal sequences or by autonomous replication of preexisting circles. Automonous replication has not been directly demonstrated for these extrachromosomal circular molecules, but three lines of evidence support its occurrence. First, human diploid fibroblasts at very late passage, undergoing little chromosomal DNA synthesis, can nevertheless incorporate ^{3}H-TdR into cccDNA (identified by buoyant density, 1.59 gm/ml) in CsCl/ethidium bromide gradients, as shown in Figure 2a. Second, both fibroblasts and normal lymphocytes can increase Inter-Alu circle numbers to levels greatly exceeding their genomic copy numbers (Figure 1; Calabretta et al., 1982; Shmookler Reis et al., 1983). This clearly cannot occur by excision alone, but would require autonomous replication of circles or perhaps a "chromosome-copy" mechanism (Brown and Blackler, 1972; Baltimore, 1981). The finding that circular Inter-Alu forms have restriction site maps which are different from the genomic map renders it difficult to envisage their origin from an integrated chromosomal copy, but does not entirely exclude that possibility (Baltimore, 1981). Third, the selective amplification of circular species with variable sizes in different fibroblast strains (Figure 1), and in different tissues or individuals, would be most easily explained by automonous replication of a specific circular form in each instance.

Replicate expansions of three fibroblast strains, derived from separate aliquots of cells in liquid nitrogen storage, produced very similar passage-dependent increases in Inter-Alu circles. For two strains, the amplified size class remained the same but in the third strain one expansion produced a single prominent extrachromosomal Inter-Alu band while the second expansion produced three size classes. This suggests that the different sizes of extrachromosomal circles appearing in different cell strains may be due to stochastic events in culture rather than donor genotype alone.

A plausible hypothesis would be that circular species containing Inter-Alu sequences arise via homologous recombination (Scherer and Davis, 1980) or gene conversion (Baltimore, 1981) between genomic Inter-Alu copies and endogenous circular species, and are subsequently amplified during aging in vitro or in vivo. An alternative possibility, that such circular forms are infectious and transmitted to cells or individuals in a time-dependent fashion, may be unlikely in view of the different circular sizes appearing in several late-passage fibroblast cultures grown concurrently. That is, the chance of infection in all four cultures, each with different viral species, seems remote. In this context it is also noteworthy that none of the aged lymphocyte donors had prior contact with members of our laboratory.

Analogy of the Inter-Alu/Alu Cluster to Prokaryote and Eukaryote Transposable Elements

Alu repeat units in human DNA possess many properties characteristic of prokaryote and eukaryote insertion sequences (Calos and Miller, 1980; Schmid and Jelinek, 1982): most units are flanked by short direct repeats; they contain promoter sequences for an RNA polymerase (pol III); they are found both in circular DNA molecules (Krolewski et al., 1982) and scattered within the genome; and they evidently have inserted into other genomic sequences, forming flanking direct repeats by duplication of a segment of the pre-insertion site sequence (Grimaldi and Singer, 1982).

The Inter-Alu sequence, together with adjacent Alu repeat units, is structurally analogous to a number of prokaryote transposons, which consist of two identical insertion sequences flanking a central region which generally encodes known gene products (Calos and Miller, 1980). Several transposable elements which have been characterized in eukaryotes share this "transposon-like" structure, e.g. Ty 1 in yeast and copia, 412 and 297 in Drosophila (Calos and Miller, 1980; Green, 1980). While the case for transposability of Alu itself is reasonably strong (Schmid and Jelinek, 1982; Grimaldi and Singer, 1982), it must be emphasized that transposition of the Inter-Alu sequence remains to be demonstrated.

CONCLUSIONS

Although many aspects of the polymorphic Inter-Alu sequence have yet to be resolved, their striking association with both in vitro and in vivo aging poses an intriguing problem. Whether they are implicated as causative agents in senescent loss of adaptive function or instead prove to be a secondary phenomenon perhaps reflecting the more general loss of genomic stability during the lifespan, they reveal a remarkable potential for structural flux in eukaryotic genomes and may provide insight into the basis of the strong age dependency of many malignant diseases.

ACKNOWLEDGMENTS

This research was supported by grants from the National Institute on Aging (AG-03314) and the Veterans Administration.

REFERENCES

Baltimore, D., 1981, Gene conversion: some implications for immunoglobulin genes, Cell, 24:592-594.

Birnboim, H. C., and Doly, J., 1979, A rapid alkaline extraction procedure for screening recombinant plasmid DNA, Nucleic Acids Res., 7:1513-1523.

Boyum, A., 1976, Isolation of lymphocytes, granulocytes and macrophages, Scand. J. Immunol. 5:9.

Brown, D. D., and Blackler, A. W., 1972, Gene amplification proceeds by a chromosome copy mechanism, J. Mol. Biol., 63:75-83.

Calabretta, B., Robberson, D. L., Barrera Saldana, H. A., Lambrou, T. P., and Saunders, G. F., 1982, Genome instability in a region of human DNA enriched in Alu repeat sequences, Nature, 296:219.

Calos, M. P., and Miller, J. H., 1980, Transposable elements, Cell, 20:579-595.

German, J., 1972, Genes which increase chromosomal instability in somatic cells and predispose to cancer, in: "Progress in Medical Genetics," Vol. 8, Grune and Stratton, Inc., New York.

Gillis, S., Kozak, R., Durante, M., and Weksler, M., 1981, Immunological studies of aging: decreased production of and response to T cell growth factor by lymphocyte from aged humans, J. Clin. Invest., 67:937-942.

Green, M. M., 1980, Transposable elements on Drosophila and other diptera, Am. Rev. Genet., 14:109-120.

Grimaldi, G., and Singer, M. F., 1982, A monkey Alu sequence is flanked by a 13 base pair direct repeats of an interrupted α-satellite DNA sequence, Proc. Natl. Acad. Sci., 79:1497-1500.

Gupta, S., and Good, R. A., 1979, Subpopulations of human T lymphocytes, J. Immunol., 122:1214-1219.

Harley, C. B., and Goldstein, S., 1978, Cultured human fibroblasts: distribution of cell generations and a critical limit, J. Cell. Physiol., 97:509.

Hayflick, L., 1977, The cellular basis for biological aging, in: "Handbook of the Biology of Aging," C. E. Finch and L. Hayflick, eds., Van Nostrand Reinhold Co., New York, p. 159.

Hayflick, L., and Moorhead, P. S., 1961, The serial cultivation of human diploid cell strains, Exp. Cell Res., 25:585-621.

Hoehn, H., Bryant, E. M., Norwood, T. H., Boman, H., and Martin, G. M., 1975, Variegated translocation mosaicism in human skin fibroblast cultures, Cytogenet. Cell. Genet., 15:282-298.

Krolewski, J. J., Berlelsen, A. H., Humayun, H. Z., and Rush, M. G., 1982, Members of the Alu family of interspersed,

repetitive DNA sequences are in the small circular DNA population of monkey cells grown in culture, J. Mol. Biol., 154:399-
415.

Martin, G. M., 1982, Syndromes of accelerated aging, Nat. Cancer
Instit., Monog. No. 60:241-247.

Norwood, T. H., Hoehn, H., Salk, D., and Martin, G. M., 1979,
Cellular aging in Werners' syndrome: a unique phenotype?, J.
Invest. Derm., 73:92-96.

Salk, D., Bryant, E., Au, K., Hoehn, H., and Martin, G. M., 1981a,
Systematic growth studies, cocultivation and cell hybridiza-
tion studies of Werners' syndrome cultured skin fibroblasts,
Human Genet., 58:310-316.

Salk, D., Au, K., Hoehn, H., and Martin, G. M., 1981b, Cytogenetics
of Werners' syndrome cultured skin fibroblasts: variegated
translocation mosaicism, Cytogenet. Cell. Genet., 30:92-107.

Scherer, S., and Davis, R. W., 1980, Recombination of dispersed
repeated DNA sequences in yeast, Science, 209:1380-1384.

Schmid, C. W., and Jelinek, W. R., 1982, The Alu family of dispersed repetitive sequences, Science, 216:1065-1070.

Shmookler Reis, R. J., and Goldstein, S., 1980, Loss of reiterated
DNA sequences during serial passage of human diploid fibroblasts, Cell, 21:739.

Shmookler Reis, R. J., and Goldstein, S., 1982, Variability of DNA
methylation patterns during serial passage of human diploid
fibroblasts, Proc. Natl. Acad. Sci., 79, in press.

Shmookler Reis, R. J., Lumpkin, C. K., McGill, J. R., Riabowol, K.
T., and Goldstein, S., 1983a, Genome instability during in
vitro and in vivo aging: amplification of extrachromosomal
circular DNA molecules containing a chromosomal sequence of
variable repeat frequency, Cold Spring Harbor Symposium on
Quantitative Biology, Vol. 47, Structure of DNA, in press.

Shmookler Reis, R. J., Lumpkin, C. K., McGill, J. R., Riabowol, K.
T., and Goldstein, S., 1983b, Extrachromosomal copies of an
inter-Alu unstable element in human DNA are amplified during
in vitro and in vivo aging, Nature, in press.

Smith, C. A., and Vinograd, J., 1972, Small polydisperse circular
DNA of Hela cells, J. Mol. Biol., 69:163.

Smith, C. A., Jordan, J. M., and Vinograd, J., 1971, In vivo
effects of intercalatory drugs on the superhelix density of
mitochondrial DNA isolated from human and mouse cells in
culture, J. Mol. Biol., 59:255-272.

Stanfield, S., and Helinski, D. R., 1976, Small circular DNA in
Drosophila melanogaster, Cell, 9:333.

Walton, J., 1982, The role of limited cell replicative capacity in
pathological age change, a review, Mech. Aging & Dev., 19:217-
244.

PROTEIN SYNTHETIC FIDELITY IN AGING HUMAN FIBROBLASTS

Samuel Goldstein [1,2,3], Roman I. Wojtyk [1,4], Calvin B.
Harley [1], Jeffrey W. Pollard [5,6], John W. Chamberlain
[5], Clifford P. Stanners [5]

1. Departments of Medicine and Biochemistry
   McMaster University
   Hamilton, Ontario, Canada

2. Departments of Medicine and Biochemistry
   University of Arkansas for Medical Sciences
   Little Rock, AR

3. Geriatric Research Educational and Clinical Center
   VA Medical Center
   Little Rock, AR

4. University of Toronto Medical School
   Toronto, Ontario, Canada

5. Ontario Cancer Institute
   Toronto, Ontario, Canada

6. Department of Biochemistry
   Queen Elizabeth College
   University of London
   Campden Hill, London, England

ABSTRACT

The fidelity of protein synthesis was measured in human diploid skin fibroblasts as a function of passage level ("aging in
vitro") and physiological age of tissue donor ("aging in vivo")
using two different test systems. First, in cell-free extracts
the ratio of Δ leu/Δ phe incorporation into peptide linkage
following in the latter case using cells derived from elderly
normal donors and from subjects with the premature aging
disorders of Hutchinson-Gilford progeria and the Werner syndrome.

Similar results were obtained using a second system of intact cells whereby histidine starvation induces quantifiable satellite spots resolved by two dimensional electrophoresis on polyacrylamide gels on the acidic side of the native actin species due to substitution of the neutral amino acid glutamine for the basic histidine. In fact, error frequencies appeared to decrease during aging in vitro, likely due to selection for clonal subpopulations with the highest fidelity of protein synthesis. The only increases were seen in the intact cell system where SV40-transformed cells showed a three-to-five fold greater error frequency compared to nontransformed fibroblasts. In total, these data fail to support the error catastrophe theory of cellular aging.

INTRODUCTION

Human diploid fibroblasts have a finite replicative lifespan when cultured in vitro (Hayflick, 1965), and the maximum number of cell doublings attained by each culture bears an inverse relation to the age of the donor (Goldstein et al., 1969; Martin et al., 1970; Schneider and Mitsui, 1976; Goldstein et al., 1978). However, the actual biological age, in contradistinction to chronological age, is the prime determinant of this replicative limit since fibroblasts derived from donors with syndromes of premature aging show curtailed lifespans (see Goldstein, 1978). Many theories have been put forward to explain this limit but its true nature has remained elusive (Hayflick, 1977). Orgel (1963) first proposed that errors in protein synthesis could lead to an increasingly error-prone translational machinery followed by an autocatalytic augmentation of errors that would kill the cell when the proportion of abnormal proteins exceeded a critical threshold. This theory has been widely tested in recent years (see Hayflick, 1977), almost exclusively by indirect means such as viral probes, but little or no evidence has been marshalled to support it (see Danner et al., 1978).

We now review our results from two different experimental systems that directly examine the fidelity of protein synthesis during cellular aging. First, we describe a cell-free system in which poly(phe) polypeptides coded for by the artificial mRNA poly(U) are synthesized since the UUU codon repeatedly orders the exclusive incorporation of phenylalanine into peptide linkage (Matthei and Nirenberg, 1961). However, other amino acids, particularly leucine (with codons UUA, UUG, and CUU) can be mis-incorporated into the poly(phe) chain if errors occur as a consequence of codon-anticodon mispairing (Davies et al., 1965). Thus, the ratio of leu/phe incorporated into poly(phe), as directed by poly(U), provides a measure of translational infidelity.

The second system utilizes intact cells such that natural mRNAs and other components of protein synthesis are preserved. Specific errors are then induced at histidine sites by starving the cells for histidine, by omitting this amino acid from the medium and by simultaneously adding histidinol, a histidine analog that competes with histidine for histidyl tRNA synthetase. Present evidence supports the idea that histidyl-tRNA becomes depleted, and glutaminyl-tRNA, most closely related in its two anticodons to those of histidyl-tRNA, binds to the specific histidine codons CAU and CAC (Parker et al., 1978; Harley et al., 1980). Therefore, glutamine, a neutral amino acid, is substituted for histidine, a basic amino acid, and this results in proteins with more acidic, i.e. decreased, isoelectric points. Such proteins can be resolved via two-dimensional gel electrophoresis on polyacrylamide gels which separates proteins according to isoelectric point and molecular weight. The result is a series of satellite spots with normal molecular weights appearing on the acidic side of the native proteins corresponding to one, two, three, etc. substitutions of glutamine for histidine.

We now review our findings comparing the accuracy of protein synthesis in normal fibroblasts at early and late passage ("young and old" cells in vitro) as well as in cells from elderly donors and others with disorders of premature aging, the Hutchinson-Gilford (progeria) syndrome and the Werner syndrome. Since one might predict as a corollary of the Orgel hypothesis that permanent lines of "immortal" cells should have lower error frequencies, we also examined SV40-transformed fibroblasts.

Cell Strains

All skin fibroblast cultures were established from biopsies of the anterior forearm of normal and prematurely aged subjects and propagated under standard conditions (Goldstein and Littlefield, 1969). MRC5 and WI38 were developed from fetal lung, and their SV40-transformed derivatives were obtained as described (Harley et al., 1980; Wojtyk and Goldstein, 1980). Cells were passaged within one or two days of achieving confluence. Young cells were subdivided at 1:8 split ratios, counting three mean population doublings (MPD) with each such manipulation. Old cells were subcultured at 1:4 or 1:2 splits counting two or one MPD, respectively, each time. The total cumulative lifespan in MPD was determined after each culture failed to reach confluence at advanced stages of passage following three weeks of incubation with fresh medium exchange weekly.

DETERMINATION OF ERROR FREQUENCY

Poly(U)-Directed System. We first preincubated 30,000g supernatants of Dounce-homogenized cells that had been augmented with
standardized components to "run off" endogenous mRNA followed by
incubation with ^{3}H-leucine or ^{3}H-phenylalanine with and without
addition of poly(U) (Wojtyk and Goldstein, 1980). Phenylalanine
incorporation into hot acid-insoluble material was very low in the
absence of poly(U) (Fig. 1A), but was stimulated approximately
1000-fold following addition of poly(U). This increment (Δphe)
averaged about 20 pmoles/hr/10^6 cells, equivalent to about 0.15
nmoles/hr/A_{260} unit. Poly(U)-directed protein synthesis was linear
with time for at least 30 minutes and was inhibited 90% by 2mM
cycloheximide and over 99% by 4mM puromycin. In parallel, low
levels of leucine were incorporated into peptide linkage in the
absence of poly(U) (Fig. 1B), but an increment (Δleu) that was
small relative to Δphe was always seen after poly(U) addition. In
order to exclude a possible effect of poly(U) on leucine
incorporation due to enhanced translation of endogenous mRNA, we
measured the incorporation of ^{3}H-lysine (coded for AAA and AAC and
thus most remote in the genetic code) with and without poly(U)
(Fig. 1C). In 82 experiments (Wojtyk and Goldstein, 1982), poly(U)
was found not to affect lysine incorporation [range $\pm$3% of no
poly(U)] and we conclude that Δleu following addition of poly(U)
was entirely coded for by poly(U).

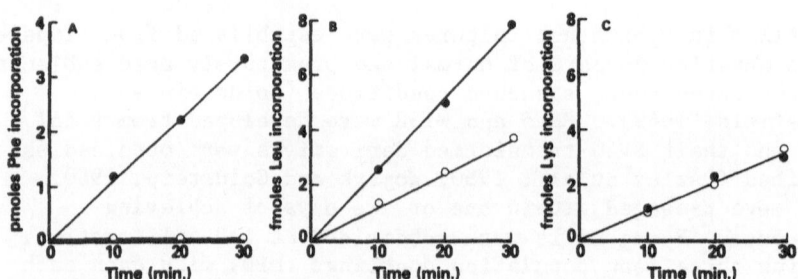

Fig. 1. Effect of poly(U)-addition on incorporation of (A)
         phenylalanine, (B) leucine and (C) lysine into hot
         trichloracetic acid-precipitable material. Note the
         incorporation of phenylalanine is in picomoles, while the
         incorporation of leucine and lysine is 1000-fold less, in
         femtomoles. [o-o, no poly(U); o-o, 0.5 mg/ml poly(U).]
         Reproduced from Wojtyk and Goldstein, 1980, with
         permission of the publisher.

These 30,000g supernatants were free of RNase activity under optimal conditions for poly(U) translation. In addition, no protease activity could be demonstrated (Wojtyk, 1981). This is important because proteolysis could mask mistranslation if there were differential degradation of normal and error-containing proteins (Goldberg and St. John, 1976).

Error frequencies varied among the normal cell strains (Table 1). By far the highest values were found in extracts of A25 at early passage. These cells have been found to be markedly resistant to diphtheria toxin, which strongly suggests that they bear a mutation in Elongation Factor 2, a key protein in protein synthesis (Gupta and Siminovitch, 1980). This in turn would lead to the high error frequencies seen in this assay which essentially measures peptide chain elongation. The next highest error frequencies were found in MRC5 fibroblasts at mid-passage. The lowest error frequency was found in late-passage A2 cells. It should be emphasized that reproducible results were observed for a given strain at a given passage level as seen in the low statistical variances. Error frequencies of strains from the 67 year old donor, from subjects with progeria or the Werner syndrome, and from the SV40-transformed counterpart of fetal lung strain MRC5 fell within this range. We were unable to find a correlation between the replicative lifespans of cell strains and their error frequencies. Indeed A25, the normal strain with the highest error frequency, did not have an abbreviated replicative lifespan. Above all, late-passage cells of all normal, postnatal, and fetal strains did not have higher error frequencies than their early-passage counterparts.

Unexpectedly, but reproducibly, early-passage cells displayed higher error frequencies than corresponding late-passage cells. This trend toward lower error frequencies was analyzed in A2 fibroblasts at 13 sequential passage levels from MPD 22 to MPD 74 (Wojtyk and Goldstein, 1982). Error frequencies declined more than 10-fold progressively over this passage interval, from 2.7×10^{-3} to 0.25×10^{-3}. Analysis of the data by the method of least squares showed that the line $y = 4.6 \times 10^{-5} x + 74.6$ fits the data with a high correlation ($r = -0.93$) that was significantly different from 0 ($p < 0.001$). The rate of decline in error frequency was -4.6×10^{-5}/MPD. It is noteworthy that the optimum for Mg^{2+} and K^+ did not vary from early to late passage of mass cultures or in clonally pure populations (below).

To determine whether decreasing growth rate was responsible for the observed decline in error frequency at late-passage, the rate of proliferation of early-passage cells was reduced by maintaining them in growth medium containing lower concentrations of fetal calf serum. Early-passage cells grown in low serum concentrations (2.0 - 2.5%) required approximately the same time to

Table 1. Error frequency of poly(U)-directed synthesis in cell-free extracts of cultured human fibroblasts as a function of passage level.

Cell Strain	Donor Age and Sex	Replicative Life Span [a]	Passage Level [b]	Error Frequency [c] $\times 10^{-3}$
Normal				
A2	10 M	65	early	2.5 $\pm$ 0.3 (3)
			late	0.5 $\pm$ 0.2 (3)
A25	9 F	50	early	11.5 $\pm$ 2.1 (2)
			late	2.4 $\pm$ 0.4 (3)
J089	67 M	55	mid	1.3 $\pm$ 0.1 (2)
			late	0.6 $\pm$ 0.1 (2)
Progeria				
P18	4 F	53	mid	2.3 $\pm$ 0.1 (3)
P5	9 M	42	mid	2.3 $\pm$ 0.3 (2)
Werner's syndrome				
WS-2	37 M	27	mid	1.7 $\pm$ 0.6 (2)
Other				
MRC5	Fetal lung M	70	mid	4.2 $\pm$ 0.4 (2)
			late	1.0 (1)
MRC5-SV40	Transformed	∞	immortal	3.0 $\pm$ 0.1 (2)

[a] Replicative life span is defined as the number of mean population doublings accruing until cultures fail to reach confluence under normal growth conditions after three weeks with weekly refeedings.

[b] Early, <50% of life span consumed; mid, 50-90% consumed; late, >90% consumed.

[c] Error frequency shown as the mean (Δleu/Δphe) $\pm$ standard deviation of fresh extract preparations from (n) separately grown lots of cells.

Reproduced from Wojtyk and Goldstein, 1980, with permission of the publisher.

growth vigor (Wojtyk and Goldstein, 1982). However, no significant correlation was found between error frequency and maximum MPD attained. Thus, the selective growth disadvantage of clones with high error frequencies is not, apparently, related to error catastrophe.

In summary, therefore, none of these clones showed the decrease in error frequency with passage seen in mass cultures, whereas terminal, post-replicative cultures, where cell selection is minimized, failed to show the predicted error catastrophe. Since the major difference is the clonal heterogeneity of the mass culture coupled to vigorous cell division, it follows that these two factors are preconditions and clonal selection the likely mechanism for the observed decrease in error frequency during passage of mass cultures.

Histidine Starvation and Error Frequencies in Intact Cells

This method has been described in detail (Parker et al., 1978; Harley et al. 1980). In brief, cells growing in plastic dishes were rinsed with medium minus histidine and methionine and incubated for 40 minutes in the same medium plus either 0.15mM histidine or 2-30mM histidinol. These media were then replaced with identical media now containing either ^{3}H-phenylalanine for measurement of protein synthetic rate or ^{35}S-methionine for labeling of proteins followed by 2-dimensional gel electrophoresis with isoelectric focusing in the first dimension (final linear pH range 4-6) followed by second dimension electrophoresis on sodium dodecyl sulfate polyacrylamide gel slabs. Gels were dried and exposed to X-ray film for varying periods to identify labeled proteins followed by scanning of autoradiograms with a microdensitometer. This allowed quantitation of both native and substituted (satellite) proteins by integrating the areas under the curves. Actin was chosen as a reference protein for three reasons: it is the major protein synthesized in human fibroblasts; it has nine histidine residues in both native actins (β and γ) synthesized by human fibroblasts; its satellite spots can be readily resolved and quantified.

Under normal (unstarved) conditions (Figs. 2A, C), no differences were evident in either charge or molecular weight of proteins from aged cells (not shown). This includes late-passage normal fibroblasts, plus cells from an old donor and subjects with progeria and the Werner syndrome. When cells were starved for histidine to induce mistranslation, satellite spots were visible on the acidic side of the native species (Figs. 2B, D). We quantified the native and satellite proteins at protein synthetic rates ranging from 2-10% of normal rates followed by normalizing induced mistranslation to the protein synthetic rate (Table 3). Late-passage cells from fetal, young or old donors

did not have greater error frequencies than early-passage cells.
As in the poly(U) assay, two young donor strains at late-passage
showed a lower error frequency than their early-passage
counterparts. In particular, cells from old donors and subjects
with progeria or the Werner syndrome did not have greater error
frequencies. In mortal strains, we found no correlation between
the in vitro lifespan and the error frequency. In striking
contrast, SV40-transformed fibroblasts showed a significantly
greater error frequency following histidine starvation than
either their own untransformed counterparts or all normal
fibroblasts combined (Fig. 2). A more detailed analysis of this
phenomenon (Pollard et al., 1982) showed that SV40 transformation
was always associated with a significant elevation in error
frequencies, in three pairs of normal and transformed human
fibroblasts and one pair of 3T3 (mouse) cells. In contrast,
other types of viral transformation failed to show an increased
error frequency. These results, therefore, do not support the
hypothesis (Harley et al., 1980) that malignant transformation
necessarily results in increased translational errors leading to
an elevated mutation rate and tumor progression. However, the
increased translational error rate induced by SV40 transformation
could provide an explanation for the reported mutagenic action of
this virus in mammalian cells (Geissler et al., 1980).

UNSTARVED   **STARVED**

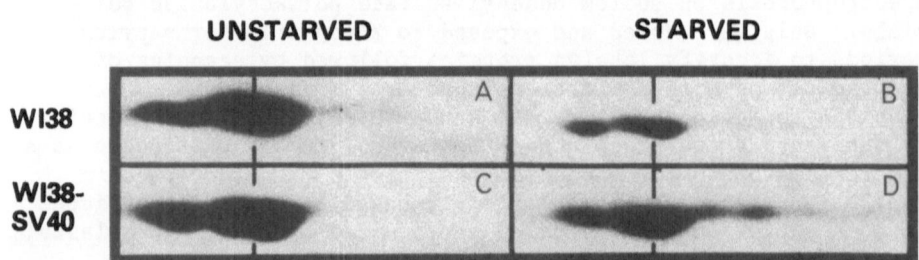

Fig. 2.   Autoradiograms of the actin regions of 2-dimensional
           gels of 35S-methionine-labeled proteins synthesized by
           WI38 (A and B) or SV40-transformed WI38 cells (C and D).

           Cells were grown in medium lacking methionine (A and C)
           or lacking methionine and histidine and containing
           histidinol at 10mM (B) or 5 mM (D). Vertical lines are
           drawn through β-actin.

           Reproduced from Harley et al., 1980, with permission of
           the publisher.

Table 3.   Error Frequencies of Cultured Human Cells as a Function
of Passage Level

Cell Type	Donor Age and Sex	Repli-cative Life Span [a]	Error Frequency x 10^{-4} [b]	
			Early Passage	Late Passage
Young Donors				
WI38	fetus F	55	0.6 ± 0.1 (7)	0.4 ± 0.1 (4)
MRC5	fetus M	65	1.5 ± 0.2 (2)	
A2	11 M	65	1.2 ± 0.2 (10)	0.9 ± 0.2 (8)
GM37	18 F	50	1.6 ± 0.1 (3)	
Mean of young donors			1.0 ± 0.1 (22)	0.7 ± 0.2 (12)
Old Donors				
J069	69 M	50	0.8 ± 0.2 (3)	0.8 ± 0.1 (3)
J088	76 F	48	1.0 ± 0.3 (4)	
Progeria				
P5	9 M	42	1.2 ± 0.2 (6)	
P18	5 F	53	1.3 ± 0.3 (4)	
Werner's Syndrome				
WS2	37 M	37	1.3 ± 0.3 (2)	
WS4	41 M	ND	0.5 ± 0.1 (3)	
Mean of old, progeria and WS Donors			1.1 ± 0.1 (22)	0.8 ± 0.1 (3)
Mean of diploid cells			1.1 ± 0.1 (44)	0.8 ± 0.1 (15)
Immortal Cells				
WI38-SV40			2.8 ± 0.2 (10) [c]	

[a]   See Table 1.
[b]   Error frequency (mean $\pm$ S.E.M.) was derived by normalizing
the fraction of substituted sites to the calculated step
time of ribosomes at the histidine codon (Harley 1979;
Harley et al., 1980).   Numbers in parenthesis are the number
of separately analyzed extracts of proteins labeled during
histidine starvation.
[c]   SV40-transformed WI38 cells have significantly greater
($p < 0.001$) error frequency than either normal WI38 cells or
all diploid cells combined at early or late passage.
ND - not determined.
Reproduced from Harley et al., 1980, with permission of the publisher.

DISCUSSION

Using two distinctly different methods to measure protein synthetic errors directly we have found data which contradict the Orgel hypothesis in several respects.

1.   Fidelity of protein synthesis measured by either technique does not decline in late-passage fibroblasts for the several strains examined. This was recently confirmed in MRC5 cells using the same poly(U)-directed system employed here (Buchanan et al., 1980).

2.   Fibroblasts derived from old donors do not show an increased error frequency.

3.   Fibroblasts from subjects with two different inherited disorders of premature aging, progeria and the Werner syndrome, which contain a diversity of altered proteins (Goldstein and Moerman, 1976) show error frequencies within the normal range. This strongly suggests that such protein alterations emanate from post-translational modifications.

4.   One might predict that escape from mortality in a permanent cell should be associated with a <u>decrease</u> in synthetic errors, but this was not observed in either assay. Indeed, error frequencies measured in SV40-transformed cells by the histidine starvation system were clearly increased. It is unclear why the cell-free system fails to reveal the greater protein synthetic infidelity of SV40-transformed cells. However, poly(U)-directed synthesis is distinctly artificial in that it does not carry out normal initiation or termination. In contrast, the histidine starvation system preserves the normal cell architecture of intact cells which presumably then utilize normal components for their protein synthetic functions. This may explain the observed discrepancy and also account for the apparently higher frequencies of errors in the poly(U)-directed system on the order of 10^{-3} versus 10^{-4} in the intact cell system. In this regard, Jelenc and Kurland (1979) have described improved accuracy of poly(U)-directed translation of E. coli extracts by optimizing the concentrations of polyamines, inorganic cations, tRNAs and nucleoside triphosphates. Another possibility, that of a differential effect of protein degradation affecting estimates of error frequency seems unlikely; the cell-free system showed no significant proteolytic activity (Wojtyk, 1981; Wojtyk and Goldstein, 1982), and we were unable to show increased turnover of the substituted actin species in the intact cell system (Harley, 1979; Harley et al., 1980). Estimates of error frequency in vivo using other means have also been reported to be about 10^{-4} (Loftfield, 1963; Loftfield and Vanderjagt, 1972; Edelmann and Gallant, 1977).

Both of the techniques employed here detect errors thought
to be the result of "ribosomal ambiguity," that is codon-
anticodon mispairing. But it is also possible that misacylation
of the relevant tRNA (tRNAPhe or tRNAhis) could be involved.
However, it is unlikely that misacylation of tRNAPhe with
leucine, or of tRNAhis with a neutral amino acid could occur to
the extent of the error frequencies observed here. Moreover,
misacylation of a cognate amino aid with noncognate tRNA is
relatively rare (Loftfield, 1972). Recent genetic evidence
overwhelmingly supports the idea of mistranslation based on
ribosomal ambiguity leading to codon-anticodon mispairing
(Gorini, 1974; Parker and Friesen, 1980; Gallant and Foley,
1980). Whatever the case may be, the comparisons between the
various cell types here would still be valid since our assays
measure errors from all causes under standardized conditions.

It is still possible that an error catastrophe occurs in
occasional cells which are then lost from the culture and do not
come to assay. This could, in fact, be responsible, at least in
part, for the diminishing plating efficiency even at high density
of late-passage cultures (Goldstein et al., 1969 and 1978), although a diminishing response to serum factors (Harley et al.,
1981) and other stochastic events could also be involved
(Shmookler Reis et al., 1980). Apropos of occasional error
catastrophe, however, Gallant and co-workers (eg., see Gallant
and Palmer, 1979) have shown in E. coli that the elevated protein
synthetic error frequency induced by streptomycin could stabilize
at a level 50 times greater than normal without extinction of
growth or increased cell wastage, although the overall cell
population grew more slowly. Additionally, both Drosophila
(Shmookler Reis, 1976) and cultured human cells (Ryan et al.,
1974) can tolerate substantial incorporation of amino acid
analogs into protein without reducing their lifespans. Finally,
in neither of our assay systems could we find a correlation
between error frequency and the replicative lifespan, although in
mass cultures where several clonal lineages with a range of
intrinsic error frequencies initially exist, cells with lower
error frequencies seem to have a selective growth advantage and
become the dominant populations (Wojtyk and Goldstein, 1982).

In conclusion, our results fail to show a decline in the
fidelity of protein synthesis during aging of human diploid
fibroblasts in vivo or in vitro or in the premature aging disorders of progeria and the Werner syndrome. It seems unlikely,
therefore, that a protein synthetic error catastrophe can be the
explanation for cellular aging.

REFERENCES

Buchanan, J. H., Bunn, C. L., Lappin, R. I., and Stevens, A., 1980,
    Accuracy of in vitro protein synthesis: Translation of
    polyuridylic acid by cell-free extracts of human fibroblasts,
    Mech. Ageing & Dev., 12:339.
Danner, D. B., Schneider, E. L., and Pitha, J., 1978,
    Macromolecular synthesis in human diploid fibroblasts, Exp.
    Cell Res., 114:63.
Davies, J., Gorini, L., and David, B., 1965, Misreading of RNA code
    words induced by aminoglycoside antibiotics, J. Mol.
    Pharmacol., 1:93.
Edelmann, P. and Gallant, J., 1977, On the translational error
    theory of aging, Proc. Natl. Acad. Sci., 74:3396.
Gallant, G. and Palmer, L., 1979, Error propagation in viable
    cells, Mech. Ageing & Dev., 10:27.
Gallant, J. and Foley, D., 1980, On the causes and prevention of
    mistranslation. in: "Ribosomes, Structure, Function and
    Genetics," G. Chambliss, G. R. Craven, J. Davies, K. Davis, L.
    Kahan and m. Nomura, eds., University Park Press, Baltimore.
Geissler, E., Scherneck, S., Theile, M., Herold, H. J.,
    Staneczetki, W., Zimmerman, W., Krause, H., Prokoph, H.,
    Vogel, F., and Platzer, H., 1980, in: "Leukaemias, Lymphomas,
    and Papillomas: Comparative Aspects. Munich Symposia on
    Microbiology," P. A. Bachmann, ed., Taylor and Francis Ltd.,
    London.
Goldberg, A. L. and St. John, A. C., 1976, Intracellular protein
    degradation in mammalian and bacterial cells, Ann. Rev.
    Biochem., 45:747.
Goldstein, S., 1978, Human genetic disorders which feature
    accelerated aging, in: "The Genetics of Aging," E. L.
    Schneider, ed., Plenum Press, New York, p. 171.
Goldstein, S. and Littlefield, J. W., 1969, Effect of insulin on
    conversion of glucose-C-14 to C-14-O$_2$ by normal and diabetic
    fibroblasts, Diabetes, 18:545.
Goldstein, S. and Moerman, E. J., 1976, Defective proteins in
    normal and abnormal human fibroblasts during aging in vitro,
    Interdiscipl. Topics Geront., 10:24.
Goldstein, S., Littlefield, J. W., and Soeldner, J. S., 1969,
    Diabetes mellitus and aging: Diminished plating efficiency of
    cultured human fibroblasts, Proc. Natl. Acad. Sci., 64:155.
Goldstein, S., Moerman, E. J., Soeldner, J. S., Gleason, R. E., and
    Barnett, D. M., 1978, Chronologic and physiologic age affect
    replicative lifespan of fibroblsts from diabetic, prediabetic
    and normal donors, Science, 199:781.
Gorini, L., 1974, streptomycin and misreading of the genetic code.
    in: "Ribosomes," M. Nomura et al., eds., Cold Spring Harbor
    Laboratory, Long Island, New York.

Gupta, R. S. and Siminovitch, L., 1980, Diptheria toxin resistance in Chinese hamster cells: Genetic and biochemical character-istics of the mutants affected in protein synthesis, Somat. Cell Genet., 6:361.

Harley, C. B., 1979, "Aging, Protein Synthesis, and Mistranslation in Cultured Human Cells," Ph.D. Thesis, McMaster University, Hamilton, Ontario, Canada.

Harley, C. B., Pollard, J., Stanners, C. P., Chamberlain, J., and Goldstein, S., 1980, Viral transformation but not aging in-creases high level mistranslation in cultured human fibro-blasts, Proc. Natl. Acad. Sci., 77:1885.

Harley, C. B., Goldstein, S., Posner, B. I., and Guyda, H., 1981, Decreased sensitivity of old and progeric human fibroblasts to a preparation of factors with insulin-like activity, J. Clin. Invest., 68:988.

Hayflick, L., 1965, The limited in vitro lifetime of human diploid cell strains, Exp. Cell Res., 37:614.

Hayflick, L., 1967, The celular basis for biological aging, in: "The Handbook of the Biology of Aging," C. E. Finch and L. Hayflick, eds., Van Nostrand Reinhold, New York.

Jelenc, P. C. and Kurland, C. G., 1979, Nucleoside triphosphate regeneration decreases the frequency of translational errors, Proc. Natl. Acad. Sci., 76:3174.

Loftfield, R. B., 1963, The frequency of errors in protein bio-synthesis, Biochem. J., 89:82.

Loftfield, R. B., 1972, The mechanism of aminoacylation of transfer RNA, Prog. Nucl. Acid. Res., 12:87.

Loftfield, R. B. and Vanderjagt, D., 1972, The frequency of errors in protein biosynthesis, Biochem. J., 128:1353.

Martin, G. M., Sprague, C. A., and Epstein, C. J., 1970, Replicative lifespan of cultivated human cells. Effect of donor's age, tissue and genotype, Lab. Invest., 23:86.

Matthei, J. H. and Nirenberg, M. W., 1961, Characteristics and stabilization of RNAase-sensitive protein synthesis in E. coli extracts, Proc. Natl. Acad. Sci., 47:1580.

Orgel, L. E., 1963, The maintenance of the accuracy of protein synthesis and its relevance to ageing, Proc. Natl. Acad. Sci., 49:517.

Parker, J. and Friesen, J. D., 1980, 'Two out of three' codon reading leading to mistranslation in vivo, Mo. Gen. Genet., 177:439.

Parker, J., Pollard, J. W., Friesen, J. S., and Stanners, C. P., 1978, Stuttering: High level mistranslation in animal and bacterial cells, Proc Natl. Acad. Sci., 75:1091.

Pollard, J. W., Harley, C. B., Chamberlain, J. W., Goldstein, S., and Stanners, C. P., 1982, Is transformation associated with an increased error frequency in mammalian cells?, J. Biol. Chem., 257:5977.

Ryan, J.M., Duda, G., and Cristofalo, V.J., 1974, Error accumula-tion and aging in human diploid cells, J. Geront., 29:616.

Schneider, E. L. and Mitsui, Y., 1976, The relationship between in
    vitro cellular aging and in vivo human age, Proc. Natl. Acad.
    Sci., 73:3584.
Shmookler Reis, R. J., 1976, Enzyme fidelity and metazoan aging,
    Interdiscip. Top. Geront., 10:11.
Shmookler Reis, R. J., Goldstein, S., and Harley, C. B., 1980, Is
    cellular aging a stochastic process?, Mech. Ageing & Dev.,
    13:393.
Wojtyk, R. I., 1981, "The Fidelity of In Vitro Protein Synthesis
    and Its Implications for the Aging of Human Cells," Ph. D.
    Thesis, McMaster University, Hamilton, Ontario, Canada.
Wojtyk, R., and Goldstein, S., 1980, Fidelity of protein synthesis
    does not decline during aging of cultured human fibroblasts,
    J. Cell Physiol., 103:299.
Wojtyk, R.I., and Goldstein, S., 1982, Clonal Selection of human
    fibroblasts: Role of protein synthetic errors, J. Cell biol.,
    95:704

ANALYSIS OF CELLULAR SENESCENCE THROUGH DETECTION AND ASSESSMENT OF
RNAs AND PROTEINS IMPORTANT TO GENE EXPRESSION: TRANSFER RNAs AND
AUTOIMMUNE ANTIGENS

Paul F. Agris[1], Andra Boak[1], Joseph W. Basler[1],
Catherine Van Voorn[1], Christine Smith[1], and Morris
Reichlin[2]

[1]Division of Biological Sciences and the Department of
  Medicine, University of Missouri, Columbia, MO 65211

[2]Oklahoma Medical Research Foundation, 825 N.E. 13th
  Street, Oklahoma City, OK 73104

INTRODUCTION

Gene expression is altered in Werner's syndrome (Salk, 1982).
Investigation of how, when, and where these alterations occur
requires fundamental understanding of the regulation of genes in
normal states--during development and aging--and in diseased organisms. Unfortunately, much of this information is lacking; therefore, only specific aspects of gene expression in Werner's syndrome
can be compared to the normal counterpart with any real understanding. However, newly designed tools in biochemistry and immunology
have opened areas of investigation previously unaccessible.

The expression of eucaryotic genetic information is no simple
matter. Gene expression is regulated at every possible level
starting from within the DNA structure itself as a control of
transcription and concluding with post-translational modifications
of some proteins in order to initiate their functions. The position of genetic information on a chromosome relative to other genes
can be regulatory. Transposition of some genes could be the primary event enabling transcription to occur (Shapiro, 1982). Such
movement of DNA sequences could also be a mechanism for inhibiting
transcription. Eucaryotic transposable genetic elements (transposons) are a reality (Spradling and Rubin, 1981, 1982). Secondary
to this event may be the juxtaposition of small, controlling
regions of DNA and the much larger structural information of the
gene. The positions of operator and promoter sequences for binding

509

of regulatory molecules and RNA polymerase, respectively, relative
to the beginning of the structural information sequence, could be
controlling factors. Modification of a uniquely situated cytosine,
in a sequence upstream of the structural information, by methylation to 5-methylcytosine possibly inhibits transcription (Shen and
Maniatis, 1980). This modification is one means by which repetitive DNA sequences may be "quieted" (Ehrlich et al., 1982).

     Interaction of histone and non-histone acidic proteins is a
mechanism that allows initiation of transcription for properly
aligned regulatory and structural sequences. The array of regulatory, chromosome-associated acidic proteins is different for
different cells and changes with organismal development and
disease. Interaction of these proteins with histones and DNA may
be contingent upon a structural rearrangement of DNA from the B to
Z form where bases are more exposed to proteins (Möller et al.,
1982). Of course, proteins that are responsible for repressing or
stimulating the transcription of particular genes are themselves
products of gene expression. Control of regulatory protein expression in eucaryotes is poorly understood; however, the procaryotic
example of self-regulation, as with control of lambda phage
lysogeny by a repressor promoting transcription of its own gene
(Johnson et al., 1981), is plausible for higher organisms as well.

     Transcription of eucaryotic genes results, in most cases, in
the synthesis of primary gene products that must undergo post-
transcriptional modifications in order to facilitate gene expression. Precursor RNAs for production of mature, functional transfer
RNA (tRNA) (Altman, 1978), ribosomal RNA (rRNA), and heteronuclear
RNA (hnRNA), the progenitor of functional messenger RNA (mRNA), all
undergo two types of post-transcriptional modifications. Primary
transcripts are both sized by specific endonucleases and derivatized by enzymes modifying nucleosides at specific locations.

     Precursor-tRNA is reduced to some 80 nucleotides in length and
elaborately derivatized at 25% of these nucleotides. Our research
on the structure and function of tRNA, in general (Agris et al.,
1982; Chan et al., 1982; Kopper et al., 1982; Munz et al., 1981),
and its alteration in Werner's syndrome and normal aging, in particular, as described here, prompts expanding review of this
molecule's contribution to gene expression. Two aspects of tRNA
synthesis are of interest here relative to its functioning as a
controller of gene expression. First, what are the functions of
the modified nucleosides in tRNA? Are they necessary prerequisites
for the proper use of aminoacyl-tRNA in ribosomal protein synthesis? Second, are particular species of tRNA potentially in control
of the synthesis of certain proteins by virtue of their concentration relative to the mRNA's demand for specific anticodons? Can
amino acid isoaccepting species of tRNA substitute for each other
through "wobble" of the first base of the anticodon?

A collection of over 200 tRNA sequences (Sprinzl and Gauss, 1983) from procaryotes and eucaryotes has shown that almost every sequence position is potentially modifiable as demonstrated in Figure 1. Functions of the more than 60 types of modified nucleosides in tRNA (Agris et al., 1983) are just beginning to be understood, particularly with regard to control of translation. Since under-modified tRNA seemed to function equally well in translation as its fully modified counterpart, identification of modified nucleoside function has eluded investigators until recently. The construction of E. coli and yeast mutants devoid of specific tRNA modifications, E. coli, yeast and Drosophila strains capable of suppressing premature termination codes with tRNA suppressors, and E. coli and yeast strains that modify the ability of suppressor tRNAs to function have all indicated that modified nucleosides within the anticodon region function in codon recognition (Kohli, 1983). These genetic studies along with biophysical investigations (Agris et al., 1983) point to modifications in the first, or wobble, position of the anticodon as being important for the absolute specificity of anticodon-codon recognition. Modification of the base adjacent to the 3'-end of the anticodon may be responsible for the strength of codon recognition, since such modifications promote base stacking, thereby enhancing the affinity of the complementary triplets. Potential functions of modified nucleosides in or near the anticodon are readily assayable as to the specificity, speed and fidelity of ribosomal protein synthesis. Other possible roles have not been as easily discerned. We have some recent evidence that the ribose methylation of guanosine in at least one tRNA, tryptophan, requires aminoacylation as a prerequisite (P. Staehli, P. F. Agris, P. Niederberger and R. Hütter, personal communication). Could this be in preparation for some function at the ribosome?

Changes in modification occurring in aging and Werner's syndrome may bear upon the cell's ability to translate specific proteins, as well as on the fidelity and rate of translation. Thus sensitive, reliable assessment of the type and quality of tRNA modifications is important for determining if changes occur in cells and tissues. We will describe some of the differences in tRNA modifications found in aging human fibroblasts in cell culture. In addition, a superior method of nucleic acid nucleoside analysis by high performance liquid chromatography (HPLC) will be reported.

Specific mRNAs do not have a random collection of codons for the amino acids constituting the protein. Particular codons are utilized in more or less amounts, thus requiring proportionate concentrations of the corresponding anticodons. A particular tRNA in low concentration could affect protein synthesis. Isoaccepting tRNA species with the potential ability to wobble at the third base of the anticodon could, in theory, substitute for a missing tRNA.

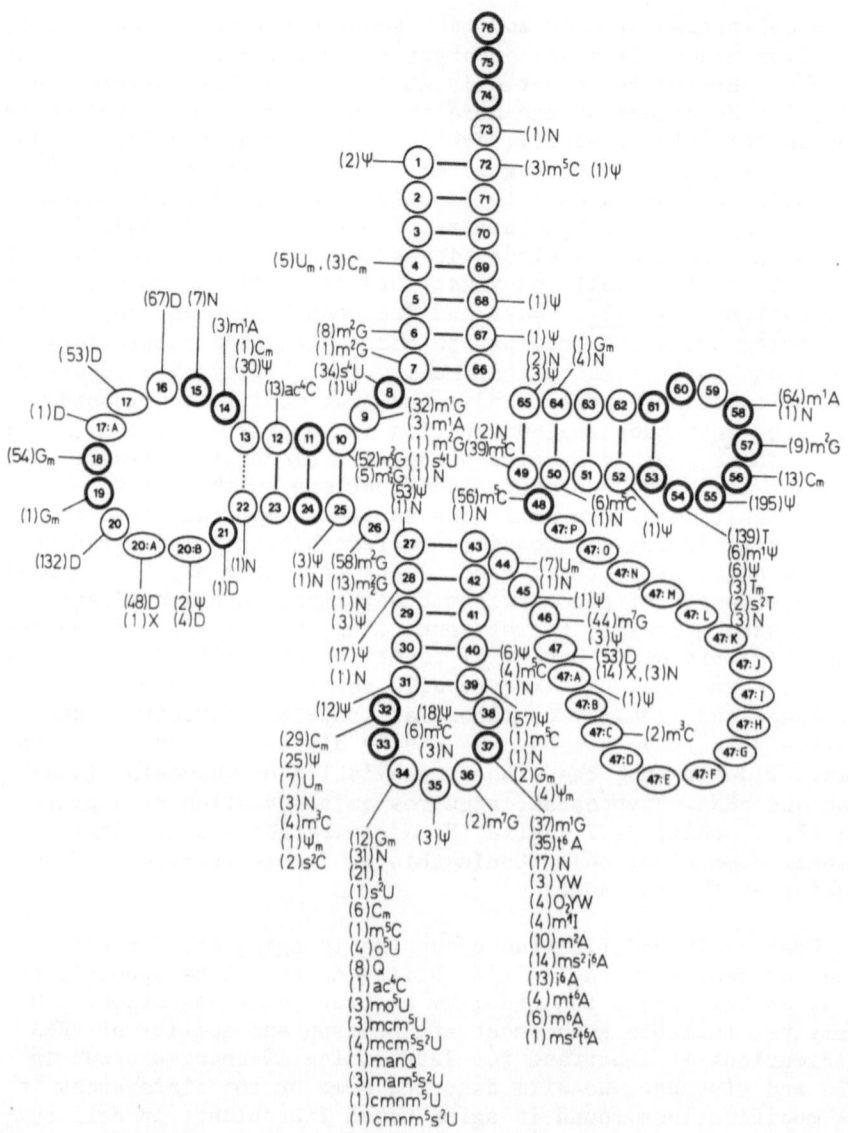

Fig. 1.   Position and occurrence of modified nucleosides in trans-
           fer RNA.   The generally accepted cloverleaf secondary
           structure of tRNA is depicted.   Nucleotides are numbered
           according to the convention based on yeast tRNA[Phe].
           Sequences of 211 tRNAs contributed to the localization
           and distribution of modified nucleosides in the struc-
           ture.   The number in parentheses preceding the modifica-
           tion denotes the number of tRNA sequences with that
           modification at the position indicated.   (The figure was
           kindly provided by Dr. Mathias Sprinzl.)

However, our research (Munz et al., 1981) indicates that wobble may not occur, rather there is an absolute requirement for the speci- fied anticodon. A particular isoaccepting species of tRNA for lysine, $tRNA_4^{Lys}$, has been shown to occur in significant amounts only in cells that are dividing or have the potential to divide (Ortwerth and Liu, 1973; Ortwerth et al., 1973). The tRNA responds to the AAG codon. We have investigated the occurrence of this tRNA in aging human fibroblasts in culture and report our results here.

The mRNA to be translated in eucaryotic cells is derived from hnRNA through sizing and modification reactions. Sizing includes the excision of intervening sequences (introns) that are tran- scribed along with and between structural information sequences (exons). Presumably, the connecting of exons occurs simultaneously with the excision of introns in an operation designated splicing. Enzymes responsible for this operation could be controlling factors in determining which genes represented in the primary transcript, hnRNA, are processed to the mature size and proper sequence as mRNA. The splicing enzymes have not as yet been identified. However, small nuclear ribonucleoprotein complexes (snRNPs) may be involved in the reaction (Lerner et al., 1980; Rogers and Wall, 1980). The snRNPs and related protein complexes have no known functions but are the object of intense investigations because they carry determinants for the autoimmune antibodies of rheumatic diseases (Sharp, 1982). We have isolated, purified and charac- terized two of the autoantigens, Sm and RNP (Takano et al., 1980, 1981). We have evidence that the antigen Sm is involved with some aspect of mRNA utilization (P. Agris, A. Boak, and S. Sarkar, personal communication). Other antigens may be involved in tRNA modification. In this research we have developed sensitive assays for the molecules bearing autoantibody determinants. This has allowed us to probe normal and Werner's syndrome fibroblasts for the presence and quantities of various autoantigens. Results of our preliminary studies are presented here.

The processing of mRNA before it reaches the cytoplasm re- quires not only splicing but two additional reactions: "capping" at the 5'-terminus and polyadenylate (polyA) synthesis at the 3'- terminus. Capping of mRNA includes the production of a 5'-5' phosphodiester linkage to a methylguanosine (m^7G). Nine different caps are found on mRNAs. They differ in the nature of the nucleo- tide to which m^7G is bound. A sensitive HPLC assay of the differ- ent caps will allow us to assess their presence and extents in normal and Werner's syndrome cells to determine differences in mRNA processing.

Thus, we have chosen to report about research on two areas of gene expression that are potentially involved in the physiological differences between human young and old fibroblast cell cultures and Werner's syndrome fibroblast cultures. The first will be

differences in tRNA modifications and the expression of tRNA^{Lys}
isoacceptors. The second will deal with the detection in normal
and Werner's syndrome cells of molecules carrying autoantibody
determinants. We will discuss briefly new HPLC and immunological
techniques that will aid in the study of altered gene expression.

MATERIALS AND METHODS

Materials

The components of Eagle's minimal essential medium (MEM) with
Earle's salts, phosphate-free MEM, and fetal bovine serum were purchased from GIBCO; (^{32}P)-orthophosphoric acid, (^{3}H)-lysine (52
Ci/mmole), (^{14}C)-lysine (292 mCi/mmole) and Omnifluor toluene
scintillation counting cocktail from New England Nuclear; Whatman
DEAE cellulose (DE52) from Scientific Products; thin layer chromatography plates from Analtech Inc.; Kodak No-Screen medical X-ray
film from Profexray; ribonucleases T$_1$, CB and bovine pancreatic
from Calbiochem Co.; eight normal human fibroblast strains derived
from a fetus and normal males ages 12, 12, 29, 32, 59, and 67 and
three Werner's syndrome strains derived from males, 19 and 60 years
old, and a female, 30 years old, from the Genetic Mutant Repository, Camden, NJ. Sera were obtained from patients with autoimmune
disease, systemic lupus erythematosus, Sjogren's syndrome, mixed
connective tissue disease, etc., with fully informed consent.

Cell Culture

Cells were grown to monolayers at 37° under 5% CO$_2$ atmosphere
in MEM supplemented with fetal calf serum (20%). Just prior to
confluency, cells were treated with saline trypsin/EDTA (0.04%/
0.02%) for 30 to 60 seconds to remove them from the flasks. They
were subcultivated at a split ratio of 1:3 or 1:4. Viability was
ascertained by trypan blue (0.1%) exclusion. Radioactive labeling
of pre-confluent monolayers was accomplished by incubating the
cells in 8 ml phosphate-free MEM with extensively dialyzed 20% FBS
and 3 mCi (^{32}P)-orthophosphoric acid for 24 to 36 hours at 37°
(Agris et al., 1975).

tRNA Isolation

Nucleic acids were extracted from cultured cells and tRNA
isolated according to previously described methods (Agris, 1975;
Agris et al., 1975).

Nucleotide Analysis

Radioactive tRNA samples were digested to mononucleotides and
dinucleoside-diphosphates with the use of a mixture of ribo -

nucleases: pancreatic, T_1 and CB (Agris, 1975; Agris et al.,
1975). Hydrolyzed tRNA was then subjected to two-dimensional thin
layer chromatography using a well-characterized system of solvents
for the separation of major and minor nucleotides (Agris, 1975;
Agris et al., 1975; Nishimura, 1972). After full development, thin
layer plates were dried and autoradiography was used to locate the
positions of the radioactive nucleotides which were then quantitated by scintillation counting. Multiple determinations were
accomplished for each cell strain at various times during their
lifespans. Transfer RNA nucleotide data throughout the lifespans
were analyzed for statistically significant changes using a
Student's t test.

High Performance Reverse-Phase Liquid Chromatography

Transfer RNA preparations, isolated from early and senescent
passage cell cultures, were aminoacylated with (^{3}H)-lysine and
subjected to reverse-phase chromatography (RPC-5) along with (^{14}C)-
lysyl-tRNA from rat liver according to previously described methods
(Lin and Agris, 1980).

Preparation of Cell Extracts

Cells were taken from culture flasks before confluency by
treatment with trypsin/EDTA and washed with minimal essential
medium (20% in fetal calf serum). Cells, collected by centrifugation in Eppendorf microcentrifuge tubes, were suspended to a volume
of 50-100 μl in phosphate-buffered saline, pH 6.8. The cells and
their nuclei were disrupted by sonication using a Heat Systems-
Ultrasonics, Inc. sonicator (W-375) which was set at maximum for
the microtip probe and four intervals of 15 seconds duration each.
Supernatant material from a 15 minute, 10,000 xg centrifugation was
assayed for autoimmune antigens or subjected to polyacrylamide gel
electrophoresis.

Polyacrylamide Gel Electrophoresis

Cell extracts were placed in a sodium dodecyl sulfate (SDS),
containing buffer, heat treated at 100°C for 1 minute, and subjected to polyacrylamide gel electrophoresis as previously described (Takano et al., 1980, 1981). Peptide bands were developed
by staining with Coomassie blue. For purposes of detecting those
bands which were antigenic, the samples were not denatured by heat
treatment prior to electrophoresis.

Western Blot for Antigen Analyses

Immediately after SDS-polyacrylamide gel electrophoresis,
peptides are transferred electrophoretically from the gel to paper
(nitrocellulose, or Gene Screen from New England Nuclear). The

blot is identical in peptide separation to that of the gel as determined from amido-black staining of the paper. However, antigenic peptides are determined by complexation with human monospecific, autoimmune antibody. The antigen-antibody complex is then detected with a secondary antibody, commercially available, rabbit anti-human IgG, conjugated with horseradish peroxidase for staining the autoantigenic components.

Ouchterlony Immunodiffusion

The Ouchterlony immunodiffusion assay is used to demonstrate and identify autoantibody specificity and to test autoantigen presence in cell extracts when high concentrations (10-12 mg protein/ml) are available (Takano et al., 1980, 1981).

Hemagglutination Inhibition Assay

Hemagglutination inhibition is a sensitive method for detection of antigen that may be present in as little quantity as a nanogram. The method is performed in microtiter plates routinely for RNP and Sm antigens as described previously (Takano et al., 1980, 1981).

Cellular Localization of Autoantigens by Immunofluorescence

Microscopy. Human normal fibroblast and Werner's syndrome fibroblasts were grown on plastic coverslips in Leighton culture tubes (Costar). The cells were fixed and stained with fluorescein-conjugated monospecific autoimmune antibody (Nakamura, 1974). Disposition of the antibody was observed by fluorescence microscopy.

RESULTS AND DISCUSSION

Cell Culture

Human diploid cell strains were cultured as described in Materials and Methods. Growth and viability data were recorded at each subcultivation throughout the cells' lifespan. Some cell strains were available only at mid or late passage levels in the lifespan. Strains derived from donors with Werner's premature aging syndrome were received during the final few passages of their lifespans. Estimates of the total number of divisions and days in culture prior to our receipt of the cultures were made from information provided by the Genetic Mutant Repository. Figures 2 through 5 describe the growth characteristics of the cell strains with respect to passage number, time, mean population doublings and the rate of division with time. From Figure 3 it can be seen that the rate of division for each strain slowed with increasing time in culture. Since both passage number and mean population doublings

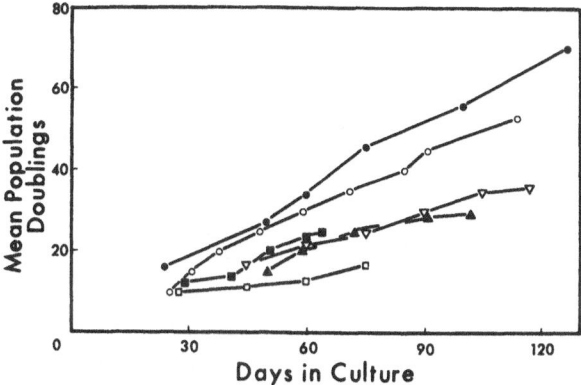

Fig. 2.   Mean population doublings vs. days in culture. The rela-
          tionship here appears to be linear with the slope of the
          curves depending on individual donor differences. Some
          leveling out of the curves for strains derived from the
          two 12-year-old and 32-year-old donors indicates a longer
          cell division time with age. Cell designations and age of
          donors is given below. A second parallel culture of the
          fetal-derived strain was begun at passage 15. Since some
          differences in behavior of this strain from the original
          were noted, it has been reported as a separate strain,
          11*.

Symbol	Cell Strain	Age of Donor	Earliest Passage
●	11	Fetus	4
○	11*	Fetus	4
▽	316	12 yr.	5
▲	442	12 yr.	8
■	103	32 yr.	5
□	274	67 yr.	6

showed nearly linear relationships with the total time in culture,
these two parameters also have linear relationships to division
rate. The inverse relation of donor age to culture lifespan is
borne out to some degree when the total time spent in culture is
considered (Figure 5). The lack of complete correlation of
calendar age in culture with donor age could be a result of differences in individual donors or to inherent variability in the culture techniques involved. However, when the correlation is made
between passage number or mean population doubling level and donor
age (Figure 6), the inverse relationship is well established.
Particularly important is the fact that the data on mean population

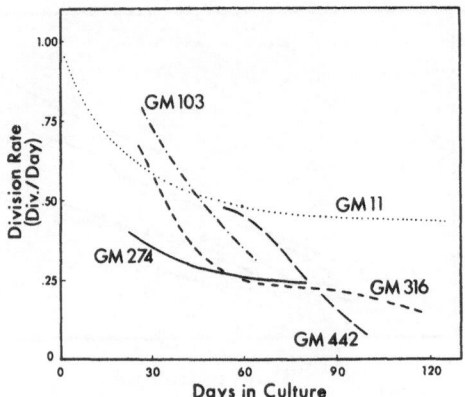

Fig. 3.   Division rate vs. days in culture. With increasing days
           in culture, cells from each donor demonstrated reduced
           rates of division. This is probably due to an increased
           number of slowly or noncycling cells in older cultures but
           may also be an indication of increased sensitivity to
           crowding with age.

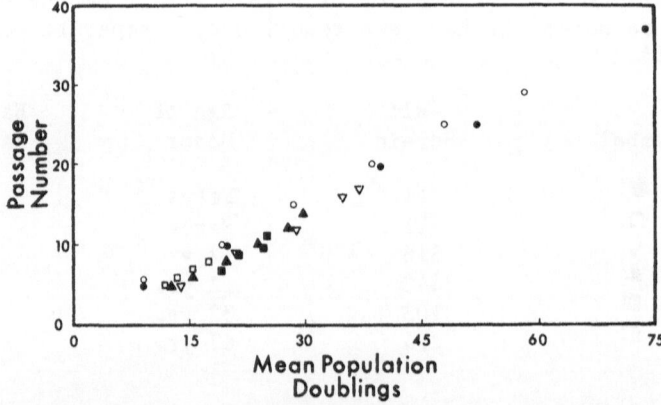

Fig. 4.   Passage number vs. mean population doublings. A linear
           relationship here reflects the subcultivation (split)
           ratio used. In this case, splits of 1:3 result in two
           population doublings between seeding and subsequent
           transfer of cells.

doublings suggest an exponentially decreasing fibroblast growth
capacity with the age of the donor. These results imply that the
total number of divisions, and not the total time spent in culture,
is the more important parameter determining a cell strain's
lifespan.

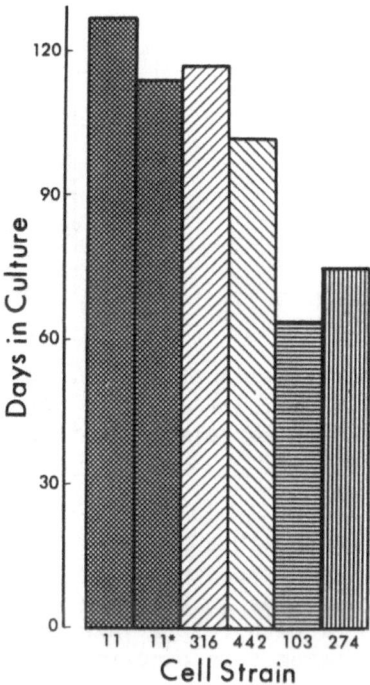

Fig. 5.   Cell strain vs. lifespan as calendar times in culture.
          While there is a downward trend with donor age, the
          results are not conclusive.

     At each subcultivation, the trypan blue exclusion test was
used to determine the percentage of cells still viable. It is
important to note that this value was then used to calculate the
total number of cells still capable of entering into divisions.
This calculation was justified because the parameter being measured
was population doublings and not individual cell doublings.

     Figure 7 shows that during the last quarter of a culture's
lifespan, measured in mean population doublings, the viability of
each strain decreased markedly. Values reported for 100% total
lifespan were obtained at the final subcultivation. Low values
during the first 50% of lifespans were obtained when vials of cells
were removed from liquid nitrogen storage. The average viability
upon thawing was 50-75%.

Transfer RNA

     Alterations in populations or subpopulations of tRNA species
could lead to both qualitative and quantitative changes in protein

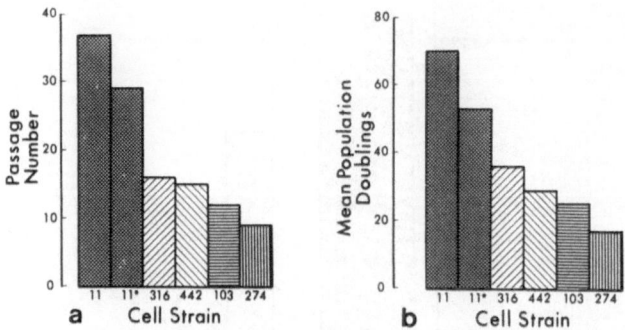

Fig. 6.   (A) Mean population doublings vs. cell strain and (B)
          passage number vs. cell strain. Both parameters demon-
          strate an inverse correlation with donor age (see text).

synthesis and thus be a possible cause of age-related deterioration
of cells. The amounts and types of major (Ap, Cp, Gp, Up) and
minor or modified nucleotides in transfer RNA were analyzed at different passage levels of each cell strain to determine if significant changes in these parameters occurred with senescence in vitro.
Whole fibroblast tRNA labeled with radioactive phosphorus was extracted, purified and digested as described previously in Materials
and Methods. The products of the digestion were mononucleotides in
all cases except those where methylation of the 2' hydroxyl group
of the ribose had occurred. These bases remained as dinucleoside
diphosphates due to the inability of the enzymes to cleave the 5'
phosphoribosyl bond. The whole digest was spotted onto a 20 cm x
20 cm, 250 μm thick microgranular cellulose thin layer chromatography plate and two-dimensional development of the chromatogram was
carried out using the isobutyric acid and isopropanol solvent
systems. The chromatograms were then photographed by exposure of
medical X-ray film to the radioactive surface and the X-ray nega-
tives were used to locate the radioactive spots. The radioactive
areas of cellulose were subsequently scraped from the plate and
counted in a liquid scintillation counter. A typical chromatogram
is shown in Figure 8. Each spot was assigned to a particular
nucleotide on the basis of the nucleotide "map" developed by Agris
et al. (1975). The correlation between the nucleotides present in
the chromatograms and the positions occupied by these bases in
typical tRNA is presented in Figure 1.

     Since extensive data reduction was necessary for this analy-
sis, we felt it may be beneficial to first discuss results from
analysis of the longest passage cell strain, that derived from a
fetal, normal male. Significant alterations were apparent for two
types of tRNA modifications as these fibroblasts entered the final
passages of the lifespan. During the final 30% of the culture

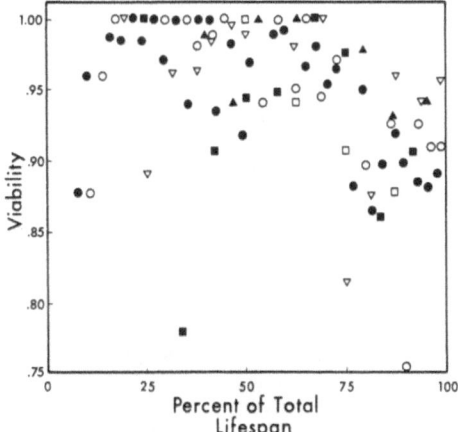

Fig. 7. Viability vs. per cent of total lifespan. Per cent of lifespan is given as a per cent of total mean population doublings undergone. Viability refers to the portion of cells that are remaining and able to exclude trypan blue (0.1%). There is a general decrease in viability throughout the final 25% of the cultures' lifespans.

lifespan, one-methyl guanosine (m^{1}Gp), a methylated cytosine [mCp(1)] and several dinucleotides (NmpNp) changed in their relative proportions in the cellular tRNA populations (Table 1A). The average percentage of radioactive (^{32}P) associated with m^{1}Gp after a 24-hour labeling period, during the first 70% of the culture's lifespan (0.67%) was more than twice the value for the final 30% (0.33%) (Figure 9). In contrast, the amount of mCp(1) increased from undetectable levels during the first 70% of the lifespan to an average value of 0.44% of the total tRNA bases present during the remaining time (Figure 9). The level of dinucleotides including GmpGp also increased significantly during the final 10% of the cells' lifetime (Figure 9). The selective increase and decrease in methylation of specific bases suggests that age-related changes may be a result of alterations in the individual species of tRNA being transcribed or due to programmed modification of species already being produced.

All of the minor and major nucleotides showed some passage variation but none, other than those mentioned, demonstrated consistent increases or decreases in their relative proportions in the tRNA preparations.

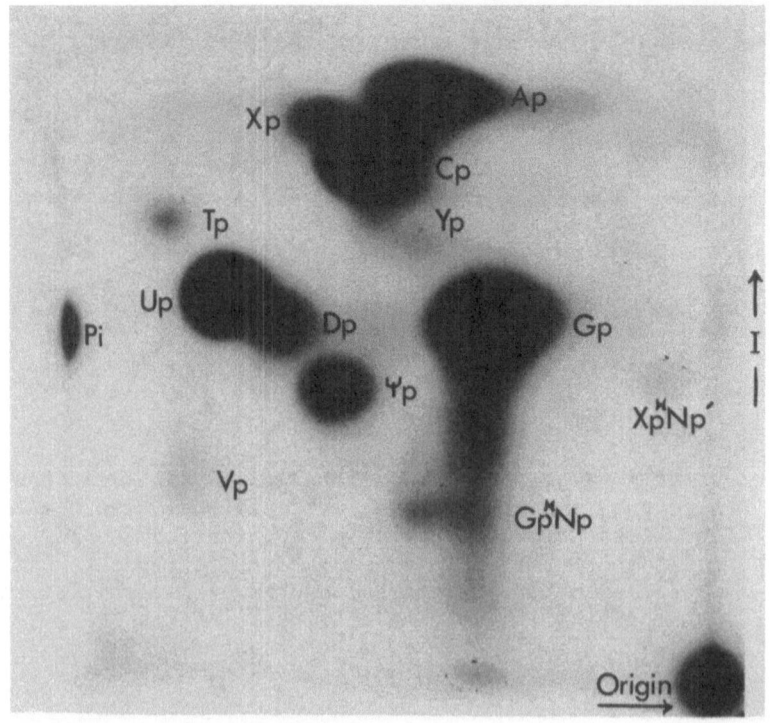

$\leftarrow$ II $\longrightarrow$

Fig. 8. Autoradiogram of chromatographically separated nucleotides. The migration of each radioactive spot was
assigned to a particular modified or unmodified nucleoside on the basis of previous work by Agris et al.
(1975). Abbreviations used in the figure are described
below.

Two nucleotides which were not identified positively but
which were tentatively designated to be methylated
cytosines, mCp(1) and mCp(2), could have been any of
three different molecules, 3-, 4-, or 5-methylcytosine.

Ap, 3' phosphoadenosine; Gp, 3' phosphoguanosine; Cp, 3'
phosphocytosine; Up, 3' phosphouridine; Ψp, 3' phospho-
pseudouridine; Tp, 3' phosphoribothymidine; Dp, 3' phos-
phodihydrouridine; m^7Ap, 3' phospho-7-methyl-adenosine;
ms^2i^6Ap, 3' phospho-2-methylthio-N^6-(Δ^2-isopentenyl)-
adenosine; m^1Gp, 3' phospho-1-methylguanosine; m^7Gp, 3'
phospho-7-methylguanosine; pGp, 3',5' diphosphoguanosine;
pUp, 3',5' diphosphouridine; NmpNp, α2'-methyl dinucleoside diphosphate; GmpGp, α2'-methylguanosine dinucleoside diphosphate; mCp-(1)(2)-methylcytosine.

Table 1A. Nucleotide analysis of fibroblast tRNA. Changes in tRNA
Nucleotide Composition for a Fetal-Derived Fibroblast
Cell Strain

Nucleotide	% lifetime completed - % lifetime remaining		
	70% - 30%	80% - 20%	90% - 10%
Ap	14.12 - 14.40[a]	13.96 - 14.97	14.25 - 14.32
Gp	28.00 - 28.84	28.72 - 27.72	28.65 - 27.50
Cp	30.27 - 30.13	30.32 - 29.91	30.16 - 30.34
Up	14.36 - 14.68	14.41 - 14.77	14.47 - 14.74
Ψp	3.30 - 3.27	3.24 - 3.38	3.26 - 3.36
Tp	0.26 - 0.38	0.29 - 0.38	0.31 - 0.37
Dp	1.84 - 2.26	2.00 - 2.17[b]	2.04 - 2.57[b]
m^7Ap	1.88 - 1.35	2.14 - 0.57[b]	2.14 - 0.57
ms^2i^6Ap	0.03 - 0.06	0.06 - 0.04	0.05 - 0.04
mCp(1)	0.03 - 0.44[b]	0.15 - 0.41[b]	0.19 - 0.41
mCp(2)	0.75 - 0.56	0.69 - 0.56	0.69 - 0.51
$m^1_{}$Gp	0.67 - 0.32[b]	0.55 - 0.32	0.52 - 0.30
m^7Gp	N.D.	N.D.	N.D.
pGp	1.08 - 1.01[b]	1.05 - 1.02	1.05 - 1.02
pUp	1.03 - 0.24	0.87 - 0.21	0.74 - 0.24[b]
All dinucleotides	0.49 - 0.82	0.53 - 0.95[b]	0.55 - 1.11
GmpGp	0.45 - 0.81	0.45 - 1.04[b]	0.50 - 1.17
NmpGp	0.54 - 0.83	0.61 - 0.86	0.60 - 1.04

[a]Amount of each nucleotide as per cent radioactive (^{32}P)orthophos-
phate incorporated during a 24-hour labeling period.

[b]Signifies that the change is significant according to the t-test
($p < 0.05$); N.D., not enough data points available to test.

This table shows the relative amounts of radioactive (^{32}P)-ortho-
phosphate incorporated into various major and minor nucleotides of
tRNA from one of the fetal-derived, diploid cell cultures at different passage levels. Cells were labeled for 24 hours. The lifespan, measured in mean population doublings, was normalized and
comparisons were made between values of incorporation prior to and
after certain percentages of the cell strains' lifetime. Of particular importance are the values for mCp(1), m^1Gp, Dp, pUp and the
combined dinucleotides, for these show significant changes in their
relative concentrations during the latter stages of culture.

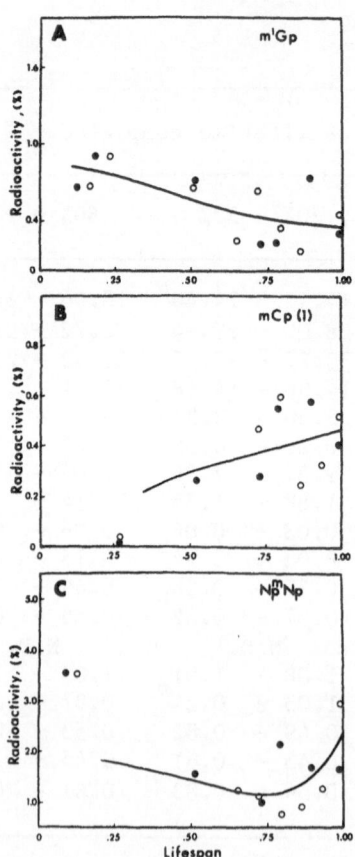

Fig. 9.   tRNA nucleotide changes with cell age for a fetal-derived
           strain. (A) The amount of incorporation of (^{32}P) into 1-
           methylguanosine decreased by nearly 50% during the life-
           span of the cells. The lifespan of the cultures has been
           normalized and values from different passages were re-
           ported as a fraction of the total lifespan. (B) Methyl-
           cytosine (1) appeared only during the latter half of the
           cultures' lifetime and increased in its proportion there-
           after. Its presence could signify the production of new
           tRNA species. (C) The level of ribose methylation was
           also shown to increase near the end of the growth phase.
           Since nucleotides, so modified, are unable to be cleaved
           by the enzyme mixture used in tRNA digestion, the amount
           of dinucleotides (NmpNp) present is a measure of the
           degree of ribose methylation.

Several late passage cultures from each of the other human cell strains were analyzed for the base content of their tRNA molecules. Unfortunately, early mid-lifespan cells were not available for these assays. However, through normalization of the lifespan of cells derived from donors of different ages, we were able to make a comparison of their tRNA nucleotide changes.

A comparison was made of the early and late lifetime tRNA nucleotide components from all cell strains combined. Changes were found in the levels of dinucleotides, dihydrouridine, 2-methylthio (Δ^6-isopentenyl)adenosine (ms^2i^6Ap) and uridine 3',5' diphosphate (Table 1B). As in the fetal-derived strain alone, the number of dinucleotides, which is an indication of the amount of ribose 2'-0-methylation, increased their average percentage of radioactive incorporation by a factor of two during the last 30% of the lifespans (Figure 10). This type of methylation is viewed as a possible protective measure applied to areas of the tRNA which are normally exposed externally through the tertiary folding of the molecule. Modification of the ribose moieties in these areas prevents cleavage of the 3'-5' phosphodiester linkage, thus possibly protecting the tRNA from endogenous nucleolytic enzymes. These, along with other lysosomal enzymes, are present in elevated levels in older cells.

An increase in dihydrouridine, which is present to a great extent in the first loop (the "D" loop, Figure 1) of mammalian tRNA, was found to occur during the final 10% of the combined lifespans (Figure 10). Since the first loop or its stem is possibly involved in aminoacyl-tRNA synthetase binding to tRNA, this increase could affect both the quality and quantity of aminoacyl-tRNA present for use in protein synthesis in older cells. The increased amount of ribose 2'-0-methylation which also occurs in this area, evidenced by the increased presence of GmpGp in digests, may have an added affect on the aminoacyl-tRNA synthetase binding activity.

Decreases in concentration of two nucleotides, ms^2i^6Ap and pUp, were also apparent in the comparison (Figure 10). The latter decreased in its proportion by a factor of approximately four during the final 30% of each cell strain's life, while the former dropped to nearly half its value during the last 20%. The isopentenyladenosine derivative is known to occupy the position adjacent to the 3' end of the anticodon and functions in the association of the tRNA with the mRNA codon (Grosjean et al., 1976, 1978) and its ribosomal binding site (Gefter and Russell, 1969). Loss of its activity could result in a slowdown in protein synthesis or a change in its quality (Agris and Söll, 1977; Agris et al., 1983).

Table 1B. Nucleotide analysis of fibroblast tRNA. Changes in tRNA
           Nucleotide Composition for All Fibroblast Strains
           Combined

| Nucleotide | % lifetime completed – % lifetime remaining | | |
	70% – 30%	80% – 20%	90% – 10%
Ap	14.37 – 13.86[a]	14.15 – 13.94	14.29 – 13.46
Gp	27.92 – 28.73	28.50 – 28.31	28.41 – 28.56
Cp	30.45 – 29.62	30.45 – 20.09	30.33 – 29.13
Up	14.48 – 14.53	14.58 – 14.42	14.65 – 14.13
Ψp	3.23 – 3.34	3.17 – 3.46	3.20 – 3.56
Tp	0.31 – 0.36	0.31 – 0.38	0.32 – 0.39
Dp	2.00 – 2.56	2.09 – 2.07	2.13 – 2.90[b]
m^7Ap	1.73 – 1.10	1.68 – 0.93	1.46 – 1.02
ms^2i^6Ap	0.05 – 0.04	0.06 – 0.03[b]	0.05 – 0.02
mCp(1)	0.18 – 0.33	0.26 – 0.30	0.26 – 0.30
mCp(2)	0.66 – 0.54	0.61 – 0.54	0.62 – 0.48
m^1Gp	0.56 – 0.45	0.49 – 0.50	0.48 – 0.52
m^7Gp	0.70 – 0.57	0.63 – 0.58	0.62 – 0.57
pGp	1.09 – 1.17	1.07 – 1.22	1.07 – 1.30
pUp	1.22 – 0.30[b]	0.89 – 0.30	0.72 – 0.35
All dinucleotides	0.53 – 1.12[b]	0.64 – 1.23[b]	0.71 – 1.36[b]
NmpUp	0.56 – 0.09	0.75 – 1.08	0.77 – 1.21
GmpGp	0.51 – 1.14[b]	0.54 – 1.38[b]	0.66 – 1.51[b]

[a]Amount of each nucleotide as per cent radioactive (^{32}P)orthophos-
phate incorporated during a 24-hour labeling period.

[b]Signifies that the change is significant according to the t-test
(p < 0.05).

The same comparisons made after combining the data from all cell
strains studied revealed some different results. In this case, the
combined dinucleotide fraction increased in its proportion as in
the fetal-derived strain, but no significant change could be found
for m^1Gp or mCp(1). Dp, pUp and one other nucleotide, ms^2i^6Ap were
altered in their amounts during the declining stages of culture.

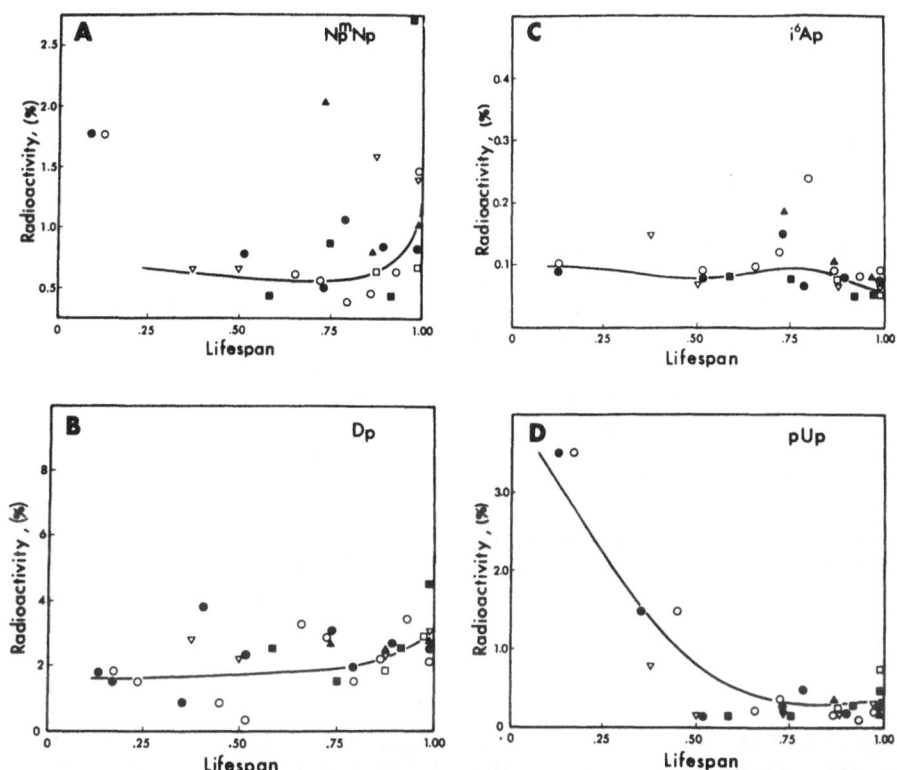

Fig. 10.   Combined data on altered nucleotides of tRNA with cell
           age. (A) The per cent of the total radioactive phosphate
           incorporated into dinucleotides was shown to increase
           near the end of the cultures' lifespan. Here all of the
           dinucleotide data from each strain was pooled and
           charted. The lifespans have been normalized for the
           comparison. (B) A gradual increase in Dp was noted when
           the data were combined, however, as can be seen in one
           case, strain 442 (▲), not all cell strains share in the
           increase. (C) Isopentenyladenosine, normally present in
           very small quantities, dropped to an even lower level
           during final passages. (D) A drastic drop in pUp
           occurred during the early stages of culture, but then the
           level remained fairly constant throughout final passages
           of all cell strains studied. Strain 11 cell nucleotides
           are denoted as ● ; 11*, ○ ; 316, ▽ ; 442, ▲ ;   103,
           ■ ; and 274, □ .

The level of the 5' terminal nucleotide, almost exclusively pGp or pUp in mature tRNA, is indicative of the species of tRNA present in the cell. It was expected that a decrease in the amount of pUp such as was observed in the final 30% of the cultures' lifetime, would result in an increase in pGp. However, the level of pGp did not change significantly during the culture period. This suggests that either pUp-beginning tRNAs were not being transcribed or some step in the sizing of tRNA precursor molecules may have been affected by senescent changes leading to the presence of incompletely processed tRNA's in the senescent cell.

It must be kept in mind that the results obtained by pooling the data from all of the normal cell strains may not be the best way of analyzing it. While species differences in tRNA composition were not a factor, individual differences in genetic makeup and physiological state of the donors could conceivably affect the types of individual tRNAs present and thus the amounts of modified nucleotides. The lack of a large number of data points from very early passages for some strains also lends difficulty to the interpretation of the results.

Theories which explain aging as a programmed phenomenon are generally supported by the results of the tRNA studies on the fetal-derived strains. Strehler's "codon restriction" hypothesis (Strehler, 1971), for instance, calls for a changing population of isoaccepting tRNAs as a control mechanism in development of a tissue or organism. Then applied to the culture situation, this theory predicts the loss of certain critical tRNA subspecies or aminoacyl-tRNA synthetase molecules, due to autogenic repression, that are needed to produce metabolically important proteins. This loss should then result in some senescent changes and cell death. The reduction in amounts of one modified nucleotide, m^1Gp, along with increases in two other types, mCp(1) and NmpNp, could, according to this theory, be the result of a change-over, from one set of tRNA species to another, which requires a slightly different pattern of modification. These methylation changes might also represent a change in modification of the same tRNAs brought on by a programmed change in the types of methylases available or a protective response brought on by the increased presence of lytic enzymes in the older cells. The protective production of methylases may also be programmed to insure that enough active tRNA remains during final passages to continue the synthesis of more lysosomal enzymes thus insuring cell death. Most theories which predict genetically programmed alterations in enzyme activities or RNA species transcribed are equally well supported by this evidence. In general, theories which explain aging in terms of random errors or mutations do not fit in well with the data. That errors will accumulate in important enzymes causing damage to their function would explain the loss in methylation of the guanosine residues but not the increased methylation of the cytosine or that noted in the case of dinucleotides, unless the errors lead to more active enzymes in these cases instead of less active ones. Another explanation is that this altered modification of the tRNA results in large amounts of inactive or partially processed molecules thus furthering senescence.

The results of the overall comparison of all strains together can also be explained in the same manner, although it is obvious that the same changes have not occurred equally in all cell strains, with the exception of the increases always noted in the amount of ribose methylation responsible for dinucleotide production.

In summary, the data have shown the following: 1) The amount of modification of certain bases is altered as cells pass from mid-passage to final passages. These alterations may be the result of transcription of different tRNA species which require modifications other than those of their predecessors or they may be due to the action of different modification enzymes produced during the late passages and effecting a steady population of tRNA species. 2) The amount of ribose methylation was increased during the final 30% of the lifespan of all cell strains, possibly as a protective measure to insure the safety of the tRNA species among the increased lyso-somal enzymes of final passage cells.

These results are now being supported by means of a more sophisticated and sensitive analysis of major and modified nucleo-sides. We have shown that HPLC analyses of any nucleic acid enzymatically hydrolyzed to nucleosides can identify and quantitate over 40 nucleosides (Gehrke et al., 1982; Zumwalt et al., 1982). Figure 11 shows an HPLC separation. Important to our analyses of modified nucleosides in tRNA of human normal and Werner's syndrome fibroblasts is the ability now to characterize some of the more esoteric nucleosides (Figure 11) occurring in very small amounts. Our methodology can identify and quantitate a nanogram of a nucleo-side occurring among 10,000-fold other nucleosides.

Early and late passage human fibroblast cultures differ sig-nificantly in their abilities to divide. Other investigators have shown that cells that are dividing or have the potential to divide have relatively high amounts of a single isoaccepting species of lysine tRNA, tRNA$^{Lys}_4$ (Ortwerth and Liu, 1973; Ortwerth et al., 1973). Some six isoaccepting species of tRNA^{Lys} have been found in mammalian cells, but only the amount of the species designated #4 by its chromatographic mobility is correlated to cell division. The analysis of lysine tRNAs is also of interest with regard to our work on fibroblast collagen synthesis (Basler et al., 1979). The debris protein produced by senescent cells and shown to have the biochemical characteristics of collagen was found by microscopic examination to have its fibers in a circular array rather than the

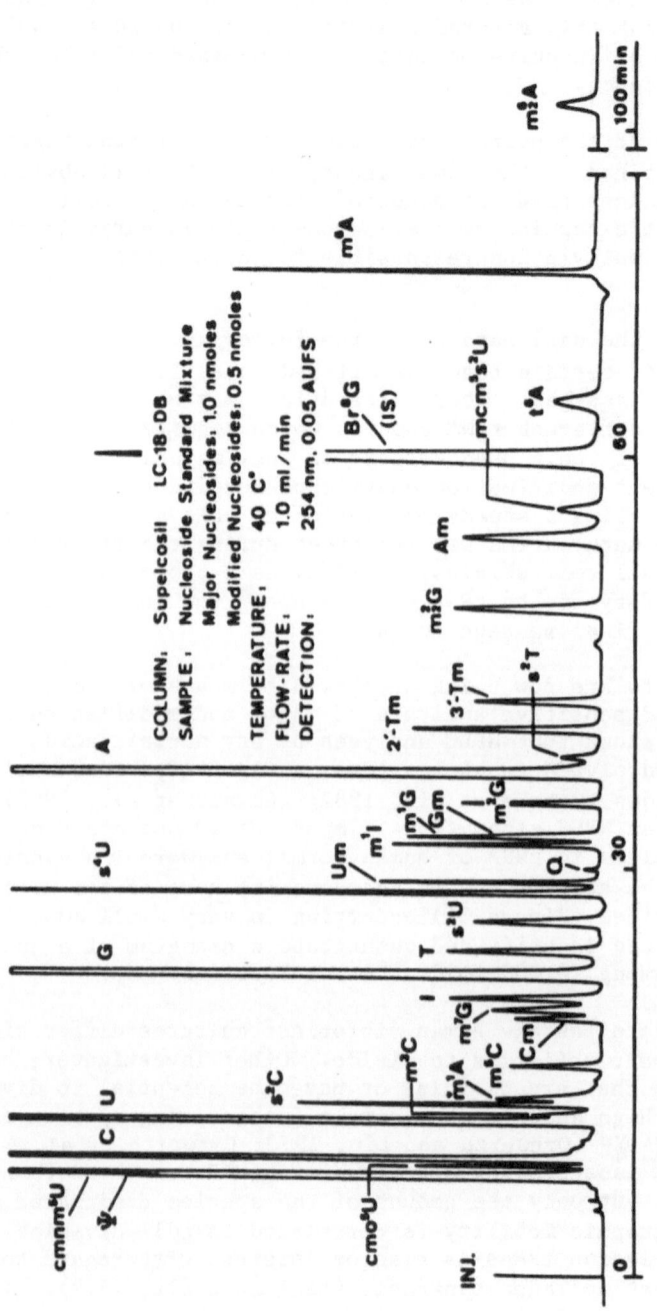

Fig. 11. High performance liquid chromatography of transfer RNA nucleosides. Nucleosides resulting from enzymatic hydrolysis of tRNA are separated and quantitated by HPLC according to Gehrke et al., (1982). The figure shows the retention times and relative responses for a variety of major and modified nucleosides.

linear arrangement of normal collagen fibers (Basler et al., 1979).
Lysine is the amino acid consistently involved in cross-linking
tropocollagen chains (Goldberg et al., 1972; Bailey, 1975). Thus,
analyses of lysine isoacceptor tRNAs in early and late passage
cells may reveal differences of interest with regard to the
collagen production by the cells, as well as differences related to
the cultures' abilities to divide.

The tRNA isoacceptor patterns for any amino acid can be compared by high performance reverse phase liquid chromatography (Lin
and Agris, 1980; Lin et al., 1980). Very little tRNA is required
because the radiolabeled aminoacyl-tRNA is subjected to chromatography and assayed by scintillation counting. An internal standard
such as aminoacylated rat liver tRNA carrying a different radio-
isotope is chromatographed along with the sample.

The isoaccepting species of tRNA^{Lys} from early and senescent
cells were compared for the two cell strains derived from fetal
tissue. Reverse phase column chromatographic separations of the
tRNA^{Lys} isoacceptors from cultures of one of the strains in the
first quarter of the lifespan are compared to that from the last
quarter in Figure 12. Isoaccepting species 1, 2 and 4 represented
7.8, 42.9 and 15.1%, respectively, of the total lysine accepting
tRNA from early passage cultures. However, the same three isoacceptors represented only 2.4, 35.6 and 10.9%, respectively, of
the total tRNA^{Lys} from senescent cells. The relative proportion of
species 5 increased correspondingly from 33.2% in early passage
cultures to 51.1% in senescent cells. Comparable changes of the
tRNA^{Lys} isoacceptors were found for tRNA from early and late passage cultures of the other strain derived from fetal tissue. The
decreased proportion of tRNA$^{Lys}_4$ late in the lifespan of the cultures coincides with decreased ability of these cells to divide.
This correlation has already been observed for tRNA$^{Lys}_4$ in other
systems, as described above. However, the dramatic decrease in
isoacceptor #1 has not been previously noted in diploid cell

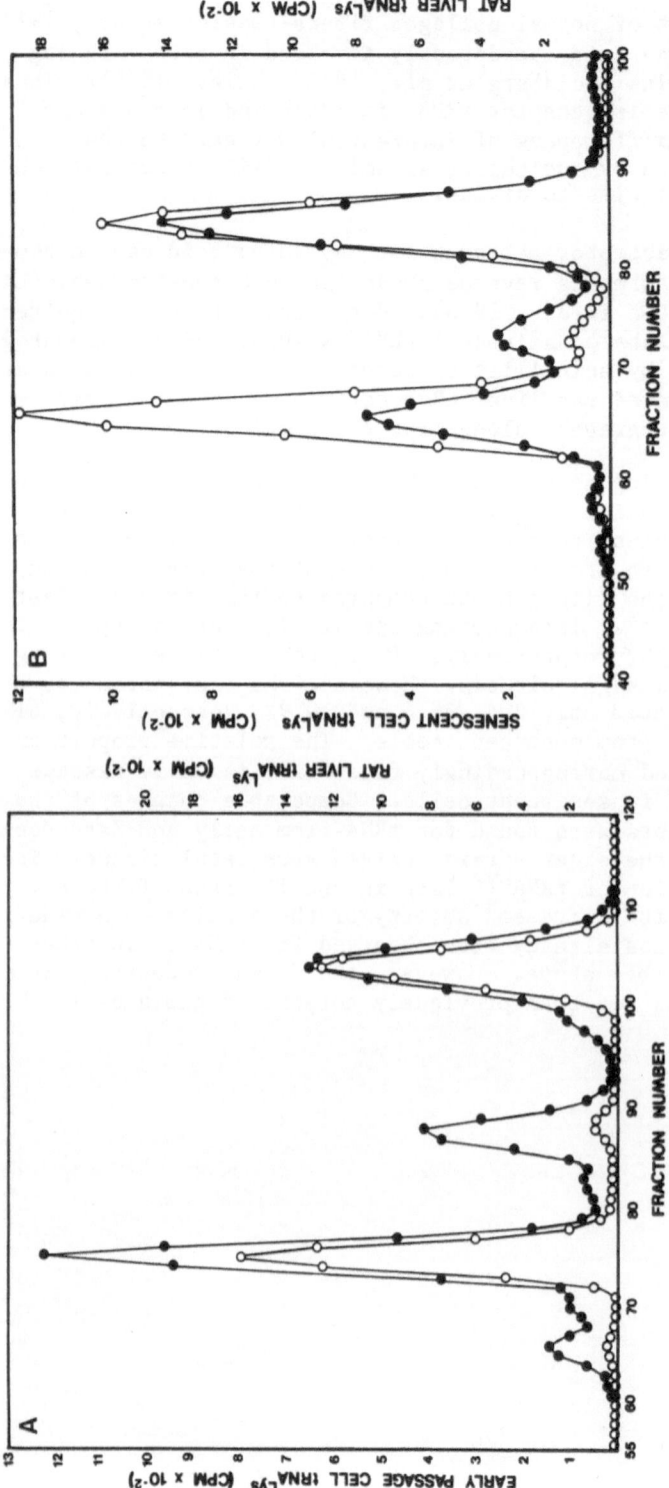

Fig. 12. Isoaccepting species of tRNA^{Lys} in early passage and senescent fibroblasts. Transfer RNA preparations that were isolated from early passage 11 and 11* cultures and from senescent cultures of 11 and 11* were aminoacylated with (^{3}H)-lysine and subjected to reverse phase chromatography. The elution profiles of tRNA^{Lys} isoacceptors from early passage 11 cells are shown in A and B, respectively. Separation of normal rat liver tRNS^{Lys} isoacceptors on the same columns is used as a control of the chromatography. No less than 85% of the radioactive lysyl-tRNA was recovered from the columns.

culture. This tRNA responds to the codon AAA for lysine. The
relationship between the amount of a particular tRNA, and therefore
its anticodon, and the efficient and correct translation of a
specific protein is of interest. We will investigate the ability
of the various proportions of tRNA^{Lys} isoacceptors from fibroblast
cultures for translating collagen mRNA in a tRNA-dependent, in
vitro translation system.

Autoimmune Antigens

Patients with rheumatic disease produce antibodies to DNA,
ribosomes, nucleolar proteins, cytoskeletal proteins, etc. However, in addition, the patients produce antibodies to a wide array
of what seem to be universal nuclear and cytoplasmic macromolecules
of unknown functions. Of recent interest is the possibility that
some of these autoantibodies are directed against the enzymes
responsible for processing mRNA from hnRNA (Lerner et al., 1980;
Rogers and Wall, 1980) and for the maturation of tRNA from its
primary transcript. Thus, there may be a relationship between gene
expression and the type and quantity of autoantigens present in a
cell. A comparison of Werner's syndrome and normal human fibroblasts with regard to these autoantigens may be informative as to
the nature and functions of the autoantigens and their relationship
to the physiological differences of these cells.

The autoantigen designated RNP is composed of RNA and protein.
This antigen is presumably involved in mRNA processing (Lerner et
al., 1980; Rogers and Wall, 1980). We have found that RNP has two
determinants for the antibodies RNP and Sm (Takano et al., 1981).
The RNP determinant is sensitive to RNase treatment of the antigen
as assayed by Ouchterlony immunodiffusion (Figure 13). The interrelationship of RNA and proteins is depicted in Figure 14 as determined by us for the RNA determinant (P. F. Agris, Y. Kikuchi, M.
Takano, H. J. Gross, and G. C. Sharp, personal communication) and
by others for the Sm determinant (Liautard et al., 1982). The 5'
terminus of the RNA is free of protein possibly allowing for
complementary base pairing with intron-exon junctions of hnRNA in
order to accomplish splicing as is hypothesized. Although RNP is
always found with Sm, Sm can be isolated and purified as a separate
antigen (Figure 13; Takano et al., 1981).

Analysis of quantity and location of the autoantigens in the
small numbers of cells available for human fibroblast cell cultures
was only possible with development of sensitive assays. Werner's
syndrome fibroblasts derived from a 30- and a 60-year-old and human
normal fibroblasts derived from 29- and 59-year-old donors were
compared as to autoantigen content and quantity by hemagglutination
inhibition, Western blot, and fluorescent antibody microscopy.

We have developed a hemagglutination inhibition assay with

antigen-coated sheep red blood cells. The assay is capable of
detecting nanogram amounts of the antigens RNP and Sm. A typical
titering of antigen is demonstrated in Figure 15. This analysis
varies no more than 10% in repeated determinations with the same or
different lots of sheep red blood cells (A. Boak, K. Ellis, and P.
F. Agris, personal communication).

Our analyses for RNP and Sm antigens in Werner's and normal
fibroblasts were conducted with whole cell extracts from approximately 10^6 cells. All four cell strains had detectable quantities
of both antigens. The amount of the antigen RNP in each of the
cell strains was similar. However, there was about 50% less Sm in
the Werner's syndrome cells in comparison to the normal
fibroblasts.

Finally, the cellular localization of various antigens was
compared for the four cell strains. This was accomplished by
fixing cells grown on plastic coverslips. The fixed cells were
then reacted with different monospecific antisera containing
fluoroscein-conjugated antibody. The locale of the resulting
antigen-antibody complex is discerned by fluorescent microscopy.
Five different known nucleolar antibodies were used. No differences in the locations of the antigens were found.

Therefore, Werner's syndrome and normal fibroblasts do contain
the same autoantigenic macromolecules as detected by Western blot
and fluorescent antibody microscopy. The latter technique also
showed that the localizations of the antigens were the same.
However, a sensitive quantitative assay for the antigens RNP and Sm
was able to detect a 50% reduction in Sm in Werner's versus normal
fibroblasts. In other work, we have found Sm peptides that asso-
ciate with mRNA during or immediately after processing are still
with mRNA in the cytoplasm and on polysomes. This indicates that
Sm may be involved in mRNA maturation, transport or translation.
In effect, Sm may be involved in mRNA utilization and therefore
gene expression. The decreased Sm content of Werner's syndrome

Fig. 13. Ouchterlony double immunodiffusion analysis of antigens.
          Antigens in cell extracts are detected by Ouchterlony
          immunodiffusion and hemagglutination inhibition. In
          parts A and B of the figure an Ouchterlony analysis shows
          the RNase sensitivity of the antigen determinant RNP and
          the insensitivity of the antigen Sm. Both determinants
          reside on the same macromolecular complex, RNP-Sm.
          Interpretation of the results as to the difference be-
          tween purified antigen (RNP) and crude extract (CTE) is
          shown in part C. Crude extract has molecules carrying
          only the Sm determinant as well as RNP-Sm molecules.

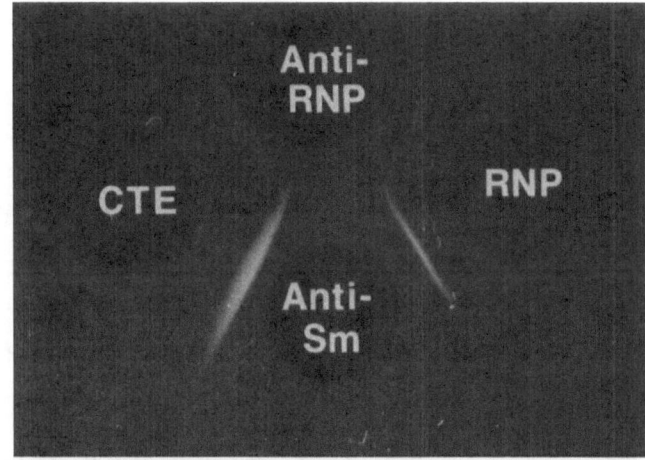

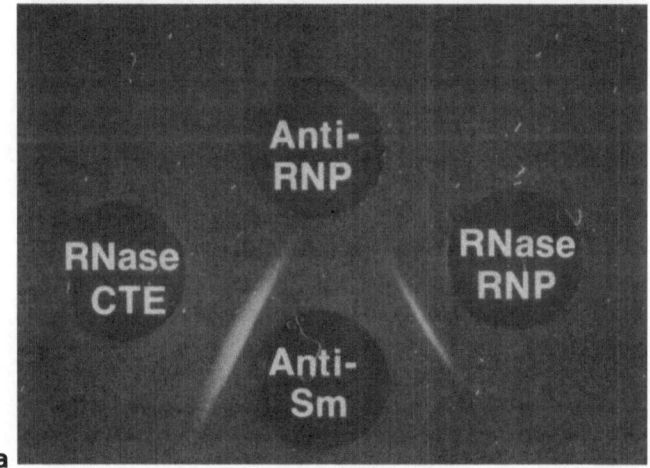

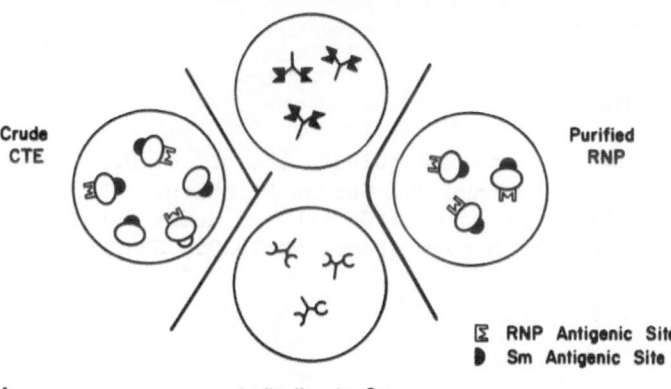

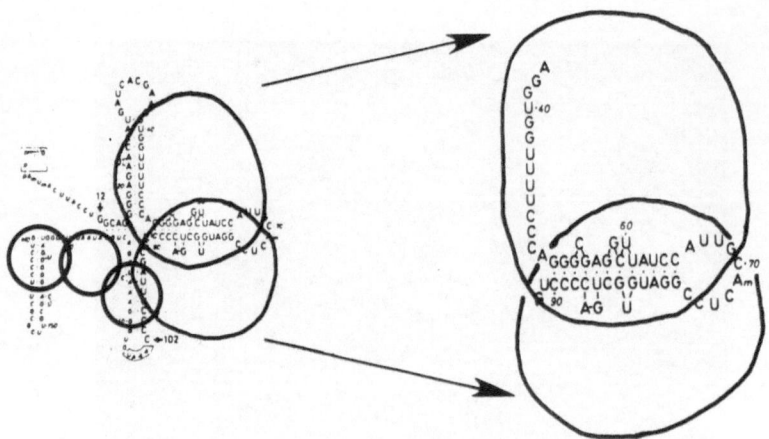

RNP / Sm ANTIGEN

   1. Ula RNA

      165 NUCLEOTIDES

   2. FIVE PEPTIDES

RNP DETERMINANT

   1. SEQUENCE OF 50 NUCLEOTIDES

   2. TWO PEPTIDES

Fig. 14. Nucleic acid-protein structure of the RNP-Sm antigen.
The figure depicts the secondary structure of the RNP
antigen containing the RNA sequence and two peptides.

cells in culture is of some interest when considering the decreased
viability and pathologic physiology of these cells compared to
normal fibroblasts.

ACKNOWLEDGMENTS

The authors wish to acknowledge the aid of Dr. Charles W.
Gehrke, Kenneth C. Kuo and Dr. Gordon C. Sharp. This work has been
supported by the Department of Health and Human Services, National
Institutes of Health through grants AM-20305, GM-27662, and
GM-23037.

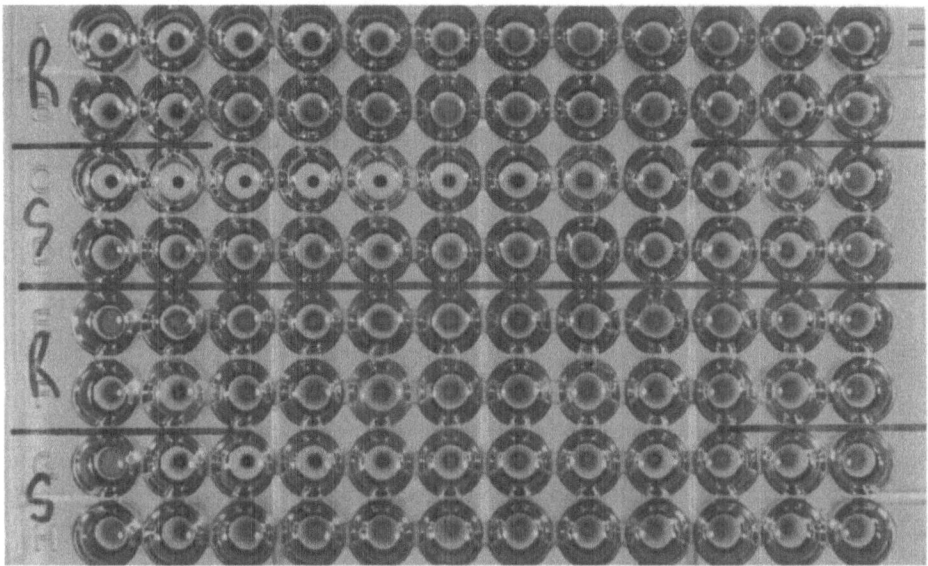

Fig. 15. Hemagglutination inhibition titer. Antigens in Werner's
          and normal fibroblasts are sensitively quantitated by
          hemagglutination inhibition. A representative titering
          of antigen extract is shown for analyses of RNP (R) and
          Sm (S) antigens using monospecific patient sera.
          Werner's fibroblasts were found to have 50% or less Sm
          antigen as their normal counterparts using this assay.
          RNP was present in Werner's and normal cells in prac-
          tically the same quantities.

REFERENCES

Agris, P. F., 1975, Arch. Biochem. Biophys., 170:114.
Agris, P. F., and Söll, D., 1977, in: "Nucleic Acid-Protein Recog-
    nition," H. Vogel, ed., Academic Press, New York, p. 321.
Agris, P. F., Powers, T., Söll, D., and Ruddle, F. H., 1975, Cancer
    Biochem. Biophys. 1:69.
Agris, P. F., Kovacs, S. A. H., Smith, C., Kopper, R. A., and
    Schmidt, P. G., 1983, Biochemistry, 22:1402.
Agris, P. F., Kopper, R. A., and Kopper, G., editors, 1983, "The
    Mofified Nucleosides of Transfer RNA II," Alan R. Liss, New
    York.
Altman, S., 1978, in: "Transfer RNA," S. Altman, ed., MIT Press,
    Cambridge, p. 48.
Bailey, A. F., 1975, in: "Inborn Errors of Skin, Hair, and Con-
    nective Tissue," J. Holton and J. T. Ireland, eds., Medical
    and Technical Publishing Co., Lancaster, England, p. 105.

Basler, J. W., David, J. D., and Agris, P. F., 1979, Exp. Cell
    Res., 118:73.
Chan, J. C., Yang, J. A., Dunn, M. J., Agris, P. F., and Wong, T.
    W., 1982, Nucleic Acids Res., 10:3755.
Erhlich, M., Gama-Sosa, M. A., Huang, L.-H., Midgett, R. M., Kuo,
    K. C., McCune, R. A., and Gehrke, C. W., 1982, Nucleic Acids
    Res., 8:2709.
Gefter, M. L., and Russell, R. L., 1969, J. Mol. Biol., 39:145.
Gehrke, C. W., Kuo, K. C., McCune, R. A., Gerhardt, K. O., and
    Agris, P. F., 1982, J. Chromatogr., 230:297.
Goldberg, B., Epstein, E. H., Jr., and Sherr, C. J., 1972, Proc.
    Natl. Acad. Sci. USA, 69:3655.
Grosjean, J., Söll, D., and Crothers, D. M., 1976, J. Mol. Biol.,
    103:499.
Grosjean, H., de Henau, S., and Crothers, D. M., 1978, Proc. Natl.
    Acad. Sci. USA, 75:610.
Johnson, A. D., Pateete, A. R., Lauer, G., Sauer, R. T., Ackers, G.
    K., and Ptashne, M., 1981, Nature, 294:217.
Kohli, J., 1983, in: "The Modified Nucleosides of Transfer RNA
    II," P. F. Agris, R. A. Kopper, and G. Kopper, eds., Alan R.
    Liss, New York.
Kopper, R. A., Schmidt, P. G., and Agris, P. F., 1982, Biochemis-
    try, 22:1396.
Lerner, M. R., Boyle, J. A., Mount, S. M., Wolin, S. L., and
    Steitz, J. A., 1980, Nature, 283:220.
Liautard, J. P., Sri-Wadada, J., Brunel, C., and Jeanteur, P.,
    1982, J. Mol. Biol., 162:623.
Lin, V. K., and Agris, P. F., 1980, Nucleic Acids Res., 8:3467.
Möller, A., Gabriels, J. E., Lafer, E. M., Nordheim, A., Rich, A.,
    and Stollar, B. D., 1982, J. Biol. Chem. 257:12081.
Munz, P., Leupold, U., Agris, P., and Kohli, J., 1981, Nature, 294,
    187.
Nakamura, R. M., 1974, "Immunopathology," Little, Brown and Co.,
Nishimura, S., 1972, Prog. Nucleic Acid Res. Mol. Biol., 12:49.
Ortwerth, B. J., and Liu, L. P., 1973, Biochemistry, 12:3978.
Ortwerth, B. J., Younschot, G. R., and Carlson, J. V., 1973,
    Biochemistry, 12:3985.
Rogers, J., and Wall, R., 1980, Proc. Natl. Acad. Sci. USA, 77:
    1877.
Salk, D., 1982, Human Genetics, 62:1.
Shapiro, J., editor, 1982, "Mobile Genetic Elements," Academic
    Press, London, in press.
Sharp, G. C., 1982, Arthritis Rheum., 25:757.
Shen, C. K. J., and Maniatis, T., 1980, Proc. Natl. Acad. Sci. USA,
    77:6634.
Spradling, A. C., and Rubin, G. M., 1981, Ann. Rev. Genet., 15:219.
Spradling, A. C., and Rubin, G. M., 1982, Science, 218:341.
Sprinzl, M., and Gauss, D. H., 1983, in: "The Modified Nucleosides
    of Transfer RNA II," P. F. Agris, R. A. Kopper, and G. Kopper,
    eds., Alan R. Liss, New York.

Strehler, B. L., Hirsch, G., Gusseck, D., Johnson, R., and Bick,
     M., 1971, J. Theor. Biol., 33:429.
Takano, M., Agris, P. F., and Sharp, G. C., 1980, J. Clin. Invest.,
     65:1449.
Takano, M., Golden, S., Sharp, G. C., and Agris, P. F., 1981,
     Biochemistry, 21:5929.
Zumwalt, R. W., Kuo, K. C. T., Agris, P. F., Ehrlich, M., and
     Gehrke, C. W., 1982, J. Liquid Chromatogr., 5:2041.

CYTOGENETIC ASPECTS OF WERNER SYNDROME

Darrell Salk*, Kam Au*, Holger Hoehn+, and George M. Martin*

* Department of Pathology, University of Washington
+ Department of Human Genetics, University of Wuerzburg

INTRODUCTION

Cultured skin fibroblast-like (FL) cells from patients with Werner syndrome display frequent pseudodiploidy involving multiple, variable structural chromosome rearrangements that are clonal (Salk et al., 1981a). This cytogenetic abnormality, which has been called variegated translocation mosaicism (VTM), has also recently been observed in peripheral blood lymphocytes (Scappaticci et al., 1982). Werner syndrome may properly be classified as a chromosome instability syndrome because, like Bloom syndrome, ataxia telangiectasia, Fanconi anemia, and xeroderma pigmentosum, it is autosomal recessive, displays chromosome instability, and is associated with an increased incidence of neoplasia.

The general cytogenetic aspects of Werner syndrome have recently been reviewed (Salk, 1982) and will only be summarized here. We present a recent analysis of the in vitro and in vivo occurrance of stable chromosome rearrangements, and a preliminary analysis of unstable rearrangements in FL cells and peripheral blood lymphocytes.

VARIEGATED TRANSLOCATION MOSAICISM

Ninety-two percent of 1,538 metaphases from 29 independent FL cell strains from five patients with Werner syndrome demonstrated multiple, variable, stable chromosome rearrangements (Salk et al., 1981a). In contrast, only eight (8.4 percent) of 95 non-Werner FL cell cultures demonstrated VTM: seven with low-grade VTM (approximately five percent of 300 metaphases) and one with VTM

541

affecting 90 to 100 percent of metaphases. Unlike the cytogenetic
abnormalities observed in the terminal stages of normal FL cell
cultures, VTM occurs throughout the entire lifespan of Werner
syndrome cultures.

Analysis of 16 major and 14 minor cytogenetically marked
clones throughout the proliferative phases of eight FL cell strains
from Werner syndrome patients indicates that clonal succession and
clonal attenuation occur in mass cultures, as predicted on the
basis of dilute plate cloning experiments using normal FL cells
(Salk et al., 1981b).

Individual chromosomes are affected approximately in
proportion to their length, but within chromosomes there is a
nonrandom distribution of rearrangement sites: four chromosomal
sites (1q12, 1q44, 5q12, and 6cen), representing only 3% of the
identifiable breakpoints in 1134 banded metaphases, account for 13%
of all definable rearrangements. The frequency distribution of
rearrangement sites is consistent with a model of specific
chromosomal hotspots overlying a Poisson-distributed background of
random rearrangement events. The chromosomal hotspots are not
reminiscent of those in other nonrandom structural chromosome
changes: eg. spontaneous, radiation induced, or chemical induced.

In comparison with the well-known chromosome instability
syndromes in man (Bloom syndrome, Fanconi anemia, ataxia
telangiectasia, xeroderma pigmentosum), chromatid aberrations,
unstable rearrangements, and chromatid exchange figures appear to
be uncommon in Werner syndrome. This suggests that the initial
structural change in VTM occurs during the G0/G1- or early S-phase
of the cell cycle, and/or that the de novo formation of aberrant
chromosomes is a rather infrequent event. To clarify these issues,
we studied the in vitro formation of chromosome rearrangements and
we quantitated chromosomal breakage and unstable chromosome
aberrations.

IN VITRO AND IN VIVO OCCURANCE OF VTM

Several observations have suggested that at least some of the
chromosome aberrations in Werner syndrome occur in vitro, but the
studies have not been conclusive. We described evolution of clonal
chromosome rearrangements (i.e. new rearrangements in a previously
recognized clone) in mass cultures of FL cells (Salk et al., 1981a;
1981b), but this finding could be explained by small numbers of
preexisting cells with these "new" rearrangements having become
evident only later in the life of the mass culture. Based on
studies of three EB virus transformed lymphoblastoid cell lines
from one patient, Schonberg et al. (1984) also suggest that
chromosome rearrangements in Werner syndrome can occur in vitro.

We have not yet observed any clonal chromosome rearrangements in preliminary studies of lymphoblastoid cell lines from three patients with Werner syndrome.

Similarly, it has not been clear if chromosome rearrangements occur in vivo in patients with Werner syndrome. Scappaticci et al. (1982) and Schonberg et al. (1984) examined Werner syndrome FL cells in the initial outgrowth from skin explants, and observed clonal chromosome rearrangements. This is suggestive, but not compelling evidence that the rearrangements had occurred in vivo; by the time the cells were analyzed they had been in culture for at least two or three weeks and had undergone an unknown number of divisions in vitro. Schonberg et al. interpret their findings as evidence of the in vitro development of chromosome rearrangements. Other evidence for the in vivo occurrence of clonal chromosome rearrangements is the observation by Scappaticci et al. of identical rearrangements in two separate blood samples from a single patient. There are other possible, although unlikely explanations for this finding, and the interpretation is made difficult by their report of four instances of apparently identical rearrangements in unrelated patients or in different tissues from the same patient.

In the present study we tested for the frequency of de novo chromosomal rearrangements in FL cells in vitro by preparing multiple skin explants from one patient with Werner syndrome and studying the cytogenetics of colonies derived from single cells. To establish colonies that would still be actively growing after seven to ten population doublings (colonies of 100 to 1000 cells), we dilute-plated cells obtained from the earliest possible stages of explant outgrowth.

We analyzed a total of thirty-one colonies derived from dilute platings of six independent primary cultures. Within each colony all of the metaphases had the same basic cytogenetic description (there was only one instance of a "foreign metaphase" contaminating an otherwise pure colony). There were ten different basic karyotypes represented, including two colonies with apparently normal metaphases.

We observed fourteen instances of cells within a colony showing a new structural rearrangement in addition to the basic clonal karyotype: a number of these variants were chromosome breaks or deletions for which an exchange of material could not be documented. Twelve cells were single instances of different rearrangements and two cells in one colony showed identical new rearrangements, thereby fitting the definition of a de novo cytogenetic clone. In view of the variety and number of structural rearrangements observed in Werner syndrome FL cell cultures, these results demonstrate remarkable stability in vitro: 90% of 139 metaphases displayed only the basic karyotype characteristic of a given colony.

Two cytogenetically identical clones appeared in more than one dilute-plated culture. These two cultures were independently derived from separate explants. Considering the stability we observed in vitro and the rarity of identical rearrangements in our previous studies, it appears that multiple cells with these two chromosome markers were already present in the piece of skin from which the explants were prepared. This observation indicates that chromosome rearrangements can occur in dermal cells in vivo in patients with Werner syndrome.

In preliminary studies of peripheral blood lymphocytes from two patients with Werner syndrome, we have examined R-banded chromosomes prepared from 48 hour cultures. At 48 hours after PHA stimulation, essentially all metaphases represent cells in their first division in vitro. We have seen instances of stable structural rearrangements in cultures from both patients, although none were clonal. These findings are compatible with either in vivo origin of chromosome rearrangments or occurrence of the initial structural change during G0/G1 or early S-phase in vitro.

Table 1. Unstable structural chromosome lesions in Werner syndrome.

Study	Cell type*	Type+ and no. of subjects	No. of cells	Aberration frequency	Relative rates
Nordenson (1977)	PBL	WS - 4	650	.136	19
		Nl - 3	300	.007	1
Scappaticci et al. (1982)	PBL	WS - 6	900	.140	4
		Hz - 4	400	.040	1
		Nl - 6	600	.040	1
Salk et al.	PBL	WS - 2	588	.061	2.5
		Hz - 1	104	.010	0.4
		Nl - 2	375	.024	1
Scappaticci et al. (1982)	FL	WS - 5	58	.260	2.6
		Nl - 5	130	.100	1
Salk et al.	FL	WS - 2	867	.283	4.6
		Nl - 2	817	.061	1

* PBL: peripheral blood lymphocytes; FL: cultured skin fibroblast-
   like cells.
+ WS: Werner syndrome; Hz: obligate Werner syndrome heterozygote;
   1: normal control.

UNSTABLE CHROMOSOME ABERRATIONS

Chromosome breakage and the formation of unstable aberrations have not been striking findings in Werner syndrome cultures when control cultures have not been simultaneously analyzed (Salk et al., 1981a; Schonberg et al., 1984). However, both Nordenson (1977) and Scappaticci et al. (1982) reported an increase in breakage in Werner syndrome cells compared with normal controls.

We analyzed both FL cells and peripheral blood lymphocytes from Werner syndrome patients and compared the results with those previously reported (Table 1). It appears that there is consistently a slight increase in the amount of gaps, breaks, and unstable chromosome aberrations in Werner syndrome cells. The amount af breakage reported by Nordenson seems much greater, but even so the increase she observed is not as large as that for the patients with Fanconi anemia in her study. We did not see a significant difference between the amount of chromatid and chromosome lesions (Table 2).

These results indicate that the chromosome instability associated with Werner syndrome is not limited to stable chromosome rearrangements in FL cells. Aberrations are observed in hematopoetic cells as well, and there is an elevated level of chromosomal breakage, albeit much less than that observed in the classical chromosome instability syndromes. It should be noted that although chromosome breakage is the most obvious manifestation of instability in the other chromosome instability syndromes, stable structural chromosome rearrangements are also seen with some frequency (Hoehn and Salk, 1984). There are distinct cytogenetic differences among the these conditions, but the factors they have in common (the association of a recessive genetic defect with chromosome instability and an increased incidence of neoplasia) present intriguing and challenging questions that may best be answered by consideration of these diseases as a group.

Table 2. Frequency of unstable chromosome lesions in Werner syndrome FL cell cultures.

	No. cells	Chromatid lesions	Chromosome lesions
Normal 1	500	.028	.034
Normal 2	317	.032	.034
Werner 1	363	.105	.190
Werner 2	504	.141	.129

REFERENCES

Hoehn, H., Salk, D. (1984) Clonal analysis of Bloom syndrome
    fibroblasts. II. Frequency and distribution of stable
    rearrangements. Cancer Genet. Cytogenet. 11:405-415.
Nordenson, I. (1977). Chromosome breaks in Werner's syndrome and
    their prevention in vitro by radical-scavenging enzymes.
    Hereditas 87:151-154.
Salk, D. (1982). Werner syndrome: A review of recent research with
    an analysis of connective tissue metabolism, growth control of
    cultured cells, and chromosomal aberrations. Hum. Genet.
    62:1-15.
Salk, D., Au, K., Hoehn, H., Martin, G. M. (1981a). Cytogenetics of
    Werner syndrome cultured skin fibroblasts: variegated
    translocation mosaicism. Cytogenet. Cell Genet. 30:92-107.
Salk, D., Au, K., Hoehn, H., Stenchever, M. R., Martin, G. M.
    (1981b). Evidence of clonal attenuation, clonal succession,
    and clonal expansion in mass cultures of aging Werner syndrome
    skin fibroblasts. Cytogenet. Cell Genet. 30:108-117.
Scappaticci, S., Cerimele, D., Fraccaro, M. (1982). Clonal
    structural chromosomal rearrangements in primary fibroblast
    cultures and in lymphocytes of patients with Werner's syndrome.
    Hum. Genet. 62:16-24.
Schonberg, S., Niermeijer, M.F., Bootsma, D., Henderson, E.,
    German, J. (1984). Werner's syndrome: Proliferation in vitro
    of clones of cells bearing chromosome translocations. Am. J.
    Hum. Genet. 36:387-397.

A POPULATION AND CYTOGENETIC STUDY OF

THE WERNER SYNDROME IN SARDINIA

M. Fraccaro, S. Scappaticci*, and D. Cerimele**

*Istituto di Biologia Generale e Genetica Medica
Università di Pavia
Pavia, Italy

**Clinica Dermatologica, Università di Sassari
Sassari, Italy

Several patients with the Werner syndrome in a group of related families in Sardinia were reported briefly by Rabbiosi and Borroni (1979). We have recently re-investigated these families, ascertained two additional families with three new patients and performed a detailed cytogenetic study on six of the living patients. These investigations are reported in detail in two papers by Cerimele et al. (1982) and by Scappaticci et al. (1982). At this symposium we give a synopsis of the main results of the population and cytogenetic studies, while for the clinical data the reader is referred to the paper by Cerimele et al. (1982).

PREVALENCE OF THE WERNER SYNDROME IN SARDINIA

The pedigrees of the three families' groups are reproduced in Figs. 1, 2 and 3. All patients were born and still reside in the three villages of Budoni (Pedigree 1), Tresnuraghes (Pedigree 2), and Bono (Pedigree 3). In 1961 the first two villages were in the administrative district of Nuoro, while Bona belongs to the administration of the province of Sassari. The resident populations of the villages at two censuses are given in Table 1. These villages have always been peripheral to the main routes of communication and they are still quite isolated.

547

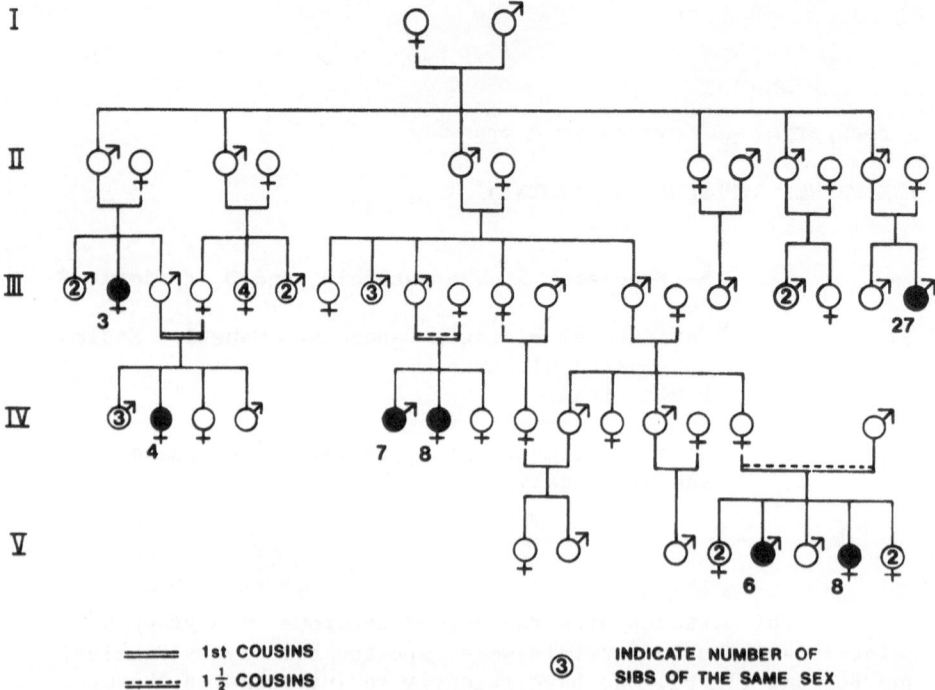

Fig. 1. Partial pedigree of Family 1. Filled circles: Patients
with the Werner syndrome.

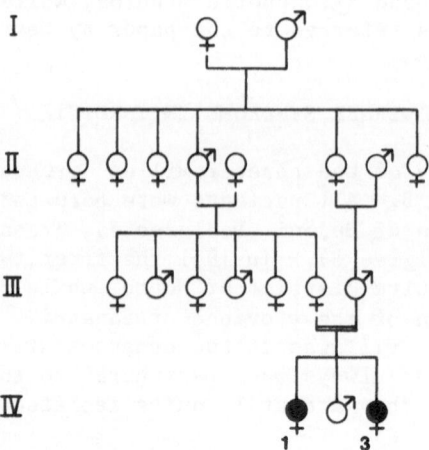

Fig. 2. Partial pedigree of Family 2. Symbols as in Fig. 1.

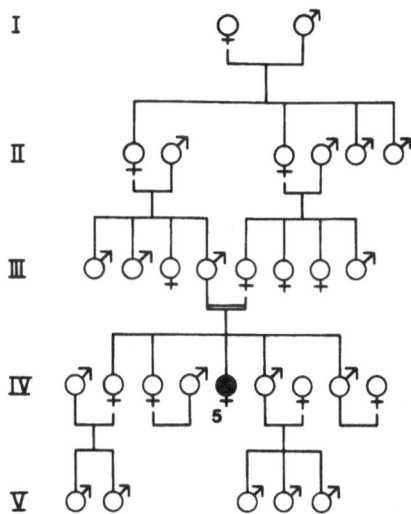

Fig. 3. Partial pedigree of Family 3. Symbols as in Fig. 1.

The resident population of the Provinces of Sassari and
Nuoro in 1961 was N = 664,397. Defining the prevalence as the
number of living cases with the trait (n) in a given area at a
given time divided by the population size (N) in the same area,
and taking n = 7 we obtain a prevalence of 1:94,914. If we take
N = 1,419,362 for the whole population of Sardinia in 1961, the
prevalence is 1:202,766.

Reported consanguinity among the seven sets of parents of
the ten subjects with the Werner syndrome included three first-
cousin and one-second cousin marriages. Reports obtained in the
field were cross-checked with the collection of consanguinous
marriages obtained from Church dispensation registers for the
whole of Italy (courtesy of Prof. A. Moroni, University of
Parma). This confirmed the three first-cousin marriages but
corrected the second-cousin marriage to first cousins once
removed and revealed a second pair with this type of
relationship. Thus, the proportion of first cousin marriages
among the parents of the Werner syndrome patient was C' (1/16) =
42.86 and that of first cousins once removed was C' (1/32) =
28.57, and the corresponding values for the whole population of
the Nuoro and Sassari district were C(1/16) = 3.624 and C(1/32) =
1.162. Using these parameters we obtained an estimate of the
gene frequency (q) using Dahlberg's formula (Dahlberg, 1950):

$$q = \frac{C(1-C')}{16C'-15-CC'} = 0.003288$$

Table 1. Population size and number of patients with the Werner
          syndrome in three Sardinian villages.

Family group (village)	Population at census of 1961	1981	No. of patients (living)
1 (Budoni)	2421	3096	7 (6)
2 (Tresnuraghes)	4024	1583	2 (2)
3 (Bono)	4906	2053	1 (1)

This yields a frequency of the syndrome (q^2) of 1:92,515.
Dahlberg's formula gives efficient estimates when the frequency
of consanguineous marriages other than those among first cousins
is negligible, but this is not the case for our sample nor for
the whole of Sardinia. An alternative estimate using a more
efficient method (see Cerimele et al., 1982) yields a value of q^2
= 1:454,505.

For the time being the small sample size precludes the use
of more refined estimates of gene frequency. Our sample is
confined to the northern part of Sardinia and, although we are
not aware of any published or unpublished case of the Werner
syndrome in the large southern province of Cagliari, an estimate
of the prevalence and gene frequency of the Werner syndrome for
the whole of the island must await further information.

With these limitations in mind, the prevalence of the Werner
syndrome in Sardinia is the highest thus far reported, much
higher than that of 1:300,000 estimated by Goto et al. (1981) for
the Japanese population.

CYTOGENETICS OF PRIMARY LYMPHOCYTE AND FIBROBLAST CULTURES

The concentration of several living patients in a few
families gave us the opportunity to investigate the cytogenetics
of the Werner syndrome with repeated sampling of blood and, in
some cases, also of skin biopsies. Thus, we were able to
investigate both the incidence of chromosome breaks and
aneuploidy in lymphocytes and also to score for the presence of
chromosomal rearrangements in primary fibroblast cultures. This
was never done before, since the discovery of extensive
translocation mosaicism and related clonal evolution was done in
fibroblasts examined after the second in vitro transfer (Norwood
et al., 1979; Salk et al., 1981a; 1981b). Primary conditions
were achieved by processing in situ the metaphases in the

outgrowth halos from primary skin explants from the patients with
the Werner syndrome.

The main results of these investigations were as follows:

1.   There is an increased frequency of chromosome breakage
in cultured lymphocytes (unbanded preparations) from the Werner
syndrome patients. The proportion of abnormalities (chromosome
and chromatid breaks, fragments and rearrangements) per cell
ranges from 0.02 to 0.23 with a mean value of 0.15. The mean
value for control is 0.04 (0-0.02) and for four of the obligate
heterozygotes 0.03 (0-0.06). These results were obtained in 100
cells for each of six patients. It is relevant that we did find
structural rearrangements also in this material. The same trend
was observed also in the primary fibroblast cultures from five
patients. In these the proportion of abnormalities per cell
ranged from 0.09 to 0.40 in the patients and from 0.09 to 0.18 in
the controls.

2.   The proportion of abnormalities per cell has a tendency
to increase with age between patients and also within the same
patient in lymphocyte cultures obtained at consecutive time
intervals. If this trend can be confirmed in a large sample of
patients, it will be a further sign of "aging" at the chromosomal
level in the Werner syndrome.

3.   Clear evidence for the existence of clonal structural
chromosome rearrangements (the "variegated translocation
mosaicism" as defined in Salk et al., 1981a) was obtained in the
necessarily limited number of metaphases analyzed directly in the
outgrowth halos of primary skin explants. This is as near as it
is possible to obtain to the in vivo condition and suggests that
the structural changes originate in fibroblast precursors in
vivo.

4.   We demonstrated for the first time that the phenomenon
of clonal structural rearrangements is present also in blood
lymphocytes cultured in vitro for 72 hours.

5.   The presence and clonal evolution of the X chromosome
abnormality known as "premature centromere disjunction" was found
in cultured lymphocytes of female patients. This abnormality was
never found before in Werner's patients and, since it is
considered characteristic of the lymphocyte cultures of old women
(Galloway and Buckton, 1978), can be also considered as a new
sign of "aging" in the Werner syndrome.

In conclusion, the finding of a high prevalence of the
Werner syndrome in Sardinia allowed us to demonstrate that
chromosome aberrations of the "variegated translocation

mosaicism" type are manifested in the same way in fibroblasts and lymphocytes and they are probably age dependent, thus confirming definitely that the Werner syndrome is indeed a chromosome rearrangement syndrome.

REFERENCES

Cerimele, D., Cottoni, F., Scappaticci, S., Rabbiosi, G., Borroni, G., Sanna, E., Zei, G., Fraccaro, M., 1982, High prevalence of Werner syndrome in Sardinia. Description of six patients and estimates of the gene frequency, Hum. Genet., 62:25-30.

Dahlberg, G., 1950, Methods for population genetics, Am. J. Biol., 25:9(104.

Galloway, S.M., Buckton, K.E., 1978, Aneuploidy and ageing: chromosome studies on a random sample of the population using G-banding, Cytogenet. Cell Genet., 20:78-95.

Goto, M., Tanimoto, K., Horiuchi, Y., Sasazuki, T., 1981, Family analys: of Werner's syndrome: A survey of 42 Japanese families with reviev the literature, Clin. Genet. 19:8-15.

Norwood, T.H., Hoehn, H., Salk, D., Martin, G.M., 1979, Cellular aging : Werner's syndrome: A unique phenotype? J. Invest. Dermatol., 78:! 96.

Rabbiosi, G., Borroni, G., 1979, Werner's syndrome: Seven cases in one family, Dermatologica, 158:355-360.

Salk, D., Au, K., Hoehn, H., Martin, G.M., 1981a, Cytogenetics of Werner syndrome cultured skin fibroblasts: Variegated translocation mosaicism, Cytogenet. Cell Genet., 30:92-107.

Salk, D., Au, K., Hoehn, H., Stenchever, M.R., Martin, G.M., 1981b, Evidence of clonal expansion in mass cultures of aging Werner's syndrome skin fibroblasts, Cytogenet. Cell Genet. 30:108-117.

Scappaticci, S., Cerimele, D., Fraccaro, M., 1982, Clonal structural chromosomal rearrangements in primary fibroblast cultures and in lymphocytes of patients with Werner's syndrome, Hum. Genet., 62:16·

PROTEOGLYCANS IN THE WERNER SYNDROME AND AGING:
A REVIEW AND PERSPECTIVE

Eileen Bryant, Darrell Salk and Tom Wight

Department of Pathology
University of Washington
Seattle, WA, USA

INTRODUCTION

The Werner syndrome (WS), like several other "segmental progeroid syndromes," provides a valuable system for investigating the genetic control of longevity and age-related pathology (Martin, 1978). In WS, except for short stature, symptoms develop in adult life and include graying and generalized loss of hair, juvenile cataracts, scleroderma-like changes in the skin, and high incidence of neoplasms. Epstein et al. (1966) noted that many of the changes in WS in vivo were suggestive of an impairment in the development and metabolism of connective tissue. Clinically, a prominent feature is atrophy of the skin over areas in which the subcutaneous adipose tissue is depleted, resulting in a shiny smooth skin which cannot be lifted or is actually adherent to the underlying tissue. There is usually atrophy of the underlying connective tissue, musculature and fat, and development of hyperkeratoses over the bony prominences. The hyperkeratoses often become ulcerated. WS patients show an increase in occurrence of mesenchymal type tumors such as fibroliposarcomas, osteogenic sarcomas, hemangiolipomas and menigiomas. Japanese researchers (Tonkunaga, et al., 1975; Goto and Murata, 1978; Zebrower et al., 1984) have identified another connective tissue-related clinical characteristic: excessive excretion of hyaluronic acid in urine. Although these clinical manifestations are reminiscent of the aging process, there is still uncertainty as to whether this syndrome is truly a caricature of aging. Part of this uncertainty arises from the paucity of information concerning the molecular events associated with aging at the tissue and cell level. More specifically, little is known about those changes that take place within specific connective tissues of patients with the Werner syndrome.

Most connective tissue is composed of at least three different types of molecules: collagen, proteoglycan (PG) and glycoprotein. Changes in collagen have been implicated in the pathogenesis of WS. For example, Fleischmajer and Nedwich (1973) reported elevated collagen content in the skin of a patient with WS. Gottesman et al. (1980) noted variable collagen fibril size and fraying of fibrils in a WS skin biopsy. Basler et al. (1979) presented evidence that fibroblasts cultured from Werner's patients produce an incompletely processed collagen molecule suggestive of defective collagen synthesis. However, it is unclear from these studies whether abnormal collagen production is a specific defect unique to cells from Werner patients or merely reflects a general abnormality in the production of other connective tissue components.

Proteoglycans and their constituent glycosaminoglycans (GAG) have also been implicated in WS. These structural macromolecules form important links between the cellular and intercellular compartments of all tissues (Wight, 1980) and influence or are influenced by many different cell processes fundamental to morphogenesis and aging.

It is the intent of this review to focus on PG and what is known about changes in these molecules with normal aging and WS. PG are defined as high molecular weight protein polysaccharides that consist of carbohydrate polymers (GAG) covalently linked to a protein backbone or core. The major type of carbohydrate protein linkage has been recognized as an O-glycosidic linkage between D-xylose of the polysaccharide and the hydroxyl group of the amino acid serine. Basically, the carbohydrate (GAG) consists of unbranched chains of repeating disaccharide units in which one of the monosaccharides is an amino sugar and the other is a hexuronic acid. There are different types of GAGs, depending upon the nature of the monosaccharides that constitute the repeating disaccharide chains. In mammalian tissues there are 5 major classes of GAG: hyaluronic acid (HA), chondroitin sulfates (CS), dermatan sulfates (DS), keratan sulfates (KS) and heparan sulfates HS). Hyaluronic acid differs from the other GAG in that it is nonsulfated, and evidence currently available indicates that HA is not covalently linked to protein. It is now established that PGs are synthesized by the same basic process with the first step being the synthesis of the core protein to which the carbohydrates are subsequently attached. The general pattern of GAG synthesis appears to be stepwise transfer of a monosaccharide unit from the appropriate nucleotide sugar to the nascent polysaccharide chain. The stepwise synthesis occurs initially in the membrane of the rough endoplasmic reticulum (RER) with chain elongation, sulfation and chain termination occurring in the membranes of the Golgi apparatus. The complexity of the molecule provides for many levels of regulation of synthesis and little is known about such critical factors regulating synthesis and carbohydrate chain termination (Roden and Schwartz, 1975).

PROTEOGLYCANS IN AGING: IN VIVO AND IN VITRO STUDIES

Proteoglycans comprise a major portion of the extracellular matrix of cartilage and the elasticity of cartilage is related to the content and structure of the PG in the matrix (Scott, 1973). Age-related changes in the structure of the sulfated PG component of cartilage matrix have been studied extensively. Most vertebrate cartilage contains chondroitin sulfate and keratan sulfate covalently attached to a central protein core. The proportion of these types, as well as their degree of sulfation, varies with species, site and age. For example, studies on composition of the costal cartilage of rats shows a decrease in chondroitin-6-sulfate (CS-6) and an increase in chondroitin-4-sulfate (CS-4) over the first 9 months of life (Kennedy, 1976). The composition of human costal cartilage changes more dramatically with age. During fetal growth, CS-4 (50%) and CS-6 (50%) comprise between 80-100% of the total GAG. After birth, the CS-6 component falls very slightly throughout life while the CS-4 fraction drops after the first 2-3 years of postnatal life, reaching 5% by 40 years of age (Mathews and Glagov, 1966). These reductions in CS species are balanced by a rise in keratan sulfate from 3-40 years. Murata and Bjelle (1980) compared the compositions of CS isomers in PG of bovine articular cartilages of three different ages. Their results indicate that with increasing age, the relative proportion of CS-4 in total GAG decreased and the CS-6 increased.

A comparison of bovine articular cartilage from immature (1-2 mos) and adult (3-5 yrs) animals indicates several age-related changes: 1) the PG became smaller due mainly to a reduction in the CS regions (i.e. fewer and shorter GAG chains) and 2) the KS rich region became larger (Sweet, et al., 1979; Inerot et al., 1978). These changes may be the result of a shortening of the protein core, but whether this change is a post-transitional modification or a change at the level of transcription awaits clarification. The physiological implications of a change in PG size and composition are not understood. Equivalent amounts of keratan sulfate influence stiffness more than chondroitin sulfate, suggesting a possible advantage of keratan sulfate rich PG in adult cartilage subject to high load.

Fleischmajer et al. (1973b) observed that the amount of GAG present in human dermis decreases steadily with age for both hyaluronic acid and dermatan sulfate. Hexosamines are present at 5.8 times the concentration of uronic acid in the newborn and at 10.2 times this concentration in the individual over 65.

Cell culture techniques have been used to study PG changes in aging. Cultured fibroblasts from lung and skin have been the predominant cell type used because this type of cell is easy to obtain and to propagate in vitro, and age-associated changes in PG and GAG have been described in these tissues during in vivo aging (Fleischmajer et al., 1973; Damle et al., 1982). Schachtschabel and Wever (1978), using WI-38 cells (lung fibroblasts), reported a gradual decline in the synthesis of GAG, as evidenced by reduced rates of incorporation of ^{35}S-sulfate and ^{14}C-glucosamine into total cellular and extracellular GAG. The decrease in radioactive precursor incorporation was not uniform. A preliminary analysis revealed a relatively stronger age-dependent reduction in ^{35}S-sulfate incorporation into extracellular CS. In further studies by this group (Sluke et al., 1981; Wever et al., 1980), WI-38 cells were treated with heparin at 20-500 g/ml. Cell proliferation was inhibited while GAG synthesis was stimulated. Characterization of the individual GAG types revealed an increased incorporation of ^{35}S-sulfate and ^{14}C-glucosamine in the HS and HA fractions of heparin-treated cells.

Vogel and colleagues (Vogel and Kendall, 1980; Vogel et al., 1981) used IMR-90 lung fibroblasts to investigate the synthesis and turnover of ^{35}S-labelled GAG in the extracellular medium, cell surface and intracellular culture compartments during in vitro cellular aging. Their results show two differences and two similarities in GAG metabolism of cultured fibroblasts during in vitro aging. The alterations are: 1) a decrease in incorporation of ^{35}S-sulfate into GAG released to the medium; and 2) delayed movement of pulse-labelled ^{35}S-GAG from cytoplasm to the cell surface and extracellular compartments. The amount of ^{35}S-GAG/mg protein at the cell surface of early and late passage cells as well as the composition of the GAG in each cell compartment did not change. Vogel and colleagues' observation of a decline in the ^{35}S incorporation into extracellular GAG is similar to the results of Schachtschabel and Weaver (1978). Decreased sulfation capability is not supported, however, by experiments with exogenous xyloside. Xyloside addition resulted in a tenfold stimulation of extracellular ^{35}S GAG production by both early and late passage fibroblast cultures. The observation that both cultures could be stimulated by the presence of exogenous initiation sites suggests that synthetic and sulfation capabilities are not limiting in late passage cells. Although there is as yet no explanation for the cause of the decline in GAG in the culture medium, the results of Vogel and his co-workers support the concept that secreted and cell surface GAG in IMR-90 fibroblasts represent different metabolic pools.

These investigators have expanded their studies by examining the native structure of the PG molecule from early and late passage

IMR-90 cells (Vogel and Peterson, 1981; Vogel and Sapien, 1982; Vogel and Pitcher, 1982). IMR-90 cells secrete at least three distinct PG populations which are unique in GAG composition and hydrodynamic size. Proteoglycans produced by early and late passage cells were similar. In medium from late passage cultures, larger components comprised an increased proportion of the total PG. Alterations of fibroblast-produced lung PG during normal aging in vivo have not been described so comparisons between possible in vivo changes and the few in vitro change described cannot be made.

Matuoka and Mitsui investigated changes in GAG during in vitro aging of lung fibroblasts. They considered the growth state of the cultures as well as the proliferative capacity. Their results demonstrate no change in GAG production in preconfluent (i.e. proliferating) cultures with increasing population doubling level (PDL). In stationary phase (confluent) cultures, the total GAG production decreased with in vitro age. This is similar to what is seen in vivo: the GAG content in human skin decreases with age. In contrast to the overall decline in GAG synthesis in in vitro aging of confluent cultures, HS on the cell surface increased as a function of PDL regardless of growth state. These investigators tested the role of cell surface HS in direct interaction in the density-dependent inhibition of cell proliferation with a new experimental system in which cells are cultivated on fixed sheets of cells degraded with various enzymes or chemicals. The cultivation of cells on gluteraldehyde-fixed cell sheets resulted in growth inhibition. The growth-inhibiting effect on the glytraldehyde fixed cell sheets was lost after heparan sulfate was degraded by heparinase or nitrous acid. This observation suggests the possibility that HS is a regulator of cell proliferation. Alterations in the cell surface during cellular aging could be determined by investigations on the physiological role of HS on the cell surface.

PROTEOGLYCANS IN WERNER SYNDROME: IN VIVO AND IN VITRO

Studies by Fleischmajer and Nedwich (1973) on skin from "scleroderma-like lesions" of WS patients, showed two important findings: (1) There was an absolute increase in the amount of hexosamines. This may reflect an increase in the total amount of connective tissue which replaces subcutaneous fat; (2) There was a marked increase in DS. In studies of autopsy-derived skin obtained from relatively normal appearing regions, we have observed a significant reduction in total GAGs per dry weight tissue in two patients compared with skin from 14 normal controls ranging in age from 20-70 years (Iozzo, Salk and Wight, unpublished). The decrease in total GAG was due to reduced amounts of HA and DS.

Recently several groups have reported changes of urinary glycosaminoslycans in WS (Murata, 1982; Zebrower et al., 1984). Since urinary GAG are one of the final products of connective tissue, these changes may relate to metabolic changes occurring in connective tissue. The most characteristic feature of urinary GAG in WS was an increased proportion of haluronic acid. This increase appeared to be specific for WS and may turn out to be useful for diagnosis, although Brown et al. (1984) have also reported increased urinary HA in patients with Hutchinson–Guilford progeria. In addition, the proportion of C-4S to total GAG was decreased. This observation corresponds' with the decrease in C-4S seen in normal aging. The composition of chondroitin sulfates in connective tissues such as cartilage shows changes with age.

Tajima and colleagues have recently reported studies of GAG production by cultured skin fibroblasts from WS patients. Their results show an increased accumulation of both HA and sulfated GAGs in intercellular, pericellular and extracellular material. The increased accumulation of GAG in WS fibroblast was not caused by differences in the growth state of the cells because the WS strains and controls had similar saturation density, population doubling level and doubling time.

Preliminary studies of WS cultured skin fibroblasts in our laboratory yield similar results. Early passage WS skin fibroblast and early and late passage age-matched, normal skin fibroblasts were used to determine whether differences existed in the synthesis and secretion of PG. One of our main concerns was to eliminate differences which might be caused by differences in growth state rather than differences that were related to in vitro age or disease states. We have incorporated a number of growth related parameters into the basic design of the experiment. The growth state of the cells was monitored by standard techniques of 24 h ^{3}H-thymidine labelling index and flow microfluorometric determination of DNA content. These techniques allow for the comparison of the remaining proliferative potential and the proliferative state (proportion of cells in different phases of the cell cycle). At the time of PG analysis, cell numbers were determined by standard hemocytometer cell counts. In addition, total DNA and protein content were measured by simultaneously staining with propidium iodide (PI) for DNA and flourescin isothiocyanate (FITC) for protein and analyzing on an Ortho dual parameter cell sorter. These different parameters for characterizing the cells at the time of PG analysis are necessary to normalize for differences in cell number, cell size and DNA and protein content (Table I).

TABLE 1

Culture	24 hr. labelling index	Cell cycle analysis (a)		Protein Content per cell (b)	
Young normal 72-166$_{T12}$	40%	G_1 79.5% G_2 13.6% S 7.4%		G_1 34.8% G_2 70.2%	
Old normal 72-166$_{T18}$	14%	G_1 76.9% G_2 15.7% S 7.3%		G_1 39.6% G_2 75.9%	
Werner 78-80$_{T4}$	18%	G_1 68.3% G_2 25.8% S 6.1%		G_1 40.0% G_2 80.3%	

a Propidium Iodide (DNA stain) flow cytometry
b FITC-PI (Protein-DNA stain) dual parameter flow cytometry; arbitrary units.

Synthesis of PG was studied by labelling the cultures for 24 h with 50 μCi/ml ^{35}S-sulfate and 5 μCi/ml ^{3}H-glucosamine and isolating the culture medium and cell layer by extraction with 4M GuHCl in the presence of protease inhibitors (Oegma et al., 1975). Medium-and cell-associated PG were analyzed by molecular sieve chromatography: three different WS strains and two different normal controls were examined. Two of the WS strains (78-80KS and 78-76A) incorporated two to three times more ^{35}S-sulfate into PG that the early and late passage control cultures. One WS strain, H81-26A, was similar to controls in terms of ^{35}S-sulfate incorporation (Table II.) The growth state and DNA content of the different cultures were equivalent at the time of biochemical analysis.

^{35}S-sulfate labelled cell-associated proteoglycans from the WS and control cultures were separated into three size classes by Sepharose CL-2B gel chromatography. The largest component (C-I) eluted in the void volume. An intermediate population (C-II and a small population C-III) eluted in the included volume. In contrast, PG of the medium were separated into two size classes. The elution position of the larger medium component (M-I) eluted at the same position as C-II (Fig. I). ^{3}H-glucosamine labelled cell associated PG from all cultures eluted in the void volume of

Table II

INCORPORATION OF ^{3}H-GLUCOSAMINE AND 35S-SULFATE INTO PROTEOGLYCANS

	^{3}H-GLN*			35S-sulfate*		
	Cell layer	Medium	Total	Cell layer	Medium	Total
EXPERIMENT III						
Young	288 + 18.5 (49%)	291 + 2.8 (51%)	578	71 + 5.5 (21%)	223 + 3.0 (79%)	294
Old	205 + 4.7 (27%)	540 + 2.8 (73%)	745	118 + 3.5 (51%)	111 + 8.7 (49%)	229
WS [a]	456 + 17.4 (36%)	788 + 37.1 (64%)	1245	155 + 9.5 (16%)	651 + 83.7 (84%)	806
EXPERIMENT IV						
Young	581 (35%)	1051 (65%)	1633	302 (50%)	312 (50%)	622
Old	408 (27.6%)	1069 (72%)	1478	255 (39%)	404 (61%)	659
WS [b]	413 (32%)	858 (67%)	1272	348 (27%)	925 (72%)	1274
HWS [c]	440 (35%)	807 (65%)	1247	269 (43%)	355 (57%)	624

*CPM x 10^3/10^6 cells

a = 78-80KS
b = 78-76A
c = H81-26A

Sepharose CL-2B

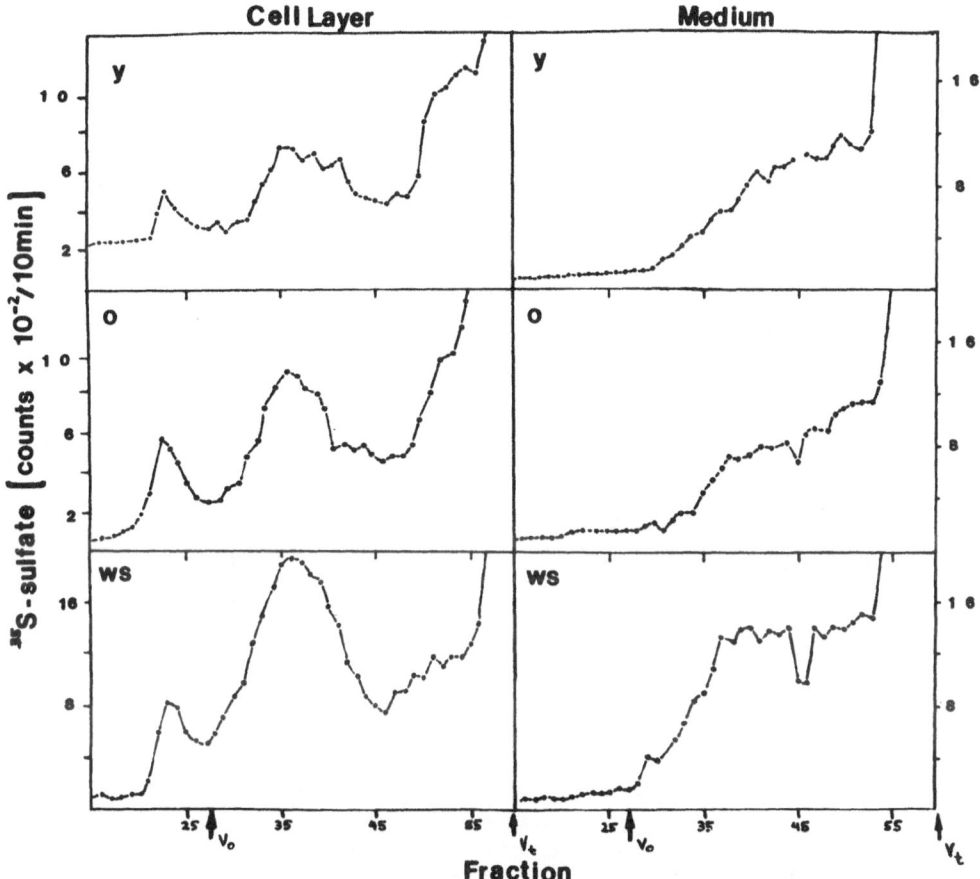

Figure 1:   Sepharose CL2B profiles of 36S-labeled proteoglycans
            from the cell layer and medium of (Y) early passage
            normal, (O) late passage normal and (WS) Werner Syndrome
            fibroblasts in culture.

Sepharose CL-2B. Cl-2B profiles of the 3H-glucosamine labelled
medium PG were similar for the H81-26 WS strain and the young and
old controls with a peak in the void volume of the medium fraction.
However, for WS 78-76A, this void volume peak was absent.

    Medium and cell associated PG from WS and normal fibroblasts
were further purified by cesium chloride (CsCl) density gradient
centrifugation and four equivalent fractions were separated and
analyzed. More than 60% of the 35S labelled material from cells

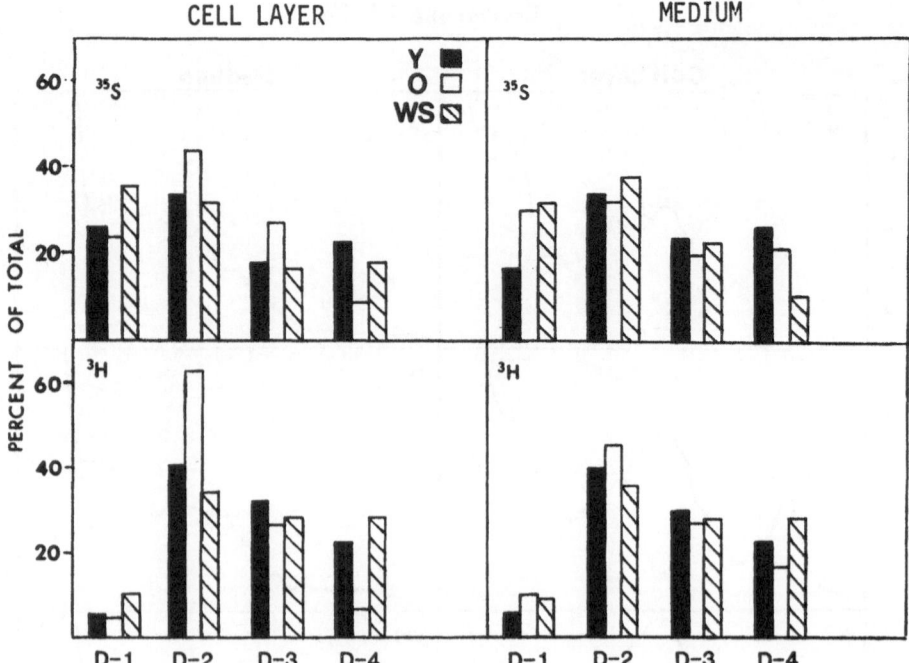

Figure 2:   Percent distribution of medium and cell associated
            proteoglycans after dissociative CsCl density gradient
            centrifugation.   (WS) Werner Syndrome, (Y) normal early
            and (O) late passage fibroblast cultures.

and medium were found in D_1 and D_2 at a density greater than 1.44
g/ml (fig. 2). Sepharose 2B profiles of the D_1 fraction showed PG
of two distinct size classes in the cells and medium. According to
their elution position, the cell-associated PG corresponded to C-II
and C-III and the medium corresponded to M-I and M-II seen before
density gradient purification. These preliminary observations
suggest that WS and normal fibroblasts produce similar RG profiles.
Further characterization of these PG populations by determining
their molecular weight and GAG composition may demonstrate
differences between WS and normal fibroblasts.

    Other investigators are beginning to do detailed characteri-
zation of PG from skin fibroblasts. Studies by Coster et al.
(1979) have concentrated on characterizing PG from human embryonic
skin fibroblasts. These results may be more relevant for
omparison with studies done on WS skin fibroblasts than studies of

PG from lung fibroblasts. The PG from the cell layer were resolved into two fractions by CL-2B gel chromatography; one, a large PG of low buoyant density was shown to be a proteoheparan sulfate and a second, smaller PG population, containing glucuronic acid rich dermatan sulfate chains. The PG from the medium were separated into two populations: one large glucuronic acid rich DS species similar to the DS found in the cell layer and a smaller iduronic acid rich species. These similar, if not identical, PG species interact specifically with HA. Thus HA present in the pericellular environment may bind this glucuronic acid rich PG. The iduronic acid-rich species has no affinity for HA and will therefore appear preferentially in the medium.

CONCLUSIONS

Proteoglycans are complex and heterogeneous molecules. Characterization of PG produced by various cell types indicates that different cell types produce proteoglycans with specific structures and functions.

In vivo and in vitro studies of the PG component of aging tissue and cells indicate that changes in the size and chemical composition of proteoglycans, and, therefore, in their functional properties occur with increased age. The results from many of the in vitro studies discussed in this paper demonstrate minor differences in PG metabolism between early and late-passage cells in vitro. The variations in PG of fibroblasts from different tissues (e.g., lung vs. skin) are greater than those related to in vitro senescence. The PG profiles of cells from some WS patients are clearly different from normal early or late passage cells. The PG of cells of more WS patients from different genetic backgrounds need to be studied to determine whether the differences in PG profiles are specific and consistent for WS.

An increased knowledge of the synthesis of different types and structural modifications of PG molecules in pathologic disorders such as Werner Syndrome will help in understanding the structural and functional changes of PG molecules in normal aging.

REFERENCES

Basler, J.W., David J.D. and Agris, P.F. (1979). Deteriorating collagen synthesis and cell ultrastructure accompanying senescence of human normal and Werner's syndrome fibroblast cell strains. Exp. Cell Res. 118:73-84.

Coster, L., Carlstedt, I. and Malmstrom, A., (1979). Isolation of [35S]- and [3H]-labelled proteoglycans from cultures of human embryonic skin fibroblasts. Biochem. J. 183:669-675.

Damle, S.P., Kieras, F.J., Tzeng, W.K. and Gregory, J.D. (1982).
    Proteodermatan sulfate isolated from pig skin. J. Biol.
    Chem. 257:5523-5527.
Epstein, C.J., Martin, G.M., Schulz, A.L., et al. (1966).
    Werner's syndrome. A review of its symptomatology, natural
    history, pathologic features, genetics and relationship to
    the natural aging process. Medicine 45:177-221.
Fleischmajer, R. and Nedwich, A. (1973). Werner's syndrome. Am.
    J. Medicine 54:111-118.
Fleischmajer, R., Perlish, J.S. and Bashey, R.I. (1973). Aging
    of human dermis. Front. Matrix Biol. 1:90-106.
Gottesman, T., Zola, L., Vogel, A., Mumen Thaler, M. (1980).
    Das Werner-Syndrome. Schweiz Med Wochenschr 110:246-250.
Inerot, S. and Heingard, D. (1978). Articular-cartilage
    proteoglycans in aging and osteoarthritis. Biochem. J.
    169:143-156.
Kennedy, J.F. (1976). Chemical and biochemical aspects of the
    glycosaminoglycans and proteoglycans in health and disease.
    Adv. Clin. Chem. 18:1-101.
Mathews, M.B. and Glagor, S. (1966). Acid mucopoly saccoride
    patterns in aging human cartilage. J. Clin. Invest.
    45:1103-1111.
Matuoka, K. and Mitsui, Y. (1981). Changes in cell-surface
    glycosaminoglycans in human diploid fibroblasts during in
    vitro aging. Mech. Ageing Dev. 15:153-163.
Murata, K., Ishikawa, T. and Ninomiya, H. (1973). Age-dependent
    changes of chondroitin sulfate isomers in normal human
    urine. Biochemical Medicine. 8:472-484.
Murata, K. and Bjelle, A. (1980). Constitutional variations of
    acidic glycosaminoglyan in normal and arthritic bovine
    articular cartilage proteoglycans at different ages.
    Connective Tissue Res. 7:143-156.
Murata, K. (1982). Urinary acidic glycosaminoglycans in Werner's
    Syndrome. Experientia. 38:313-314.
Oegma, T.R., Hascall, V.C. and Dziewiatkowsky, D.D. (1975).
    Isolation and characterization of proteoglycans from the
    swarm rat chondrosarcama. J. Biol. Chem. 250:6151-6159.
Oohira, A. and Nogami, H. (1980). Age-related changes in
    physical and chemical properties of proteoglycens
    synthesized by costal and matrix-induced cartilages in the
    rat. J. Biol. Chem. 255:1346-1350.
Rodin, L., and Schwartz, N.B. (1975). Biosynthesis of connective
    tissue proteoglycans, in Whelan, W.J. (ed): Biochemistry of
    carbohydrates. MTP International Review of Science.
    Biochemistry Series One, vol. 5, London, Butterworths, p.
    95.
Schachtschabel, D.O. and Wever, J. (1978), Age-related decline in
    the synthesis of glycosaminoglycans by cultured human
    fibroblasts (WI-38). Mech. Ageing Dev. 8:257-264.
Scott, J.E. (1973), in Current Developments in Rheumatology, eds:

Lovgren, O., Bostrom, H., Olhagen, B. and Sannerstedt, R., pp 10-29, A. Lindgren, Molndal.

Sluke, G. Schachtschabel, D.O. and Wever, J. (1981). Age-related changes in the distribution pattern of glycosaminoglycens synthesized by cultured human diploid fibroblasts (WI-38). Mech. Ageing Dev. 16:19-27.

Sweet, M.B.E., Thonar, E.J.M.A. and Marsh, J. (1979). Age-related changes in proteoglycan structure. Arch. Biochem. and Biophys. 198:439-448.

Tajima, T., Iyima, K. and Watanabe, T. (1978). Collagen synthesis of cultured fibroblast from Werner's syndrome of premature aging. Experientia. 34:10-11.

Tajima, T., Watanabe, T., Iyima, K., Ohshika, Y. and Yamaguchi, H. (1981). The increase of glycosaminoglycans synthesis and accumulation on the cell surface of cultured skin fibroblasts in Werner's syndrome. Exp. Path. 20:221-229.

Tokunago, M., Futami, T., Wakamatsu, E., Endo, M., Yosizawa, Z. (1975). Werner's syndrome as hyaluronuria. Clin. Chim. Acta. 62:89-96.

Wever, J., Schachtschabel, D.O., Sluke, G., Wever, G. (1980). Effect of short or long term treatment with exogeneous glycosaminoglycans on growth and glycosaminoglycan synthesis of human fibroblasts (WI-38) in culture. Mech. Ageing Dev. 14:89-99.

Vogel, K.G. and Kendall, V.F. (1980). Cell-surface glycosaminoglycans: Turnover in cultural human embryo fibroblasts (IMR-90). J. Cell Physiol. 103:475-487.

Vogel, K.G. and Peterson, D.W. (1981). Extracellular, surface, and entra-cellular proteoglycans produced by human embryo lung fibroblasts in culture (IMR-90). J. Biol. Chem. 256:13235-13242.

Vogel, K.G., Kendall, V.F. and Sapien, R.E. (1981). Glycosaminoglycan synthesis and composition in human fibroblasts during in vitro cellular aging (IMR-90). J. Cell Physiol. 107:271-281.

Vogel, K.G. and Sapien, R.E. (1982). Production of proteoglycans by human lung fibroblasts (IMF-90) maintained in a low concentration of serum. Biochem. J. 207:369-379.

Vogel, K.G. and Pitcher, D.E. (1982). Sulfated proteoglycans produced by human lung fibroblasts during in vitro cellular aging. European J. Cell Biol. 29:61-67.

Zebrower, M., Kieras, F.J. and Brown, W.T. (1984). Glycosaminoglycan (GAG) and hyaluronic acid (HA) elevation in genetic aging syndromes. Am. J. Hum. Genet. 36:845

CELL SURFACE CHANGES IN SENESCENT AND WERNER'S SYNDROME

FIBROBLASTS: THEIR ROLE IN CELL PROLIFERATION

Youji Mitsui, Kiyotaka Yamamoto, Mari Yamamoto, and
Koji Matuoka

Fermentation Research Institute*
Chief, Division of Cell Science and Technology
Agency of Industrial Science and Technology
Higashi 1-1-3, Yatabe-machi
Ibaraki, 305
Japan

INTRODUCTION

Werner's syndrome (WS) has segmental progeroid features and
pedigree analysis suggests its autosomal recessive inheritance
(Epstein et al., 1966). Two of the clinical characteristics of
Werner's syndrome are hyperkeratinized skin and an excessive
excretion of hyaluronic acid into the urine (Tokuraga et al., 1975,
Goto and Murata, 1978) suggesting some disorder(s) of connective-
tissue metabolism. Cultured fibroblasts from human skin have been
used for characterization of genetic defects in many inherited
diseases. Epstein et al. (1966) cultured fibroblast-like cells
from the skin of patients with WS and noted that they grew very
poorly. Since then, WS fibroblasts have been used to find the
explanation for the shortened lifespan in vivo and in vitro (Martin
et al., 1970). However, the primary molecular defect that retards
cell growth has remained elusive. Recently, Salk (1982) published
an extensive review article summarizing 15 years of research since
that of Epstein et al.

Cell surface is known to have some role in the regulation of cell proliferation and cell communication through interaction with adjacent cell surfaces, with the intercellular matrix, or both (Matuoka and Mitsui, 1981b). Glycosaminoglycans (GAGs), such as hyaluronic acid, chondroitin sulfate, dermatan sulfate, and heparan sulfate, make up the cell-surface peripheral coat and give a negative charge on the cell surface; they are excreted into the extracellular space, changing the environment for the neighboring cells. Thus, any altered GAGs produced by fibroblasts may play a critical role in cell communication and cell proliferation.

We report here alterations of cell-surface GAGs in conjunction with changes in surface (negative) charge and cell proliferation capacity in fibroblasts from young and old patients with and without Werner's syndrome.

MATERIALS AND METHODS

Cell strains and cell cultures

The cell strains used were TIG-1 human fetal lung fibroblasts (Mitsui et al., 1980, Ohashi et al., 1980), GRC-series skin fibroblasts (Schneider and Mitsui, 1976) from 13 men (aged 0-89 years), and WS-series skin fibroblasts from 5 male patients aged (1961 years) with WS. WS fibroblats WS TY01 and WS TY02 at 5 population doubling levels (PDL) were a gift from Matsumura (Matsumura et al., 1980) and WS 12KO at 6 PDL from Fujiwara (Fujiwara et al., 1977). Primary cultures of the other skin fibroblasts were obtained by outgrowth as described before (Schneider and Mitsui, 1976; 1978). The cells were cultured in Eagle's minimum essential medium containing nonessential amino acids, supplemented with 10% fetal bovine serum, in an environment of 5% CO_2 and 95% air by 37°C. A routine subcultivation was achieved by harvesting cells with 0.25% trypsin solution in CA^{++}, Mg^{++}-free phosphate buffered saline [PBS(-)]; the cells were inoculated at 1:4 or 1:2 split ratio.

Cell elecrophoresis

Confluent cells, 99% of which were in the G_1 phase of cell growth as determined with a cytofluorometer, were rinsed and dispersed with 0.05% EDTA containing PBS (-) solution. The cells were centrifuged and resuspended in M/15 phosphate buffer containing 5.4% glucose (pH 7.30). The electrophoretic mobility (EPM) of each cell suspended in this buffer was measured using Cell Electrophoresis Microscope Systems (Sugiura Laboratory). A mean value and standard deviation were calculated from the EPM of 50-100 cells. The values were expressed as μm/sec/V/cm. EPM reflects a negative charge density on a unit area of cell surface within a depth of about 10 Å.

Radioisotope Incorporation

Confluent cells were cultured in medium containing D-3H glucosamine hydrochloride (specific radioactivity 38 Ci/mmole, 5 μCi/ml x 10 ml) under normal conditions for 48 hours. After being washed, the cell layer was treated with 0.25% trypsin solution for 30 minutes to isolate the cell-surface GAGs fractions.

Isolation of GAGs and Two-Dimensional Electrophoresis Analysis

Cell-surface GAGs were precipitated by cetylpyridinium chloride after removal of the protein fraction and the purified cellulose acetate membrane. For quantitative determination, each spot on the mebrane was cut off and transferred to a scintillation vial to measure the radioactivity in each glycosaminoglycan. Details were described in a previous paper (Matouka and Mitsui, 1981a).

Cell Culture on the Fixed Cell Sheets with Enzyme Treatment

Confluent cells were fixed with 2.5% glutaraldehyde for 30 minutes. After thorough washing and incubation in serum-free medium overnight, the cell layer was treated with Streptomyces hyaluronidase (0.03 TRU per cm2) at 50°C, chondroitinase ABC (0.0015 units per cm2) at 37°C, or Flavobacterium heparitinase (87 units/mg, 11 μg per cm2) at 43°C for 4 hours. Nitrous acid (0.2 ml per cm2, as 18% NaNO2 aqueous solution) was also used to remove heparan sulfate. The details were described before (Matouka and Mitsui, 1981b). To see the effect of cell sheets on the fibroblast proliferation, fibroblasts were inoculated into dishes with the fixed cell sheets on which the GAGs were treated with degradation enzymes.

RESULTS

Cell Growth

Fibroblast-like cells were obtained by outgrowth from skin fragments of normal donors and patients with WS. Although migration and outgrowth of fibroblasts were very slow from WS skin fragments, selective outgrowth of keratinocytes was sometimes discernible. Serial cultivations of fibroblasts were performed at 1:4 or 1:2 split ratio to the end of their lifespans in vitro. A typical cell-growth characteristic of WS fibroblasts is seen in Fig. 1. The proliferative capacity of WS fibroblasts

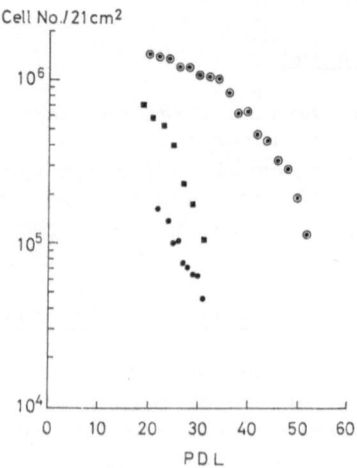

Fig. 1. Cell number at harvesting time throughout life span of
         normal and Werner fibroblasts. Cell number density at
         confluent was counted on the 7th day after the
         inoculation at 1:4 or 1:2 split ratio. Skin fibroblasts
         from normal subjects of 56 years old (⊙) and 88 years
         old (■), and skin fibroblasts from a Werner syndrome
         patient of 56 years old (●).

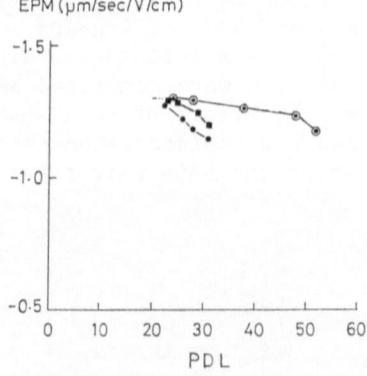

Fig. 2. Decrease in electrophoretic mobility (EPM) during in
         vitro aging. Confluent state of cell at each harvesting
         time (Fig. 1) was dispersed with 0.05% EDTA solution and
         EPM of 50-100 cells were measured by Cell
         Electrophoresis Microscope System. The cells used are
         of the same origins as shown in Fig. 1.

was markedly less than that of the age and sex-matched normal
control fibroblasts. An increase in cell size, characteristic of
senescent cultures (Mitsui and Schneider, 1976a), was also
evident in the WS fibroblasts.

Electrophoretic Mobility (EPM)

At each time of cell harvesting (Fig. 1), usually one week
after the subcultivation, confluent cells in the parallel
cultures were dispersed in 0.05% EDTA solution without using
enzymes and subjected to cell electrophoresis. Cell EPM was
found to decrease with passage number in vitro (Fig. 2). On the
other hand, cell-size distribution has been found to increase and
to become more heterogenous with aging in vitro (Mitsui and
Schneider 1976a,b,c) and EPM, which reflects the amount of
negative charge per unit area of cell-membrane surface, declines
when cells are enlarged by hypotonic treatment. Determination of
the EPM of different size cells in the young and senescent
cultures confirmed that a decrease in charge density noted in
senescent cultures occurred even in the small-cell populations of
heterogeneous senescent cultures.

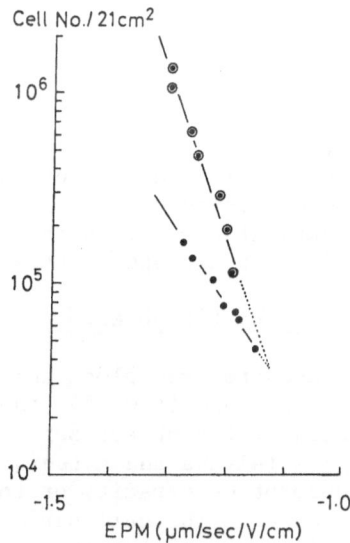

Fig. 3. Relationship between confluent cell number and
         electrophoretic mobility at each passage. As shown in
         Fig. 1 and 2, cell number and EPM at harvesting time of
         each passage declined with aging. Their linear
         relationships were confirmed in all the cell strains
         examined. Skin fibroblasts from 56-year-old normal (⊙)
         and Werner syndrome (●) subjects.

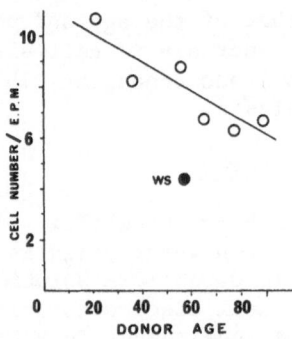

Fig. 4.   Donor age effect on slope of linear regression between
          cell number and EPM.   Slope of line in Fig. 3 and other
          similar data were plotted as a function of donor age.
          (○): skin fibroblasts from different ages of normal
          donors. (●): cell from a Werner syndrome patient.

When EPM was plotted as a function of numerical density at
harvesting time throughout the life span, a strict linear
relationship between them was found in all the cell strains
examined.   Figure 3 demonstrates two typical examples of these
linear relations in WS and normal control fibroblasts and
suggests a decline in the slope in WS fibroblasts.   When slopes
were plotted for fibroblasts from donors of different ages
against donor age, an age-related decline in slope was found
(Fig. 4).   The same figure also suggests that the patient with WS
had older characteristics for his age in this index.

Haemadsorption Capacity in WS Fibroblasts

When Concanavalin A-coated red blood cells were adsorbed
onto the fibroblast cell surface (Fig. 5), the amount of red
blood cells per unit area of fibroblast surface increased in
vitro with cellular aging (Aizawa and Mitsui, 1979).   Also, the
increase in the haemadosorption capacity of the fibroblasts was
found to reflect a decrease in the cell-surface negative charge
on the senescent cells (Aizawa et al., 1980a).   Examination of
the haemadosorption capacity of fibroblasts from normal subjects
(13 men) and WS patients (5 men)(Fig.6) suggested that WS
patients have older characteristics for their age in this index
(Aizawa et al., 1980b).   This increase in haemadsorption capacity
in WS cells was well correlated with the above-mentioned decrease
in the slope of EPM per cell, suggesting a decrease in the
density of the negative charges on the cell surface.

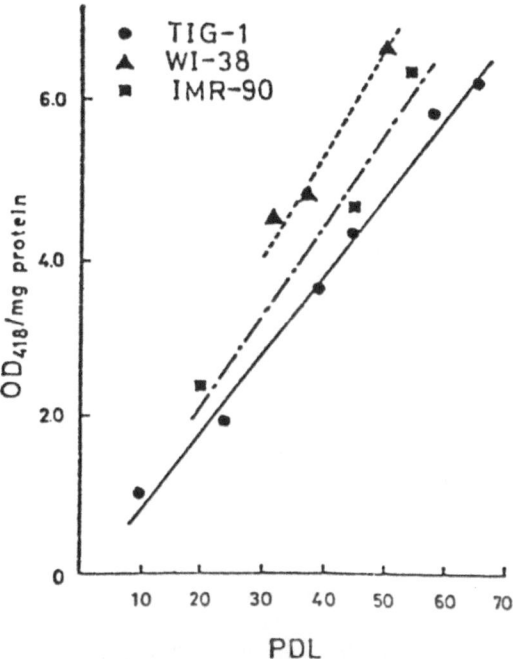

Fig. 5. Adsorption of Con-A treated red blood cells on cell surface of senescent fibroblasts. Note the linear increases in haemadsorption activity with cellular aging of WI-38, IMR-90 and TIG-1 cells.

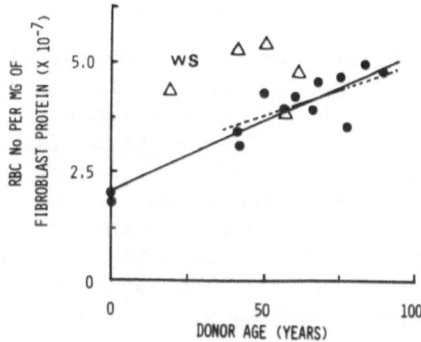

Fig. 6. Haemadsorption activity of fibroblasts as a function of donor age. Skin fibroblasts (20 PDL) from normal subjects (●; 0-88 years old) and fibroblasts from Werner patients (△; 29-56 years old) were examined for the Con-A treated red blood cell adsorption capacity. Data from Aizawa et al. (1980b) were redrawn.

Role of Cell-Surface Glycosaminoglycans (GAGs) and Sialic Acid in Electrophoretic Mobility

Negative charges on the cell surface are thought to be due mainly to the sialic acid and sulfate in the GAGs in a thin layer (10 Å) of the cell-surface coat. In order to know the contribution of each GAG and sialic acid on age-related changes in negative charge, EPMs of young and senescent cells were examined after treatment of the cell surface with various degradation enzymes. Summarized data are shown in Table 1. A decrease in EPM after treatment with neuraminidase, hyaluronidase, chondroitinase ABC, or heparitinase indicates the contribution in negative charge of neuraminic acid, hyaluronic acid, chondroitin sulfates and heparan sulfate, respectively. It is apparent that the degree of contribution of each anion changes with aging. In early passaged cells, hyaluronic acid had the greatest contribution (28% of the total negative charge), but only a small contribution (12%) in late passaged cells. During cell aging in vitro, a definite decrease in negative charge was observed (1.242 - 1.658 = -.416). During the same period, hyaluronic acid contents of the surface coat decreased markedly (.149 - .471 = -.322), chondroitin sulfates mildly (.087 - .288 = -.201), and neuraminic acid slightly (.206 - .297 = -.081). On the other hand, heparan sulfate seems not to have decreased but rather to have increased slightly.

Thus, it is noteworthy that the age-related decrease in the negative charge in vitro would be due to mainly a decrease in hyaluronic acid and that the proportion of heparan sulfate became greatest (31%) in senescent cells.

Glycosaminoglycans on Cell Surface Coat

Human diploid fibroblasts produce hyaluronic acid, chondroitin 4-sulfate, chondroitin 6-sulfate, dermatan sulfate, and heparan sulfate, which are excreted mostly into medium (Matuoka and Mitsui, 1981a). The amount of each GAG on the cell surface, however, can be examined by prolonged incubation with labeled precursors. Glycosaminoglycans on the cell surface at the confluent state of growth were released by treatment with trypsin after incubation for 48 hours in a medium containing ^{3}H-glucosamine. The purified GAGs were subjected to two-dimensional electrophoresis to quantitate each fraction of GAGs. Figure 7 demonstrates the amounts of radioactivity in hyaluronic acid (HA), chondroitin sulfates plus dermatan sulfate (CS) and heparan sulfate (HS) per mg protein in young, middle, and late passage cells. It is quite clear that with cell aging in vitro hyaluronic acid and chondroitin sulfates dramatically decline and that heparan sulfate gradually increases during the same period. Thus, heparan sulfate becomes a main component of GAGs in the

Table 1

Electrophoretic Mobility
Decrease in Senescent Cells and Role of GAGs

(μm/sec/V/cm)

| | | TREATMENT | | |
PDL Control	Neuraminidase	Hyaluronidase	Chondroitinase	Heparitinase
15 -1.658 ±.108	-1.361 ±.103 -.297*	-1.187 ±.106 -.471*	-1.371 ±.128 -.288*	
(25 -1.605)				-1.218 ± .079 -.387
65 -1.242 ± .113	-1.036 ± .138 -.206*	-1.093 ± .130 -.149*	-1.135 ± .137 -.087*	-0.851 ± .059 -.391*
Diff. -.416**	-.081**	-.322**	-.201**	+.004*

*   Difference in EPM between control and enzyme-treated cells at each passage.

**   Difference in EPM between young (15 PDL) cells and old (65 PDL) cells in control and enzyme-treated populations.

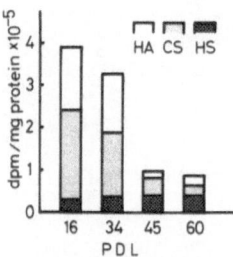

Fig. 7.   Changes in glycosaminoglycans on the cell surface with
          in vitro cellular aging. 48-hour incorporation of 3H-
          glucosamine into hyaluronic acid (HA), chondritin
          sulfate (CS) and heparan sulfate (HS) on the cell
          surface examined as a function of in vitro passage of
          TIG-1 fibroblasts.

cell-surface coat of the senescent cells. These findings
correlate with the observations obtained from measuring the
enzyme-treated cell EPM.

Retardation of Cell Growth on the Fixed Cell Surface Sheets

    The numerical saturation density in vitro of cells at the
confluent stage of growth declines steadily with age, in spite of
repeated changes of medium. Because contact inhibition of cell
growth in normal fibroblasts is thought to be mediated by cell-
surface interaction (Dulbecco et al., 1970) and age-related cell
surface changes have been found, we pursued the possibility that
the cell-surface constituents, such as glycosaminoglycans,
contributed to the regulation of cell proliferation.

    To find out the effect of direct contact of the cell
surface, avoiding metabolic communication, we treated the cells
with fixatives and made cell-surface sheets onto which another
cell strain was inoculated and left to grow. Glutaraldehyde was
the best fixative, seemingly preserving the natural configuration
of cell-surface coat as described before (Matuoka and Mitsui,
1981b). Cell growth and saturation density were lower when the
cells were inoculated onto fixed cell-surface sheets. As seen in
Table 2, a greater inhibition of cell growth was observed when
the cells were inoculated onto the cell sheet surface from older
cultures. Increased synthesis and accumulation of heparan
sulfate on the cell surfaces of senescent cultures were
accompanied by an enhanced inhibitory effect on cell growth
(Figure 7 and Table 2).

Table 2

Heparan sulfate content and growth-inhibitory effect
of fixed cell-surface sheets: Changes with aging.

Age (PDL)	HS contents (pg / cell)	Age (PDL)	Growth inhibition (%)
17	1.5	12	16
38	1.8	31	35
55	2.5	47	45

Note that senescent fibroblasts accumulated more heparan sulfate
(HS) on the cell surface and experienced greater growth-inhibition.

To confirm the role of heparan sulfate in cell growth
regulation, we treated the fixed cell sheet surface with GAG
degradation enzymes or agents and examined their effect on
recovery from growth inhibition. Table 3 demonstrates that cell-
surface chondroitin sulfates had no contribution on the observed
cell-growth inhibition, and that removal of heparan sulfate
completely restored cell growth. Although hyaluronidase
treatment resulted in 50% recovery of cell growth, it removed
about 6% of the heparan sulfate in addition to 75% of the
hyaluronic acid. As the most superficial layer of the cell
surface is more easily removed, hyaluronidase may have removed
the most effective part of the heparan sulfate for the cell-
growth manipulation. Since the amount of hyaluronic acid on cell
surface became small and relative amount of heparan sulfate
became very high in senescent cells (Fig. 7), it is evident that
heparan sulfate has the most effective role in inhibiting the
cell growth on senescent cultures. The cell-growth inhibiting
effects of fixed cell surface coats from WS fibroblasts and from
age-matched normal fibroblasts were compared. As seen in Figure
8, WS fibroblast surface coat was found to have the greater
inhibitory effect on cell growth.

Examination of ^{3}H-glucosamine incorporation into WS
fibroblasts and normal fibroblasts from donors of different ages
confirmed that the total amount of heparan sulfate on the cell
surface was higher in WS fibroblasts (Table 4).

Thus, we conclude that there is a possibility that changes in cell-surface GAGs may be a cause of the retarded cell growth of WS cells and also of senescent fibroblasts.

DISCUSSION

Although cellular changes at the nuclear level have been examined in WS fibroblasts as well as senescent fibroblasts in vitro (Mitsui and Schneider, 1976a,b,c; Fujiwara et al., 1977; Mitsui et al., 1979, 1980a,b, 1981; Takeuchi et al., 1982; Ide et al., 1983; Mitsui and Sakagami, 1983), cell-surface changes also should be regarded as possible primary causes of changes in cell-proliferation capacity. There have been several reports of cell-surface (membrane) defects in WS fibroblasts. These include reduced expression of HLA antigens (Goldstein and Singal, 1974), increased procoagulant activity of tissue factor (Goldstein and Niewiarowski, 1976), resistance to insulin (Nakao et al., 1978,

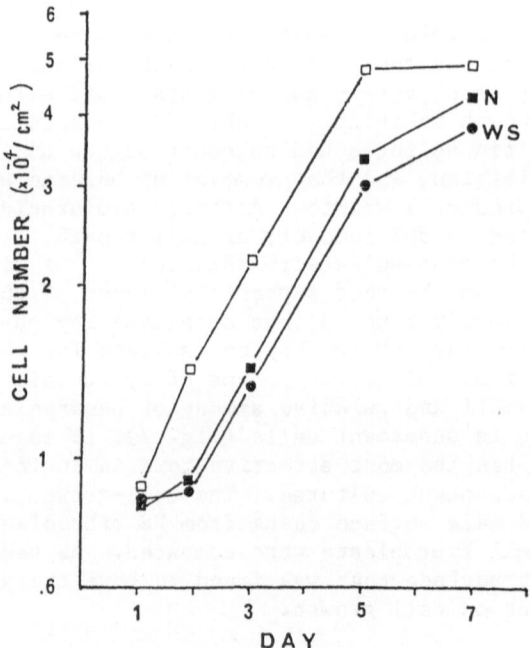

Fig. 8.   Cell growth on the fixed cell sheets of normal and Werner fibroblasts. Fixed cell sheets were prepared from Werner fibroblasts (●, 5 PDL) and donor age-matched normal fibroblasts (■, 25 PDL). Normal cells were grown on the fixed cell sheets.

Table 3

Cell Growth Recovery After Removal of GAGs

	Removal of GAGs	Recovery of Cell Growth
Normal Control		(100%)
Treatment		
Chondroitinase ABC	78% (CS)	-7%
Hyaluronidase	75% (HA), 6% (HS)	50%
Heparitinase	75% (HS)	95%
Nitrous Acid	88% (HS)	100%

Fixed cell sheets were treated with enzymes to remove GAGs and tested for cell growth recovery. Untreated cell sheets inhibited cell growth by 40%. When the enzyme-treated cell sheet lost the inhibitory effect completely, recovery of cell growth was assessed as 100%.

Smith et al., 1980) and a decrease in insulin receptors (Beadle et al., 1978). However, their relation to shortened replicative life span in WS fibroblasts has not been examined.

A decrease in total glycosaminoglycans production (Weber et al., 1980; Matuoka and Mitsui, 1981a), changes in hyaluronidase sensitivity (Yamamoto et al., 1977), and an increase in accumulation of heparan sulfate on cell surface (Matuoka and Mitsui, 1981a, b; Sluke et al., 1981) in senescent cultures have been reported, as has a marked increase in the accumulation of sulfated GAGs in Werner fibroblasts (Tajima et al., 1981; Salk, 1982). In our previous paper, we claimed that cell-surface heparan sulfate is involved in the density-dependent inhibition of cell proliferation in senescent fibroblasts (Matuoka and Mitsui, 1981b).

In the present study, we showed that WS cells had a poorer cell growth ability and a lowered negative-charge density as revealed by the retarded EPM. A strict linear relationship

Table 4

GLYCOSAMINOGLYCANS IN NORMAL AND WS FIBROBLASTS

Cell strain	Distribution of ^{3}H-GAGs (%)			Hep. Sulf. (%) in surface GAGs	Hyal. Acid in Medium dpm x 10^{-5}/dish
	Surface	Medium	Cell		
Normal					
29 years	6.5	73.8	19.7	21.3	1.60
56 years	6.1	72.6	21.2	42.5	2.91
88 years	3.7	71.7	24.6	54.5	5.26
WS					
19 years	13.9	74.0	12.2	34.6	6.90
29 years	5.8	82.3	11.9	33.0	9.47
46 years	12.6	74.8	12.6	37.9	6.64

between EPM and cell number at confluency in several passages was found in WS fibroblasts as well as in normal donor cells. The slope of this line (cell number change per EPM change) was lower in WS fibroblasts, depicting older characteristics for the donor age of the cells. This lower slope reflects a greater inhibition of cell growth in early-passage cultures compared with the changes in negative-charge density on surface coat, as evidenced by the other series of experiments. A lower negative-charge density in WS cells than in normal controls was confirmed by their increased red blood cell adsorption capacity. A decreased negative-charge density during the aging of normal lung fibroblasts in vitro was ascribed to decreases in the hyaluronic acid and chondroitin sulfates at the cell surface, as revealed by EPM changes after treatment with GAG degradation enzymes and by changes in the amount of GAGs produced. These experiments also demonstrated that heparan sulfate slightly increased with cell aging and became the main component of the cell surface coat. Involvement of cell-surface heparan sulfate in the lowered ability of senescent cells to proliferate is shown by the growth inhibition of cells inoculated onto the fixed cell-surface sheet with various heparan sulfate contents. WS fibroblasts had a greater inhibition effect than cells from an age-matched donor. Cell surface plays an important role in the regulation of function and cell growth through direct interaction with the cell surfaces or with the environment. Thus, changes in cell-surface properties should be extensively examined to discover the mechanisms of aging in WS and normal cells.

SUMMARY

Cell surface is known to participate in the regulation of cell proliferation through interaction with adjacent cell surfaces or the extracellular matrix, or both. A clinical survey of the Werner syndrome suggests some disorders in glycosaminoglycan metabolism. Also, the skin fibroblasts derived from the patients with WS have a reduced proliferation capacity. We here examined, in vitro and in vivo, alterations of the cell-surface properties of WS cells and aging human fibroblasts.

Cell-surface negative charges, examined by electrophoretic mobility of dispersed single cells in buffer, were seen to decline steadily as a function of cumulative population doublings. A strict linear relationship was found between electrophoretic mobility ($\mu m/sec/V/cm$) and number of cells harvested at each passage in all cell lines examined. The slope of this line in cells from donors of different ages indicated that WS fibroblasts resemble cells from much older normal controls. The same conclusion was drawn from our previous study of Con A-mediated red cell adsorption, which was confirmed as

reflecting an alteration of cell-surface coat negative charge.
Electrophretic mobility after treatment of cell surface with
degradative enzymes showed that the cell-surface negative charges
were attributable to sialic acid, chondroitin sulphates,
hyaluronic acid, and heparan sulphate. Two-dimensional
electrophoresis of ^{3}H-glucosamine incorporated glycosaminoglycans
(GAGs) revealed that heparan sulphate was the main component of
GAGs on the fibroblast cell surface and that the relative amount
of heparan sulphate among GAGs on the cell surface increased in
vitro with the number of passages. Growth kinetics of
fibroblasts on sheets of fixed cells treated with a fixative
(glutaraldehyde) and degradative enzymes were examined to
elucidate the role of cell-surface GAGs in the regulation of cell
proliferation. Cell growth was inhibited 40% when the
fibroblasts were cultured on the fixed sheets of late passage
cells. Treatment of the fixed cell sheets with heparitinase or
nitrous acid resulted in complete recovery from the growth
inhibition. Cell growth on sheets of fixed cells derived from
young, middle, and senescent fibroblasts showed that the surface
of the senescent cells had the greatest inhibitory effect. These
inhibitory effects of fixed cell sheets correlated well with both
the amount of heparan sulphate relative to the total GAGs on the
surface and to the saturation density of cell growth at each
passage. These findings strongly suggest that heparan sulphate,
or its complex, on the cell surface is involved in the regulation
of cell proliferation.

Examination of ^{3}H-glucosamine incorporation into the cell-
surface GAGs of skin fibroblasts from donors of different ages
and from WS patients showed that heparan sulfate accumulates on
the cell surface more rapidly in the WS cells and that more
hyaluronic acid was excreted from WS cells into the medium. By
using the fixed cell sheet assay, WS fibroblasts were confirmed
to have a greater inhibitory effect on cell growth than age-
matched normal fibroblasts. Thus, the role of cell-surface
changes in the regulation of cell proliferation in normal aging
and in the Werner syndrome should be given greater emphasis.

REFERENCES

Aizawa, S., and Mitsui, Y. (1979), A new cell surface marker of
    aging in human diploid fibroblasts. J. Cell. Physiol.
    100:383.
Aizawa, S., Mitsui, Y., Kurimoto, F., and Nomura, K. (1980a),
    Cell surface changes accompanying aging in human diploid
    fibroblasts. V. role of large major cell surface protein
    and surface negative charge in aging and transformation
    associated changes in Con-A mediated red blood cell
    adsorption. Exp. Cell Res. 127:143.

Aizawa, S., Mitsui, Y., Kurimoto, F. and Matuoka, K. (1980b),
    Cell surface changes accompanying aging in human diploid
    fibroblasts: Effects of tissue, donor age and genotype.
    Mech. Age. Dev. 13:297.
Aizawa, S., and Mitsui, Y. (1982), Cell surface and clonal
    proliferative properties of aging human diploid fibroblasts.
    Exp. Cell Res. 139:416.
Beadle, G.F., Mackay, I.R., Whittingham, S., Taggert, G.,
    Harris, A.W., and Harrison, L.C. (1978), Werner's syndrome,
    a model of premature aging? J. Med. 9:377.
Dulbecco, R., and Stoker, M.G.P. (1970), Conditions determining
    initiation of DNA synthesis in 3T3 cells. Proc. Natl. Acad.
    Sci. (USA), 66:204.
Epstein, C.J., Martin, G.M., Schultz, A.L., and Motulsky, A.G.
    (1966), Werner's syndrome: A review of its symptomatology,
    natural history, pathologic features, genetics and
    relationship to the natural aging process. Medicine 45:177.
Fujiwara, Y., Higashikawa, T., and Tatsumi, M. (1977), A retarded
    rate of DNA replication and normal level of DNA repair in
    Werner's syndrome fibroblasts in culture. J. Cell. Physiol.
    92:365.
Goldstein, S., and Singal, D.P. (1974), Alternation of fibroblast
    gene products in vitro from a subject with Werner's
    syndrome. Nature 251:719.
Goldstein, S., and Niewiarowski, S. (1976), Increased
    procoagulant activity in cultured fibroblasts from progeria
    and Werner syndromes of premature aging. Nature 260:711.
Goto, M., and Murata, K. (1978), Urinary excretion of macro-
    molecular acidic glycosaminoglycans in Werner's syndrome.
    Clin. Chim. Acta. 85:101.
Martin, G.M., Sprague, C.A., and Epstein, C.J. (1970),
    Replicative life span of cultivated human cells: Effects of
    donor's age, tissue and genotype. Lab. Invest. 23:86.
Matsumura, T., Mitsui, Y., Fujiwara, Y., Ishii, T., and Shimada,
    H. (1980), Cell, tissue and organ banks in Japan with
    special references to the study of premature aging. Jpn. J.
    Exp. Med. 50:321.
Matuoka, K., and Mitsui, Y. (1981a), Changes in cell surface
    glycosaminoglycans in human diploid fibroblasts during in
    vitro aging. Mech. Age. Devel. 15:153.
Matuoka, K., and Mitsui, Y. (1981b), Involvement of cell surface
    heparan sulfate in the density-dependent inhibition of cell
    proliferation. Cell. Struc. Func. 6:23.
Mitsui, Y., Aizawa, S., and Matuoka, K. (1979), The relation of
    cell nuclei and surface membranes to the capacity of cell
    proliferation in human diploid fibroblasts. In Recent
    Advances in Gerontology, ed. by Orimo, H., Shimada, K.,
    Iriki, M., Maeda, D., Excepta Medica, Amsterdam, 108.

Mitsui, Y., Sakagami, H, Murota, S, and Yamada, M. (1980a), Age related decline in H1 histone fraction in human diploid fibroblast cultures. Exp. Cell. Res. 126:289.

Mitsui, Y., Matuoka, K., Aizawa, S., and Noda, K. (1980b), New approaches to the characterization of aging human diploid fibroblasts at individual cell level. Adv. Exp. Med. Biol. 129:5.

Mitsui, Y., and Schneider, E.L. (1976a), Relationship between cell replication and volume in senescent human diploid fibroblasts. Mech. Age. Dev. 5:45.

Mitsui, Y. and Schneider, E.L. (1976b), Increased nuclear sizes in senescent human diploid fibroblast cultures. Exp. Cell. Res. 100:147.

Mitsui, Y., and Schneider, E.L. (1976c), Characterization of fractionated human diploid fibroblast cell populations. Exp. Cell. Res. 103:23.

Mitsui, Y., Smith, J.R., and Schneider, E.R. (1981), Equivalent proliferation potential of different size classes of human diploid fibroblasts. J. Gerontology 36:416.

Mitsui, Y., and Sakagami, H. (1983), Histone H1 depletion with human cellular aging. Acta Histochem. Cytochem.

Nakao, Y., Kishihara, M., Yoshimi, H., Inoue, Y., Tanaka, K., Sakamoto, N., Matsukura, S., Imura, H., Ichihashi, M. and Fujiwara, Y. (1978), Werner's syndrome: In vivo and in vitro characteristics as a model of aging. Am. J. Med. 65:919.

Ohashi, M., Aizawa, S., Ooka, H., Oosawa, H., Kaji, K., Kondo, H., Kobayashi, T., Noumura, Y., Matsuo, M., Mitsui, Y., Murota, S., Yamamoto, K., Ito, H., Shimada, H. and Utakoji, T. (1980), A new human diploid cell strain, TIG-1, for the research on cellular aging. Exp. Geront. 15:121.

Salk, D. (1982), Werner's syndrome: A review of recent research with analysis of connective tissue metabolism, growth control of cultured cells and chromosomal aberrations. Hum. Genet. in press.

Schneider, E.L., and Mitsui, Y. (1976), Relationship between in vitro cellular aging and in vivo human age. Proc. Natl. Acad. Sci. (USA) 73:3584.

Schneider, E.L., and Mitsui, Y. (1978), The effect of serum batch on the in vitro life spans of cell cultures derived from old and young human donors. Exp. Cell. Res. 115:47.

Sluke, G., Schachtschabel, D.O., and Werver, J. (1981), Age-related changes in the distribution pattern of glycosaminoglycans synthesized by cultured human diploid fibroblasts (WI-38). Mech. Age. Devel. 16:19.

Smith, J.C., Singh, J.P, Lillquist, J.S., Goon, D.S. and Stiles, C.D. (1982), Growth factors adherent to cell substrate are mitogenically active in situ. Nature 296:154.

Tajima, T., Watanabe, T., Iijima, K., Ohshika, Y. and Yamaguchi,
    H. (1981), The increase of glycosaminoglycans synthesis and
    accumulation on the cell surface of cultured skin
    fibroblasts in Werner's syndrome. Exp. Path. 20:221.
Takeuchi, F., Hanaoka, F., Goto, M., Akaoka, I., Hori, T.,
    Yamada, M., and Miyamoto, T. (1982), Altered frequency of
    initiation sites of DNA replication in Werner's syndrome
    cells. Hum. Genet. 60:365.
Tokunaga, M., Futami, T., Wakamatsu, E., Endo, M. and Yoshizawa,
    Z. (1975), Werner's syndrome as "hyaluronuria", Clinica
    Chim. Acta. 62:89.
Wever, J., Schachtshabel, D.O., Sluke, G. and Wever, G. (1980),
    Effect of short-or long-term treatment with exogenous
    glycosaminoglycan synthesis of human fibroblasts (WI-38) in
    culture. Mech. Age. Devel. 14:89.
Yamamoto, K., Yamamoto, M., and Ooka, H. (1977), Cell surface
    changes associated with aging of chick embryo fibroblasts in
    culture. Exp. Cell. Res. 108:87

ACIDIC GLYCOSAMINOGLYCANS IN WERNER'S SYNDROME:

STUDIES ON LEVELS IN TISSUE, ORGAN, CELL, AND FLUID

Katsumi Murata[1], Ryoichi Hiwatari[2], and Toshiharu Matsumura[3]

1   Department of Medicine and
    Physical Therapy Faculty of Medicine
    University of Tokyo, 7-3-1 Hongo
    Bunkyo-ku, Tokyo, Japan 113

2   The Third Department of Medicine
    Kagoshima University School of Medicine
    Kagoshima, Japan

3   Institute of Medical Science
    University of Tokyo

    Supported in part by Grants-in-aid from the Ministry of
    Education, Science and Culture of Japan, and grants from
    the Life Science Section of the Institute of Physical and
    Chemical Research and from the Adult Disease Clinic
    Memorial Foundation, Tokyo.

INTRODUCTION

The clinical manifestations of Werner's syndrome resemble
those of the normal aging process (Werner, 1904; Epstein et al.,
1966; Murata and Nagashima, 1982). Scleroderma-like features and
cataracts are the main symptoms of Werner's syndrome in the
original description (Werner, 1904). It is a genetic disorder
disease affecting the mesodermal connective tissues of the whole
body (Fleischmajer and Nedwich, 1973) of which acidic
glycosaminoglycans (AGAG) are one component. Some of the degraded
components of these AGAG are excreted in urine as catabolic
products. In normal subjects, urinary AGAG comprise small amounts
of chondroitin 4-sulfate (C-4S), chondroitin 6-sulfate (C-6S), and
heparan sulfate (HS) and even smaller amounts of other chondroitin
sulfate (CS) isomers (Varadi, 1967; Murata et al., 1971; Wessler,

587

1971; Taniguchi, 1972). Hyaluronic acid (HA) is absent or in trace amounts (Varadi et al., 1967).

The components of urinary AGAG in Werner's syndrome were investigated by using an enzymatic assay method with chondroiti-nases and hyaluronidase, with which they can be analyzed at the constitutional level (Saito et al., 1968; Murata et al., 1968; Murata, 1980), and by other chemical assays.

Approximately 10 litres each of pooled urine were collected from 4 patients with Werner's syndrome. Urinary AGAG were prepared by a modification of the method reported previously (Murata et al., 1971; Murata and Takeda, 1980). The urinary AGAG were precipitated by adding 5% cetylpyridinium chloride. After the specimens were digested with pronase, trichloroacetic acid was added at a final concentration of 10%. The supernatants were dialyzed against water in dialysis tubing with reduced pore size. The nondialyzable AGAG that remained in the tube were concentrated and 4 vol of ethanol was added. The crude AGAG were applied to Dowex 1-X2 columns (Cl-form, 200-400 mesh), and eluted with 0.25 M and 3.0 M NaCl, and the latter eluate was desalted before use (Murata, 1980).

The purified AGAG thus prepared were then subjected to an enzymatic assay using chondroitinase-ABC and -AC to identify the constitutional disaccharide units of CS isomers after separating them from the other macromolecular AGAG (Saito et al., 1968; Murata, 1980), as described below. The AGAG, approximately 400 ug as uronic acid, were digested with chondroitinase-ABC (1.0 unit) in 0.1 M tris buffer, pH 8.0, and the other halves were digested with chondroitinase-AC (1.2 units) in 0.1 M acetate buffer, pH 6.0, at 37°C for 120 min (Murata 1980). The macromolecular AGAG undigested by both enzymes were characterized by electrophoresis (Murata, 1980). The unsaturated disaccharides were then applied to Whatman No. 1 filter paper and separated in 1-butyric acid - 0.5 M ammonia (5:3, v/v) for 60 h (Saito et al., 1968; Murata, 1980). The separated unsaturated disaccharides as well as the origin were cut out and eluted for measurement by the borate carbazole reaction.

The AGAG amount daily excreted in urine of the patients with Werner's syndrome (1-4 samples of urine pooled from each individual) was higher than that of the normal individuals, when the amount was expressed on the basis of kg body weight. The constitution of urinary AGAG in Werner's syndrome at the disaccharide unit after digestion by chondroitinase-ABC and -AC is summarized in Table 1. Detected HA accounted for 10-13% of total AGAG in the urine of the WS patients. In contrast, very little HA is present in normal individuals. In Werner's syndrome, the proportion of C-4S to total AGAG was found to be less than the normal, but that of C-6S was the same as the normal. Thus, the ratios of C-4S to C-6S in Werner's syndrome were less than those in normal subjects. HS amounted to approximately one-third of total

Table 1: Composition of urinary glycosaminoglycans in Werner's syndrome and normal subjects

Age in years, sex and number of samples	Werner's syndrome				Normal
	Case 1 5IM (N=4)	Case 2 28F (N=1)	Case 3 38F (N=3)	Case 4 43F (N=3)	5 cases (N=5) (27-51M & F)
Glycosaminoglycans	0.112±0.018²	0.073	0.081=0.014	0.085±0.015	0.055±0.07
Hyaluronic acid ¹ (%)	11.9±0.8	9.9	11.0±1.9	13.4±2.8	1.1±1.2
Chondroitin (%)	15.7±2.8	18.6	13.1±1.7	13.1±2.2	19.4±2.1
Chondroitin 4-sulfate (%)	15.5±0.9	16.0	16.5±1.1	15.3±4.3	28.5±1.5
Dermatan sulfate (%)	3.2±1.9	1.8	2.6±0.8	2.3±0.5	0.4±0.3
Chondroitin 6-sulfate (%)	15.6±1.2	17.2	15.7±0.8	15.1±1.9	17.4±4.2
Oversulfated chondroitin sulfate (%)	5.2±1.5	3.5	5.6±0.9	3.4±0.3	4.4±1.0
Heparan sulfates (%)	33.0±1.2	33.0	35.6±3.4	37.5±2.8	28.8±1.8

All values were determined by the borate carbazole reaction and expressed as %. Numbers indicate the mean and standard deviation.

1. Yield of glycosaminoglycans was determined by the borate carbazole reaction and expressed as mg/kg body weight. Hyaluronic acid, chondroitin and chondroitin 6-sulfate were calculated from the mean values of the unsaturated unsulfated and 6-sulfated disaccharides derived from hyaluronic acid, chondroitin and chondroitin 6-sulfate by digestion with chondroitinase-ABC and -AC. The yield of dermatan sulfate was estimated by subtraction of the value for the unsaturated 4-sulfated disaccharide from digestion with chondroitinase-AC from that with chondroitinase-ABC. Oversulfated chondroitin sulfate was estimated from the value for the unsaturated disulfated disaccharide after digesting with chondroitinase-ABC. Heparan sulfates were calculated from the value of glycosaminoglycans undigested with chondroitinase-ABC.

AGAG. The proportion of HS in Werner's syndrome was relatively greater than the normal. Therefore, the increased urinary AGAG in Werner's syndrome may result from the increased amount of HA and HS. By electrophoretic characterization, the band corresponding to standard HA was detected in the urinary AGAG of all 4 cases of Werner's syndrome. The HA band was not detected after digestion with Streptomyces hyaluronidase, a specific HA-lyase.

The urinary AGAG reflect the metabolism of connective tissue with aging. An increased ratio of HS to total AGAG with aging was reported by Taniguchi (1972). The proportion of C-4S to total AGAG decreased with aging, while that of C-6S tended to increase (Murata et al., 1973; Murata and Takeda, 1980). The ratios of C-4S to C-6S decreased from 1.53 during childhood to nearly or below 1.0 with aging (Murata et al., 1973). Also, the presence of HA in urinary AGAG in Werner's syndrome has been detected. The constitution of the other individual urinary AGAG in Werner's syndrome remain to be defined. The present study shows that the most characteristic feature of urinary AGAG in Werner's syndrome is the increase in the proportion of HA, followed by that of HS. This is clearly shown on electrophoresis, after fractionation by Dowex 1-X2 column chromatography (Fig. 1). It has been proposed that the increased urinary HA in Werner's syndrome may be used for diagnosis (Murata, 1982; Murata and Nakashima, 1982). In addition, the decreased proportion of C-4S to C-6S with aging in normal subjects corresponded to those in Werner's patients. Thus, the composition of urinary AGAG in this syndrome appeared to relate to the normal aging changes of connective tissue of the whole body.

Another attempt was made to ascertain in more detail the molecular-weight-dependent distribution of urinary AGAG in Werner's syndrome by focusing on enzymatic approaches, together with gel filtration, electrophoretic separation, and other chemical methods.

Approximately 20 litres of urine each were obtained from 2 patients with Werner's syndrome (Case 1, 48-year-old man; Case 2, 28-year-old woman). The urinary AGAG were prepared and purified by the methods described in previous papers (Murata et al., 1971; Murata and Takeda, 1980). The specimens were first purified by passing them through a Dowex 1-X2 column. After fractionation by gel filtration on a Sephadex G-100 column, the AGAG were subjected to enzymatic assay as mentioned above.

The amount of urinary excretion of AGAG in Werner's syndrome was 2.5 mg and 3.8 mg/24-h urine in Cases 1 and 2, respectively; both corresponded to 0.07 0.10 mg/24-h urine/kg body weight. The quantity of urinary excretion of AGAG during a 24-h period was within normal limits or a little lower than that of a healthy person of the same age, but the daily urinary excretion of AGAG per kg body weight was a little higher, as described above.

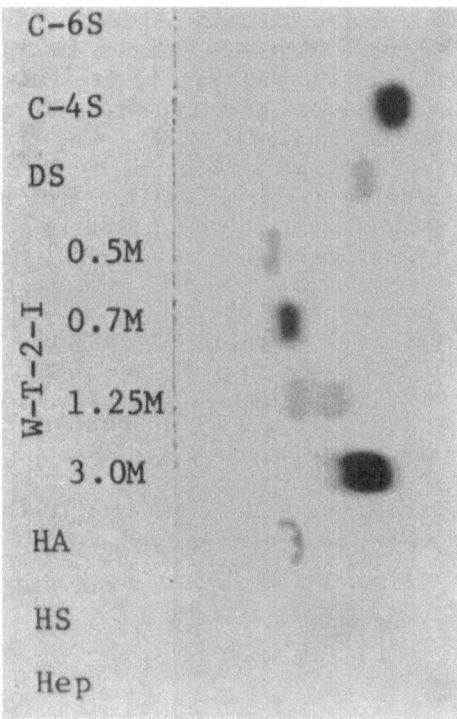

Fig. 1:   Electrophoretic characterization of urinary AGAG of a
           patient with Werner's syndrome (50 years, male)
           fractionated previously by a Dowex 1-X2 column (Cl- form,
           200-400 mesh, 1 x 35 cm) with stepwise elution at
           different CaCl molarities. Electrophoresis was carried
           out in 0.1 M pyridine formic acid buffer at pH 3.0 for 50
           min. Note that the single band at 0.5 M and 0.7 M NaCl
           fraction and the slower band at 1.25 M NaCl moved like
           the standard HA. The bands were digested with
           Streptomyces hyaluronidase.

    The crude urinary AGAG obtained from the patients with
Werner's syndrome were then subjected to Sephadex G-100 column
chromatography. The elution profiles showed two main peaks which
were fractionated to Fr. I to V and characterized by
electrophoresis and enzymic procedure (Fig. 2). The
electrophoretic mobility of AGAG shows that the faster moving
bands, corresponding to the HS standard, stained with high optical
density. As the slower bands were digested with Streptomyces
hyaluronidase, they were judged to be HA. The presence of HA and
HS in the higher-molecular-weight fractions and with wider
distribution was supported by the electrophoresis study using
barium acetate and calcium acetate buffers.

The profile of separated unsaturated disaccharides was derived from the fractionated AGAG after digestion with chondroitinase-AC. Under these conditions, HA was degraded by treatment with chondroitinase-AC. This enzyme gave two spots of non-sulfated disaccharides (Murata and Nakazawa, 1976). The data on the separated disaccharides that were obtained by the borate carbazole reaction are summarized in Table 2. The ratio of HS or HA to the total AGAG in the fraction fell in proportion to the moleclar weight. Conversely, CS isomers such as C-4S and C-6S were predominant in the low-molecular-weight fraction, C-4S in particular. In the urinary AGAG of Case 1, HA accounted for 10.2% of total AGAG, whereas 34.6% of total AGAG assumed to be HS remained undigested. Chondroitin, C-4S, and C-6S accounted for 17.1%, 17.8%, and 15.0%, respectively, or total AGAG. In Case 2, very similar results were obtained by the enzymic assay as well as by gel filtration and electrophoresis.

The question whether the AGAG components in the urine in WS patients are dependent on molecular weight has yet to be answered.

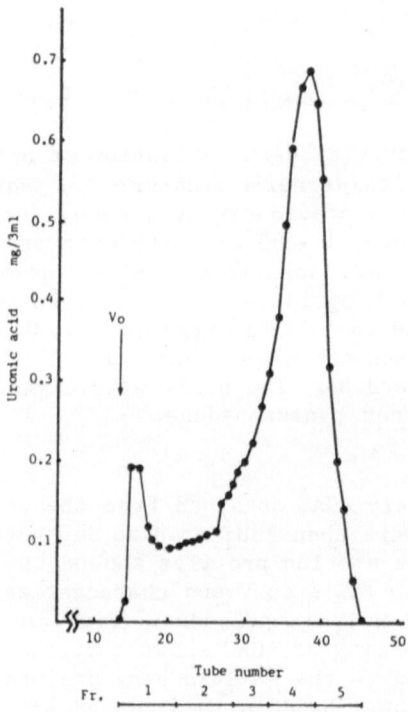

Fig. 2:   Gel chromatographic fractionation on Sephadex G-100
           column (1 x 88 cm) of urinary AGAG prepared from a
           Werner's patients (28 years female). Elution was collected
           3 ml each.

Table 2: Percent distribution of Acidic Glycosaminoglycans of Werner's syndrome by gel-chromatography on Sephadex G-100.

Acidic glucosaminoglycans	Unsaturated disaccharide	I	II	III	IV	V	Total
Hyaluronic acid	Unsulfated	18.6	10.4	7.7	7.1	8.0	10.2
Chondroitin	Unsulfated	1.9	19.6	27.7	21.4	11.1	17.1
Chondroitin 4-sulfate	4-sulfated	3.6	15.6	19.8	24.2	27.0	17.8
Chondroitin 6-sulfate	6-sulfated	5.7	17.8	17.1	16.8	16.4	15.0
Oversulfated chondroitin sulfate	Di-sulfated	1.0	4.5	5.3	6.6	10.0	5.3
Heparan sulfates	Undigested with chondroitinase-ABC	69.2	32.2	22.4	24.0	27.5	34.6
Recovery (%)		19.0	22.2	22.1	22.5	14.2	100
Chondroitin 4-sulfate / Chondroitin 6-sulfate		0.63	0.88	1.16	1.44	1.64	1.13

Fraction

This enzymic study provides a detailed description of the
composition of urinary AGAG in Werner's syndrome. It was found
that (1) HS was the major AGAG component, followed by CS isomers,
(2) HA composed about 10% of total AGAG, (3) both HA and HS were
predominant in the macromolecular fraction, (4) CS isomers such as
chondroitin, C-4S, and C-6S were prominant in the low-molecular-
weight fractions and (5) the ratio of C-4S/C-6S was higher for low-
molecular weight fractions and the average ratio was over 1.0.
Numerous studies reported that the major AGAG in normal human urine
are C-4S and C-6S (Murata et al., 1971). The ratio of C-4S/C-6S is
decreased to less than 1.0 in adults after adolescence (Murata et
al., 1973). However, a proportion of HA as high as 10% has only
been detected in Werner's syndrome. Thus, in this syndrome, the
composition of urinary AGAG, other than HA, was similar to that of
the normal aged human. Both findings implied that Werner's syndrome
is not simply a process of accelerated aging, but also suggest that
it may represent a new type of mycopolysaccharidosis. HS and HA are
known as the major AGAG in the renal connective tissue (Van Praag et
al., 1972; Murata 1976, 1980). However, it has never been
considered that HA is excreted in appreciably large amounts (over 1%
of total urinary AGAG) into normal human urine because of its high
molecualr weight (Varadi et al., 1967). In WS patients, however,
macromolecular HA and HS were both detected in the urine.
Therefore, on the basis of our results, it might be assumed that
there is some metabolic disorder in renal connective tissue, and
that laboratory examination might be expected to reveal some renal
dysfunction. Some of the HA appears to be derived from the blood
stream because HA with a lower molecular weight was detected in
urine after HA was injected intravenously (Yamada et al., 1980). In
Werner's syndrome, urinary AGAG composition may reflect some
pathological degenerative processes in the renal connective tissue,
as well as a metabolic dysfunction of the other connnective tissue
components as reflected by sclerodermatous skin changes, cataracts,
arteriosclerosis, and osteoporosis.

To study the passage through glomerulus membrane and tubes, HA
was injected intravenously in rabbits. The AGAG excreted in rabbit
urine were collected for 72 hr after the injection and purified by
the methods described above (Murata, 1979).

The HA was excreted during the first 24 h after injection.
Their molecular weight was widely distributed from 30 x 10^3 (Yamada
et al., 1980); this was estimated from the elution pattern on the
Dowex 1-X2 column. The major AGAG of the excreted urine was found
to be HA, judging from the susceptibility to Streptomyces
hyaluronidase. This finding indicates that the HA that appeared in
the urine was not only a product of kidney connective tissue but
also derived from elsewhere and passed through the glomerular
membranes. Although a small amount of HA was present in the blood
plasma (Murata and Horiuchi, 1976), it could not be detected in the

AGAG in urine. This may be due to its degradation by HA-lyase. A detectable amount of HA was also present in the plasma of a patient with Werner's syndrome.

REPORT OF AN AUTOPSIED CASE OF WERNER'S SYNDROME

The patient (A.F.) was a 50-year-old Japanese woman. Her parents were first cousins. At 15 years of age, she was of short stature and emaciated. At the age of 18, she was operated on for bilateral cataracts. Greying and loss of hair were noted at age 30. At age 43 she injured her left patellar region, the skin of which healed with difficulty. Later, she was admitted to the institute for physically handicapped persons for a severe gait disturbance and given a diagnosis of Werner's syndrome. Since age 48, she suffered from gangrene of the left toes and the heel; this then extended to the right foot and bilaterally to the knee joints. On physical examination, she was 140 cm in height and 23 kg in weight. The skin was dry and hard. It was especially thin, taut, and shiny over the extremities. There was slight pigmentation. The hair on the scalp was white and very sparse as was axillarly and pubic hair. An eyebrow had disappeared. The chest and the abdomen had no remarkable abnormalities. The extremities were slender; the knee and elbow joints showed contrictures. Blood pressure was 150/60 mmHg. She died at the age of 50 of cardial arrest.

At autopsy, the tissues and organs were analyzed for the AGAG components. Fresh tissues were obtained 8 h after death: they consisted of skin, heart (left ventricle and atrium), aorta, cerebral artery, iliac artery, vertebrae, lung alveoli, esophagus, duodenum, liver, spleen, and kidney (cortex and medulla). These specimens were kept at $-20°C$ until the chemical analysis was performed. The wet tissue weight was measured at least twice until the weight maintained constant. Approximately 20 vol of acetone and of chloroform was added to the specimen to extract contaminating lipids overnight. The AGAG were extracted and purified by the method reported previously (Murata and Yokoyama, 1982).

The specimens were cut into pieces and were homogenized and dried by lypholization. The specimens were heated in a water bath. Protein digestion was performed with pronase (1,000,000 tyrosine unit/g, Kaken Kagaku Co., Tokyo) at a rate of 20 mg/g dry tissue weight three times. β-elimination was followed at 0.4 N NaOH at 5°C overnight. Both procedures were repeated three times to complete degradation. Cold trichloroacetic acid was added at a 10% concentration and kept at 5° overnight. After centrifugation, the supernatant was dialyzed against water in a dialyzing tube at 5°C overnight. After the non-dialyzable portion was condensed, 3 vol of ethanol was added and kept at 5°C overnight to precipitate the extracted-AGAG. The AGAG were dissolved with a small amount of water and electropheretic characterization was carried out in buffer systems as reported previously (Murata et al., 1974; Seno et al., 1972; Wessler, 1968). Two-dimensional electrophoresis was also performed (Murata and Yokoyama, 1982). Uronic acid content was measured by the borate carbazole reaction of Bitter and Muir (1962). The yield of macromolecular AGAG that stained metachromatically was measured densitometrically by means of a successive sliding at 2 mm width. The amount of individual AGAG was estimated by correction on the basis of the grade of density of the standard AGAG.

The highest content of AGAG was obtained from vertebral bone, which accounted for 5.1 mg/g of defatted dry tissue weight (DFTW) when it was expressed as uronic acid unit (Table 3). The AGAG contents of the vascular tissues ranged from 2.0 to about 3.9 mg/g (DFTW) and they were relatively higher than in the other organs.

Table 3. Glycosaminoglycan Content in Various Organs and Tissues of a Patient with Werner's Syndrome

Organ & tissue		Werner's patient (mg/g DFTW)	Normal (mg/g DFTW)
Bone (vertebral)		5.1	5 - 10
Aorta		3.9	3.0-5.5
Iliac arteries	Intima	3.2	3.1
	Externa	1.9	
Cerebral arteries		2.5	2.5
Kidneys	Cortex	1.6	1.1-1.2
	Medulla	2.1	1.6-1.7
Heart	Ventricle	1.2	
	Atrium	1.6	
Esophagus		1.7	0.75
Duodenum		1.5	
Lung		1.4	0.17-0.84
Abdominal skin		1.2	0.52-0.72
Liver		0.6	0.2-0.3

All values were determined by the carbazole reaction.

In iliac arteries, a higher content of AGAG was found in the intima than in the externa. This agrees with our previous data on human aorta (Nakazawa and Murata, 1975).

Analysis of the contents of AGAG in the circulatory connective tissues such as kidneys and heart followed those of the arteries. The AGAG content in the renal medulla (2.1 mg/g DFTW) was higher than that in the cortex (1.6 mg/g DFTW). This accords also with our previous report on age-matched controls (Murata, 1980). The atrium and ventricle contained 1.6 annd 1.2 mg/g DFTW, which was lower than the values of age-matched normal control hearts (Murata, 1980). The digestive organs and tissues contained smaller amounts of AGAG. The esophagus had 1.7 mg/g DFTW, which was somehow higher than that of the normal value reported previously: 0.75 mg/g DFTW between 30 and about 59 years of age (Sekino and Murata, 1978). The AGAG content of the duodenum was less than that of esophagus. The lung alveoli contained 1.3 mg/g DFTW, which was higher than the previously reported amount (Arai et al., 1979). This may have been due to the comopositional differences in the lungs used for analysis. The AGAG content of the liver was 1.8 times normal (Murata et al., 1973). The abdominal skin in the disease contained a higher amount of 1.2 mg/g DFTW: AGAG content in normal skin was reported as 0.527 mg/g DFTW (Masuda et al., 1977), and 0.72 mg/g DFTW. The urinary AGAG of the patients was within normal limit.

The qualitative study of the AGAG was carried out by electrophoresis, either one-dimensional in various electrophoretic solutions or two-dimensional. The selective specimens of iliac arteries, which were severely affected by arteriosclerosis with calcification, was subjected to Dowex column chromatography. The AGAG in the bone contained mainly CS isomer (90%) with a minor amount (10%) of HA.

In the vascular tissue, the AGAG in the normal aorta consisted of, in the order of decreasing quantity, CS isomer, HS, DS, and HA (Table 4). This order was the same as in the intima of the iliac arteries. The cerebral arteries contained a somewhat larger HS and DS, as reported in the previous paper (Murata and Nakazawa, 1976). The AGAG constitution in the intima of the iliac artery was different from that of the externa. CS isomer predominated in the intima, whereas DS and HA were prominant in the externa. This is in accord with our previous study of the aorta (Nakazawa and Murata, 1975). However, DS was proportionally increased in the iliac artery in a Werner's patient (Fig. 4). In general, the proportion of DS in the arterial AGAG was predominantly increased in a patient with Werner's syndrome (Table 4). The main AGAG in the cerebral arteries in a Werner's syndrome patient was DS, followed by HS and CS isomers; there was a small amount of HA. In the cerebral arteries, the proportion of DS in the WS patient was 1.8 times that in the normal (Murata and Nakazawa, 1976). In the aorta and iliac arteries of the WS patients, the proportion of DS was much greater than that in the normal human aorta (Murata et al., 1975), whereas that of HS was only half that in the normal (Table 4). Thus, in the WS patient, the increased proportion of DS and the decreased

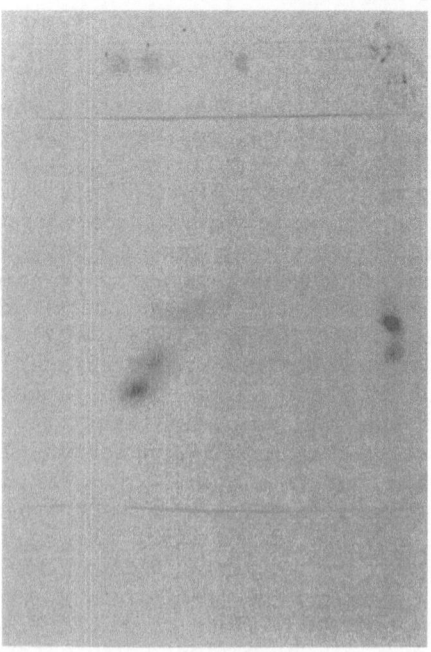

Fig. 3: Two dimensional electrophoresis of AGAG prepared from the
intima of iliac artery of a patient with Werner's syndrome.
Note a relative increase of the density of migrated like
standard DS. The staining density of the separated AGAG
consisted of, in the decreasing amount, CS isomer, DS, HS and
HA. 1st run, in 0.1 M pyridine formic acid, pH 3.0, at
0.5mA/cm, for 60 min; 2nd run, in 0.1 M calcium acetate, pH
6.8, at 0.5mA/cm, for 180 min (Murata and Yokoyama, 1982).

proportion of HS were detected in the aorta, iliac arteries, and
cerebral arteries.

The major AGAG of the kidneys was HS, which accounted for more
than half the total AGAG, and HS was more prominent in the cortex
than in the medulla (Murata, 1980). The ratio of DS to HS in the
normal medulla was 0.16, whereas that in the WS patient was 0.55.
In the cortex, the ratios were 0.39 and 0.55, respectively. The
proportion of DS to total AGAG increased markedly in the WS
patient, particularly in the medulla. A smaller amount of HA was
present in the WS patient than in the normal.

The AGAG in the atrium and ventricle consisted of HA, DS, CS
isomers, and HS. The proportion of HA in Werner's syndrome was
less than that in the normal (66% of total AGAG) whereas that of DS
was greater than normal (20% of total AGAG) (Murata, 1980).

In the lung, esophagus, and duodenum of the patient with Werner's syndrome, DS was the major AGAG followed by a moderate amount of HA. Since HA in gastrointestinal tracts decreased greatly with age (Sekino and Murata, 1978), the actual change of HA in Werner's syndrome cannot be estimated. However, the increased amount of DS in gastrointestinal tracts of this syndrome seems to be noteworthy. In the liver, DS accounted for half the total AGAG, far exceeding HA. Attention should be paid to the much higher content of DS in the syndrome because the proportion of DS to total AGAG were nearly 20% in normal liver (Murata et al., 1984). The skin AGAG in the disease consisted of DS and HA at a ratio of 71% to 22%. Since the ratio for normal skin was nearly 1:1 (Shetler et al., 1972, Masuda et al., 1977), this indicates that there is a greater proportion of DS than in the normal, and that the soft abdominal skin in the Werner's patient had undergone an imbalance of the AGAG constituents.

Werner's syndrome is a disease affecting the connective tissue. Information, however, is limited on the AGAG composition of the tissues and organs in this syndrome. The present study revealed that the AGAG content in the various organs tended to reflect the severity of the changes in the fibrous proteins. In comparative studies of AGAG constituents, the ratios of DS to total AGAG increased in these tissues and organs, whereas that of HS to total AGAG tended to decrease.

In the vascular tissues, the AGAG of the arteriosclerotic portion of the iliac arteries contained more DS than did the normal portion, whereas the amount of HA was moderate (Table 4). This observation agrees with proportionally higher DS content and moderate HA content, the DS increasing with the degree of severity of arteriosclerosis (Murata annd Yokoyama, 1982). The ratio of collagen type I to type III and their proportion to collagen type V increased in the arteriosclerotic iliac arteries in Werner's syndrome. The AGAG in the externa was unchanged in relation to those in the interna. The AGAG in the cerebral arteries and aorta still had a higher ratio of DS to HA in Werner's syndrome than in normal possibly because of the fibrous changes in situ (Table 4). In the AGAG in the renal medulla, the proportion of DS increased to 29% of total AGAG in Werner's syndrome in comparison to the age-matched control (6.2% of total AGAG), either reflecting kidney dysfunction or pathological changes in the disease. The decreased proportion of HA in the medulla in WS may be related to the release of HA into the urine. This may suggest a certain destructive change in the medulla constitution in Werner's syndrome. There is also an evidence that normal kidney medulla cells produce HA (Takeuchi et al., 1974).

The present study showed an increase in total AGAG and in the proportion of DS to total AGAG in the digestive organs (liver,

Table 4: Distribution of glycosaminoglycan composition in various arteries in a patient with Werner's syndrome.

	Cerebral arteries		Aorta		Iliac Arteries	
	Werner's patient	Normal	Werner's patient	Normal	Werner's patient	Normal
Hyaluronic acid	14	5	14	10	14	8
Chondroitin sulfates	20	36	49	55	44	45
Dermatan sulfate	41	24	27	12	25	17
Heparan sulfates	25	35	11	24	18	30

Determination was made by the borate carbazole reaction.
The values were expressed as % to total AGAG.

esophagus, duodenum) and in the lung and heart (Table 3), indicating that certain fibrous changes occur in situ, because fibrous change in these organs which appear to be associated with aging resulted in the increase of the proportion of DS to total AGAG (Murata, 1980). The AGAG content was also increased in the macroscopically non-sclerotic skin in the patient with Werner's syndrome (Table 3), which was somewhat higher than the normal values reported previously [527 ug/DFTW (Masuda et al., 1977), 720 ug/DFTW (Shelter et al., 1972)] and higher than that reported by Fleischmajer and Nedwich (1973), who analyzed the AGAG content of the induratively sclerotic portion of a patient with the syndrome. Some difference in the AGAG composition seemed to be the different degree of sclerotic change between our case and this. Similarly, the ratio of DS to HA was 2.8 times normal in his case, whereas that of our case 2.1 times normal. Our study showed that the ratio of DS to HA was 67:33, indicating the increase in the DS component in WS even in the absence of sclerosis. The same was true for all the organs and tissues studied.

Skin fibroblasts prepared from biopsy specimens from WS patients and from normal subjects were cultured in Eagle's minimum essential medium (MEM) supplemented with non-essential amino acids and with 10% fetal calf serum. As an initial approach, the fibroblasts were cultured as a monolayer in 2-ml culture flasks in MEM to which was added 0.5% or 10% calf serum for 72 h at 3 different temperatures, e.g. 34°C, 37°C and 39°C. Under the various conditions, the AGAG content was persistently higher in the medium cultured in 10% (average, 11.6 ug/2 ml) than in 0.5% (average 5.1 ug/2 ml) serum. In normal fibroblasts, the AGAG content increased with increasing temperature, when either the cells were incubated in 0.5% or 10% serum. Temperature had little effect on the AGAG content of WS fibroblasts either in 0.5% or in 10% serum. It should be noted that when WS fibroblasts were transformed by SV40, the AGAG content in the medium decreased 30% 40% in each or in serum used. This was more noticeable when both temperature and serum content were higher. Also, the decreasing effect of cell transformation on the AGAG content was observed in normal fibroblasts. Although the reduction in the amount of AGAG in the culture medium by transformed cells was related to the small number of cells (see chapter by Matsumura et al.), the reduction in the amount of AGAG was far greater than that in the number of cells. Thus, cell transformation changed the AGAG content not only quantitatively but also qualitatively.

Next, the qualitative change of AGAG was examined electrophoretically. AGAG in skin fibroblasts of the WS patient was compared with those of the normal subject. The AGAG components, in the normal skin fibroblasts were HA plus a small amount of HS and CS, but HA predominated in the confluent WS fibroblasts (Fig. 4). The normal fibroblasts contained other AGAG in addition to HA,

whereas the WS fibroblasts contained mainly HA. Furthermore, when
the WS fibroblasts were transformed, the predominant AGAG
constituent was HA (Fig. 5). This finding was observed in repeated
determinations.

DISCUSSION

We do not know why cell transformation reduces the AGAG
content and increases the proportion of HA in fibroblasts, WS skin
fibroblasts in paticular. It may be explained in vivo by the
findings that an appreciable amount of HA is excreted in urine of
WS patients. In vitro, the HA content was proportionately higher
in the culture medium (100%) than synthesized in the fibroblasts
(46%) (Fig. 4).

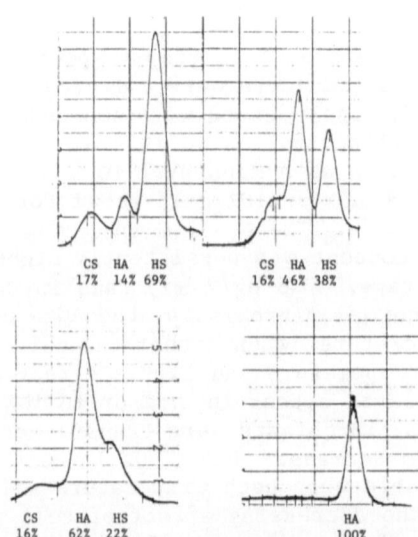

Fig. 4: Electrophoretic comparison of the constituents of
intracellular and extracellular AGAG in Werner's
fibroblast (1216) and normal fibroblast (WI-38). Both
cells were cultured for 72 h in Eagle's minimum essential
medium added 0.5% fetal calf serum and obtained at
confluent state. Electrophoresis was performed in 0.1 M
pyridine - formic acid solution at 0.5 mA/cm for 60 min.
Upper, intra-cellular AGAG; lower, in culture medium;
Left, normal; right, Werner's fibroblast. Note the
increased proportion of HA in Werner's fibroblast both in
intracellular and extracellular AGAG. Higher proportion
of HA was detected in the culture medium than in cells.

In summary, the recent data mentioned above regarding AGAG composition in Werner's syndrome, in various specimen levels (cells, tissues, organs, and body fluids) indicated that the fibroblasts in Werner's syndrome intracellularly produce predominantly HA, followed in decreasing amounts by HS and CS isomers. In the tissues or organs in this disease, HA content was unchanged or increased somewhat, but DS content constantly increased. In cell cultures, the HA was released extracellularly after being synthesized in the cells.

Reflecting metabolism in vitro, the HA was predominantly excreted in urine in patients with Werner's syndrome. This study suggests that in vivo HA, which is proportionally higher in fetal, new-born, and young ages, degrades and is released from the body's connective tissues. This phenomenon in Werner's syndrome may be interpreted as the disorder of AGAG metabolism and used for diagnosis of the disease. To date we do not know from where HA is derived. However, it could be produced partly in the cells of the renal medulla and partly by fibroblasts in connective tissue throughout the body.

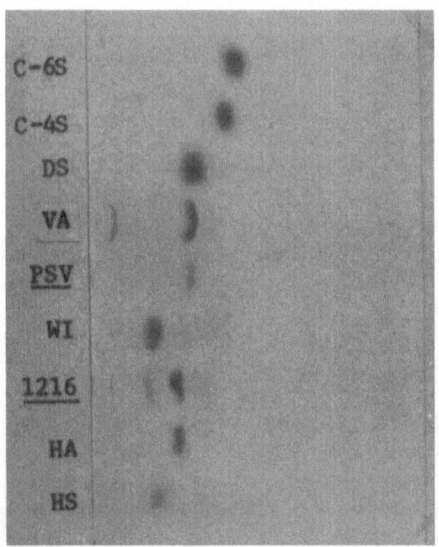

Fig. 5:   Electrophoretic profile of cellular AGAG in 0.1 M barium acetate buffer. They were prepared from normal fibroblast (WI 38) and transformed normal fibroblast (VA 13), Werner-fibroblast (1216) and and transformed Werner's fibroblast (PSV, 1216). Note that HA was predominant in Werner's fibroblasts.

PSV mostly HA, VA, HA 68%, HS 14%, CS 18%, WI, HA 14%, HS 69%, CS 17%, 1216, HA 47%, HS 38%, CS 15%.

REFERENCES

Arai, H., Kang, K., Saito, H., Nagai, H., Motomiya, M., and Konno,
    K., 1979, Significance of the quantification and demonstration
    of hyaluronic acid in tissue specimens for the diagnosis of
    pleural mesothelioma, Am. Rev. Resp. Dis., 120:529.
Bitter, J., and Muir, H., 1962, A modified uronic acid carbazole
    reaction, Analyt. Biochem., 4:330.
Epstein, C.J., Martin, G.M., Schultz, A.L., and Motulsky, A.G.,
    1966, Werner's syndrome. A review of its symptomatology,
    natural history, pathologic features, genetics and
    relationship to the natural aging process, Medicine, 45:177.
Fleischmajer, R., and Nedwich, A., 1973, Werner's syndrome, Am. J.
    Med., 54:111.
Fleischmajer, R., Perlish, J.S., and Bashey, R.I., 1972, Human
    dermal glycosaminoglycans and aging, Biochim. Biophys. Acta,
    279:265.
Fleischmajer, R., Perlish, J.S., and Gaisin, A., 1973, Comparative
    study of dermal glycosaminoglycans, J. Invest. Derm., 61:1.
Goto, M., and Murata, K., 1978, Urinary excretion of macrolomecular
    acidic glycosaminoglycans in Werner's syndrome, Clin. Chim.
    Acta, 85:101.
Kojima, J., Nakamura, N., Kanatani, M., and Ohmori, K., 1975, The
    glycosaminoglycans in human hepatic cancer, Cancer Res.,
    35:542.
Laurent, T.C., 1970, Structure of hyaluronic acid, in: "Chemistry
    and Molecular Biology of the Intercellular Matrix," E.A.
    Balaazs, ed., Academic Press, New York, p. 703.
Masuda, H., Shichijo, S., and Takeuchi, M., 1977, Comparative
    studies on the distribution of the glycopeptide and
    glycosaminoglycans in the human abdominal wall, Int. J.
    Biochem., 8:633.
Murata, K., 1979, Differences in acidic glycosaminoglycans in
    cortical and medullary tissue in human kidney, Renal Physiol.,
    2:346.
Murata, K., 1981, Acidic glycosaminoglycans in human heart values,
    J. Mol. Cell. Cardiol., 13:281.
Murata, K., 1980, Enzymic assay of acidic glycosaminoglycans, in:
    "Methods in Carbohydrate Chemistry," R.L. Whistler and J.N.
    BeMiller, eds., Academic Press, New York, p. 79.
Murata, K., 1982, Glycosaminoglycans in kidney normal and
    pathological aspects, in: "Glycosaminoglycans and
    proteoglycans in Physiological and Pathological Processes of
    Body System," R.S., Varma, R. Varma, eds., Karger, Warren Pa.
Murata, K., Akashio, K., and Ochiai, Y., 1984, Changes in acidic
    glycosaminoglycan components at different stages of human liver
    cirrhosis, Hepato-Gastroent., in press.
Murata, K., and Horiuchi Y., 1977, Molecular weight-dependent
    distribution of acidic glycosaminoglycans in human plasma,
    Clin. Chim. Acta, 75:59.
Murata, K., and Nakazawa, K., 1976, Composition of acidic

glycosaminoglycans in human cerebral arteries,
Atherosclerosis., 25:31.

Murata, K., Nakazawa, K., and Hamai, A., 1975, Distribution of
acidic glycosaminoglycans in the intima, media and adventitia
of bovine aorta and their anticoagulant properties,
Atherosclerosis, 21:93.

Murata, K., and Nakashima, H., 1982, Werner's syndrome: Twenty-
four cases with a review of the Japanese medical literature,
Am. Geriat. Soc., 30:303.

Murata, K., Ishikawa, T., and Ninomiya, H., Age-dependent changes
of chondroitin sulfate isomers in normal human urine, Biochem.
Med., 8:472.

Murata, K., Ogura, T., and Okuyama, T., 1974, The acidic
glycosaminoglycAns in leukocytes: an application of enzymatic
methods, Connect. Tiss. Res., 2:101.

Murata, K., Okudaira, M., and Adashio, K., 1973, Mast cells in
human liver tissue: Increased mast cell number in relation to
the components of connective tissue in cirrhotic process, Acta
Dermatoverner, 73:157.

Murata, K., and Takeda, M., 1980, Compostional changes of urinary
acidic glycosaminoglycans in progressive systemic sclerosis,
Clin. Chim. Acta, 108:49.

Murata, K., and Yokoyama, Y., 1982, Acidic glycosaminoglycan, lipid
and water content in human coronary arterial branches,
Atherosclerosis, 45:53.

Nakazawa, K., and Murata, K., 1975, Acidic glycosaminoglycans in
three layers of human aorta: their different constitution and
anticoacul and function, Arterial Wall, 2:203.

Praag, D.V., Stone, A.L., Richter, A.J., and Farber, S.J., 1972,
Composition of glycosaminoglycans (mucopolysaccharides) in
rabbit kidney. II Renal cortex, Biochim. Biophys. Acta,
273:149.

Reichel, W., Garcia-Bunnel, R., and Dilallo, J., 1971, Progeria and
Werner's syndrome as models for the study of normal human
aging, J. Am. Geriatr. Soc., 19:369.

Saito, H., Yamagata, T., and Suzuki, S., 1968, Enzymatic methods
for the determination of small quantities of isomeric
chondroitin sulfates, J. Biol. CHem., 243:1536.

Sekino, T., and Murata, K., 1978, Age dependent chostitutional
change of acidic glycosaminoglycans in human esophagus,
Digestion, 18:319.

Seno, N., Anno, K., Kondo, K., Nagase, S., and Saito, S., 1970,
Improved method for electrophoretic separation and rapid
quantitation of isomeric chondroitin sulfates on celllulose
acetate strips, Analyt. Biochem., 37:197.

Shelter, M.R., Shetler, C.L., Chien, S.F., Linares, H.,
Dobrokowsky, M., and Larson, D.L., 1972, The hypertrophic
scar. Hexosamine containing components of burn scars, Proc.
Soc. Biol. Med., 139:544.

Takeuchi, J., Sobue, M., Shimamoto, M., Yoshida, M., Sato, E., and
Leighton, H., 1977, Cell surface glycosaminoglycans of cell

line MDCK derived from canine kidney, Cancer Res., 37:1507.

Taniguchi, N., 1972, Age differences in the pattern of urinary glycosaminoglycan excretion in normal individuals, Clin. Chim. Acta, 37:225.

Tokunaga, M., Futami, T., Wakamatsu, Endo, M. and yoshizawa, Z., 1975, Werner's syndrome as hyaluronuria, Clin. Chim. Acta, 62:89.

Varadi, D.P., Cifonelli, J.A., and dorfman, A., 1967, The acid mucopolysaccharides in normal human urine, Biochim. Biophys. Acta, 141:103.

Werner, C.W.O., 1904, Uber Katarakt in Verbindung mit sklerodermie, Thesis, Schmidt and Klauning, Kiel, Doctoral dissertation.

Wessler, E., 1968, Analytical and preparative separation of acid glycosaminoglycans by electrophoresis in barium acetate, Analyt. Biochem., 26:439.

Wessler, E., 1971, The nature of the non-ultrafiltrable glycosaminoglycans of normal human urine, Biochem. J., 112:373.

Yamada, Y., Murata, K., Miyamoto, Y., and Horiuchi, Y., 1979, 2 cases of Werner's syndrome with hyaluronuria, Metabolism, (Tokyo), 16:1215 (in Japanese)

ACIDIC GLYCOSAMINOGLYCANS OF

SV40-TRANSFORMED WERNER'S SYNDROME CELLS

Katsumi Murata, Mieko Kudo*, and Toshiharu Matsumura**

*Department of Medicine and Physical Therapy
Faculty of Medicine
University of Tokyo
Bunkyo-ku, Tokyo 113

**Department of Pathobiochemical Cell Research
Institute of Medical Science
University of Tokyo
Shirokanedai, Minato-ku
Tokyo 108

INTRODUCTION

Patients with Werner's syndrome (WS) excrete in their urine a relatively high content of hyaluronic acid (HA) among acidic glycosaminoglycan (AGAG) species (Tokunaga et al., 1975, Murata, 1982). Recently a permanent cell line (PSV811) of WS skin cells was established by SV40-transformation (Matsumura et al., in this issue). It is of interest, therefore, to study the release of AGAGs by this cell line. We isolated AGAGs from the culture fluids of PSV811 and of VA13 cells (WI-38 VA13 2RA, i.e., and SV40-transformed permanent cell line of human lung cells established by Girardi et al., 1966), and compared them by electrophoresis and desitiometry with respect to the relative contents of AGAGs. We used VA13 cells for comparison because we kept this cell line in our laboratory together with PsV811 and therefore needed to compare them to check the possibility of cell contamination and because we had no more suitable control lines (SV40-transformed permanent line of normal skin fibroblasts) on hand. The relative composition of the AGAGs differed in the two lines. We describe this preliminary

607

difference between the two lines and suggests the possibility of
PSV811 carrying a WS trait.

MATERIALS AND METHODS

VA13 cells and PSV811 cells were grown in a modified Eagle's
MEM supplemented with 10% fetal bovine serum (FBS) as described
(Matsumura et al., in this issue) and transferred routinely by
trypsinization. To determine the relative composition of AGAGs
released from cells into culture fluid, we grew cells in either a
confluent monolayer or in a subconfluent monolayer in the growth
medium, and further incubated them for addiditonal 3 days in MEM
supplemented with 0.5% FBS and non-essential amino acids. After
the 3-day incubation, the culture fluid of 24 ml or more for one
sample (from more than six 6 cm-dishes) was collected. AGAGs
were prepared by a procedure modified from that described
previously (Murata, 1974). Briefly, AGAGs were precipitated from
the culture fluid by the addition of ethanol. The AGAG-
containing precipitate was freed from proteins by pronase
digestion and dialyzed. Some AGAG preparations were further
freed from peptides by -elimination, removal of 10% cold
trichloroacetic acid-precipitable materials, and subsequent
dialysis. AGAG preparations and authentic AGAGs (from Dr. M. B.
Mathews, Chicago Univ., Ill. and Seikagaku Kogyo Co., Tokyo) were
separated by electrophoresis on slips of acetate membrane either
one-dimensionally or two-dimensionally in a barium acetate-buffer
solution (Wessler, 1968), a calcium acetate-buffer solution (Seno
et al., 1978), or a pyridine-formic acid solution (Murata et al.,
1974). Some AGAG preparations were digested by Streptomyces
hyaluronidase (Seikagaku Kogyo Co.) before they were
electrophoretically characterized. The slips were then stained
with Alcian blue solution. The relative contents of AGAGs on
them were densitometrically measured.

RESULTS AND DISCUSSION

Both the spent culture fluid from the PSV811 cells and that
from the VA13 cells contained HA, heparan sulfate (HS), and
chondroitin sulfates (CSs) identifiable by electrophoresis. They
contained dermatan sulfate (DS) below the level of the
sensitivity of desitometry. Spots from the fresh medium were
very weak in comparison with those from an equal volume of spent
culture fluid, and did not seriously disturb the semiquantitative
determination of AGAGs. The culture fluid of PSV811 contained
HA, but only small amounts of other AGAGs. This was confirmed by
two-dimensional electrophoreses (Fig. 1). On the other hand, the
culture fluid of VA13 contained certain amounts of AGAGs, which

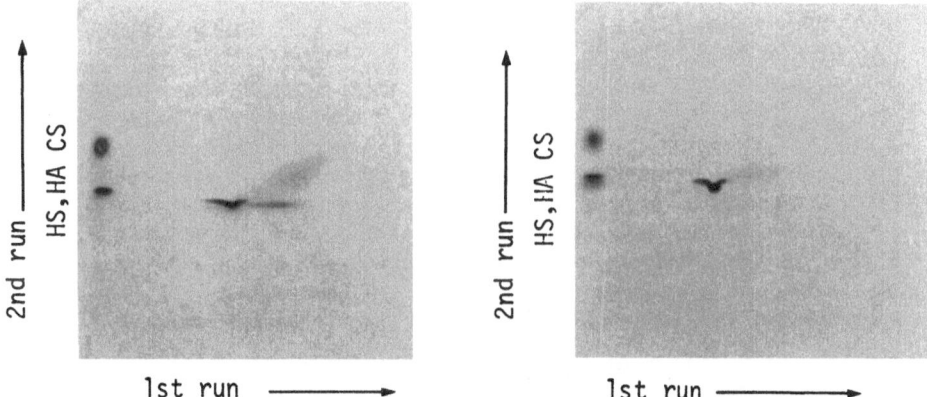

Fig. 1:   Two-dimensional electrophoretograms of AGAGs released in
culture fluid from VA13 (left) and PSV811 (right). Note
the higher proportion of HA in PSV811 than in VA13.   The
first run, pyridine-formic acid solution; the second
run, barium acetate buffer solution. The arrow
indicates the origin of the sample.

were not digested by <u>Streptomyces</u> hyaluronidase (Fig. 2).   The
relative composition of AGAGs in the culture fluid is shown in
Table 1.   The AGAG composition fluctuated among the experiments
using different samples and different electrophoretic conditions.
The composition also fluctuated between samples from a confluent
culture and from a nearly confluent culture. However, we found
in any pair of the culture-fluid samples of PSV811 and VA13 that
the proportion of HA to total AGAG was higher in that of PSV811
than is that of VA13. We also examined cell-bound AGAGs. Again
PSV811 cells contained a higher proportion of HA than VA13
(Murata et al., in this issue). These results suggest that
PSV811 and VA13 differ in their capacities of AGAG production and
excretion. This difference adds evidence that PSV811 is not a
contaminant of VA13 and that PSV811 can possibly reflect the
association of WS with abnormal HA metabolism.

ABSTRACT

    Acidic glycosaminoglycans (AGAGs) were isolated from the
culture fluids of a SV40-transformed permanent line (PSV811) of
the Werner syndrome skin cells and of a SV40-transformed
permanent line (VA13) of WI-38 normal lung cells. The relative
composition of component AGAGs was estimated by acetate membrane

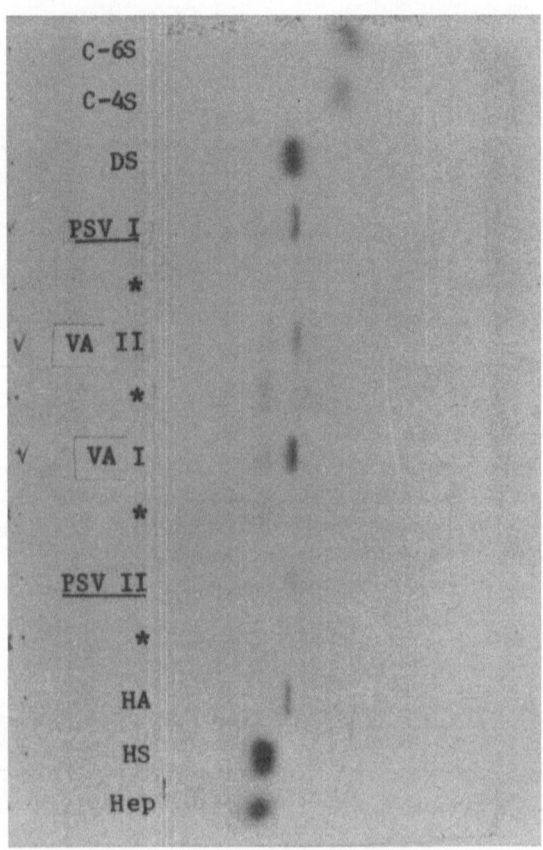

Fig. 2: Effects of <u>Streptomyces</u> hyaluronidase treatment on the
AGAG composition of culture fluids. From top to bottom:
C-6S, authentic chondroitin 6-sulfate; C-4S, authentic
chondroitin 4-sulfate; DS, authentic DS; PSVI, an AGAG
preparation from a nearly confluent PSV811 culture; *,
the above, after a <u>Streptomyces</u> hyaluronidase treatment:
VAII, an AGAG preparation from confluent VA13; *, the
above, after a hyaluronidase treatment; VAI, an AGAG
preparation from nearly confluent VA13; *, the above,
after a hyaluronidase treatment; PSVII, an AGAG
preparation from a confluent PSV811 culture; *, the
above, after a hyaluronidase treatment; HA, authentic
HA; HS, authentic HS; hep, authentic heparin.
Electrophoresis was run in barium acetate buffer
solution. This profile and the data of Exp. 1-2 in
Table 1 are from the same experiment.

Table 1. Relative Composition of Glycosaminoglycans released into the culture medium.

Exp. No.	Electro-phoresis[a]	Sample (condition)[b]	Relative composition (1%)		
			Hyaluronic acid	Heparan Sulfate	Chrondroitin Sulfate
1-1[c]	Ba	VA13(sub)	68	31	1
		VA13(conf)	68	21	11
		PSV811(sub)	100	ND	ND
		PSV811(conf)	100	ND	ND
1-2[c]	Ba	VA13(sub)	58	35	7
		VA13(conf)	42	34	24
		PSV811(sub)	67	23	10
		PSV811(conf)	100	ND	ND
2	P-F, Ca	VA13(conf)	38	21	41
		PSV811(conf)	59	13	28
	Ba	VA13(conf)	72	9	18
		PSV811(conf)	77	8	14

aElectrophoresis in: Ba, barium acetate buffer;Ca, calcium acetate buffer; P-F, puridine-formic acid solution

bsub, nearly confluent cell culture;conf, confluent cell culture. A confluent culture contained ca. 10⁷ cells per 6 cm dish. One ml of culture fluid after 3-day incubation contained 1.5-4 μg/ml uronic acid as determined by carbozole method.

cresults of two independent runs.

ND: not detected

electrophoresis followed by Alcian blue staining and desitometry.
Hyaluronic acid (HA) was the major AGAG component in all the
preparations tested. The relative content of HA fluctuated
considerably among the preparations obtained in independent
experiments and among the results using three different buffer
systems. However, the proportion of HA was persistently greater
in PSV811 culture fluid than in VA13 culture fluid. VA13 cells
released an appreciable amount of heparan sulfate as the second
major AGAG component, but PSV811 released only a small amount.
These results show a difference between the two cell lines, and
suggest that PSV811 may possibly reflect the association of the
Werner syndrome with abnormal HA metabolism.

ACKNOWLEDGEMENT. This work was in part supported by a grant from
Institute of Physical and Chemical Research.

REFERENCES

1.   A.J. Girardi, D. Weinstein, and P.S. Moorhead, SV40
      transformation of human diploid cells. A parallel study of
      viral and karyologic parameters, Ann. Med. Exp. Fenn. 44:242
      (1966).
2.   T. Matsumura, M. Nagata, R. Konishi, and M. Goto, Studies of
      SV40-infected Werner's syndrome fibroblasts, in this issue.
3.   K. Murata, Acidic glycosaminoglycans in human platelets and
      leukocytes: The isolation and enzymatic characterization of
      chondroitin 4-sulfate, Clin. Chim. Acta. 57:115 (1974).
4.   K. Murata, Urinary acidic glycosaminoglycans in Werner's
      syndrome, Experientia. 38:313 (1982).
5.   K. Murata, R. Hiwatari, and T. Matsumura, Acidic
      glycosaminoglycans in the Werner syndorme: Studies on
      tissue, organ, cell and fluid levels, in this issue.
6.   K. Murata, T. Ogura, and T. Okuyama, The acidic
      glycosaminoglycans in leukocytes: An application of enzymatic
      methods, Connect. Tissue Res. 2:101 (1974).
7.   N. Seno, K. Anno, K. Kondo, S. Nagase, and S. Saito, Improved
      method for electrophoretic separation and rapid quantitation
      of isomeric chondroitin sulfates on cellulose acetate strips,
      Analyt. Biochem. 37:197 (1970).
8.   M. Tokunaga, T. Futami, E. Wakamatsu, M. Endo, and Z.
      Yosizawa, Werner's syndrome as "Hyaluronuria". Clin. Chim.
      Acta., 62:89 (1975).
9.   E. Wessler, Analytical and preparative separation of acidic
      glycosaminoglycans by electrophoresis in barium acetate,
      Analyt. Biochem. 26:439 (1968).

GLYCOSAMINOGLYCAN SYNTHESIS IN UNTRANSFORMED AND TRANSFORMED

WERNER SYNDROME FIBROBLASTS: A PRELIMINARY REPORT

Yoshisada Fujiwara[1] and Masamitsu Ichihashi[2]

Department of Radiation Biophysics[1],
and Department of Dermatology[2]
Kobe University School of Medicine, Kusunoki-cho 7-5-1,
Chuo-ku, Kobe 650, Japan

ABSTRACT

    Glycosaminoglycan (GAG) synthesis was studied in
untransformed and transformed normal and Werner syndrome (WS)
fibroblasts, because WS manifests pleiotropic abnormalities in
connective tissue. Continuous labelling of cells with [3H]
glucosamine and [35S] sulfate for 48 hours revealed enhanced
synthesis of cellular GAG, more rapid transfer of these into the
pericellular fraction, and more accumulation of GAG in the medium
in cultures of untransformed WS fibroblasts compared with
cultures of normal diploid cells. Total GAG in the 24 hour
medium from confluent cultures was composed of 80-90% hyaluronic
acid (HA) and 10-20% sulfated GAG (S-GAGs) in both untransformed
normal and WS fibroblasts, whereas it was approximately 50% each
HA and S-GAG in transformed normal and WS cells. The
proportional enhancement of [35S] GAG synthesis in response to
exogenous beta-D-xylopyranosides was similar in normal and WS
cells, although transformed cells demonstrated only approximately
one-half the enhancement observed in non-transformed cells.
Thus, the overall activity of GAG synthesis is not grossly
altered by the WS gene mutation. Enhanced synthesis and
accumulation of HA and dermatan sulfate (DS) in the medium was
characteristic of untransformed WS fibroblasts, but appeared to
be normalized in an SV40-transformed WS cell line (PSV811), as in
transformed normal cells (WI38CT-1). We need more experiments to
determine whether aberrant GAG metabolism in WS cells is a direct
or indirect expression of the primary gene defect.

INTRODUCTION

The Werner syndrome (WS) manifests a wide spectrum of age-related symptoms, as a segmental progeroid condition (Martin, 1978). WS also demonstrates pleiotropic impairments in the development, morphology, and metabolism of connective and mesenchymal tissues, as revealed by skin atrophy, atherosclerosis, cataracts, hypogonadism, osteoporosis, high incidence of mesenchymal tumors (Epstein et al., 1966; Nakao et al., 1978; Salk, 1982) and excess excretion of GAGs in urine (Goto and Murata, 1978; Murata, 1982). The life span in vitro of cultured skin fibroblasts from WS patients is shortened (Martin et al., 1970; Higashikawa and Fujiwara, 1978; Goldstein, 1979; Salk et al., 1981; Fujiwara, 1982; Salk, 1982). Such age-related abnormalities appear to result from an autosomal recessive mutation, but the basic molecular defect of WS is not known.

The matrix of skin connective tissue consists of collagen, proteoglycans, and their complex links. Compared with the inconsistent abnormalities of collagen, the aberrant components and metabolism of GAG may be of greater importance to the clinically observed skin changes (Fleishmajor and Nedwich, 1973; Salk, 1982). Study of cultured skin fibroblasts suggest there is altered metabolism of GAG, especially in increased accumulations of HA and S-GAGs in WS cells (Tajima et al., 1981). However, the detailed kinetics and mechanism of disturbed GAG metabolism in WS are not yet known.

We have studied the synthesis and accumulation of specific GAG components in untransformed WS skin fibroblasts in vitro at the middle of their life span in vitro. Cell transformation has been known to change GAG synthesis (Cohn et al., 1976; Hopewood and Dorfman, 1977), and if transformation normalizes GAG metabolism in WS cells, then the genetic effect on GAG synthesis would appear to be secondary. Thus, we also compared GAG synthesis in an SV40-transformed WS strain with those of transformed normal cells and untransformed normal and WS cells.

MATERIALS AND METHODS

Cell Strains and Cultures

Two normal untransformed fibroblast strains (NHSF46, TIG-1) and three WS strains were used (Table 1; see also Fujiwara et al., this volume). Cells were routinely cultured in Eagle's MEM supplemented with 1 x non-essential amino acids and 15% fetal calf serum (FCS; Flow Lab.), as described previously (Fujiwara and Satoh, 1981).

Incubation of Cells with [35S] Sulfate and [3H] Glucosamine

For labelling, untransformed cells grown in 60- or 100-mm
Corning culture dishes were made contact-inhibited and
transformed cells were made confluent. Cells were then fed
overnight with medium containing 10% or 0.1% FCS, and labelled
with 5.44 μCi/ml [35S] sulfate (sp. act., 40-63.6 Ci/mole; The
Radiochemical Centre) or with 13.4-20 μCi/ml D-[3H] glucosamine

Table 1. The Fibroblast Strains Used and Their Characteristics.

Strains	Origin	MPD(a)	PDs used	Sources
Untransformed				
NHSF46	46 yr-old male skin (normal)	48	12-25	Authors
TIG-1	Fetal lung (female)	82	28-40	Ohashi,M.(b)
WS5KO	45-yr-old male Werner skin	28	10	Authors
WS11KO	37-yr-old male Werner skin	26	6-15	Authors
WS12KO	46-yr-old male Werner skin	28	7-18	Nakao,Y.(c)
Transformed				
WI38CT-1	WI38 (fetal lung) gamma ray transformed	unlimited	430-440	Namba,M.(d)
PSV811	WS2JTO Werner skin SV40 trans- formed	unlimited	415-420	Matsumura, T.(e)

a Maximum population doubling
b Tokyo Metropolitan Institute of Gerontology, Tokyo
c Kobe University School of Medicine, Kobe
d Kawasaki Medical School, Kurashiki
e Institute of Medical Science, University of Tokyo, Tokyo

(sp. act., 2.17 Ci/mmole; The Radiochemical Centre) or both, in 5
and 15 ml of high or low-serum medium per 60 and 100 mm dish,
respectively, for the desired lengths of time, up to 48 hours.
To see if xylotransferases abnormally stimulate the incorporation
of [^{35}S] sulfate in WS and transformed cells, either 0.5 mM p-
nitrophenyl-beta-D-xylopyranoside or 1 mM 4-methylumbellyferryl-
beta-D-xylopyranoside (P-L Biochemicals) was added to the
confluent cultures (0.1% FCS) for 36 hrs.

Fractionation of Labelled Cells

     The culture medium, the materials released by the EDTA-
trypsin treatment, and the remaining cell residue from the
labelled cultures were fractionated as the extracellular,
pericellular, and intracellular compartments, according to a
minor modification of the method of Glimelius et al. (1978a).
The three cellular compartments were digested with pronase (1-2
mg/ml, 3 hrs, 37°C) or papain (100-500μ g/ml, 18 hrs, pH 6.0, 60°
C) to avoid protein precipitation with the addition of acid.
When further fractionation of GAG species was not required, the
GAG were precipitated as total GAG for 3 hrs with 1%
cetylpyridinium chloride (CPC) in 0.2 M NaCl (Saani and Tammi,
1977) for the filter assay of total [^{3}H] GAG and [^{35}S] GAG. When
treated with chondroitinase or hyaluronidase, soybean trypsin
inhibitor (100 µg/ml) was added to the trypsin-containing
fractions.

Determination of GAG in the Medium

     We employed the following methods to determine the GAG
species and their distribution in the medium fraction.
Hyaluronic acid (HA) and total S-GAG were separated either by the
rapid method of Saani and Tammi (1977), which involves the
selective elution of HA from the loaded, papain-digested CPC-
precipitate with 0.5 N HCl through a membrane (S-GAG were
retained on the membrane) or by the specific digestion with
Streptomyces hyalurolyticus hyaluronidase (3 units/0.1 ml sample,
1 hr, 60°C; Sekagaku Kogyo Co., Tokyo), followed by CPC
precipitation. The relative amounts of heparan sulfate (HS),
chondroitin sulfate (CS), and dermatan sulfate (DS) in the [^{35}S]
GAG in the medium fraction were determined by differential
degradations with nitrous acid, chondroitinases AC and ABC (0.1-
0.5 unit/0.1-0.5 ml sample; Sekagaku Kogyo Co.) (Malström et al.,
1975; Glimelius et al., 1978a; 1978b), followed by the CPC
precipitation for the membrane assay.

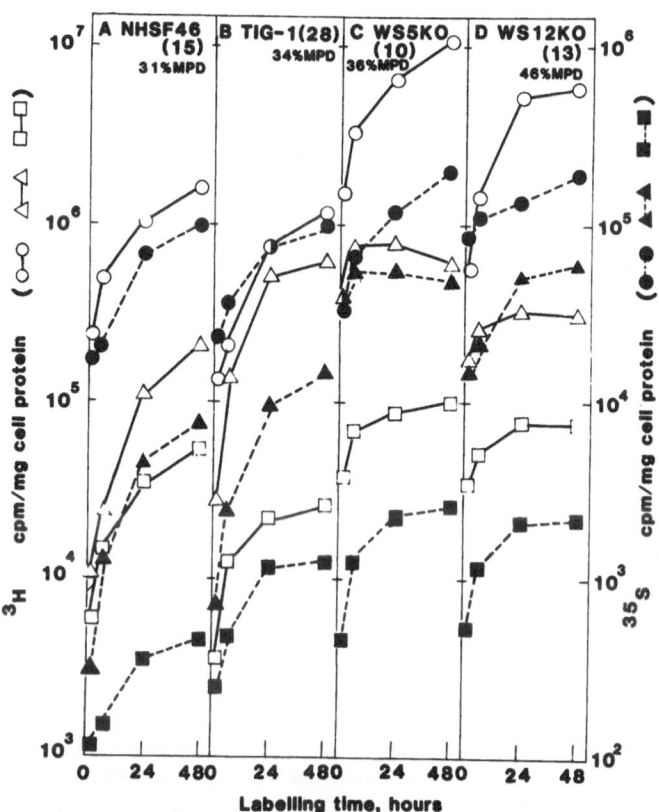

Figure 1. Total GAG synthesis in untransformed normal and WS
          fibroblasts. Cells at the indicated population
          doublings (PD) were made confluent and contact-
          inhibited, incubated overnight in fresh 10% FCS medium,
          and then double-labeled with 5.44 µ Ci/ml [35S] sulfate
          and 13.4 µ Ci/ml of [3H] glucosamine up to 48 hrs. At
          the indicated times, the extracellular, pericellular
          and intracellular fractions were prepared, treated with
          pronase (heat inactivated). [3H] GAG and [35S] GAG
          were precipitated with CPC, collected on membrane
          filters, washed exhaustively with CPC, and assayed for
          radioactivity per 1 mg cell protein. O, ● :
          extracellular, △, ▲: pericellular, □, ■:
          cellular. (Open and closed symbols indicate 3H and 35S,
          respectively.)

RESULTS

Synthesis of Total GAG in Normal and WS Fibroblasts

Confluent normal and WS cells were double-labelled
continuously in medium containing 10% FCS, 5.44 μCi/ml [35S]
sulfate, and 13.4 μCi/ml [3H] glucosamine for the desired lengths
of time up to 48 hrs. Figure 1 displays the radioactivity
profiles (cpm/mg cell protein) of [3H] GAG and [35S] GAG
synthesized in the separated extracellular, pericellular, and
cellular fractions of the cells at the middle passage of 31-46%
maximum population doubling (MPD). Synthesis of the total [3H]
and [35S] GAG in the cellular fractions of WS5KO and WS12KO cells
was somewhat faster than that in NHSF46 and TIG-1 cells over the
whole period. Transfer of total GAG to the pericellular
compartment fraction and then their excretion or shedding into
the extracellular compartment were in greater amount and more
rapid in the two WS strains than in the normal strains. As a
result, more [3H] GAG (5-10 fold) and [35S] GAG (approximately 2
fold) accumulated in the media of the two WS strains than in
normal cultures.

Analysis of GAG Synthesized in Untransformed and Transformed Normal and WS Cells

Contact-inhibited confluent untransformed cells and densely
confluent transformed cells were labelled separately with 20μ
Ci/ml of either [3H] glucosamine or [35S] sulfate, in 0.1% FCS.
Table 2 shows the analysis of the GAG in 24 hr culture medium.
There was a substantial difference between the untransformed and
transformed cells in the proportions of HA and S-GAG as estimated
from [3H] GAG. In untransformed normal and WS cells, total GAG
consisted of 80-90% HA and 12-21% S-GAG, which agrees with the
normal human skin fibroblast (NHSF) data of Saani and Tammi
(1977). However, in transformed WI38CT-1 and PSV881 (WS) cells
the distribution was approximately 50%. Thus, transformation
depressed the synthesis activity of HA in human fibroblasts under
these culture conditions.

The specific and differential degradations of the [35S] GAG
in the medium by chondroitinase AC or ABC; or by treatment with
nitrous acid revealed relative amounts of [35S] HS, [35S] CS and
[35S] DS as shown in Table 2. Untransformed WS11KO and WS12KO
cells in vitro at middle cellular age contained a greater
proportion of DS (approximately 50% of total [35S] GAG), and less
CS than did untransformed NHSF46 and TIG-1 cells; there was no
difference in percent HS (Table 2). This suggests that a larger
DS content is characteristic of these WS strains. However,

Table 2. Relative amounts of GAG Synthesized in the 24 hr medium

| Cells | PD used | %MPD | [^{3}H] GAG[a] | | [^{35}S] GAG[b] | | |
			HA	S-GAG	HS	CS	DS
Untransformed cells							
NHSF46	24	50	87 ± 1.9	13 ± 1.6	34.7	33.7	30.6
TIG-1	30	37	79 ± 1.1	21 ± 2.2	30.5	31.3	38.4
WS11KO	12	46	88 ± 2.4	12 ± 0.8	31.7	13.3	54.9
WS12KO	18	64	88 ± 1.3	13 ± 0.7	34.0	21.2	44.9
Transformed cells							
WI38CT-1	433 passages		49 ± 3.8	51 ± 1.4	27.8	45.6	26.6
PSV811	426 passages		47 ± 2.1	53 ± 1.6	26.9	47.5	25.6

[a] Combined results obtained by the methods of Saani and Tammi
    and by the treatment with Streptomyces hyalurolyticus
    hyaluronidase.

[b] Single determination

----

transformed WI38CT-1 and PSV811 cells were alike in their
distributions of HS, CS and DS (Table 2), which differed from the
distributions in the untransformed cells.

To test a possibility that the enhanced synthesis and
accumulation of S-GAG in the WS culture medium (Fig. 1) may arise
from the abnormal synthesis activity of xylosyltransferases, we
examined the effects of beta-D-xylopyranosides, which are known
to stimulate the synthesis of free GAG by providing initiation
sites for GAG-chain elongation without core protein acceptors
(Hopewood et al., 1977; Vogel et al., 1981). Beta-D-
xylopyranosides were added to confluent cultures in the presence
of 20 µCi/ml [^{35}S] sulfate in 0.1% FCS for 36 hrs, and the
radioactivity of total [^{35}S] GAG released to the medium was
analyzed. Without the pyranosides, synthesis in the WS cultures
was again approximately twice that in the NHSF46 cultures, an

Table 3. Stimulation of [35S] sulfate incorporation into
          extracellular GAG of confluent cultures by beta-D-
          xylopyranosides.

| | | | [35S] GAG, cpm/10^5 cells | | |
| | | | | | |
Cells	PD Used	% MPD	None	p-nitrophenyl-β-D-xylopyrano-side, 0.5 mM	4-methylumbelly-ferryl-β-D-xylo-pyranoside, 1mM
Untransformed					
NHSF46	12	25	1,430	19,000	19,500
WS11KO	6	23	2,970	47,000	35,500
WS12KO	12	43	2,250	38,700	31,700
Transformed					
WI38CT-1			1,070	7,700	6,710
PSV811(WS)			910	7,160	6,840

less accumulated in the medium of WI38CT-1 and PSV811 cultures
(Table 3). However, the addition of either 0.5 mM p-nitrophenyl-
beta-D-xylopyranoside or 1 mM 4-methylumbellyferryl-beta-D-
xylopyranoside caused very similar, 13-17 fold stimulations of
the total [35S] GAG synthesis in terms of cpm/10^5 cells in
NHSF46, WS11KO and WS12KO fibroblasts. On the other hand, both
pyranosides produced a similar, but less (6-8 fold) stimulation
in transformed WI38CT-1 and PSV811 cells under such conditions
(Table 3). Thus, it appears that the synthesis activity, or
overall GAG polymerization, is unaltered in WS cells. A lower
rate of synthesis of total GAG in transformed cells suggests that
the level of xylosyltransferases is lower or that other unknown
factors may be involved.

Characteristics of Enhanced GAG Synthesis in Untransformed WS Cells

Untransformed normal (TIG-1, NHSF46) and WS (WS11KO, WS12KO)
cells at the confluent phase were incubated as described above
with 20 μCi/ml of either [3H] glucosamine or [35S] sulfate under
the low-serum conditions. . The medium was withdrawn at 6 and 24
hrs for analysis of incorporations in terms of cpm/cell into [3H]
HA, total [35S] GAG, and the fractionated species [35S] HS, [35S]
CS and [35S] DS.

In WS11KO (PD,15; MPD, 58%) and WS12KO (PD,7; MPD, 25%) cells synthesis of [3H] HA (Fig. 2a) and total [35S] GAG (Fig. 2b) was 2-3 times faster than in NHSF46 (PD, 25; MPD, 52%) and TIG-1 (PD, 40; MPD, 50%) cells. However, since the HA fraction appears to occupy 80-90% of the total [3H] GAG synthesized during the 24 hr incubation (Table 2), the absolute amount of HA in WS cells must be more abundant than in the amount of S-GAG in WS cells. In addition, the extent of increased synthesis differed between WS11KO and WS12KO at different cellular age.

Synthesis of [35S] DS (Fig. 2e) is enhanced most in these WS strains despite similar rates of synthesis of [35S] HS (Fig. 2c) and [35S] CS (Fig. 2d) in both normal and WS cells. Therefore, the stimulated cellular synthesis and accumulation of the HA and DS fractions in the medium compartment are characteristic of WS cells.

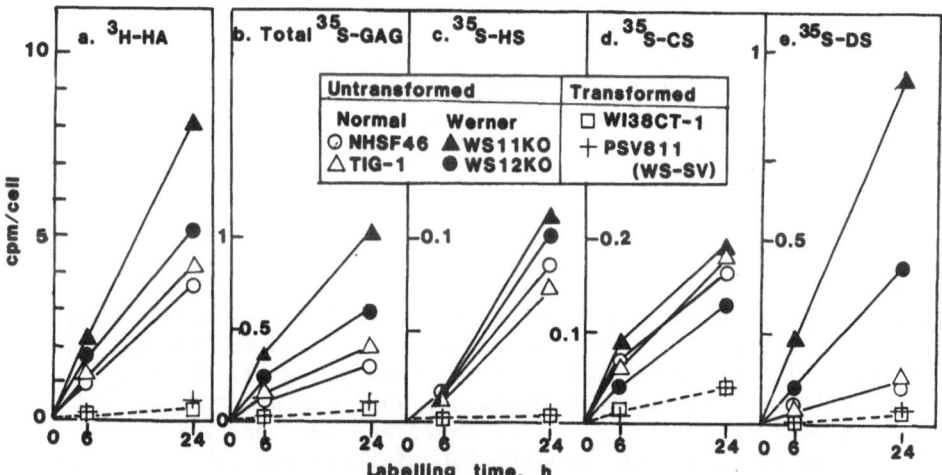

Fig. 2. The GAG synthesis in untransformed and transformed normal and WS cells. Confluent cultures of untransformed (NHSF46; 25 PDs = 52% MPD, TIG-1; 40 PDs = 50% MPD, WS11KO; 15 PDs = 58% MPD, WS12KO; 7PDs = 25% MPD) fibroblasts were incubated overnight in 0.1% FCS medium, and labelled with either 20 µCi/ml of [3H] glucosamine or or 20 µCi/ml [35S] sulfate for 24 hrs in the low-serum medium. Similarly, confluent WI38CT-1 and PSV811 cells were labelled. HA and S-GAGs (HS, CS, DS) were fractionated, and radioactivity was measured by the membrane assay after the CPC precipitation and expressed by cpm/cell. O ; NHSF46, △ ; TIG-1, ▲ ; WS11KO, ● ; WS12KO, □ ; WI38CT-1, † ; PSV811.

Change in the GAG Synthesis in Transformed WS Cells

In the same series of GAG experiments, we compared the
specific synthesis of GAG in SV40-transformed PSV811 cells of
skin origin and gamma ray transformed WI38CT-1 cells of fetal
lung origin (Table 1). The low serum, confluent condition and
transformation suppressed the synthesis of all the GAG species in
both PSV811 and WI38CT-1 cells to a comparably greater extent
(Fig. 2). A remarkable contrast to untransformed fibroblasts is
that PSV811 cells and transformed wild type WI38CT-1 cells
synthesized similar amounts of HA and DS (Figs. 2a; 2e).
Therefore, this finding implies that transformation of WS cells,
despite only a single strain, may normalize the characteristic
property of enhanced HA and DS synthesis in untransformed cells.
This phenomenon should be investigated and generalized using many
lines of tranformed WS cells and strains from different patients.

DISCUSSION

Our results presented above indicate the abnormally enhanced
synthesis and accumulation of HA and S-GAG, especially DS, in WS
fibroblasts in vitro at the middle cellular age compared with
that of normal skin and lung fibroblasts (Figs. 1 and 2). Most
of the [3H] and [35S] GAGs synthesized in the cells moved rapidly
to the surface and were excreted into the medium (Glimelius et
al., 1978b; Vogel and Kendall, 1980). Accumulation in the medium
of the WS cultures did not appear to be due to decreased
degradation of GAGs, because the accumulation kinetics were
similar to those in normal cells (Fig. 1), but rather to enhanced
synthesis (or modification) in the WS cells. These findings seem
to agree with those of Tajima et al. (1981) and Bryant et al.
(this volume). Also, our results may well explain the increased
urinary excretion of HA (Murata, 1982) and the increased
deposition of DS in the skin (Fleishmajor and Nedwich, 1973) and
other tissues (Murata, this volume). Such a feature may enhance
the development of atherosclerosis in the patients.

By studying the relation between cellular aging and GAG
metabolism in vitro, Vogel et al. (1981) showed that in IMR-90
normal human fibroblasts, the 48 hr incorporation of [35S]
sulfate into [35S] GAGs in the medium decreased with increasing
PD. Further, they suggest that cellular aging has the primary
effect on the only secreted pool of GAGs in IMR-90 cells. The
results of Vogel et al. (1981) in normal cells disagree with our
present WS cell findings of enhanced HA and DS accumulations
(Figs. 1 and 2) and a shortened life span in vitro (Table 1)
(Fujiwara et al., this volume). Cell surface HS, which increases

in amount with human cellular aging (Matsuoka and Mitsui, 1981; Sluke et al., 1981), may regulate cell growth (Matsuoka and Mitsui, 1981), but the specific HA and DS increases with no alteration of HS in the present WS strains (Table 2; Fig. 2) are not consistent with the above view. Thus, the WS condition is unique. There is still another possibility that increased S-GAGs might affect the cell and DNA replicative potential in WS cells (Fujiwara et al., this volume). In this regard, it has been recently reported that some GAG components may inhibit DNA synthesis in isolated nuclei (Furukawa and Bhovanandan, 1982). Therefore, the aberrant GAG metabolism in WS cells may be a manifestation of the WS gene mutation, but neither the specific enzyme nor the aberrant mechanism have yet been elucidated.

The enhancing effect of beta-D-xylopyranoside was similar in both normal and WS fibroblasts, and even in the transformed PSV811 and WI38CT-1 cells (Table 3). This implies that WS cells may have no grossly altered capacity of polymerizing free GAG chains. A finding that untransformed WS cells synthesized a larger amount of S-GAGs in the absence of exogenous xylosides (Figs. 1 and 2; Table 3) suggests the existence of more initiation sites for GAG chains in WS cells. However, we need further precise experiments to find out the possibly aberrant post-synthetic, polymer-level modification in WS cells, since DS, which contains the $IdU-GalNAc-SO_4$ or IdUA $(-SO4)$-GalNAc repeats in the galactosaminoglycans of the DS/CS copolymers in human fibroblasts (Malstrom et al., 1975), predominates in the present WS cells (Fig. 2; Table 2).

Under the low-serum conditions, synthesis of all the GAG species in transformed PSV811 and WI38CT-1 cells at confluence was somewhat decreased during 24 hr (Fig. 2). It has been reported that the GAG synthesis in transformed human cells is enhanced under the high-serum conditions (Hopewood and Dorfman, 1977). Although our present comparative study was done under limited conditions using only a single PSV811 line, permanent transformation appears to normalize the aberrant GAG metabolism (Fig. 2). We still cannot eliminate the possibility of masking by suppression under these conditions. This particular normalization is, however, difficult to understand, because WS is a recessive mutation, assuming that such an aberration is directly linked to the genotype. Otherwise, the aberrant gene expression for GAG metabolism in WS cells may be phenotypic and secondary. In this regard, DNA synthesis is also abnormal in WS fibroblasts (Fujiwara et al., 1977; Fujiwara et al., this volume), but such an abnormality can be normalized in transformed PSV811 cells as in WI38CT-1 cells (Fujiwara et al., this volume). We should await further experimentation.

REFERENCES

Cohn, R.H., Cassiman, J-J., and Benfield, M.R., 1976, Relationship
     of transformation, cell density and growth control to the
     cellular distribution of newly synthesized glycosaminoglycan,
     J. Cell Biol., 7:280.
Epstein, C.J., Martin, G.M., Schultz, A.L., and Motulsky, A.G.,
     1966, Werner syndrome: a review of its symptomatology,
     natural history, pathologic features, genetics, and
     relationship to the natural aging process, Medicine, 45:177.
Fleishmajor, R., and Nedwich, A., 1973, Werner's syndrome, Am. J.
     Med., 54: 111.
Fujiwara, Y., 1982, Progeroids: Genetic aspects of life span and
     cell senescence (in Japanese). Pathophysiology, 1:614.
Fujiwara, Y., and Satoh, Y., 1981, Age-dependent changes in
     fibroblast cultures from xeroderma pigmentosum variant. J.
     Invest. Dermatol., 76:215.
Fujiwara, Y., Higashikawa, T., and Tatsumi, M., 1977, A retarded
     rate of DNA replication and normal level of DNA repair in
     Werner's syndrome fibroblasts in culture, J. Cell Physiol.,
     92:365.
Furukawa, K. and Bhovanandan, V.P., 1982, Influence of
     glycosaminoglycans on endogenous DNA synthesis in isolated
     normal and cancer cell nuclei: differential effect of
     heparin, Biochim. Biophys. Acta, 697:344.
Glimelius, B., Norling, B., Westermark, B., and Wasteson, A.,
     1978a, Composition and distribution of glycosaminoglycans in
     cultures of human normal and malignant glial cells, Biochem.
     J., 172:443.
Glimelius, B., Norling, B., Westermark, B., and Wasteson, A.,
     1978b, Turnover of cell surface associated glycosaminoglycans
     in cultures of human normal and malignant glial cells, Exp.
     Cell Res., 117:179.
Goldstein, S., 1979, Studies on age-related diseases in cultured
     skin fibroblasts, J. Invest. Dermatol., 73:19.
Goto, M. and Murata, K., 1978, Urinary excretion of macromolecular
     acidic glycosasminoglycans in Werner's syndrome, Clin. Chim.
     Acta, 85:101.
Higashikawa, T. and Fujiwara, Y., 1978, Normal level of unscheduled
     DNA synthesis in Werner's syndrome fibroblasts in culture,
     Exp. Cell Res., 113:438.
Hopewood, J.J. and Forfman, A., 1977, Glycosaminoglycan synthesis
     by cultured human skin fibroblasts after transformation with
     simian virus 40, J. Biol. Chem., 252:4777.
Malstrøm, A., Carlstedt, I., Aberg, L., Fransson, L.A., 1975, The
     copolymeric structure of dermatan sulfate produced by cultured
     human fibroblasts: different distribution of induronic acid-
     and glucuronic acid-containing units in soluble and cell-
     associated glycans, Biochem. J., 151:477.

Martin, G.M., 1978, Genetic syndromes in man with potential relevance to the pathobiology of aging, Birth Defect Orig. Art. Ser., 14:5.

Martin, G.M., Sprague, C.A., and Epstein, C.J., 1970, Replicative life span of cultivated human cells: effects of donor's age, tissue and genotype, Lab. Invest., 23:86.

Matsuoka, K., and Mitsui, Y., 1981, Changes in cell-surface glycosaminoglycans in human diploid fibroblasts during in vitro aging, Mech. Age. Devel., 15:153.

Murata, K., 1982, Urinary acidic glycosaminoglycans in Werner's syndrome, Experimentia, 38:313.

Nakao, Y., Kishihara, M., Yoshimi, M., Inoue, Y., Tanaka, K., Sakamoto, N., Imura, H., Ichihashi, M., and Fujiwara, Y., 1978, Werner's syndrome: in vivo and in vitro characteristics as a model of aging, Am. J. Med., 65:919.

Saani, H. and Tammi, M., 1977, A rapid method for separating and assay of radiolabelled mucopolysaccharides from cell culture medium, Anal. Biochem., 81:40.

Salk, D., 1982, Werner syndrome: A review of recent research with analysis of connective tissue metabolism, growth control of cultured cells, and chromosomal aberrations, Hum. Genet., 62:1.

Salk, D., Au, K., Hoehn, H., Stenchever, M.R., and Martin, G.M., 1981, Evidence of clonal attenuation, clonal succession and clonal expansion in mass cultures of aging Werner's syndrome skin fibroblasts, Cytogenet. Cell Genet., 30:108.

Sluke, G., Schachtschabel, D., and Wever, J., 1981, Age-related changes in the distribution pattern of glycosaminoglycans synthesized by cultured human diploid fibroblasts (WI-38), Mech. Age. Devel., 16:19.

Tajima, T., Watanabe, G., Iijima, K., Ohshiba, Y., and Yamaguchi, H., 1981, The increase of glycosaminoglycan synthesis and accumulation on the cell surface of cultured skin fibroblasts of Werner's syndrome, Exp. Pathol., 20:221.

Vogel, K.G., and Kendall, V.F., 1980, Cell-surface glycosaminoglycans: turnover in cultured human embryo fibroblasts (IMR-90), J. Cell Physiol., 103:475.

Vogel, K.G., Kendall, V.F., and Sapien, R.E., 1981, Glycosaminoglycan synthesis and composition in human fibroblast during in vitro cellular aging (IMR-90), J. Cell Physiol., 107:271

THE NOTION OF PRIMORDIAL BUILDING BLOCKS IN CONSTRUCTION OF GENES AND TRANSCRIPTIONAL AND PROCESSING ERRORS DUE TO RANDOM OCCURRENCE OF OLIGONUCLEOTIDE SIGNAL SEQUENCES

Susumu Ohno

City of Hope Research Institute
Duarte, CA 91010

ABSTRACT

Contrary to the currently popular belief, genes (flanking and internal noncoding sequences included) that specify beta-sheet and alpha-helical proteins are not unique sequences, rather they are degenerate repeats of short primordial building block sequences that are 45 to 48 bases long in the case of genes belonging to the beta-2-microglobulin superfamily. Accordingly, a large number of base decamers, nonomers, octamers, heptamers and hexamers recur within every gene.

One consequence of the above is the random and inadvertent occurrence within genes of various oligonucleotide signal sequences for initiation and termination of transcription as well as for processing of transcripts by removal of intervening sequences. Inadvertent transcription of nonsense sequences and missplicing of transcripts may increase with age and contribute to the aging process.

There is little doubt that the life span, being one of the species' characteristics, is genetically programmed. The question remains, however, as to whether or not such a program is embodied in each and every somatic cell type. If the cessation of cell proliferation is regarded synonymous with senescence, one is placed in the awkward position of having to state that most neurons of the central nervous system enter the state of senescence at the neonatal stage. An alternative to the above is the assumption of

central control; e.g., the programmed secretion of an aging peptide
hormone by the pituitary.

To be sure somatic cells accumulate randomly sustained
mutations as do germ cells and whatever other genetic mishaps
(e.g., deletions, duplications) that may affect somatic cells also
occur in germ cells. Yet, the monophyletic germ line on this
earth has persisted for three billion years and has the potential
of being immortal. Furthermore there can be no direct cause-and-
effect relationship between the process of differentiation and the
loss of immortality, for spermatozoa are one of the most, if not
the most, differentiated cell types that can be found in the body.

Nevertheless, if one's scope is confined to the types of
genetic mishaps that may afflict somatic cells in their given life
span, the one particular type that has hitherto escaped notice
should be considered.

Genes are not unique sequences but rather they are degenerate
repeats of the primordial building block

In spite of the fact that some of the genes such as that for
Callagen (Yamada et al., 1980) are obvious repeats of the short
primordial sequence, the mistaken notion of genes being comprised
of unique sequences is still wide-spread. The roughly 1,000-base-
long coding sequence for mouse H-2K^b class I MHC antigen shown in
Figures 1 and 2, destroys the mistaken notion mentioned above once
and for all, since within this intermediate sized coding sequence,
there recurred one base decamer, 4 octamers, 12 heptamers and 29
hexamers; these hexamers identified as numbers 23, 25 and 26
recurred not twice but thrice. In addition, the nonomeric portion
identified as No. 1' of the only decamer (No. 1) recurred three
times within the most conserved 3rd domain coding sequence (Figure
2, left column). Similarly, the hexameric portion identified as
numbers 5', 6' and 9', of one octamer (No. 5) and two heptamers
(Nos. 6 and 9) also recurred three times. If the coding sequence
for the class I MHC antigen is unique sensu stricto, a given base
octamer is expected to occur only once every 65,550 bases or so and
even a given base hexamer only once every 1,000 bases (Ohno et al.,
1982). These recurring base oligomers are individually identified
in Figures 1 and 2. Similarly, mouse Ig C mu (immunoglobulin mu-
class heavy-chain constant region) gene totaling in length 2,168
base4s that included three intervening sequences and the 299-base-
long 3' noncoding region (Kawakami, et al., 1980) yielded 2
recurring base decamers, 8 nonomers and 39 octamers, recurring base
heptamers and hexamers were too numerous to merit individual
identification (Yazaki and Ohno, 1983). Of these recurring base
decamers, nonomers and octamers, the situation of one copy residing
within one of the coding sequences, whereas the other copy being
found within one of the noncoding sequences was encountered with

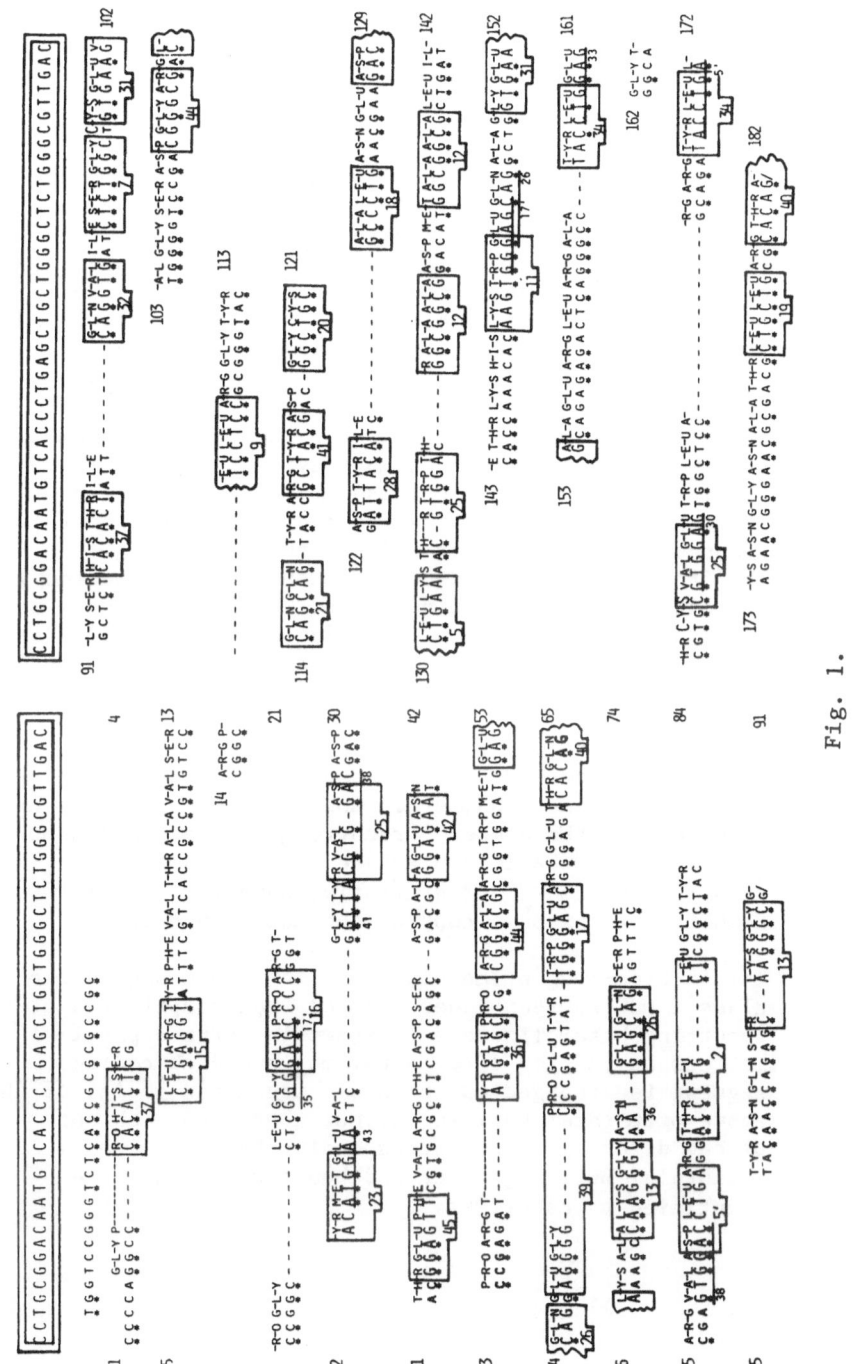

Fig. 1.

Figures 1 and 2:   The 1,088-base-long coding sequence for mouse
                   class I MHC antigen H-2K^b is shown arranged in four
                   columns.   The first three columns correspond to the
                   coding segments that specify the first three domains,
                   each roughly 90 amino acid residues long, of H-2K^b
                   antigen.   The third domain (Figure 2, left column) is the
                   most conserved in that it maintains the original
                   characteristics of the 2-microglobulin-like domain
                   faithfully.   The second domain (Figure 1, right column)
                   is a considerably degenerate copy of the third domain,
                   and the degeneracy is even more evident in the first
                   domain (Figure 1, left column).   The fourth column
                   (Figure 2, right) contains the coding segment for the 4th
                   transmembrane domain, as well as two coding segments for
                   the 5th intramembrane domain.   Each spliced junction is
                   indicated by a distinctive slash.   Coding sequences are
                   accompanied by corresponding amino acid residues.   Bases
                   of recurring base oligomers are shown in large capital
                   letters, and each of them is boxed in and identified by
                   numbers.   1 decamer (1), 4 octamers (2 to 5), 12
                   heptamers (6 to 17) and 28 hexamers (18 to 45) recurred.
                   In fact, numbers 23, 25 and 26 hexamers recurred not
                   twice but thrice.   Number 1' nonomer TCACCCTGA is a nine-
                   base copy of the number 1 recurring decamer, and number
                   5' hexamer ACCTGA is a six-base copy of number 5
                   recurring octamer, and similarly, number 9' hexamer
                   CTCCTC is a six-base copy of the number 9 heptamer.

                   The 45-base-long primordial building block sequence of
                   class I MHC antigen genes deduced from compilation of
                   recurring base oligomers is shown in large capital
                   letters at the top of each column, and each coding
                   segment is arranged as variously truncated copies of the
                   above primordial building block.   Bases of each copy are
                   placed directly below corresponding bases of the
                   primordial building block and homologous bases are
                   identified by asterisks.

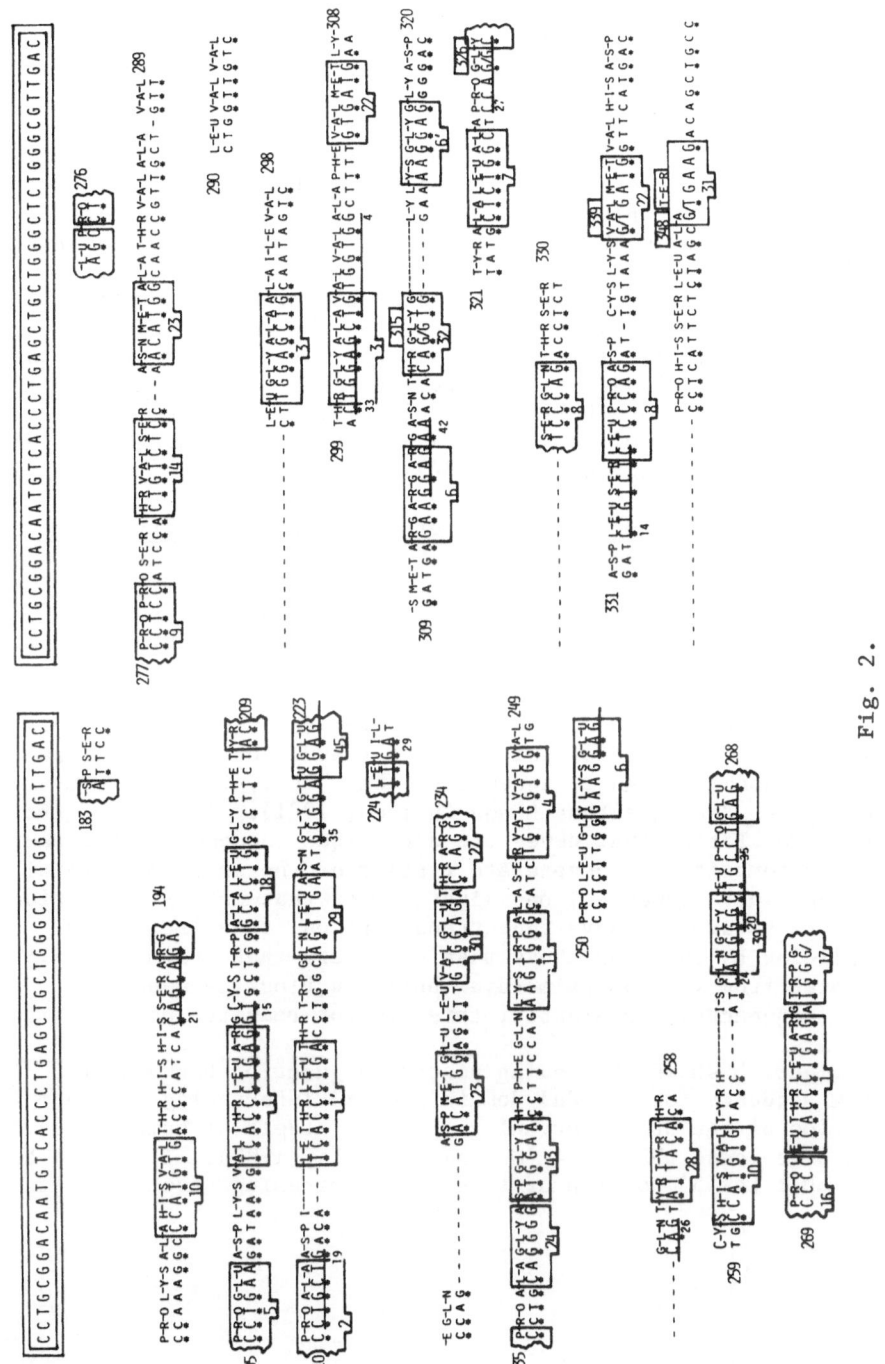

Fig. 2.

regard to one decamer, 2 nonomers and 4 octamers (Yazaki and Ohno, 1983). From the above, it was deduced that individual genes (noncoding sequences included) of the beta-2-microglobulin family evolved from tandem repeats of 45-to-48-base-long primordial building block sequences that were similar but individually distinct. It was thought that these primary building blocks originally specified 15-to-16-amino-acid-residue-long primordial arms of loops that form the beta-sheet structure. The 45-base-long primordial building block sequence characteristic of the class I MHC antigen genes is shown at the top of Figure 1 as well as Figure 2. The entire coding sequence is shown as variously truncated copies of the above primordial building block. Such cryptic repetitiousness has also been reported on the insulin gene (Douthart and Norris, 1982), and that the polytenic Balbiani ring 2 gene in salivary glands of the dipteran insect (_Chironomus tentans_) specifying a very long polypeptide of one million in molecular weight is comprised of tandem repeats of the 9-base-long primordial building block (Sumegi et al., 1982).

Recurring base oligomers and inadvertent (random) occurrence of signal base sequences

The proper functioning of genomic DNA within the nucleus depends upon the exact placing of various oligonucleotide signal sequences in the vicinity of genes. These signal sequences include RNA polymerase II promotor sequence (TATAATAT, etc.). Splicing signal sequences at the coding/intervening functions (CACAG/GUGAG, etc.), the 5' cap site signal sequence (GACCT, etc.) as well as poly-A attachment signal sequence (AATAAA, etc.) for the formation of messenger RNA (Breathnach and Chambon, 1981). In view of the present revelation that genes are not unique sequences but rather they are comprised of degenerate repeats of the short primordial building block sequences, one might expect that natural selection took care to avoid inadvertent transcription, translation and missplicing by choosing those base oligomers that are not easily generated from various primordial building block sequences as signal sequences. Apparently, this has not been the case.

Figure 3 shows the coding-noncoding junction between the coding sequence for the 2nd domain and 3rd intervening sequence and a portion of the 3rd intervening sequence itself of human class I MHC antigen gene pHLA 12.4 (Malissen et al., 1982). It should be noted that the 5' portion of this 3rd intervening sequence contains

the octameric sequence TATAATAT which can serve as a respectable
RNA polymerase II promotor site, and that 52 bases further
downstream is found the hexameric sequence GACTC which might
function as the 5' cap site signal sequence. Whether or not the
transcription is inadvertently initiated from this promotor site at
all ages of individuals is not known. If man has developed the
mechanism to suppress such an inadvertent transcription, such a
mechanism might deteriorate with age, if so, such an inadvertent
transcription might contribute to the disfunctioning of aged cells.

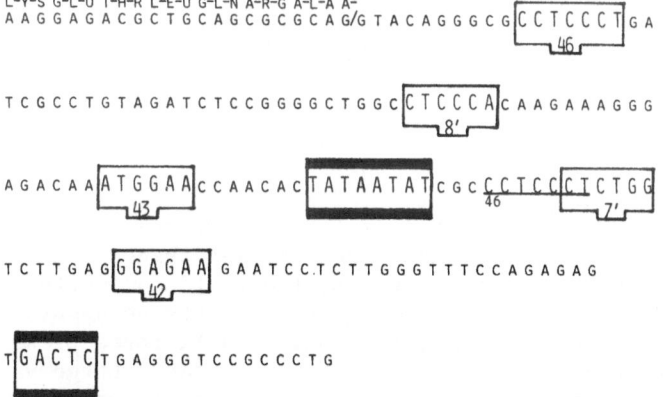

Figure 3:   A segment of human class I MHC antigen HLA 12.4 gene
            containing a 3' terminal portion of the coding segment
            for the 2nd domain and a 5' portion of the adjacent
            intervening sequence. The inadvertent occurence of the
            octameric signal sequence TATAATAT that serves as the RNA
            polymerase II promotor site within the intervening
            sequence is indicated; boxed in large capital letters.
            Fifty-two bases further downstream, there occurs the
            pentameric sequence GACTC (boxed in large capital
            letters) that may serve as the 5' cap site signal. A
            number of base oligomers that recurred within Figures 1
            and 2 are so identified, and so are a new heptamer that
            recur within this segment; i.e., No. 46.

More alarming are numerous opportunities for missplicing that recurring base oligomers offer during the processing of nuclear transcripts to mature messenger RNA. The tendency of recurring base oligomers to occupy splicing junctions is already evident in Figures 1 and 2, for the junction between the 2nd and 3rd domain coding sequences (bottom row, Figure 1, right), as well as that between the 3rd and 4th domain coding sequences (bottom row, Figure 2, left) and that between the 4th and 5th domain coding sequences (sixth row, Figure 2, right) are straddled by recurring base oligomers identified as numbers 40, 17 and 32. Figure 4 shows an example of recurring base oligomers offering ample opportunities for missplicing with regard to the splicing between the 3rd and 4th domain coding sequences of the human class I MHC antigen gene pHLA 12.4 (Malissen et al., 1982). It should be noted that the end of the 3rd domain coding sequence is marked by the nonomeric sequence GAGATGGG/G, but the same nonomer recurs only 8 bases further downstream within the 4th intervening sequence. Looking at each immediate surroundings, there appears to be no a priori reason why the first and not the second copy of the same nonomeric sequence should always serve as the upstream splicing signal. Figure 4 also shows that the end of the 4th intervening sequence is marked by the base heptamer TTCCCAG, but only 7 bases further downstream the same heptamer recurs within the 4th domain coding sequence specifying the amino acid residues Ser and Gln. Again each copy's immediate surroundings reveal no a priori reason why the 1st and not 2nd copy of the same heptameric sequence should always serve as the downstream splicing signal. Thus, there appear to be four different ways of splicing the 3rd and 4th coding sequences of human class I MHC antigen HLA 12.4. While there is little doubt that most of this human class I MHC antigen transcript is processed properly in the manner indicated by the solid connection between the 1st and 3rd rows in Figure 4, there exists no assurance that the three alternative splicings, indicated by three broken line connections in Figure 4, do not occur. In fact, three variant class I MHC antigen heavy chains may normally be produced as minorities. Furthermore, if the splicing function becomes increasingly infidelous with advancing age, they might become significant minorities to hinder proper function of the immune system. It should be noted that the first illicit splicing between the 1st and 4th rows of Figure 4 causes a frame-shift in translation after the deletion of five amino acid residues (Glu-Pro-Ser-Ser-Gln). Since any frame-shift is bound to create a new chain terminating codon in the immediate downstream, such a frame-shift is expected to cause a premature chain termination. The second illicit splicing between the second and third rows of Figure 4 merely inserts 6 extra amino acid residues (Gly-Lys-Glu-Gly-Asp-Gly) without causing a frame-shift, whereas the third illicit splicing between the 2nd and 4th rows of Figure 4 also causes a frame-shift in addition to the above-noted insertion of 6 amino acid residues.

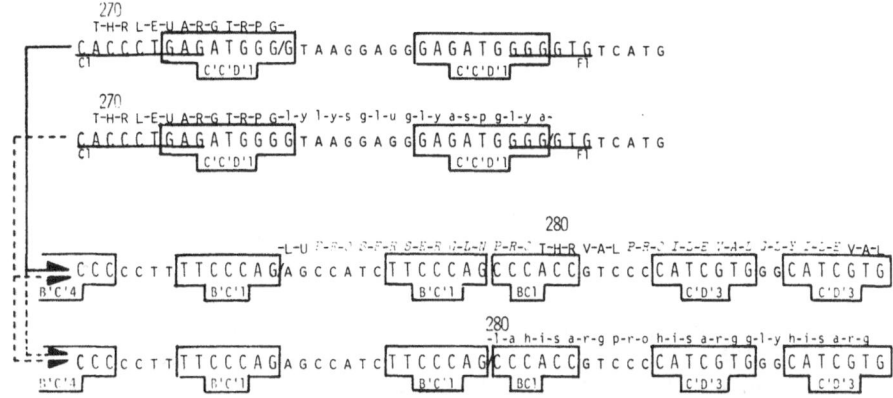

Figure 4: The successive recurrence of the base nonomer GAGATGGGG
identified as C'C'D'1 at the coding-intervening junction
between the coding segment for the most conserved 3rd
domain and the subsequent intervening sequence of human
class I MHC antigen HLA 12.4 gene (top two rows) as well
as the similarly successive recurrence of the base
heptamer TTCCCAG identified as B'C'1 at the intervening-
coding junction between the already noted intervening
sequence and the coding segment for the 4th transmembrane
domain (bottom two rows) is shown. Thus, the splicing
between the coding segment for the most conserved 3rd
domain and that for the hydrophobic transmembrane 4th
domain may involve two sets of upstream and downstream
splicing signals. The proper splicing is indicated by
the solid connection, whereas three alternative splicings
are indicated by broken line connections.

The clonal recurrence with age of serum albumin production
in the liver of analbuminemic rats reported in this symposium by
Esumi and Sugimura may indeed indicate increased utilization of
alternative splicing sites by the degenerating splicing
mechanism.

ACKNOWLEDGEMENT

This work was supported in part by the Frank W. Denny
Research Fund.

REFERENCES

Breathnach, R., and Chambon, P., 1981, Organization and expression
    of eukaryotic split genes coding for proteins, <u>Ann. Ref.</u>
    <u>Biochem.</u>, 50:349.
Douthart, R. J., and Norris, F. H., 1982, Events in the evolution
    of pre-proinsulin, <u>Science</u>, 217:729.
Kawakami, T., Takashima, N., and Honjo, T., 1980, Complete
    nucleotide sequence of mouse immunoglobulin gene and
    comparison with other immunoglobulin heavy chain genes, <u>Nucl.</u>
    <u>Acid. res.</u>, 8:3933.
Malissen, M., Malissen, B., and Jordan, B. R., 1982, Exon/intron
    organization and complete nucleotide sequence of an HLA gene,
    <u>Proc. Natl. Acad. Sci., USA</u>, 79:893.
Ohno, S., Matsunaga, T., Epplen, J. T., Itakura, K., and Wallace,
    R. B., 1982, Identification of the 45-base-long primordial
    building block of the entire class I major histocompatibility
    complex antigen gene, <u>Proc. Natl. Acad. Sci., USA</u>, 79:6342.
Sumegi, J., Wieslander, L., and Daneholt, B., 1982, A hierachic
    arrangement of the repetitive sequences in the Balbiani ring 2
    gene of <u>Chironomus</u> tentans, <u>Cell</u>, 30:579.
Yamada, Y., Avvedimento, V. E., Murdryj, M., Ohkubo, H., Vogeli,
    G., Irani, M., Pastan, I., and Crombrugge, B. de, 1980, The
    collagen gene: Evidence for its evolutionary assembly by
    amplification of a DNA segment containing an exon of 54 BP,
    <u>Cell</u>, 22:287.
Yazaki, A., and Ohno, S., 1983, The recurrence of 49 base decamers,
    nonomers and octamers within mouse Ig Cmu$_H$ genes and its
    primordial building block, <u>Proc. Natl. Acad. Sci., USA</u>,
    80:(in press).

APPEARANCE OF ALBUMIN-PRODUCING CELLS IN THE LIVER OF ANALBUMINEMIC RATS ON AGING AND ADMINISTRATION OF MUTAGENS

Hiroyasu Esumi,[1] Yuri Takahashi,[1] Reiko Makino,[2]
Shigeaki Sato,[2] and Takashi Sugimura[2]

Virology Division[1] and Biochemistry Division[2]
National Cancer Center Research Institute, 5-1-1,
Tsukiji, Chuo-ku, Tokyo, Japan

ABSTRACT

The lack in serum albumin in analbuminemic rats, a strain derived from Sprague-Dawley rats, was found to be due to deficient synthesis of albumin in the liver caused by a disturbance in the processing of albumin mRNA. The serum albumin gene was cloned from analbuminemic rats and from parental normal Sprague-Dawley rats. Analyses of the nucleotide sequences of these albumin genes revealed that there is a seven base pair deletion in the HI intron of the albumin gene of analbuminemic rats. This deletion extends from the 5th to the 11th base of the 5'-end of the intron causing change in the nucleotide sequence of the 5'-end of the HI intron from GTAGGTT to GTAGCGA. The HI intron sequence was found to be accumulated in the nuclear RNA of analbuminemic rat liver indicating blocking of mRNA splicing.

Although analbuminemic rats are almost completely deficient in serum albumin, a small but appreciable amount of "albumin" was detected in their serum. This protein was purified by immunoprecipitation and SDS-gel electrophoresis and shown to have the same immunological crossreactivity and digestion patterns with V8 protease and papain as those of normal rat serum albumin. The concentration of "albumin" increased slightly upon aging of analbuminemic rats. The existence of serum albumin in hepatocytes of analbuminemic rats was studied immunohisto-chemically by the peroxidase anti-peroxidase method. There were about $1/10^5$ albumin-positive cells, presumably albumin-producing hepatocytes at birth, and their number increased gradually to

637

100~200/10^4 about 24 months after birth. When the
hepatocarcionogenic mutagen 3'-methyl-4-dimethylaminoazobenzene was
administered to analbuminemic rats, the number of albumin-positive
cells in the liver increased 8-fold in 5 weeks and 10-fold in 15
weeks. A similar increase was observed after administration of
acetylaminofluorene, but not after partial hepatectomy or
administration of diethylnitrosamine.

INTRODUCTION

Analbuminemic rats were accidentally discovered in a stock
of Sprague-Dawley rats (Nagase et al., 1979) and found to lack
serum albumin genetically. The trait of analbuminemia was
autosomally recessive (Nagase et al., 1980). Although
analbuminemic rats showed hyperlipidemia (Nagase et al, 1979;
Ando et al., 1980) and slight growth retardation, their longevity
and fertility.were normal (Nagase et al., 1980). A similar
disorder of serum albumin, namely analbuminemia, was found in
humans (Benhold et al., 1954; Boman et al., 1976). In
analbuminemia in both humans and rats, no serious disorder other
than slight hyperlipidemia was found. It is very interesting that
serum albumin, which constitutes about 50% of the total serum
protein, does not have any indispensable function.

The molecular mechanism of the lack of serum albumin in rats
is interesting. Since serum albumin is synthesized in the liver
(Peters, 1962), there are three possible explanations for the
lack of serum albumin: lack of its synthesis in the liver,
deficiency in secretion of albumin from the liver, and increased
clearance of albumin from the blood. Results showed that the
clearance rate of serum albumin was prolonged in this mutant
(Esumi et al., 1979) and serum albumin was found not to be
synthesized in the liver (Esumi et al., 1980). Further analysis
of the reason for lack of albumin synthesis showed that albumin
mRNA precursor is transcribed but not processed correctly in this
mutant rat (Esumi et al., 1982). Analbuminemic rats were found
to have a mutation that blocks correct processing of albumin mRNA
precursors, resulting in lack of synthesis of serum albumin in
the liver. More recently, we cloned albumin genes from
analbuminemic and parental normal Sprague-Dawley rats and found a
seven base pair deletion in the HI intron (Esumi et al., 1983).
The mechanism of deficiency in synthesis of albumin in this
mutant rat is very similar to that of β-globin in β+-thalassemia
(Westaway and Williamson, 1981; Spritz et al., 1981.) In β+-
thalassemia, a reduced but appreciable amount of albumin is found
in the serum (Makino et al., 1982). Moreover, the amount of
serum albumin was found to increase on administration of a
hepatocarcinogen, 3'-methyl-4-dimethylaminoazobenzene (3'-Me-
DAB), and also on aging (Makino et al., 1982). These findings

suggested that some mutation induced by aging or mutagen relieved the blockade of mRNA splicing in analbuminemic rats. This paper presents data suggesting induction of somatic mutation in hepatocytes by mutagens and aging.

MATERIALS AND METHODS

Animals. Analbuminemic rats, derived from Sprague-Dawley rats maintained in CLEA, Japan, were kindly provided by Dr. S. Nagase, Sasaki Institute, Tokyo. Normal Sprague-Dawley rats were obtained from the same stock of rats in CLEA, Japan, from which the analbuminemic rats had been isolated (Nagase et al., 1979).

Chemicals. α-[^{32}P]dNTP was from the Radiochemical Centre, Amersham, England. DNA polymerase I and a large fragment of DNA polymerase I were purchased from Boehringer Mannheim, GmbH, West Germany. Restriction endonucleases, EcoRI, Hind III, BamHI, PstI, SalI, HinfI, Sau3AI and Hae III were obtained from Takara Shuzo, Kyoto, Japan. T4 DNA ligase was from Bethesda Research Laboratory, Bethesda, Md., USA. Nitrocellulose paper and aminobenzyloxymethyl cellulose were products of Schleicher & Shuell, USA. All other chemicals were commercial products of reagent grade.

Albumin gene cloning. Rat genomic libraries were made essentially by the method of Maniatis et al. (1978) using Charon 4A as a vector. Approximately 15-20kb DNA fragments, generated by partial digestion with EcoRI of DNAs from analbuminemic and normal Sprague-Dawley rats, were purified by sucrose density gradient contrifugation twice. The resulting purified DNA fragments were ligated to Charon 4A arms in vitro under the conditions described by maniatis et al. (1978). Rat albumin genes were identified by plaque hybridization (Benton and Davis, 1977) using cloned rat albumin cDNA, prAlb-1 (Kioussis et al., 1979), which was kindly provided by S.M. Tilghman, Fels Institute, as a probe. Subcloning of rat albumin genes was performed with pKH47 (Hayashi, 1980) as a vector.

DNA sequence determination. The DNA sequences of subcloned albumin genes were determined by the method of Maxam and Gilbert (1977).

DNA and RNA blot hybridization analyses. DNA blot hybridization analysis was performed by the method of Southern (1975), and RNA blot hybridization analysis by the method of Alwine et al. (1977). Hybridization conditions were as described by Wahl et al. (1979). The procedures used were described in detail elsewhere (Esumi et al., 1983).

Immunohistochemical staining of albumin-producing cells in the
liver. Livers were perfused with saline and then with 4%
paraformaldehyde in 0.1 M sodium phosphate buffer (pH 7.5)
containing 2% sucrose. Perfused and fixed liver tissue was cut
into 2-3 mm thick slices, which were rinsed extensively with 0.1 M
sodium phosphate buffer (pH 7.5) and dehydrated in ethanol and
xylene. Fixed liver slices were embedded in paraffin and
sectioned; sections 3 microns thick were stained for albumin
immunohistochemically by the peroxidase anti-peroxidase (PAP)
method (Taylor, 1978) using rabbit anti-rat serum albumin antiserum
(Esumi et al., 1980). Briefly, paraffin was removed with xylene
and ethanol and the slices were incubated for 30 min at room
temperature in 1% H_2O_2 in methanol and then in 5% normal swine
serum. Then they were incubated successively with 0.1% rabbit
anti-rat serum albumin antiserum, 5% swine anti-rabbit IgG and
horse radish peroxidase-rabbit anti-horse radish peroxidase
complex. The peroxidase-antibody-albumin complex was located by
the diaminobenzidine reaction.

Biocontainment. All procedures involving recombinant DNA were
carried out in P3 biocontainment at the National Cancer Center
Research Institute, Tokyo.

RESULTS

RNA·cDNA hybridization kinetics

    Since the lack in serum albumin in analbuminemic rats has been
found to be caused by lack of its synthesis, the albumin mRNA
concentration was examined by RNA·cDNA hybridization kinetics. As
clearly demonstrated in Fig. 1, the amount of albumin mRNA in liver
cytoplasm of analbuminemic rats was found to be less than 0.2% of
the normal amount. However, Fig. 1 shows that the nuclear RNA
fraction of analbuminemic rat liver contained almost the same
concentration of albumin mRNA sequence as that of normal liver,
presumably as mRNA precursors. The specificity of the
hybridization of albumin cDNA to RNA was examined by S1 nuclease
mapping and RNA blot hybridization (Esumi et al., 1982). From
these data, analbuminemic rats seemed to be mutants with a
disturbance of albumin mRNA processing.

Albumin gene structure

    First, we examined the structure of the albumin gene of
analbuminemic rats by Southern blot hybridization of total genomic
DNA. As shown in Fig. 2, the digestion patterns with EcoRI, Hind
III and Pst I of the albumin genes of analbuminemic and normal rats
were indistinguishable upon electrophoresis on 1% agarose gel.
Digests with Bam HI and Sal I also showed no difference between the

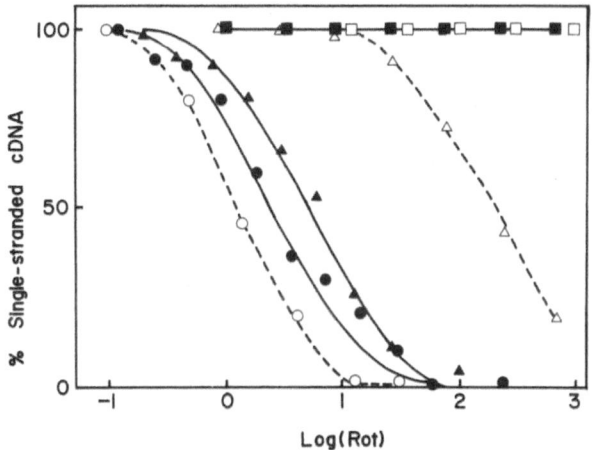

Fig. 1:   RNA·cDNA hybridization kinetics of cytoplasmic and
           nuclear RNAs using albumin cDNA as a probe. Total
           cytoplasmic and nuclear RNAs from normal and
           analbuminemic rat liver and normal rat kidney were
           hybridized to [^{3}H]-cDNA. The S_1 nuclease resistant
           fraction of cDNA was assayed as described (Esumi et al.,
           1980). O‑O, normal rat liver cytoplasmic RNA; △‑△,
           analbuminemic rat liver cytoplasmic RNA; □‑□, normal rat
           kidney cytoplasmic RNA; ●‑●, normal rat liver nuclear
           RNA; ▲‑▲, analbuminemic rat liver nuclear RNA; ■‑■,
           normal rat kidney nuclear RNA.

two albumin genes. These results indicate that there is no large
deletion, insertion or rearrangement in the gene in analbuminemic
rats.

    Therefore, the albumin genes of analbuminemic and normal rats
were molecularly cloned in E. coli phage Charon 4A. Of about 1.2 x
10^6 independent clones screened, 15 and 16 containing the albumin
gene from the analbuminemic and normal rat library, respectively,
were picked up by plaque hybridization using prAlb-1 as a probe.
Three representative clones of each type were selected for detailed
study.

    Restriction maps of these 6 clones are shown in Fig. 3. The
results again indicated that there is no large structural change in
the albumin gene of analbuminemic rats. All the bands of the
albumin gene detected on Southern blot hybridization of total
genomic DNA are found to be present in the cloned albumin gene and
to be contiguous in one gene. So far, there is no indication of
the existence of a pseudogene of the albumin gene. Moreover, we
recently found restriction fragment length polymorphism in the 3'-
flanking sequence of the albumin gene and applied it in a genetic

segregation study. Results clearly indicated that the rat serum albumin gene is unique (Esumi et al., 1982).

Organization of albumin genes

The structural organization of the rat albumin gene was first reported by Sargent et al. (1979) and later revised (Sargent et al., 1981). Cloned albumin genes from analbuminemic and normal

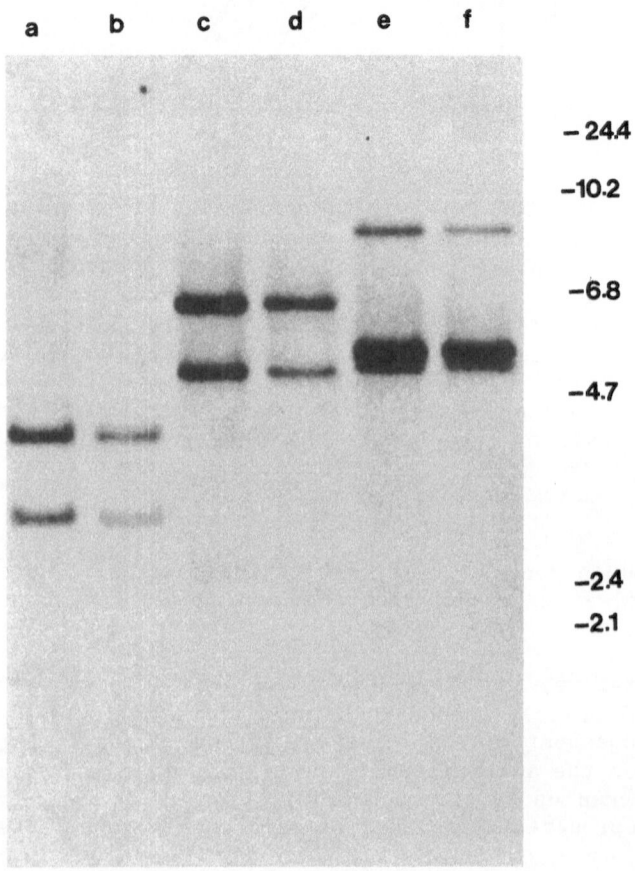

Fig. 2:   Digestion pattern of the albumin gene with Eco RI, Hind III and Pst I. DNA fragments generated by restriction enzyme digestions were separated on 1% agarose gel and transferred to nitrocellulose paper by the method of Southern. The probe was nick-translated cloned albumin cDNA. a, c and e, normal rat; b, d and f, analbuminemic rat; a and b, EcoRI digestion; c and d, Hind III digestion; e and f, Pst I digestion.

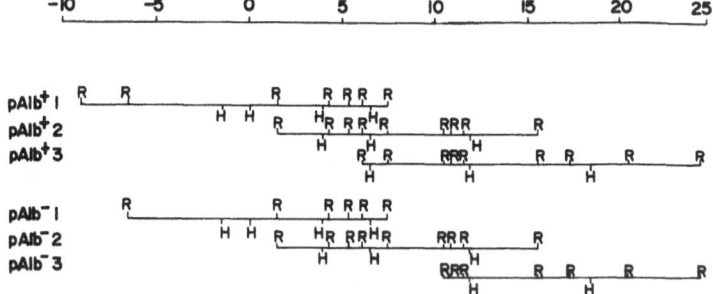

Fig. 3:   Restriction maps of cloned albumin genes. pAlb+1, pAlb+2
           and pAlb+3 were clones from the normal rat genome and
           pAlb-1, pAlb-2 and pAlb-3 were from analbuminemic rat
           genome. R, EcoR I site; H, Hind III site. Length is
           expressed in k bases.

rats had similar structures to that reported (Esumi et al., 1983),
as shown in Fig. 4.   The rat albumin gene extended approximately
16kbp and was split into 15 exons.   Like many other eukaryotic
genes, it has a TATA box and a CCAAT box in its putative promoter
region and an AATAAA sequence as a poly(A)-addition signal at its
3'-end.   All these structures were identical in the albumin genes
of analbuminemic and normal rats.   However, partial nucleotide
sequence determination revealed a 7 bp deletion in the 5'-splicing
junction region of the HI intron of the gene from analbuminemic
rats.   As shown in Fig. 5, all introns start with the GT sequence
and end with the AG sequence as previously reported for many

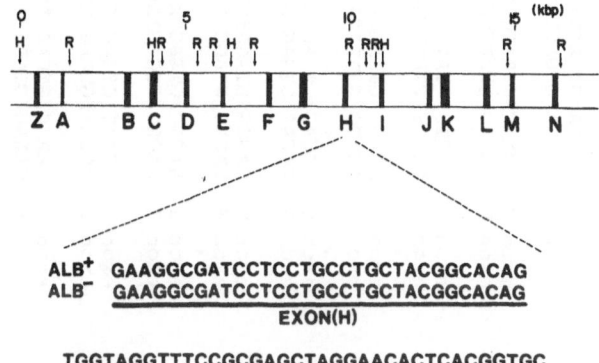

Fig. 4:   Organization of albumin genes. Black portions designated
           Z to N are exons. R, EcoR I site; H, Hind III site. The
           upper and lower genomes are normal and analbuminemic rat
           albumin genes, respectively.

Alb+	exon Z	AGCAC/GTAAGCATCTTATGTTT	intron ZA	CTCCCCATTCCCACAG/ACAAG	exon A
Alb-	exon Z	AGCAC/GTAAGCATCTTATGTTT	intron ZA	CTCCCCATTCCCACAG/ACAAG	exon A
Alb+	exon A	GGCCT/GTAAGTTAAGAGGCTGA	intron AB	TTCTGCCTGTCTTTCAG/AGTCC	exon B
Alb-	exon A	GGCCT/GTAAGTTAAGAGGCTGA	intron AB	TTCTGCCTGTCTTTCAG/AGTCC	exon B
Alb+	exon B	CCATT/GTGAGTACATTCTGATT	intron BC	TTCTGTCTTCCACTTAG/CACAC	exon C
Alb-	exon B	CCATT/GTGAGTACATTCTGATT	intron BC	TTCTGTCTTCCACTTAG/CACAC	exon C
Alb+	exon C	GGACA/GTGAGTACATTCTGATT	intron CD	CTCTTCCCATAATTCAG/CTATT	exon D
Alb-	exon C	GGACA/GTGAGTACATTCTGATT	intron CD	CTCTTCCCATAATTCAG/CTATT	exon D
Alb+	exon D	CGAAG/GTAATCCTTGGAAAGAC	intron DE	TGGATTTCTTTTGGTAG/CTTGA	exon E
Alb-	exon D	CGAAG/GTAATCCTTGGAAAGAC	intron DE	TGGATTTCTTTTGGTAG/CTTGA	exon E
Alb+	exon E	GCCTG/GTATATGAATTTTCTTT	intron EF	CTTTTTTCCTTTTTCAG/GGCAG	exon F
Alb-	exon E	GCCTG/GTATATGAATTTTCTTT	intron EF	CTTTTTTCCTTTTTCAG/GGCAG	exon F
Alb+	exon F	ACAGG/GTAAAGAGGGGGATGC	intron FG	GCCTTCCATTCTCACAG/GCAGA	exon G
Alb-	exon F	ACAGG/GTAAAGAGGGGGATGC	intron FG	GCCTTCCATTCTCACAG/GCAGA	exon G
Alb+	exon G	GGCAC/GTGAGTAGATGCCTTCT	intron GH	TGTTTCGCCTCAATTAG/GTTTT	exon H
Alb-	exon G	GGCAC/GTGAGTAGATGCCTTCT	intron GH	TGTTTCGCCTCAATTAG/GTTTT	exon H
Alb+	exon H	CAGTG/GTAGGTTCCGCGAGCT	intron HI	TTACTTTATCTTGCAG/CTTGC	exon I
Alb-	exon H	CAGTG/GTAGCGAGCTAGGAGCT ◄	intron HI	TTACTTTATCTTGCAG/CTTGC	exon I
Alb+	exon I	AACGC/GTGAGTAGTTTTTTTTC	intron IJ	AACTTTTTGTTACACAG/CGTTC	exon J
Alb-	exon I	AACGC/GTGAGTAGTTTTTTTTC	intron IJ	AACTTTTTGTTACACAG/CGTTC	exon J
Alb+	exon J	ACTAT/GTGAGTCTTTAAACAA	intron JK	GCTGTCTCTTCTTTAG/CTGTC	exon K
Alb-	exon J	ACTAT/GTGAGTCTTTAAACAA	intron JK	GCTGTCTCTTCTTTAG/CTGTC	exon K
Alb+	exon K	CAAAC/GTGAGAGATATATTCTTT	intron KL	TTTCTGTCCTGCTGCAG/GGCTC	exon L
Alb-	exon K	CAAAC/GTGAGAGATATATTCTTT	intron KL	TTTCTGTCCTGCTGCAG/GGCTC	exon L
Alb+	exon L	CTGAG/GTAACAAATGTCTCTC	intron LM	CAATTTTCCTGTTCAG/GGGCC	exon M
Alb-	exon L	CTGAG/GTAACAAATGTCTCTC	intron LM	CAATTTTCCTGTTCAG/GGGCC	exon M
Alb+	exon M	CTCAG/GTAACTATACTCGGAA	intron MN	/GCTAC	exon N
Alb-	exon M	CTCAG/GTAACTATACTCGGAA	intron MN	/GCTAC	exon N

Fig. 5 (legend on next page)

eukaryotic genes (Breathnach et al., 1978). The GT sequence at the 5'-end of introns is followed by a $\frac{G}{A}$ AGT sequence in many eukaryotic genes (Mount, 1982), and this was also the case in most of the introns of the rat albumin gene. However, since a 7 bp deletion in the analbuminemic rat gene extended from the 5th to the 11th base of the 5'-end of the HI intron, the nucleotide sequence normally located at the 5'-end of the HI intron, GTAGGTT, was replaced by the sequence GTAGCGA. So far we have sequenced approximately 12,000 bp of the albumin genes of analbuminemic and normal rats, and found that these genes are identical except for the 7 bp deletion in the HI intron.

RNA blot hybridization analyses

Because we detected a mutation in the splicing junction region of the albumin gene of analbuminenic rats and the rest of the gene so far examined was normal, we postulated that this 7 bp deletion blocks albumin mRNA processing, presumably splicing. To test this possibility, we examined by RNA blot hybridization analyses whether the HI intron sequence accumulated and persisted in the nuclear RNA fraction of analbuminemic rats. Samples of 10 µg of each RNA of cytoplasmic and nuclear RNAs of normal and analbuminemic rat liver were subjected to electrophoresis on a 1% agarose gel and transferred to DBM-paper by the method of Alwine et al. (1977). The DBM-paper was then hybridized with cDNA (Fig. 6a). After autoradiography, the paper was heat-treated to remove hybridized cDNA and hybridized to HI intron probe (Fig. 6b). As shown in Fig. 6, the HI intron sequence was accumulated in the nuclei of analbuminnemic rat liver. In analbuminemic rat liver the HI intron sequence was present even in mature mRNA-sized or smaller nuclear RNA. These data clearly indicate that a 7 bp deletion in the HI intron blocks albumin mRNA splicing in the liver of analbuminemic rats.

Immunohistochemical examination of albumin-producing cells in the liver of analbuminemic rats

As mentioned earlier, a tiny but appreciable amount of RNA that could hybridize to cloned albumin cDNA was observed in the cytoplasm of analbuminemic rat liver (Fig. 1) and a very small amount of albumin which reacted specifically with anti-rat albumin antiserum was present in the serum of analbuminemic rats (Makino et

Fig. 5:   Nucleotide sequences around exon-intron junctions. All exons were determined by sequencing of cloned rat albumin genes and GT/AG rule (Breathnach et al., 1978). Exons are named by the designation of Sargent et al. (1981). ▲, location of the deletion in the albumin gene of analbuminemic rats.

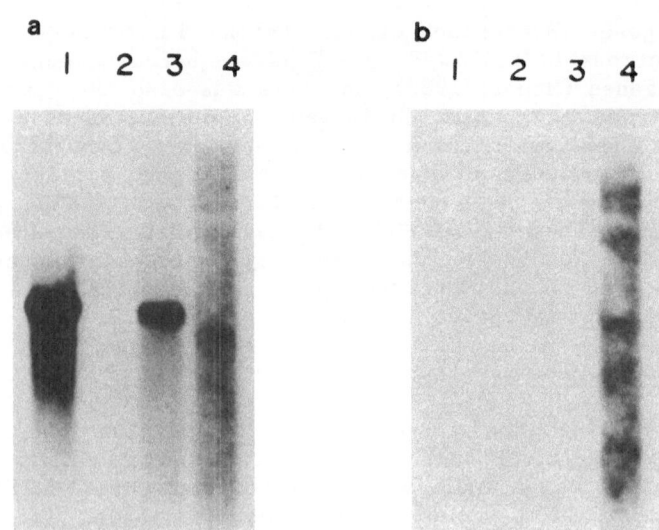

Fig. 6:   RNA blot hybridization analyses. a, RNA blot
           hybridization using cDNA as a probe. b, RNA blot
           hybridization using the DNA fragment of the HI intron as
           a probe. 1, 10 μg of normal rat liver cytoplasmic RNA;
           2, 10 μg of analbuminemic rat liver cytoplasmic RNA; 3,
           10 μg of normal rat liver nuclear RNA; 4, 10 μ g of
           analbuminemic rat liver nuclear RNA.

al., 1982). Therefore, we wondered if all hepatocytes of
analbuminemic rats synthesized albumin at a very low level or
whether only a limited number of hepatocytes did so. To answer
this question, we stained liver for albumin immunohistochemically
by the PAP method. As shown in Fig. 7, only a limited number of
hepatocytes stained with anti-rat serum albumin antiserum.

     It is interesting that the number of albumin-positive
hepatocytes increased during aging. The frequencies of albumin-
positive hepatocytes were, respectively, $1.4/10^4$, $6/10^4$ and $100/10^4$
at 4, 9 and 100 weeks after birth. Moreover, the number of
albumin-positive hepatocytes also increased on administration of
3'-Me-DBA (our unpublished data.). A similar increase was observed
on treatment with acetyl-aminofluorene. These results indicate
that some mutations that accumulated on aging or administration of
a hepatocarcinogenic mutagen relieved the blockade of albumin mRNA
splicing caused by the 7 bp deletion in the HI intron.

     It is essential to know if functional albumin mRNA also
increases in the liver of analbuminemic rats upon aging and
treatment with 3'-Me-DBA and AAF. In preliminary analyses of the

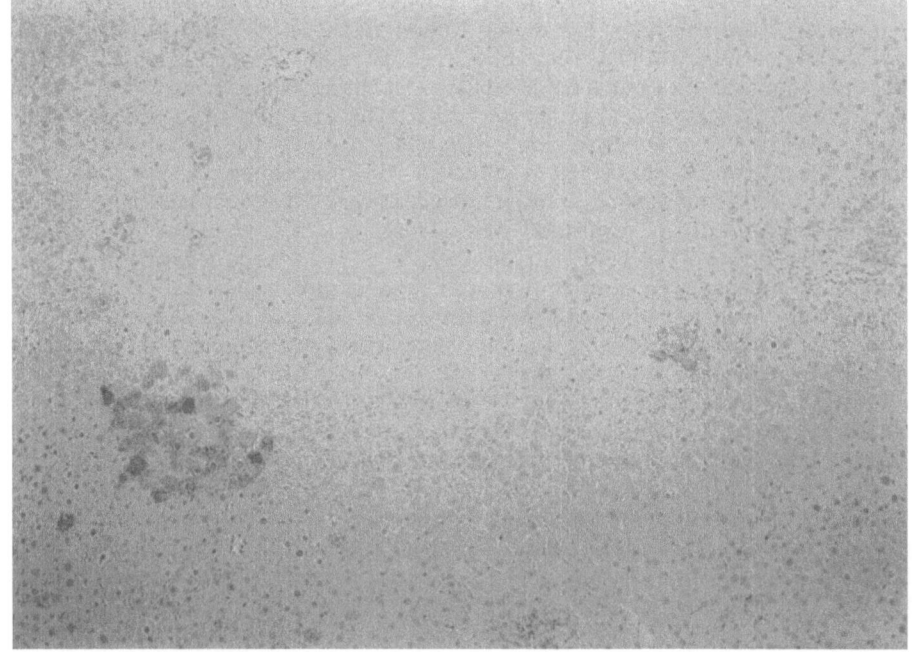

Fig. 7:   Immunohistochemical staining of analbuminemic rat liver.
           A thin section of liver of an analbuminemic rat treated
           with 0.03% 3'-methyl-4-dimethylaminoazobenzene for 8
           weeks was stained for albumin by the PAP method using
           rabbit anti-rat serum albumin antiserum.

total amount of cytoplasmic albumin mRNA sequence in the liver of
analbuminemic rats, several-fold increase in the mRNA sequence was
detected by dot hybridization analysis of RNA.

DISCUSSION

    There are at least two possible explanations for the
heterogeneity of albumin content of hepatocytes found in
analbuminemic rats. One is that in some hepatocytes of
analbuminemic rats the ability to synthesize serum albumin is
restored as a result of some sort of somatic reverse mutations
induced by mutagens or aging. The other possibility is that all
hepatocytes can synthesize albumin but at an extremely reduced
level due to the 7 bp deletion in the HI intron and that aging or
treatment with a mutagen causes alteration in the process of
albumin secretion, resulting in accumulation of albumin in some
hepatocytes. The first possibility is supported by finding that
the serum albumin concentration also increased, although less

than expected from the increase in number of albumin-positive
hepatocytes (Makino et al., unpublished data). Moreover, the total
cytoplasmic albumin mRNA sequence also increased similarly,
although again less than the number of albumin-positive
hepatocytes. This discrepancy between the extents of increases of
serum albumin concentration and of albumin-positive hepatocytes
favors the second possibility. But we do not necessarily have to
postulated 100% suppression of the mutation. If suppression takes
place in a cis-acting fashion, the final product will be decreased
by a factor of two to four because most of the hepatocytes are
diploid or tetraploid. Moreover, if the suppression is
insufficient to restore full production of albumin irrespective of
whether it is cis-or trans-acting, the level of product will not
correspond directly to the number of hepatocytes with restored
ability to synthesize albumin. For examination of these
possibilities, it is essential to isolate cell lines synthesizing
albumin from hepatocytes of analbuminemic rats.

Since many eukaryotic genes coding protein have been found to
have a chimeric structure, exon-intron, mRNA splicing is an
obligatory step in mRNA synthesis (Crick, 1979). Moreover, mRNA
splicing was found to play an important role in regulation of gene
expression in several gene systems (Maki et al., 1981, Amara et
al., 1982). However, information on the molecular mechanism(s) of
mRNA splicing is still only limited. Breathnach et al. first
reported that all introns start with the GT sequence and end with
the AG sequence (Breathnach et al., 1978). From data on the
nucleotide sequences of a large number of intron-exon junctions,
Lerner et al. proposed a model of mRNA splicing (Lerner et al.,
1980) in which U1 RNA or U1 RNP (ribonucleoprotein) plays a key
role in mRNA splicing; hybrid formation of U1 RNA with both ends of
the intron results in close proximity of two exons. This model was
supported in part by results with an adenovirus mRNA splicing
system (Yang et al., 1981). In addition to the above findings, a
systematic study on the nucleotide sequence requirement for mRNA
splicing in the globin gene system supports the view that the
nucleotide sequence of the 5'-end of the intron in important in
splicing (Wieringa et al., 1982). More recently, in β+thalassemia,
β°-thalassemia, α-thalassemia and analbuminemia in rats, alteration
of the 5'-consensus sequence of the intron or generation of a
consensus sequence-like sequence was found to alter the pattern of
splicing (Felber et al., 1982, Treisman et al., 1982). In
thalassemia, mutations break a strictly conserved sequence, GT
(Mount, 1982), but in analbuminemia in rats, the mutation breaks
only a part of the consensus sequence which is not well conserved in
many eukaryotic genes. Therefore the questions arise of what the
function of the consensus sequence is and what extent of sequence
at the 5'-end of introns is functionally indispensable. A
systematic study of the functional role of the 5'-end sequence of
introns using directed-mutation is required to answer this

question. But at present we can state that a "not well conserved portion of consensus sequence" at 5'-end of introns is also important for splicing. For clarifying the functional importance and minimal requirement of the nucleotide sequence of the 5'-end of introns, the "reverse mutant" observed in the liver of analbuminemic rats will be useful. We are now attempting to isolate cells lines from analbuminemic rat liver that have restored ability to synthesize albumin.

Acknowledgements

We thank Dr. Sumi Nagase, Sasaki Institute, Tokyo, Japan, for providing analbuminemic rats. This work was partly supported by grants from the Ministry of Health and Welfare, and the Ministry of Education, Science and Culture of Japan, the Princess Takamatsu Cancer Research Fund, the Yamada Science Foundation and the Research Foundation for Cancer and Cardiovascular Diseases.

REFERENCES

Alwine, J.C., Kemp. D.J. and Stark, G.R. (1977), Proc. Natl. Acad. Sci., USA, 74:5350.

Amara, S.G., Jonas, V., Rosenfeld, M.G., Ong, E.S. and Evans, R.M. (1982), Nature, 298:240.

Ando, S., Kon, K., Tanaka, T., Nagase, S. and Nagai, Y., (1980), J. Biochem., 87:1859.

Benhold, H., Peters, H. and Poth, E., (1954), Verh. Deut. Ges. Inn. Med., 60:630.

Benton, W.D. and Davies, R.W. (1977), Science, 196:180.

Boman, H., Hermodson, M., Hammond, C.A. and Motulsky, A.G. (1976), Clinical Genetics, 9:513.

Breathnach, R. Benoist, C., O'Hare, K., Gannon, F. and Chambon, P. (1978), Proc. Natl. Acad. Sci., USA, 75:4853.

Crick, F. (1979), Science, 204:264.

Esumi, H., Sato, S., Okui, M. Sugimura, T. and Nagase, S. (1979), Biochem. Biophys. Res. Commun., 87:1191.

Esumi, H., Okui, M., Sato, S., Sugimura, T. and Nagase, S., (1980), Proc. Natl. Acad. Sci., USA, 77:3215.

Esumi, H., Takahashi, Y., Sekiya, T., Sato, S., Nagase, S. and Sugimura, T. (1982), Proc. Natl. Acad. Sci., USA, 79:734.

Esumi, H., Takahashi, Y., Sato, S., Nagase, S. and Sugimura, T. (1983), Proc. Natl. Acad. Sci., USA, 80:95.

Felber, B.K., Orkins, S.H. and Hamer, D.H. (1982), Cell, 29:895.

Hayashi, K. (1980), Gene, 11:109.

Houseman, D., Forget, B.G., Skoultchi, A. and Benz, E.J. (1973), Proc. Natl. Acad. Sci., USA, 70:1809.

Kioussis, D., Hamilton, R., Hanson, R.W., Tilghman, S.M. and Taylor, J.M. (1979), Proc. Natl. Acad. Sci., USA, 76:4370.

Lerner, M.R., Boyle, J.A., Mount, S.M., Wolin, S.L. and Steitz, J.A. (1980), Nature, 283:220.

Maki, R., Roeder, W., Traunecker, A., Sidman, C., Wabl, M., Raschke, W. and Tonegawa, S. (1981), Cell, 24:353.

Makino, R., Esumi, H., Sato, S., Takahashi, Y., Nagase, S. and Sugimura, T. (1982), Biochem. Biophys, Res. Commun., 106:863.

Maniatis, T., Hardison, R.C., Lacy, E., Laur, J., O'Connell, C. and Quon, D. (1978), Cell, 15:687.

Maxam, A.W. and Gilbert, W. (1977), Proc. Natl. Acad. Sci., USA, 74:560.

Mount, S.M. (1982), Nucleic Acids Res. 10:459.

Nagase, S., Shimamune, K. and Shumiya, S., (1979), Science, 205:590.

Nagase, S., Shimamune, K. and Shumiya, S., (1980), Exp. Anim. 29:33.

Peters, T. Jr., (1962), J. Biol. Chem. 237:1181.

Sargent, T.D., Wu, J., Sala-Trepat, J.M., Wallace, R.B., Reyes, A.A. and Bonner, J., (1979), Proc. Natl. Acad. Sci., USA, 76:3256.

Sargent, T.D., Jagodinski, L.L., Yang, M. and Bonner, J. (1981), Mol. Cell. Biol., 1:871.

Southern, E.M. (1975), J. Mol. Biol. 98:503.

Spritz, R.A., Jagadeeswaran, P., Choudary, P.V., Biro, P.A., Elder, J.T., deRiel, J.K., Manley, J.L., Gefter, M.L., Forget, B.G. and Weissman, S.M. (1981), Proc. Natl. Acad. Sci., USA, 78:2455.

Taylor, C.R. (1978), J. Histochem. Cytochem. 26:496.

Tresman, R., Proudfoot, N.J., Shander, M. and Mantiatis, T. (1982), Cell, 29:903.

Wahl, G.M., Stern, M. and Stark, G.R., (1979), Proc. Natl. Acad. Sci., USA, 76:3683.

Westaway, D. and Williamson, R. (1981), Nucleic Acids Res., 9:1777.

Wieringa, B., Meyer, F., Reiser, J. and Weisman, C. (1982), Proc. Cetus-UCLA Symposium on Gene Regulation, (in press).

Yang, V.W., Lerner, M.R., Steitz, J.A. and Flint, S.J. (1981), Proc. Natl. Acad. Sci., USA, 78:1371

INDEX